DATE

Functional Rehabilitation
of Sports and Musculoskeletal
Injuries

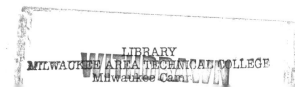

THE REHABILITATION INSTITUTE OF CHICAGO PUBLICATION SERIES

Don A. Olson, PhD, Series Coordinator

Spinal Cord Injury: A Guide to Functional Outcomes in Physical Therapy Management

Lower Extremity Amputation: A Guide to Functional Outcomes in Physical Therapy Management, Second Edition

Stroke/Head Injury: A Guide to Functional Outcomes in Physical Therapy Management

Clinical Management of Right Hemisphere Dysfunction, Second Edition

Spinal Cord Injury: A Guide to Functional Outcomes in Occupational Therapy

Spinal Cord Injury: A Guide to Rehabilitation Nursing

Head Injury: A Guide to Functional Outcomes in Occupational Therapy Management

Speech/Language Treatment of the Aphasias: Treatment Materials for Auditory Comprehension and Reading Comprehension

Speech/Language Treatment of the Aphasias: Treatment Materials for Oral Expression and Written Expression

Rehabilitation Nursing Procedures Manual

Psychological Management of Traumatic Brain Injuries in Children and Adolescents

Medical Management of Long-Term Disability

Psychological Aspects of Geriatric Rehabilitation

Clinical Management of Dysphagia in Adults and Children, Second Edition

Cognition and Perception in the Stroke Patient: A Guide to Functional Outcomes in Occupational Therapy

Spinal Cord Injury: Medical Management and Rehabilitation

Clinical Management of Communication Problems in Adults with Traumatic Brain Injury

Rehabilitation of Persons with Rheumatoid Arthritis

Functional Rehabilitation of Sports and Musculoskeletal Injuries

W. Ben Kibler, MD, FACSM
Medical Director, Lexington Clinic Sports Medicine Center
Associate Clinical Professor, University of Kentucky School of Medicine
Lexington, Kentucky

Stanley A. Herring, MD, FACSM
Puget Sound Sports and Spine Physicians
Clinical Associate Professor
Department of Rehabilitation Medicine and Orthopaedics
University of Washington
Team Physician, Seattle Seahawks
Seattle, Washington

Joel M. Press, MD
Medical Director
Center for Spine, Sports, and Occupational Rehabilitation
Rehabilitation Institute of Chicago
Assistant Professor, Physical Medicine and Rehabilitation
Northwestern University Medical School
Chicago, Illinois

With
Patricia A. Lee
Consulting Editor and Writer
Past President, American Medical Writers Association
Greater Chicago Area Chapter
Chicago, Illinois

AN ASPEN PUBLICATION®
Aspen Publishers, Inc.
Gaithersburg, Maryland
1998

The authors have made every effort to ensure the accuracy of the information herein. However, appropriate information sources should be consulted, especially for new or unfamiliar procedures. It is the responsibility of every practitioner to evaluate the appropriateness of a particular opinion in the context of actual clinical situations and with due considerations to new developments. Authors, editors, and the publisher cannot be held responsible for any typographical or other errors found in this book.

Library of Congress Cataloging-in-Publication Data

Functional rehabilitation of sports and musculoskeletal injuries /
edited by W. Ben Kibler, Stanley A. Herring, Joel M. Press, with Patricia A. Lee.
p. cm.—(The Rehabilitation Institute of Chicago publication series)
"Rehabilitation Institute of Chicago."
Includes bibliographical references and index.
ISBN 0-8342-0612-9
1. Sports injuries—Patients—Rehabilitation. 2. Sports physical therapy.
3. Musculoskeletal system—Wounds and injuries—Patients—Rehabilitation.
I. Press, Joel M. II. Kibler, W. Ben. III. Rehabilitation Institute of Chicago.
IV. Series.
[DNLM: 1. Athletic Injuries—rehabilitation. 2. Musculoskeletal System—
injuries. 3. Rehabilitation—methods. QT 261 F979 1998]
RD97.F86 1998
617.1'027—dc21
97-41935
CIP

Orders: (800) 638-8437
Customer Service: (800) 234-1660

About Aspen Publishers • For more than 35 years, Aspen has been a leading professional publisher in a variety of disciplines. Aspen's vast information resources are available in both print and electronic formats. We are committed to providing the highest quality information available in the most appropriate format for our customers. Visit Aspen's Internet site for more information resources, directories, articles, and a searchable version of Aspen's full catalog, including the most recent publications: **http://www.aspenpub.com**
Aspen Publishers, Inc. • The hallmark of quality in publishing
Member of the worldwide Wolters Kluwer group.

Editorial Services: Ruth Bloom
Library of Congress Catalog Card Number: 97-41935
ISBN: 0-8342-0612-9

Printed in the United States of America

1 2 3 4 5

Table of Contents

Contributors

Bruce E. Becker, MD
Assistant Professor
Department of Physical Medicine and Rehabilitation
Rehabilitation Institute of Michigan
Detroit, Michigan

Krystal Chambers, MD
Associate
Georgia Spine and Sports Physicians, PC
Marietta, Georgia

Jeffrey Chandler, EdD
Lexington Clinic Sports Medicine Center
Lexington, Kentucky

Andrew J. Cole, MD
Director, Education and Research
Puget Sound Sports and Spine Physicians
Medical Director
Overlake Hospital Medical Center
Spine Center
Bellvue, Washington
Clinical Assistant Professor
Department of Physical Medicine and
    Rehabilitation
Department of Physical Therapy
University of Texas Southwestern
    Medical Center
Dallas, Texas

Joseph P. Farrell, MS, PT
Redwood Orthopaedic Physical Therapy, Inc.
Castro Valley, California

Steve R. Geiringer, MD
Professor
Wayne State University
Director, Outpatient Services
Director, Electrodiagnostic Services
Rehabilitation Institute of Michigan
Detroit, Michigan

Michael C. Geraci, Jr., MD, PT
Clinical Assistant Professor
Department of Medicine and Rehabilitation
State University of New York
Buffalo, New York and
Michigan State University College of Osteopathic Medicine
East Lansing, Michigan
Fellowship Program Director and Medical Director
Buffalo Spine and Sports Medicine, PC
Williamsville, New York

Stanley A. Herring, MD, FACSM
Puget Sound Sports and Spine Physicians
Clinical Associate Professor
Departments of Rehabilitation Medicine and Orthopaedics
University of Washington
Team Physician, Seattle Seahawks
Seattle, Washington

Richard J. Herzog, MD
Associate Professor of Radiology
Section Chief—Teleradiology
Department of Radiology
University of Pennsylvania Medical Center
Philadelphia, Pennsylvania

Matthew Kaul, MD
Clinical Assistant Professor
Department of Rehabilitation Medicine
University of Washington
Seattle, Washington
Rehabilitation Medicine Staff
Portland Veteran's Affairs Medical Center
Portland, Oregon

W. Ben Kibler, MD, FASCM
Medical Director
Lexington Clinic Sports Medicine Center
Associate Clinical Professor
University of Kentucky School of Medicine
Lexington, Kentucky

Beven Pace Livingston, PT
Clinical Specialist
Physical Therapist, Athletic Trainer
Lexington Clinic Sports Medicine Center
Lexington, Kentucky

Daniel J. Mazanec, MD, FACP
Director, The Spine Center
The Cleveland Clinic Foundation
Cleveland, Ohio

Joel M. Press, MD
Medical Director
Center for Spine, Sports, and Occupational Rehabilitation
Rehabilitation Institute of Chicago
Assistant Professor
Physical Medicine and Rehabilitation
Northwestern University Medical School
Chicago, Illinois

David B. Richards, MD
Orthopaedic Surgeon
Lexington Clinic Sports Medicine Center
Lexington, Kentucky

Joel S. Saal, MD
SOAR, The Physiatry Medical Group
Menlo Park, California

Steven A. Stratton, PhD, PT, ATC
Alamo Physical Therapy Resources, Inc.
Associate Clinical Professor
University of Texas Medical Center
San Antonio, Texas

Robert P. Wilder, MD
Director, Sports Rehabilitation Services
Department of Physical Medicine and Rehabilitation
Tom Landry Sports Medicine and Research Center
Baylor University Medical Center
Dallas, Texas

Robert E. Windsor, MD
Assistant Clinical Professor
Department of Physical Medicine and Rehabilitation
Emory University
Atlanta, Georgia
President
Georgia Spine and Sports Physicians, PC
Marietta, Georgia

Jeffrey Young, MD, MA
Associate Director of Spine and Sports Rehabilitation
Beth Israel Medical Center
Associate Professor
Physical Medicine and Rehabilitation
Albert Einstein College of Medicine
New York, New York

Preface

PURPOSES FOR WRITING THIS BOOK

Rehabilitation of all types of problems—not just sports medicine injuries—is at a crossroads. Economic and medical pressures are being applied to the rehabilitation process, its physicians, and its therapists, with the emphasis on providing the most cost-effective care. Some pressures are occurring that focus on eliminating the rehabilitation process altogether because of its perceived ineffectiveness in changing the natural history of recovery after injury. Others feel that directed rehabilitation is too costly to be cost-effective and that formal physical therapy should be replaced by a series of home programs based on sheets that are handed out to patients with minimal instruction.

Further pressures include the necessity for having a system of accountability for the results of the rehabilitation process so that resulting benefits can be compared to the rehabilitation effort and cost. Peer review has been instituted to evaluate the appropriateness of the use of different methods of rehabilitation ranging from modalities to whirlpools, rest, and exercise. Demand is high for a series of specific protocols that will define the most effective pathway for rehabilitation of specific injuries so that the rehabilitation process can be standardized across populations or across therapy groups. Finally, there has been the emphasis on home-based programs to cut the cost of physical therapy services and the cost of actually going to a physical therapy office.

Medical pressures on rehabilitation include the need to demonstrate that rehabilitation does affect the natural history of recovery from an injury and that performance is enhanced and repeat injury risk is reduced as a result. In addition, athletes demand to have the most up-to-date rehabilitation programs so that they can return to as nearly normal performance as soon as possible.

All of these pressures are occurring at a time when the amount of money that is available for medical care and rehabilitation is fluctuating. Unless rehabilitation is proven to be cost-effective and shown to positively affect the natural history of tissue healing, repair, and function, it will not receive funding for treatment or research.

This combination of circumstances has required that the older methods of rehabilitation be reexamined for their appropriateness and that a scientific basis and rationale for rehabilitation be established. Rehabilitation practitioners may use this base to answer some of the questions and problems posed by the changing health care situation. Among the major issues under examination is the question of whether the symptom-based, modality-based form of physical therapy that emphasizes visits to the physical therapist is cost-effective.

Basic science studies are being conducted to allow a better understanding of the process of healing from injury and surgery, and a better understanding of the mechanical and physiologic alterations that occur as a result of the injury and its subsequent treatment. More basic science studies are appearing in the literature that document that the healing process occurring after microtrauma injury is relatively similar for different anatomic areas of the body and that there are associated alterations in physiology and mechanics that may alter functional recovery after injury. These alterations should be recognized and rehabilitated, in addition to the actual injury site and symptoms. A large body of literature exists that shows the advantage of aggressive rehabilitation of injuries around the knee, the ankle, the elbow, and the shoulder. These benefits include earlier restoration of range of motion, decreased pain, decreased neural inhibition, quicker return of muscle function, more appropriate return of muscle function, and earlier return to performance with decreased injury risk. This has led to the newest concepts in rehabilitation that emphasize functional restoration rather than symptomatic resolution, early motion within the limits of tissue tolerance after injury or after surgery, rehabilitation of the entire kinetic chain of the activity in which the athlete competes, the need for closed-chain rehabilitation of most joints, and loading of joints and tissues within safe tolerance as early as possible. These new programs, though still being developed, offer the promise of cost-effective, performance-oriented rehabilitation that will allow safe healing and will emphasize the importance of rehabilitation in altering the natural history of functional recovery from injury. A suitable framework for evaluation and rehabilitation that is based on scientfic rationale is the foundation for implementation of these types of programs. This framework would allow a complete understanding of the pathologic process and the development of a consistency of rehabilitation across different injuries and different parts of the body.

The bottom line for rehabilitation specialists is that we need to know *why* we are rehabilitating a joint or muscle, *what* parameters we are rehabilitating, and, finally, *how* we are rehabilitating. Unless the first two questions are answered, the answer to the third question becomes inconsistent and inefficient.

Functional Rehabilitation of Sports and Musculoskeletal Injuries is organized to answer all three questions. The first part of the book answers the question, Why are we rehabilitating? This section summarizes information about the pathophysiology, abnormal biomechanics, and physiologic alterations that exist as a result of an injury and addresses how to evaluate them. The second section of the book emphasizes what we are rehabilitating. This part discusses the specific alterations that exist and how to evaluate them using physical and radiologic exams. One chapter discusses the negative feedback vicious cycle, which is the framework for evaluating all the parameters that are occurring as a result of the injury. This description of the pathologic process includes all of the parameters that require rehabilitation and sets up a priority framework of which parameters require rehabilitation and in what order.

The third and largest part of the book describes the how of rehabilitation and lists specific protocols for the rehabilitation process. This section first shows how to formulate the exercise prescription, which will be specific for the individual, the sport, and the area of injury. It then describes the phases of rehabilitation that require resolution to allow the athlete to return to play. These phases include the acute phase, the recovery phase, and the functional phase. Each phase has specific goals to be accomplished during that phase and specific criteria that must be met for advancement to the next phase. Also, specific criteria have been determined for return to activity or sport.

Most of the variations in the rehabilitation process between different pathologic problems in the same joint will be in the acute phase. Each of the specific injuries will be treated initially according to their specific tissue injury. The recovery and functional phases usually are fairly similar for problems around the joint because, at this time, the rehabilitation process is concerned with the physiologic and biomechanical alterations, and the functional return to activity instead of tissue injury.

In conclusion, we present a unified framework for evaluation, exercise prescription, and rehabilitation that will allow the rehabilitation practitioner to have a consistency of approach and treatment for the athlete and will focus on restoration of function as the major guide for rehabilitation. Because of this consistency, outcome studies can be based on this type of framework. We expect that these studies will eventually serve as the backbone of the rehabilitation process, allowing rehabilitation practitioners to understand how well they are implementing specific rehabilitation processes and providing further scientific evidence of the role of rehabilitation.

This work is based on several years of study and evaluation and is the result of the effort of many dedicated rehabilitation practitioners. By giving the scientific rationale for the *why* and the *what,* rather than just the implementation of the *how* of rehabilitation, we provide a useful, broad-based tool for addressing the rehabilitation needs that occur in a sports medicine practice.

CHAPTER 1

A Framework for Rehabilitation

Stanley A. Herring and W. Ben Kibler

INTRODUCTION

The clinical practice of sports medicine is a growing concern. The September 1980 issue of *The Physician and Sports Medicine* published its first directory of sports medicine centers, listing 176 facilities. By September 1982, the directory had 410 entries[1]; by 1988, over 1,000 independent sports centers were operating. Also by 1988, 18 million American patients spent approximately 10 billion dollars rehabilitating sports injuries.[2]

The number of free-standing and institution-based sports medicine centers and the funds dedicated to rehabilitation of sports injuries no doubt continues to rise. Professional interest also continues to grow. Forty-seven sports medicine organizations, 23 groups and committees that generate sports medicine information, and 12 statistics-gathering groups are catalogued in the January 1995 issue of *The Physician and Sports Medicine*. The common denominator of all of these sports injuries and a large component of sports treatment and education is the rehabilitation of the injured patient. A rehabilitation framework can be organized around four principles[3]: (1) discovery of the type of injury that is present, (2) determination of the method of presentation of the injury, (3) complete and accurate diagnosis of the injury, and (4) plan of treatment of the injury and return to play of the athlete. Within this framework, the focus is first on *why* rehabilitate and *what* should be rehabilitated. The issue of *how* to rehabilitate then becomes much more manageable and orderly.

WHY REHABILITATE?

The burgeoning field of sports medicine reflects the injured athlete's search for specialized care. The sports participant is frequently significantly involved in his or her activity.

An injury is viewed as a real disability. The first and immediate reason for rehabilitation is to resolve the clinical symptoms and signs that exist at the time of the injury. Appropriate medication, physical modalities, relative rest, or even appropriate periods of splinting and/or immobilization are employed in this phase of rehabilitation. If the pathology is significant enough, surgical intervention may be necessary to treat the acute problem.

However, an athlete demands more than just relief of symptoms; return to activity is a goal. The issue is not simply treatment of symptoms; it is restoration of function. This is a second reason for rehabilitation to occur. Restoration of function should address both the local and general effects of an injury. Muscle strength may decrease up to 17% within the initial 72 hours of immobilization. That rate of decline slows after five to seven days, but losses of up to 40% of muscle strength are still seen after 6 weeks of casting.[4–6] Immobilization of the knee joint causes significant local biochemical and biomechanical alterations. Joint capsule, subchondral bone, bone ligament complex, and cartilage are all markedly affected within six to eight weeks of immobilization.[7] Prolonged rehabilitation of greater than one year may be necessary to regain flexibility and strength about the knee joint,[8] whereas articular cartilage may never return to normal after as little as eight weeks of immobilization.[9,10]

In addition to the local effects of an injury, general fitness can be affected as well and should be addressed in order to restore athletic function. Cardiovascular fitness can decrease very rapidly with inactivity. Maximum volume of oxygen utilization ($\dot{V}o_2$ max) decreases by up to 25% after three weeks of bed rest.[11,12] The positive effects of a seven-week endurance training program are almost completely lost within eight weeks of discontinuation of training. Approximately half of that loss occurs within the first two weeks.[13,14]

Along with cardiovascular fitness, strength is affected when training is interrupted by injury. If the athlete can maintain some form of strength training, even if it is reduced to one time per week, strength can still be fairly well maintained over a three-month period.[15,16] Indeed, a program to specifically address restoration of strength, power, flexibility, balance, and performance for both local and general deficits assures optimum treatment. The absence of symptoms does not mean normal function.

By developing a complete functional restoration program, the practitioner hopes to comprehensively treat the injury. This will limit the extent of the present injury and will also decrease the chance for recurrent injury. This is the third reason for rehabilitation to be undertaken. Injuries in sports are remarkably common. For instance, there are an estimated 1.2 million football-related injuries annually.[17] Even at the high school level of American football, injury rates of 50–80% have been reported.[18–19] Noncontact sports also result in frequent injury. Thirty percent to 50% of all sports injuries have been related to overload.[20–23] Whereas a variety of intrinsic and extrinsic factors have been analyzed to predict who will become injured,[24] the single best predictor for a new injury during sporting activity is the history of a previous injury.[17,25–27] The Lysens et al.[28] study of a group of students showed that those with previous injury were at relatively high risk for recurrence. Twenty-seven percent of the injuries in the study were reinjuries, 16% of which occurred within one month of returning to activity. Eighteen percent of these reinjuries were to exactly the same body part, and 82% of the reinjuries involved the same body segment at a different site. When considering why to place a patient in a rehabilitation program, it appears that the history of a previous injury carries significant risk for recurrent injury. Comprehensive rehabilitation may be necessary to break the cycle.

The final reason for a rehabilitation program to be considered is that a *re*habilitation program may lead eventually into a *pre*habilitation program.[29] The benefits gained from a rehabilitation program can be continued and generalized into an overall fitness program that extends throughout the year. As the patient progresses through rehabilitation to more sports-specific exercises, the training regimen can then be continued. This maintains physiologic and biomechanical fitness and, it is hoped, decreases the occurrence of future injury.

WHAT IS BEING REHABILITATED?

Construction of a complete treatment program requires the identification of what type of injury has occurred, as well as the fashion in which that injury presents. These issues are two of the four basic principles that make up the framework of a rehabilitation program.

Type of Injury

Two major types of sports injuries—*macrotrauma* and *microtrauma*—can occur.[3,29] Macrotrauma injuries occur due to a specific event. The time, place, and mechanism of injury is usually quite clear. This single event results in previously normal (or nearly normal) anatomic structures becoming suddenly and distinctly abnormal after the injury. Anterior cruciate ligament tears, fractures, or acute traumatic dislocations serve as examples.

Microtrauma injuries are chronic, repetitive injuries. These injuries are actually a process that results from the failure of homeostasis of the cellular mechanisms and tissue constituents to maintain integrity of the structures subjected to the demands of physical activity.[30,31] Cellular repair mechanisms appear to be disrupted by repetitive tensile overload. The cells cannot produce the proper matrix for the reparative process of injured muscle, tendon, ligament, or other tissue. Instead, the healing process produces scar. This is often a fairly long process, and clinically evident adaptive changes in flexibility, balance, strength, biomechanics, and performance occur in the athlete who continues to participate in sports. Achilles tendinitis, plantar fasciitis, medial and lateral epicondylitis, rotator cuff tendinitis, and other such problems represent chronic repetitive microtrauma injuries.

Method of Injury Presentation

When an injury occurs due to macrotrauma or microtrauma, the symptoms can present in several methods. The injury can be classified as (1) *acute*, (2) *chronic*, (3) *an acute exacerbation of a chronic injury*, and (4) *subclinical adaptation to athletic activity*.[3]

Acute injuries usually are the result of acute macrotrauma, as described above. The injury episode is easily recalled, and the usual athletic activity is halted or significantly curtailed immediately postinjury.

Chronic injuries usually result from microtrauma, with a gradual onset of symptoms. The pain may be fairly widespread, due to secondary adaptations and resultant injuries to other tissues. Athletic activity may still be ongoing, although at a reduced level of performance.

An athlete often has a history of a previous injury—apparently successfully treated because the symptoms have improved. However, absence of symptoms does not mean normal function. When the athlete returns to activity, an acute exacerbation of the previous injury occurs. Knowledge of the history of the previous injury and of the details of the previous rehabilitation plan provides clues that underlying problems (inflexibilities, strength deficits and imbalances, and biomechanical faults) may remain. A subacromial bursal injection takes away the shoulder pain until the player returns to tennis, for example. Indeed, the entire kinetic chain may be at risk. A seemingly acute injury may not occur at the exact site of previous injury; however, the same limb is frequently injured soon after return to physical activity.[28]

Acute injury, chronic injury, and acute flares of chronic problems all produce symptoms in athletes. The fourth method of presentation of injury is actually subclinical. Sporting activity can cause subclinical adaptations in lieu of actual signs or symptoms of injury. Whereas exercise has many helpful adaptations to the cardiovascular and musculoskeletal systems, some of the adaptations that occur to the musculoskeletal system, in particular, are, in reality, *mal*adaptations. There are asymptomatic strength, flexibility, and biomechanical changes that may predispose the athlete to future injury. Strength imbalances[32–34] and posterior shoulder inflexibilities[35] in overhead throwing and racquet athletes without current shoulder pain serve as examples. These subclinical adaptations demonstrate the continuum between rehabilitation and prehabilitation. A knowledgeable preparticipation examination can identify and treat these potential pain generators.[36]

Determination of what type of injury has occurred and the method of presentation of that injury helps delineate what requires rehabilitation. This task is completed by making a complete and accurate diagnosis of the injury—the third principle of rehabilitation mentioned in the introduction.

When an athlete is injured and symptoms develop, a clinical alteration occurs. This clinical alteration frequently occurs in the presence of subclinical alterations in anatomy, physiology, and mechanics, as noted above. This is particularly true with chronic injuries and acute exacerbation of chronic injuries. These alterations may be present with acute injuries as well, or they may be produced as consequences of the acute injury.

The clinical alterations produced by an injury include pain, swelling, decreased range of motion, and similar findings, producing a *clinical symptom complex*. The anatomic alterations from an injury include the actual tissue that has been damaged—the *tissue injury complex*—as well as tissues that have been stressed or overloaded and are contributing to, or exacerbating, the injury—the *tissue overload complex*.

The physiologic and mechanical alterations include abnormalities in strength, strength balance, and flexibility that alter the mechanics of performance of athletic activities— the *functional biomechanical deficit complex*. There are substitute motions and/or activities that the athlete utilizes to compensate for the injury and associated mechanical problems. Such changes in sports motions are referred to as the *subclinical adaptation complex* (see Table 1–1).

Clinical symptoms with their associated injured tissue, overloaded tissue, functional biomechanical deficits, and

Table 1–1 Areas of Alteration and Their Associated Complexes

Alteration	*Complex*
Clinical alteration	Clinical symptom complex
Anatomic alteration	Tissue injury complex
	Tissue overload complex
Physiologic and mechanical alteration	Functional biomechanical deficit complex
	Subclinical adaptation complex

subclinical adaptations can produce a negative feedback cycle, perpetuating or causing recurrences of an injury. A complete and accurate diagnosis that addresses all of these areas is necessary to provide for comprehensive and thorough rehabilitation (see Figure 1–1). This is true for acute injuries, chronic injuries, and acute exacerbations of chronic injuries (see Tables 1–2 and 1–3).

Table 1–2 Complete Diagnosis of Rotator Cuff Tendinitis/ Impingement—Chronic Injury and/or Acute Exacerbation of Chronic Injury

Tissue overload complex	Tensile load on posterior shoulder capsule structures Tensile load on posterior shoulder muscles Tensile load on scapular stabilizers
Tissue injury complex	Tears in posterior capsule Rotator cuff impingement Glenoid labral attrition
Clinical symptom complex	Rotator cuff impingement pain Anterior-superior glenohumeral instability Decreased ball or service velocity
Functional biomechanical deficit complex	Internal rotation inflexibility External rotation strength imbalance Lateral scapular slide
Subclinical adaptation complex	Alteration of shoulder throwing position or motion Decreased velocity

Source: Reprinted with permission from S.A. Herring, Rehabilitation of Muscle Injuries, *Medicine and Science in Sports and Exercise,* Vol. 22, p. 455, © 1990, Williams & Wilkins.

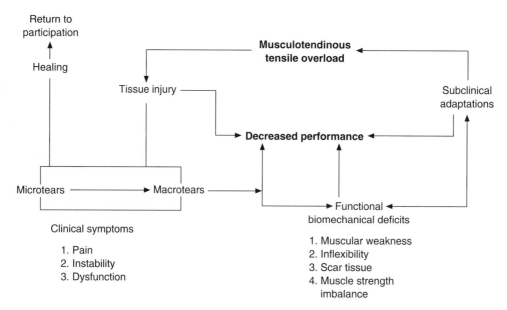

Figure 1–1 Injury cycle with negative feedback. *Source:* Reprinted with permission from W.B. Kibler, T.J. Chandler, and B.K. Pace, Injury Cycle with Negative Feedback, from Principles of Rehabilitation after Chronic Tendon Injuries, *CI Sports Medicine,* Vol. 11, p. 663, © 1992, W.B. Saunders.

Table 1–3 Complete Diagnosis of an Acute Quadriceps Contusion

Tissue overload complex	Same as tissue injury complex
Tissue injury complex	Direct trauma to muscle with tissue disruption, hemorrhage, acute inflammatory reaction
Clinical symptom complex	Pain Swelling Decreased range of motion Decreased ability to bear weight
Functional biomechanical deficit complex	None Decreased hip extension* Decreased knee flexion* Quadriceps/hamstrings strength imbalance*
Subclinical adaptation complex	None Gait alteration* Decreased speed*

* Will develop if rehabilitation is incomplete.

Source: Reprinted with permission from S.A. Herring, Rehabilitation of Muscle Injuries, *Medicine and Science in Sports and Exercise,* Vol. 22, pp. 453–456, © 1990, Williams & Wilkins.

HOW TO REHABILITATE

Once the type of injury has been determined and a complete and accurate diagnosis has been made, the plan for treatment and eventual return to play can be developed. This is the fourth principle of rehabilitation, as discussed in the introduction to this chapter.

The rehabilitation plan progresses through stages as biologic healing and repair occur. Appropriate tools are utilized in each of these treatment stages. Criteria can be developed for advancement from one stage of rehabilitation to the next. The clinical symptom complex, tissue injury complex, tissue overload complex, functional biomechanical deficit complex, and subclinical adaptation complex (see Table 1–1, Figure 1–1) make up the components of each phase of rehabilitation.[29] Three broad stages can be used to guide the rehabilitation of the injured athlete. These stages are: (1) *the acute stage*, (2) *the recovery stage*, and (3) *the functional stage*.[3,37]

In the acute stage of rehabilitation, the clinical symptom complex and tissue injury complex are the focus of treatment. During this stage of rehabilitation, goals are oriented toward decreasing the signs and symptoms of the injury. Pain, swelling, stiffness, and other clinical findings are addressed with relative rest, physical modalities, and medications. These measures also provide physiologic benefit for the damaged tissue by controlling the exuberant inflammatory response. Therapeutic cold, for example, decreases pain and spasm, and causes blood flow to diminish. The time for application to cool an injured muscle is directly dependent upon the depth of overlying fat. The addition of compression and elevation increases efficacy of treatment.[38–40] High-frequency electrical stimulation may also be used at this point to decrease muscle spasm and increase circulation while helping to remove inflammatory waste products.[41]

Superficial heat also relieves pain and muscle spasm, but it increases blood flow.[39] Deep-heating modalities (diathermy), such as ultrasound, are usually reserved for subacute or chronic problems.[15,40] Physical modalities can be utilized based on an understanding of their biophysical principles. Contraindications also exist for the use of these modalities and should be known to the practitioner. These physical modalities can be used acutely and occasionally in the subacute phases of tissue healing when repair and remodeling occur.[42–44] If tissue injury and clinical symptoms are severe, immobilization and/or surgery may be necessary.

Preserving as much mobility and strength as possible in the injured limb, as well as trying to maintain general strength and cardiovascular fitness, are also goals of the acute stage of rehabilitation. Soft tissue and articular mobilization and directed local and general strength and fitness training as tolerated are prescribed.

Criteria for advancement to the next stage of rehabilitation include adequate pain control and tissue healing. This allows for normal or near-normal painless range of motion and initial strengthening of the injured joint or limb (Exhibit 1–1).[3,29,45]

In the recovery stage of rehabilitation (Exhibit 1–2), treatment emphasis shifts from resolution of clinical signs and symptoms to restoration of function. Tissue healing is complete or nearly complete. The remodeling tissue can now be appropriately loaded to regain local flexibility, proprioception, and strength. Also, other tissue subjected to chronic overload prior to the injury and/or as a result of the injury itself is treated. These secondary biomechanical deficits in flexibility, strength, and strength balance at sites other than that of the clinical injury itself are now addressed. Along with these goals of the recovery stage, general fitness is also maintained.

While some manual therapy for myofascial and articular mobilization may continue, treatment emphasis shifts away from passive modalities and medications. Active interventions become more focused and aggressive. Carefully selected treatment is important. For example, muscle training effects are specific to limb position, joint angle, limb velocity, and type of contraction.[14,46–48] As rehabilitation progresses, such activities as running, jumping, throwing, and others are introduced.

The recovery stage may be the longest stage of the rehabilitation process. Criteria for advancement to the next stage of rehabilitation include complete pain control and tissue healing with essentially full painless range of motion and good flexibility. The athlete should be able to demonstrate strength of approximately 75–80% or greater as compared with the uninjured side. There should also be good strength balance.[3,29,45]

The final stage of rehabilitation is the functional stage. During this phase of treatment, residual biomechanical defi-

---

Exhibit 1–1 Acute Stage of Rehabilitation

Focus of treatment
 clinical symptom complex
 tissue injury complex

Tools
 rest and/or immobilization
 physical modalities
 medications
 manual therapy
 initial exercise
 surgery

Criteria for advancement
 pain control
 adequate tissue healing
 near-normal ROM
 tolerance for strengthening

 ROM, range of motion.

Exhibit 1–2 Recovery Stage of Rehabilitation

Focus of treatment
 tissue overload complex
 functional biomechanical deficit complex

Tools
 manual therapy
 flexibility
 proprioception/neuromuscular control training
 specific, progressive exercise

Criteria for advancement
 no pain
 complete tissue healing
 essentially full pain-free ROM
 good flexibility
 75–80% or greater strength, as compared with uninjured
  side, and good strength balance

cits continue to receive attention. Restoration of strength and strength balance allows for proper force generation and absorption. Regained flexibility and proprioception no longer impede motion. Normal movement patterns and sports-specific skills with the eventual return to athletic competition are the goals of treatment as the subclinical adaptation complex is addressed.

Using a lower-extremity injury in a tennis player for illustration, the athlete would continue to work on running, emphasizing symmetric weight-bearing during stance, coordinated push-off and landing, and proper force transfer for jumping or serving motions. Treatment for the entire kinetic chain necessary for tennis would have started during the recovery stage of rehabilitation. Treatment would continue and expand. Trunk, shoulder, and upper-extremity mobility and strength work would continue as the tennis player's mechanics are reviewed and corrected. Sports-specific progressions would be added, such as spider agility drills.

Criteria for return to competition include no signs or symptoms of the clinical injury, full painless range of motion, normal flexibility, normal strength and strength balance, good general fitness, normal sports mechanics, and the ability to demonstrate sports-specific skills (Exhibit 1–3). This rehabilitation period is indeed a maintenance stage; it is continued as an ongoing injury protection program for the athlete.[3,29,45]

CONCLUSION

Sporting activities commonly lead to injury. The type of injury and how that injury presents should be identified.

Exhibit 1–3 Functional Stage of Rehabilitation

Focus of treatment
  functional biomechanical deficit complex
  subclinical adaptation complex

Tools
  power and endurance exercise
  sports-specific functional progression
  technique/skills instruction

Criteria for return to play
  no pain
  full pain-free ROM/normal flexibility
  normal strength and strength balance
  good general fitness
  normal sports mechanics
  demonstration of sports-specific skills

ROM, range of motion.

Also, a complete, accurate diagnosis of the injury is essential. The practitioner can then develop a rehabilitation plan that progresses rationally and is based on restoration of function, not just relief of symptoms. Such a program will give the athlete the best chance to make a full recovery, to return to competition, and to avoid future injury. The rehabilitation plan must be specific for each injury and individualized for each athlete. A representational comprehensive treatment program for a rotator cuff problem is presented in Exhibit 1–4.

Exhibit 1–4 Comprehensive Rehabilitation for Rotator Cuff Tendinitis/Impingement

---

I. Acute Phase
   A. Goals
      1. Reestablish nonpainful range of motion
      2. Retard muscle atrophy of entire upper extremity
      3. Neuromuscular control of scapula in neutral glenohumeral position
      4. Reduce pain and inflammation
   B. Range of motion
      1. Dependent
         a. Mobilization of glenohumeral, clavicle, and scapulothoracic joints
         b. Manual capsular stretching and cross-friction massage
      2. Independent
         a. Codman's and/or pendulum exercises

         b. Ropes and pulleys
         c. T-bar
   C. Muscle atrophy/neuromuscular control
      1. Local
         a. Isometrics
         b. Scapular control
         c. Closed chain activities
      2. Distant
         a. Open chain—nonpathologic areas (elbow, back)
            i. Concentrics
            ii. Eccentrics
      3. Aerobic/anaerobic activities
   D. Pain and inflammation
      1. NSAIDs 48–96 hrs

continues

Exhibit 1–4 continued

2. Modalities 2–3 wks
3. Joint mobilization
4. Joint protection
E. Range of motion
  1. Passive flexibility
  2. Active flexibility
F. Criteria for advancement
  1. No swelling
  2. Minimal to no pain
  3. Manual muscle testing strength 75% of strength in other muscles
  4. Scapular control in neutral position

II. Recovery Phase
  A. Goals
    1. Regain and improve upper extremity muscle strength
    2. Improve upper extremity neuromuscular control
    3. Normalize shoulder arthrokinematics in single planes of motion
    4. Improve active/passive range of motion flexibility
  B. Strengthening
    1. Dependent
      a. Scapular proprioceptive neuromuscular facilitation
      b. Glenohumeral proprioceptive neuromuscular facilitation
    2. Independent single-plane motions
      a. Concentric and eccentric isotonics
      b. Isokinetics
      c. Tubing
      d. Rotator cuff isolation exercises (Jobe)
  C. Neuromuscular control
    1. Proprioceptive neuromuscular facilitation
    2. Emphasis on force couples
      a. Scapular retractors/protractors

      b. Glenohumeral elevators/depressors
      c. Glenohumeral internal/external rotators
  D. Arthrokinematics
    1. Joint mobilization
    2. Kinetic chain movement patterns
  E. Criteria for advancement
    1. Full nonpainful scapulothoracic motion
    2. Almost full nonpainful glenohumeral motion
    3. Normal scapular stabilizer strength (lateral slide asymmetry < 0.5 cm)
    4. Rotator cuff strength 75% of normal
    5. Normal throwing motion

III. Functional Phase
  A. Goals
    1. Increase power and endurance in upper extremity
    2. Increase normal multiple-plane neuromuscular control (eliminate subclinical adaptations)
    3. Sports-specific activity
  B. Power and endurance
    1. Multiple plane motions
    2. Plyometrics
      a. Wall push-ups
      b. Ball throws
      c. Tubing or other elastic resistance
      d. Medicine ball
    3. Conditioning based on principles of periodization
  C. Sports-specific functional progression
    1. Long toss–short toss
    2. Throwing
    3. Pitching

IV. Criteria for Return to Play
  A. Normal arthrokinematics in multiple planes
  B. Isokinetic strength 90% of normal
  C. Negative clinical examination

Source: Reprinted with permission from W.B. Kibler, T.J. Chandler, and B.K. Pace, Principles of Rehabilitation after Chronic Tendon Injuries, *Cl Sports Medicine,* Vol. 11, pp. 668–669, © 1992, W.B. Saunders.

REFERENCES

1. Hage P. Sports medicine clinics: are guidelines necessary? *Phys Sports Med.* 1982;10:165.
2. Behar R. Medicine's $10 billion bonanza. *Forbes.* June 13, 1988:107.
3. Kibler WB. A framework for sports medicine. *Phys Med Rehabil Clin North Am.* 1994;5:1.
4. Booth FW. Physiologic and biochemical effects of immobilization on muscle. *Clin Orthop.* 1987;219:15.
5. Lindboe CF, Platou CS. Effect of immobilization of short duration on the muscle fibre size. *Clin Physiol.* 1984;4:183.
6. MacDougall J, Ward G, Sale D, Sutton J. Biomechanical adaptation of human skeletal muscle to heavy resistance training and immobilization. *J Appl Physiol.* 1977;43:700.
7. Akeson W, Woo SL-Y, Amiel D. The connective tissue response to immobility: biomechanical changes in periarticular connective tissue of the immobilized rabbit knee. *Clin Orthop.* 1973;93:356.
8. Zarins B. Soft tissue injury and repair—biomechanical aspects. *Int J Sports Med.* 1982(suppl 1):319.
9. Finsterbush A, Friedman B. Reversibility of joint changes produced by immobilization in rabbits. *Clin Orthop.* 1975;111:290.
10. Paulos LE, Payne FC, Rosenberg TD. Rehabilitation after anterior cruciate ligament surgery. In: Jackson D, Drew D, eds. *The Anterior Cruciate Deficient Knee.* St. Louis: Mosby; 1987:291.
11. American College of Sports Medicine. *Guidelines for Exercise Testing and Prescription.* 4th ed. Philadelphia: Lea & Febiger; 1991.

12. Grimby G, Saltin B. Physiological effects of physical training. *Scand J Rehabil Med.* 1971;3:6.

13. Orlander J, et al. Low intensity training, inactivity and resumed training in sedentary men. *Acta Physiol Scand.* 1977;101:351.

14. Winter D. Moments of force and mechanical power in jogging. *J Biomech.* 1983;16:91.

15. Cole AJ, Eagleston RA. The benefits of deep heat. *Phys Sports Med.* 1994;22(2):77.

16. Graves JE, Pollock SH. Effect of reduced training frequency on muscular strength. *Sports Med.* 1988;9:316.

17. Robey JM, Blyth CS, Mueller FD. Athletic injuries: application of epidemiologic methods. *JAMA.* 1971;217:184.

18. DeLee JC, Farney WC. Incidence of injury in Texas high school football. *Am J Sports Med.* 1992;20:575.

19. Garrick JG, Regua RK. Injuries in high school sports. *Pediatrics.* 1978;61:465.

20. Herring SA, Nilson KL. Introduction to overuse injuries. *Clin Sports Med.* 1987;6:225.

21. Orava S. *Exertion injuries due to sports and physical exercise. A clinical and statistical study of nontraumatic overuse injuries of the musculoskeletal system of athletes and keep-fit athletes.* Oulu, Finland: University of Oulu, 1980. Thesis.

22. Renstrom P, Johnson RJ. Overuse injuries in sports: a review. *Sports Med.* 1985;2:316.

23. Sperryn PN, Williams JGP. Why sports injury clinics? *Br Med J.* 1975; 5966:364.

24. Taimela S, Kujalu U, Osterman K. Intrinsic risk factors and athletic injuries. *Sports Med.* 1990;9:205.

25. Bende et al. Factors affecting the occurrence of knee injuries. *J Assoc Phys Ment Rehabil.* 1964;18:130.

26. Blyth CS, Mueller FU. Football injury survey. 1: When and where players get hurt. *Phys Sports Med.* 1974;2:45.

27. Ekstrand J, Gillquist J. Soccer injuries and their mechanisms: a prospective study. *Med Sci Sports Exerc.* 1983;15:267.

28. Lysens, et al. The predictability of sports injuries. *Sports Med.* 1984;1:6.

29. Kibler WB, Herring SA. Formulating a rehabilitation program. In: Griffin LY, ed. *Rehabilitation of the Injured Knee.* 2nd ed. St. Louis: Mosby; 1995.

30. Kibler WB. Physiology of injury. In: Schafer MA, ed. *AAOS Instructional Course Lectures,* vol 43. In press.

31. Leadbetter WB. Physiology of tissue repair. In: *Athletic Training and Sports Medicine.* Park Ridge, IL: American Academy of Orthopaedic Surgeons; 1991:43.

32. Chandler TJ, Kibler WB, Kiser AM, et al. Shoulder strength power, and endurance in college tennis players. *Am J Sports Med.* 1992;20:455.

33. Cook EE, Gray UL, Savinar-Nogue E, et al. Shoulder antagonistic strength ratios: a comparison between college level pitchers and non-pitchers. *J Orthop Sports Phys Ther.* 1987;8(9):451.

34. Hinton RY. Isokinetic evaluation of shoulder rotational strength in high school baseball pitchers. *Am J Sports Med.* 1988;16:274.

35. Chandler TJ, Kibler WB, Uhl TL, et al. Flexibility comparisons of junior elite tennis players to other players. *Am J Sports Med.* 1990;18: 134.

36. Kibler WB, Chandler TJ, Uhl TL. A musculoskeletal approach to the preparticipation physical examination preventing injury and improving performance. *Am J Sports Med.* 1989;17:525.

37. Kibler WB. Concepts in exercise rehabilitation. In: Leadbetter W, Buckwalter JA, Gordon SL, eds. *Sports Induced Inflammation.* Chicago: American Academy of Orthopaedic Surgeons; 1990:759.

38. Herring SA. Rehabilitation of muscle injuries. *Med Sci Sports Exerc.* 1990;22:453.

39. Kaul MP, Herring SA. Superficial heat and cold. *Phys Sports Med.* 1994;22(12):65.

40. Lehmann JF, DeLateur B. Diathermy and superficial heat and cold therapy. In: Koltke EJ, Stillwell GK, and Lehmann JF, eds. *Krusen's Handbook of Physical Medicine and Rehabilitation.* 3rd ed. Philadelphia: W.B. Saunders; 1982:275.

41. Windsor RE, Lester JP, Herring SA. Electrical stimulation in clinical practice. *Phys Sports Med.* 1993;21(2):85.

42. Kellett J. Acute soft tissue injuries—a review of the literature. *Med Sci Sports Exerc.* 1986;18:489.

43. Oakes BW. Acute soft tissue injuries: nature and management. *Aust Fam Physician.* 1982;10(suppl):3.

44. VanDerMeulin JHC. Present state of knowledge on processes of healing in collagen structures. *Int J Sports Med.* 1982;3(suppl):4.

45. Kibler WB, Chandler TJ, Pace BK. Principles of rehabilitation after chronic tendon injuries. *Clin Sports Med.* 1992;11:661.

46. McConnell J. The management of chondromalacia patellae: a long-term solution. *Aust J Physiother.* 1986;32:215.

47. Moffroid M, Whipple R. Specificity of speed of exercise. *Phys Ther.* 1970;50:1692.

48. Sale D, MacDougall D. Specificity in strength training: a review for the coach and athlete. *Can J Appl Sports Sci.* 1981;6:87.

CHAPTER 2

The Physiologic Basis of Sports Rehabilitation

Jeffrey Young and Joel M. Press

Understanding the principles and applications of exercise physiology is critical for the quickest and best rehabilitation of sports-injured athletes. Appropriate application of exercise training principles by skilled professionals enables injured athletes to recover and prepares healthy athletes for higher levels of sports performance. This chapter focuses on the basic physiologic principles of sports rehabilitation.

TYPES OF MUSCULAR CONTRACTION

Depending on the external resistance applied to the musculotendinous unit and the specific demands of the athletic activity, muscular contraction may be described in several ways.

Concentric

During this type of contraction, the muscular force generated overcomes an applied external resistance, and the whole muscle length is reduced.[1] As a result, at least one of the two limb segments spanned by the contracting muscle moves, with the assigned origin and insertion brought closer to one another. For example, the combined concentric contractions of the middle deltoid and rotator cuff muscles produces elevation (abduction) of the humerus. Concentric contractions are also important because they accelerate the more distal link segments in the kinetic chain. For instance, combined concentric contractions of the pectoralis major and the latissimus dorsi enable a quarterback to rapidly accelerate, in sequence, the upper arm, the lower arm and wrist, and the football. Healthy muscle and, for that matter, the entire musculotendinous unit, is not usually injured when the muscles contract in a concentric manner. This may be because the muscle length is moving toward a protected (shortened) state, and the muscle is both at a lower absolute tension and at a lower point on the force-tension curve. Muscle that is acutely injured or that has been repeatedly injured but not rehabilitated may also demonstrate a lesser load-to-failure and receive further injury under high-resistance concentric contraction conditions.

Eccentric

A contraction is considered to be eccentric when development of increased muscle tension is accompanied by muscle lengthening.[1] Motion occurs, but the assigned origin and insertion move away from one another. The slow lowering of an abducted humerus to the side of the body is an example of an eccentric contraction.

Muscles are capable of generating greater forces under eccentric conditions than under either isometric or concentric conditions, and more under isometric conditions than under concentric conditions.[2–5] Thus, it is easier to hold a weighted barbell still than to actually lift it, and it is even easier to gradually lower the barbell than to hold it still. Muscle contractions are further modified by their speed of contraction. Rapid eccentric contractions generate more force than do slow ones (slower eccentric work approximates isometric), and slower concentric contractions generate more force than do rapid ones.[2,3,6] Eccentric contractions are also more efficient than are concentric contractions (i.e., require less oxygen) at the same tension and contraction velocity.[7,8] The time to reach peak tension is also faster during eccentric contractions than during concentric contractions.[8,9]

Eccentric contractions are essential for deceleration of kinetic link segments that have acquired large amounts of kinetic energy. For example, once a quarterback's arm has accelerated forward and the football is released, the eccentric firings of scapular stabilizer muscles and rotator cuff muscles are necessary to retain normal glenohumeral relationships and to prevent the humerus from flying toward the receiver with the ball.

The large tensile forces that typically occur with sudden eccentric contractions in sports (i.e., the football defensive back who has to rapidly stop running toward the line of scrimmage and reverse direction because he had mistakenly taken the cue to run instead of to pass), or the microtraumatic tensile forces that occur with repetitive eccentric contractions (such as those within the gastroc-soleus complex of an ultramarathon runner) both render muscle vulnerable to injury. Eccentric muscle overload can be associated with both early- and delayed-onset muscle soreness.[1] Muscle that is unprepared for eccentric work is injured more readily because of the absolute tension being higher and the muscle-tendon length being closer to load-to-tensile failure. Traditional athletic and sports rehabilitation programs have often omitted eccentric training as the final preparatory step before the athletes resume their sports. Although no definitive study exists supporting the premise that eccentric training is a prerequisite for safe resumption of activity, the authors suggest that, given the growing body of literature indicating the vulnerability of the musculotendinous unit under eccentric contraction conditions and the nature of skeletal muscle's response to overload (see section related to specificity of training), it makes sense to incorporate this type of exercise into a functionally based sports rehabilitation program.

Isometric

Under this condition, the length of the whole muscle is unchanged, and there is no net movement of the link segments spanned by the contracting muscles. While a gymnast holds himself in an L position on the parallel bars, the shoulder depressors, pectoralis major, latissimus dorsi, and triceps contract isometrically to stabilize the upper body, while the abdominal muscles, hip flexors, and knee extensors isometrically contract to maintain the 90-degree angle between the legs and the torso. Although the forces generated during isometric contractions are potentially greater than during concentric work, muscles are rarely injured during isometric contractions.

This is presumably due to the lack of change in muscle length, so that although the absolute tension is higher, the muscle does not move any closer to its failure length. Furthermore, if there are multiple muscles around a joint that are isometrically contracting together, there may be less chance of injury because the multimuscle cocontractions serve to stabilize the joint. Isometric exercises are often prescribed during the early phases of rehabilitating a musculotendinous injury because the intensity of contraction and the muscle length at which it contracts can be controlled.

Isotonic versus Dynamic

When originally used, the term *isotonic* encompassed contractions of both the eccentric and concentric types.[6] This term implies that either the tension within the muscle or the torque generated by the muscle is constant throughout the arc of motion. Because muscle tension changes constantly with alteration of joint angle, even when the speed of the contraction is kept constant, this is an imprecise term.[5,6,10] Therefore, it is more appropriate to use the term *dynamic* when categorizing contractions such as those associated with limb motion.

Isokinetic

This is a contraction that takes place at a constant velocity. Computerized machines that can calculate external torque generation by a muscle group within a predetermined arc of motion and at a predetermined velocity are necessary to evaluate isokinetic strength. Although it is common for therapists, trainers, and researchers to refer to isokinetic data when evaluating strength and performance, it is important to recognize that isokinetic contractions do not occur in real life, which renders extrapolation from isokinetic data to clinical situations limited. Furthermore, training athletes on isokinetic equipment should probably be reserved for the injured or postsurgical athlete, whose range of motion or exercise intensity needs to be more carefully monitored.

Plyometric

This type of exercise is designed to use the viscoelastic properties of the whole muscle to produce greater forces than those created by sarcomere shortening alone. A rapid overload (prestretch) is placed upon the muscle immediately before a concentric contraction. This both stretches the connective tissue (tendon as well as muscle) and places an eccentric load upon the muscle that facilitates subsequent concentric force generation.[4,5,11] Plyometric exercises emphasize explosive motions and are a valuable component of skill and agility training. They are also among the most sports-specific of all the types of contractions reviewed in this section. For example, high jumpers first lower their bodies toward the ground, placing a prestretch upon the gastroc-soleus complex, quadriceps, upper hamstrings, and gluteal muscles before the shortening contractions of these muscles, which propels the athletes up and over the bar.

Closed versus Open Kinetic Chain Exercises

The difference between closed kinetic chain (CKC) and open kinetic chain (OKC) exercises is important. If, for instance, during knee extension or flexion, the foot is allowed to move freely through space, the system is called *open*. In an OKC system, the hamstrings are predominant in knee flexion, whereas extension is dominated by the quadriceps. During CKC exercises for the lower limbs, the foot is kept immobile or maintains contact with a ground reactive force, and a multiarticular closed chain is created. Rather than the near isolation of the large muscle groups seen during OKC exercises, performance of CKC knee flexion and extension results in coactivation of both hamstrings and quadriceps groups.[12,13] An example of a CKC lower limb exercise (leg press) is shown in Figure 2–1. Both agonists and antagonists are simultaneously strengthened via cocontraction, which occurs in lower limb sports such as running. An OKC knee extension is depicted in Figure 2–2. Closed kinetic chain and OKC conditions exist for the upper limbs as well. Closed kinetic chain upper limb exercises are particularly useful during the early recovery period from shoulder surgery as there is less shear force imparted across the glenoid labrum, whereas multiple muscles around the scapula and glenohumeral joint can be simultaneously activated.[14] An example of a rehabilitation technique that alternates between OKC and CKC exercise for the upper limbs is shown in Figure 2–3.

PRESCRIPTION OF EXERCISE

Exercise prescription for developing strength, power, or endurance is based upon a relatively simple principle called the *specific adaptation to imposed demand* (SAID) principle. It recognizes that the human body will respond to given demands with specific and predictable adaptation.[15] An important corollary is that although muscle is extremely adaptable and can "learn" to do many different things, it can probably do only one thing best. Although an athlete can improve in more than one area of fitness at a time (i.e., cross-training), he or she cannot attain maximal gains in both strength and marathon-type endurance at the same time.[2,16–18] Therefore, when designing conditioning programs, it is important to identify what the specific goals of the particular program are and then select exercises that maximize the likelihood that the desired training effect will be achieved. The basic components of the exercise prescription follow:

Intensity

Essentially, this describes the difficulty level of the exercise. For aerobic training, the exercise should be carried out at 40–85% maximal aerobic power (maximum volume of oxygen utilization [V_{O_2}max]) or 55–90% of maximal heart rate.[19] Lower intensities may promote a training effect, but the exercises must be carried out for lengthy periods of time to do so.[2,11,19] For recreational exercisers, use of the rating of perceived exertion (RPE) scale may be a convenient method of ensuring that approximately the same intensity is achieved on a day-to-day basis.[20,21] However, RPE is also related to the "familiarity" the athlete has with the given type of exercise, and an RPE of 14 on one mode of exercise does not necessar-

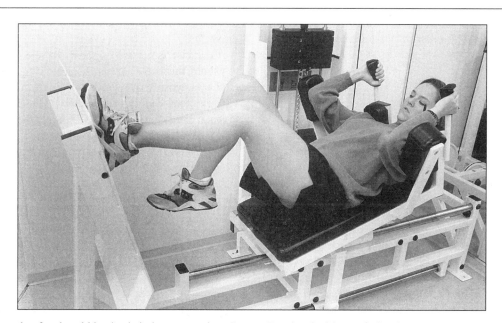

Figure 2–1 Example of a closed kinetic chain knee extension. *Source:* Reprinted with permission from J. Young, N. Olsen, and J. Press, Musculoskeletal Disorders of the Lower Limb, in R.L. Braddom, *Physical Medicine and Rehabilitation,* pp. 787–788, © 1996, W.B. Saunders.

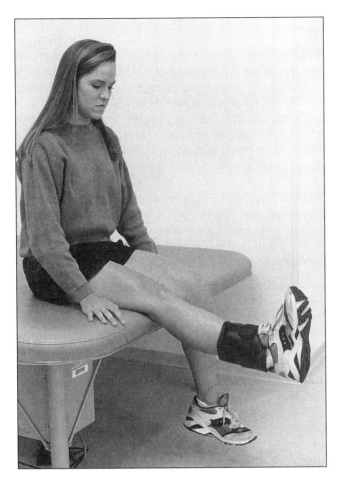

Figure 2–2 Example of an open kinetic chain knee extension. *Source:* Reprinted with permission from J. Young, N. Olson, and J. Press, Musculoskeletal Disorders of the Lower Limb, in R.L. Braddom, *Physical Medicine and Rehabilitation,* pp. 787–788, © 1996, W.B. Saunders.

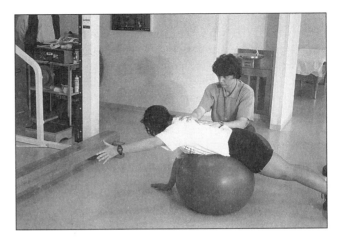

Figure 2–3 Combination of open kinetic chain condition for athlete's left upper limb and closed kinetic chain for the right upper limb. Note that the therapist is able to incorporate truncal control training as well. *Source:* Copyright © Rehabilitation Institute of Chicago.

Duration

This indicates the exercise session's length. Exercise should be carried out for between 15 and 60 minutes to develop an aerobic training effect and may be performed continuously or discontinuously.[19] Continuous training can have different outcomes, depending on the exercise intensity selected. Specificity dictates that if the athlete trains at high intensities for shorter time periods, a tolerance for lactate will be built up, and $\dot{V}O_2$max will likely improve.[2,5,22]

If exercise is carried out near the intensity of the lactate threshold, this is the parameter most influenced.[22,24] Exercise at lower intensities carried out for more than one hour allows for large total energy expenditure without exposure to high levels of stress and promotes more efficient utilization of free fatty acid (FFA) stores.[1,5,11] In general, there is an inverse relationship between the intensity of exercise and the length of time it can be sustained.

Interval training is a method of discontinuous training that alternates "work" and "relief" periods.[2] The work interval typically consists of exercise that is a very high percentage of maximum for a short time period, followed by the relief period that is of low intensity. The relief interval allows for resynthesis of phosphagens and decreases the need for glycolytic metabolism when the high-intensity work interval is started again.[2,5] When the cumulative exercise time is examined, it becomes apparent that this scheme potentially enables the individual to work for long periods at an intensity that would normally cause fatigue in a few minutes.[2,5] Daniels recommends that a 1:1 work:relief ratio be used,

ily equate to the same power output or caloric expenditure on another. For example, a recreational exerciser who is a runner will perceive bicycle exercise requiring an equivalent oxygen uptake demand to be more intense. This sense of increased effort will be accompanied by a greater heart rate and metabolic response as well.

For sprint or anaerobic training, the absolute work intensity needs to be "supramaximal," i.e., the athlete must exercise at work rates in excess of that necessary to elicit $\dot{V}O_2$max during a progressive exercise test.[3,19,22] Intensities that promote endurance training effects do not have an effect on anaerobic capacity.[22] However, if the Fartlek ("speed play") type of training is employed in which short, fast bursts of running are interspersed within the running workout, there may be development of some anaerobic qualities as well.[23]

with the work bouts kept less than 5 minutes for aerobic-type training.[23]

Frequency

This tells how often the exercise is performed and is typically 3–5 days per week for the majority of recreational exercisers.[19] Competitive athletes' training schedules vary, depending on whether it is "preseason," during competition, or "off season." During preseason training, high-level athletes may train up to six or seven days per week and may complete more than one session per day. The focus of these workouts varies, as the athlete may need to improve endurance, strength, and skill all at the same time. During the competitive season, the number of formal workouts per week often drops. In contact sports such as football, the athlete may take days off to recover from acute and subacute musculotendinous injury. In sports such as tennis, for instance, a three- or five-set singles match may more than substitute for a session on a treadmill or bike ergometer.

Mode of Exercise

If improvement in fitness is desired, the athlete should be tested in a manner that approximates the mode of training as much as possible. A bicycle-trained athlete should be tested on a bike, a runner on a treadmill, and a swimmer in a flume. Failure to conduct these tests will often result in underprediction of the training effect. From a general conditioning standpoint, varying the mode of exercise from session to session can be extremely useful by potentially increasing the number of muscle groups trained, reducing the likelihood of musculotendinous overload without adequate time for tissue healing and repair, and decreasing the athlete's likelihood of boredom.

MUSCULAR OVERWORK AND OVERTRAINING

Exercise that is too intense or that involves a significant amount of eccentric overload may induce excessive postexercise muscular soreness, which reflects a condition of acute muscular overwork. In general, if exercise results in elevation of blood levels of creatine phosphokinase (CPK), lactate dehydrogenase (LDH), or myoglobin, some level of rhabdomyolysis has occurred.[25] This is apparent within 24 hours of exercise. Extremes of either intensity or duration are both capable of producing these enzymatic changes, although intensity appears to be the more critical factor.[25,26]

Intense eccentric exercise is associated with numerous disturbances of muscle ultrastructure. Forced lengthening of contracted muscle produces damage that includes sarcolemmal rupturing, degeneration, and disorganization of myofibrils, and increased numbers of inflammatory cells.[7,27–29] Eccentric exercise that induces delayed-onset muscle soreness (24–72 hours postexercise) is also associated with decreased ability to resynthesize glycogen during this time frame.[28,30] Despite a more than 50-fold greater tensile strength than muscle, tendon—which represents the conduit between muscle and bone—can also become deformed and injured with either sudden high force or repetitive eccentric loads.[2] If the athlete is not allowed adequate recovery following eccentric overload, microscopic breakdown occurs, and the nidus of both the tissue injury and tissue overload complexes (see later discussion) is created. This then increases the likelihood that a maladaptive response to exercise will occur, with ultimate worsening of performance or injury.

Overtraining is the product of an imbalance between overload (training) and recovery. The athlete who overtrains exhibits symptoms and findings of muscular and systemic breakdown (maladaptation), which are, unfortunately, frequently overlooked until athletic performance begins to decline. From a subjective standpoint, the person who is overtraining may complain of feeling "stale," of not being as motivated, or of being generally fatigued.[31] Sleep patterns may be disturbed, and the athlete may report that he or she is always tired upon waking in the morning. The school-age or college-age athlete may admit having a difficult time completing assignments in classes or receiving poorer grades. In addition, teammates or family members may note that the athlete is more irritable or difficult to talk to. Loss of appetite is common.[32] Complaint of pain and soreness of muscles and joints, often in the absence of overt cause, is another clue that the person is overtraining and that a "chronic athletic fatigue" syndrome is present.[32]

Objective findings of overtraining include elevation of the AM resting heart rate by more than five beats per minute, immune suppression with an increased frequency of respiratory illnesses, and weight loss.[2,32,33] In addition, testosterone levels tend to drop whereas cortisol levels tend to rise, suggesting hypothalamic dysfunction.[31,34] Glycogen depletion, which can be caused by repeated lengthy bouts of exercise accompanied by inadequate ingestion of carbohydrates, may also contribute to muscular fatigue.[32] Certain muscle enzyme concentrations (creatine phosphokinase, lactate dehydrogenase, transaminase) and myoglobin rise rather dramatically following single bouts of heavy exertion, signifying muscle damage, but in and of themselves are not reliable markers of chronic overtraining.[25,26,32] Recurrent stress fractures indicate some repetitive biomechanical overload. Although full discussion of this issue is beyond the scope of this chapter, when stress fractures are discovered in a lean female athlete, her dietary habits and menstrual history should be investigated. Consultation with a sports psychologist and a formal endocrinologic evaluation may be required as well.

Ultimately, preventing overtraining is more critical than are its detection and treatment. Prudent recommendations include ensuring that the athlete matches energy expenditure with caloric intake, encouraging the athlete to obtain adequate sleep every night, and increasing training frequency, duration, or intensity by small increments. Periodization of training (i.e., varying the volume and intensity of training sessions) at different times of the year so that the athlete "peaks" near competitions but does not have to maintain peak form year-round is critical. Tapering the volume of training in the weeks prior to competition allows for reduction of muscular soreness, recovery from injury, and restoration of metabolic stores.[11]

THE APPLICATION OF PHYSIOLOGIC PRINCIPLES TO SPORT-SPECIFIC TRAINING

For the sports medicine professional to create a meaningful sports-specific training program, he or she needs an understanding of the relative contributions of the different energy systems combined with recognition of the muscular demands of a given athletic activity An excellent method of characterizing different sports in this manner is provided by Kibler.[35] For each activity, five critical parameters (flexibility, strength, power, anaerobic endurance, aerobic endurance) are rated on the basis of how critical they are for performance of that sport. A rating of 1 indicates that the parameter is minimally needed, a rating of 2 implies that it is necessary for injury reduction, a rating of 3 identifies the parameter as being synergistic for optimum performance, and a rating of 4 designates the parameter as being maximally required for optimum performance.[35] Some profiles follow.

Basketball

Players may be on the court for just a few seconds or for as much as 40 minutes per game. Although there are many breaks, the action is of high intensity, with running, jumping, and quick changes of direction. The participant needs an aerobic base with superimposed anaerobic power and endurance. This sport has been rated as flexibility 3, strength 3, power 4, anaerobic endurance 4, and aerobic endurance 4.[35] This profile clearly shows that basketball is a demanding sport in many areas. It is also clear that an athlete cannot train in all these areas during the course of the season and play ball as well. Therefore, implementation of a vigorous aerobic training program, out of season, is essential. Maximum volume of oxygen utilization should be evaluated during the off season as well. Strength and flexibility can be actively addressed during the season. Regular participation in the sport,

augmented by additional preseason conditioning, facilitates development of anaerobic endurance and power. If testing of anaerobic power and endurance is desired, the Wingate Test may be used.[2,5]

Long-Distance Running

This is a somewhat more straightforward profile, as the most important parameter, by far, is aerobic endurance. The profile is flexibility 3, strength 2, power 2, anaerobic endurance 2, and aerobic endurance 4.[35] Other than having to remember to stretch appropriate muscle groups, this athlete can spend almost all training time in one area. If this were a "middle-distance runner" instead, anaerobic work (or at least high-intensity aerobic work) and strength training would be encouraged. Measurement of $\dot{V}o_2max$ and the ventilatory breakpoint (work intensity during incremental exercise, at which minute ventilation increases disproportionately to oxygen consumption but not to carbon dioxide production) or the onset of peripheral blood lactate accumulation during an incremental treadmill exercise test may be beneficial.

Similar profiles can be established for other sports.[1] Montgomery analyzed ice hockey and found that the on-ice heart rate (HR) was 85–90% HRmax and on-ice oxygen consumption 70–80% $\dot{V}o_2max$ with bursts in excess of 90% maximum for both parameters.[36] Given the fast pace of the sport and the need for upper-body strength, the need for development of power, strength, and anaerobic endurance was identified. The $\dot{V}o_2max$ values for forward were between 55 and 60 mL/kg/min, indicating the need for an aerobic base.[36] Therefore, a battery of tests, including a skating $\dot{V}o_2max$ test, would be appropriate. Interestingly, it was reported that an on-ice training program during the season did not induce an increase in $\dot{V}o_2max$ in professional skaters.[36] This further emphasizes the need for preseason conditioning programs to improve aerobic fitness in a skill sport. Applying the Kibler system to hockey, it can be rated as flexibility 3, strength 3, power 4, anaerobic endurance 3, and aerobic endurance 3 or 4, depending on position requirements (i.e., goalie vs. forward).[1]

Incorporation of Kinetic Chain Principles

Muscles rarely act in isolation. Sports-specific movements are combinations of muscle cocontractions—the working of agonist and antagonist muscles in a finely tuned, timed manner. To rehabilitate specific musculotendinous structures, understanding of which other structures work with the injured part to perform a specific function is required. For example, numerous muscles around the lower limbs, trunk, shoulder girdle, and arm work together when an athlete pitches a baseball. Although the supraspinatus tendon may be the critical tissue injured in rotator cuff disease, rehabilitation that neglects the importance of the scapular stabilizers and trunk and extremity muscles will be incomplete and often inadequate.

A complete understanding for the biomechanics of specific sports-related motions, i.e., pitching, kicking a ball, hurdling, etc., are useful in sports rehabilitation. Addressing all of the components of the "kinetic chain" will allow more physiologic training to be added to the rehabilitation program. Examples include addressing shoulder internal/external rotation mobility and strength in lateral epicondyli-tis and hamstring, and hip flexor flexibility in plantar fasciitis.

CONCLUSION

Exercise physiologic principles are the basis of sports rehabilitation. Understanding of the specific type of musculotendinous injury and the response of muscles and tendons to training, along with the intensity and intervals of training, is essential for prescribing a complete rehabilitation program.

REFERENCES

1. Young JL, Press JM. The physiologic basis of sports rehabilitation. *Phys Med Rehabil Clin North Am.* 1994;5:9–36.

2. Astrand PO, Rodahl K. *Textbook of Work Physiology.* New York: McGraw-Hill; 1986.

3. Guyton AC. *Textbook of Medical Physiology.* 8th ed. Philadelphia: WB Saunders; 1991.

4. Komi PV, ed. *Strength and Power in Sport.* London: Blackwell Scientific Publications, 1992.

5. McArdle WD, Katch FI, Katch VL. *Exercise Physiology: Energy, Nutrition and Human Performance.* 3rd ed. Philadelphia: Lea & Febiger; 1991.

6. Lehmkuhl LD, Smith LK. *Brunnstrom's Clinical Kinesiology.* 4th ed. Philadelphia: FA Davis; 1985.

7. Friden J, Sjostrom M, Ekblom B. Myofibrillar damage following intense eccentric exercise in man. *Int J Sports Med.* 1983;4:170–176.

8. Knuttgen HG, Bonde Petersen F, Klausen K. Oxygen uptake and heart rate responses to exercise performed with concentric and eccentric contractions. *Med Sci Sports.* 1971;3:1–5.

9. Cavanagh PR, Komi PV. Electromechanical delay in human skeletal muscle under concentric and eccentric contractions. *Eur J Appl Physiol.* 1979;42:159–163.

10. DiNubile N. Strength training. *Clin Sports Med.* 1991;10:33–62.

11. Sharkey BJ. Training for sport. In: Cantu RC, Michelli LJ, eds. *ACSM's Guidelines for the Team Physician.* Philadelphia: Lea & Febiger; 1991:34–47.

12. Draganich LF, Jaeger RJ, Kralj AR. Coactivation of the hamstrings and quadriceps during extension of the knee. *J Bone Joint Surg* Am. 1989;71:1075–1081.

13. Shelbourne KD, Wilckens JH, Mollabashy A, et al. Accelerated rehabilitation after acute anterior cruciate ligament reconstruction. *Am J Sports Med.* 1990;18:292–299.

14. Sobel J, Pettrone FA, Nirschl RP. Prevention and rehabilitation of racquet sports injuries. In: Nicholas JA, Hershman EB, eds. *The Upper Extremity in Sports Medicine.* St. Louis: Mosby Yearbook; 1995:805–823.

15. Allman FL. Exercise in sports medicine. In: Basmajian JV, ed. *Therapeutic Exercise.* 9th ed. Baltimore: Williams & Wilkins; 1984:277–315.

16. Dudley GA, Djamil R. Incompatibility of endurance- and strength-training modes of exercise. *J Appl Physiol.* 1985;59:1446–1451.

17. Hickson RC. Interference of strength development by simultaneously training for strength and endurance. *Eur J Appl Physiol.* 1980;45:255–263.

18. Sale DG, MacDougall JD, Jacobs I, et al. Interaction between concurrent strength and endurance training. *J Appl Physiol.* 1990;68:260–270.

19. American College of Sports Medicine. *Guidelines for Exercise Testing and Prescription.* 4th ed. Philadelphia: Lea & Febiger; 1991.

20. Borg GAV, Linderholm H. Perceived exertion and pulse rate during graded exercise in various age groups. *Acta Med Scand Suppl.* 1967;472:194–210.

21. Ceci R, Hassmen P. Self monitored exercise at three different RPE intensities in treadmill vs field running. *Med Sci Sports Exerc.* 1991;23:732–738.

22. Medbo JI, Burgers S. Effect of training on the anaerobic capacity. *Med Sci Sports Exerc.* 1990;22:501–507.

23. Daniels J. Training distance runners—a primer. *Sports Science Exchange.* Gatorade Sports Science Institute. 1989;1(11).

24. Pate RR, Branch JD. Training for endurance sport. *Med Sci Sports Exerc.* 1992;24(9):S340–S343.

25. Evans WJ. Exercise-induced skeletal muscle damage. *Physician Sports Med.* 1987;15(1):89–100.

26. Tiidus PM, Ianuzzo CD. Effects of intensity and duration of muscular exercise on delayed soreness and serum enzyme activities. *Med Sci Sports Exerc.* 1983;15:461–465.

27. Costill DL, Pascoe DD, Fink WJ, et al. Impaired muscle glycogen resynthesis after eccentric exercise. *J Appl Physiol.* 1990;69:46–50.

28. Russell B, Dix DJ, Haller DL, et al. Repair of injured skeletal muscle: a molecular approach. *Med Sci Sports Exerc.* 1992;24:189–196.

29. Waterman-Storer CM. The cytoskeleton of skeletal muscle: is it affected by exercise? A brief review. *Med Sci Sports Exerc.* 1991;23:1240–1249.

30. O'Reilly KP, Warhol MJ, Fielding RA, et al. Eccentric exercise-induced muscle damage impairs glycogen repletion. *J Appl Physiol.* 1987;63:252–256.

31. Barron GL, Noakes TD, Levy W, et al. Hypothalamic dysfunction in overtrained athletes. *J Clin Endocrin Metab.* 1985;60:803–806.

32. Sherman WS, Maglischo EW. Minimizing chronic athletic fatigue among swimmers: special emphasis on nutrition. *Sports Science Exchange.* Gatorade Sports Science Institute. 1991;4(35).

33. Keast D, Cameron K, Morton AR. Exercise and the immune response. *Sports Med.* 1988;5:248–267.

34. O'Connor PJ, Morgan WP, Raglin JS, et al. Selected pseudoendocrine responses to overtraining. *Med Sci Sports Exerc.* 1989;21(2):S50.

35. Kibler WB. *The Sport Preparticipation Fitness Examination.* Champaign, IL: Human Kinetics Books; 1990.

36. Montgomery DL. Physiology of ice hockey. *Sports Med.* 1988;5:99–126.

CHAPTER 3

Determining the Extent
of the Functional Deficit

W. Ben Kibler

Every athletic activity involves movements of joints and limbs in coordinated ways to perform an athletic task. These activities include running, jumping, throwing, stopping, or kicking. The tasks may include throwing a ball, hitting a ball, kicking a ball, jumping over an object, or propelling a body through air or water. Individual body segments and joints, collectively called the *links*, must be moved in certain specific sequences to allow efficient accomplishment of the tasks.

The sequencing of the links is called the *kinetic chain* of an athletic activity. Each kinetic chain has its own sequence, but the basic organization includes proximal to distal sequencing, a proximal base of support or stability, and successive activation of each segment of the link and each successive link. The net result is generation of force and energy in each link, summation of the developed force and energy through each of the links, and efficient transfer of the force and energy to the terminal link. A graphic example of the kinetic chain of the tennis serve is illustrated in Figure 3–1, and some sequenced links are described in Table 3–1.

This sequencing is accomplished by specific motor control patterns that allow link stabilization, force generation, joint positioning, and link motion. These physiologic patterns depend on feedback about joint and limb position and motion, and are intimately linked with the biomechanical chain so that alteration in either the physiology or the biomechanics alters the other.

Athletic injury can affect the biomechanical chain in several ways. Direct injury to the joint, such as a fracture, internal derangement, or ligamentous injury, can alter the joint's ability to move or to be stable. Examples would include torn menisci and ankle ligament tears. Injury to nerves or muscles can affect force generation or joint stabilization due to weakness or muscle imbalance. Examples include rotator cuff tear or acute or chronic hamstring strain. Physical inactivity due to injury can lead to disuse atrophy, either locally or in other areas of the kinetic chain that are also not being used. Examples would include cast-induced atrophy or quadriceps weakness after ankle sprain. Microtrauma injury may lead to mild subclinical tensile overload in specific tissues, causing inflexibility and mild muscle weakness. Examples include posterior shoulder inflexibility in throwers and hamstring tightness in runners. Finally, injuries or adaptations in some areas of the kinetic chain can cause problems not only locally but distantly, as other distal links have to compensate for the lack of force or energy delivered through the more proximal links. This phenomenon, called *catch-up*, is both inefficient in the kinetic chain and dangerous to the distal link because it may create more load or stress than the link can safely handle. Catch-up can be achieved only by manipulating the variables in the equations for kinetic energy (KE = $\frac{1}{2}$ mass $\times$ velocity^2) and force (F = mass $\times$ acceleration). If kinetic energy or force is decreased, either mass, velocity, or acceleration must be increased. The "catch-up" phenomenon for the next most distal link in a tennis serve is illustrated in Figure 3–2 and presented mathematically in Exhibit 3–1. As can be seen, absolute or percentage changes in mass, velocity, or acceleration can be quite large. These changes may result in anatomic or biomechanical situations that increase injury risk, perpetuate injury patterns, or decrease performance. Examples of these kinetic chain adaptations include back inflexibility—seen with rotator cuff tendinitis—and posterior shoulder strength deficit—seen in tennis players with lateral epicondylitis.

The kinetic chains of athletic activity operate with a high degree of efficiency in most athletes. They play a major role in what is called *skill*, or function, in sporting activities. Small degrees of alterations in the kinetic chain, by any of the previously mentioned problems, have been demonstrated to have major effects on the kinetic chains and on the skills

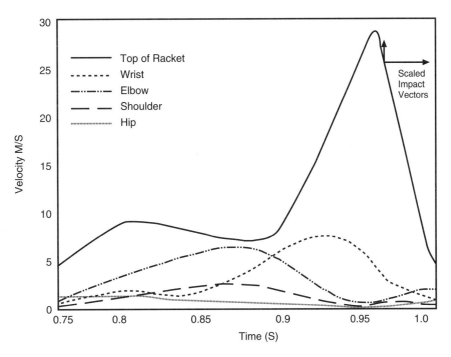

Figure 3–1 Analysis of the tennis serve. *Source:* Reprinted by permission from B. Elliot, T. Marsh, and B. Blanksby, 1986, "A three-dimensional cinematographic analysis of the tennis serve," *International Journal of Sports Biomechanics,* 2 (4): 269.

Table 3–1 Kinetic Chains of Sports Activities

Sporting Activity	Kinetic Chain
Baseball Pitch	Ground → Plant Leg → Hip and Trunk → Landing Leg
	Ground → Plant Leg → Hip and Trunk → Shoulder → Elbow → Wrist → Hand
Running	Ground → Plant Leg → Pelvis → Landing Leg
Freestyle Swimming	Hand, Wrist, and Elbow → Shoulder → Hip and Trunk → Opposite Shoulder → Hand, Wrist, and Elbow
Soccer Kick	Ground → Plant Leg → Plant Pelvis and Trunk → Kicking Hip → Knee → Foot

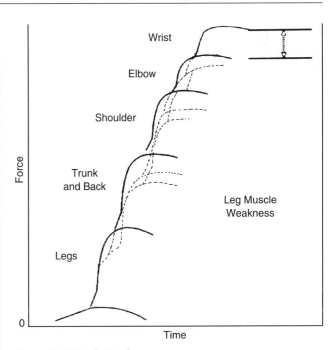

Figure 3–2 Catch-Up phenomenon

that are based on the chains. Because the major goal of rehabilitation is functional restoration, identification and normalization of the biomechanical deficits that result directly or indirectly from the athletic injury are major components of the rehabilitation process.

These biomechanical deficits may be of two types. Anatomic biomechanical deficits occur as a result of overt tissue injury and are present in all activities. Examples would include physiologic pes planus, with "navicular drop" of greater than 1.5 cm between weight-bearing and non–

Exhibit 3–1 Normal and "Catch-Up" Values for the Next Distal Link for an Average Elite Tennis Player

	Normal	"Catch-Up"	% Change
• 10% ↓ back and trunk kinetic energy to shoulder			
Shoulder Mass			
Shoulder Velocity			
• 20% ↓ back and trunk kinetic energy to shoulder			
Shoulder Mass (kg)	9	16.25	80
Shoulder Velocity (m/sec)	3.3	4.43	34
• 20 % ↓ back and trunk force to shoulder			
Shoulder Mass (kg)	9	12.2	35.5
Shoulder Acceleration (m/sec^2)	33	44.75	35.6
• 10% ↓ shoulder force to elbow			
Elbow Mass (kg)	4	4.56	14
Elbow Acceleration (m/sec^2)	53	60.4	14

weight-bearing conditions; rotator cuff or biceps tendon tear, with diminished active shoulder abduction or elbow flexion; or torn medial meniscus with a locked knee. However, most deficits are considered functional biomechanical deficits. These occur from subclinical or overt tissue injury but become biomechanically abnormal only when specific athletic activities put certain stresses on the joint or body. Examples would include functional pes planus due to heel cord inflexibility and weak gastrocnemius muscles; quadriceps inflexibility, causing increased contact pressures with jumping and anterior knee pain; anterior cruciate ligament (ACL) deficiency, creating the pivot shift phenomenon upon cutting or deceleration; and posterior shoulder internal rotation inflexibility, which results in anterior shoulder translation as the glenohumeral joint internally rotates during throwing or serving.

The effects of the biomechanical deficits, regardless of cause, are widespread in the athlete. In chronic microtrauma injury, the cumulative process of injury results in many adaptations, which cause the deficits. In acute macrotrauma injuries, effects of the injury or subsequent immobilization and/or surgery create deficits. These deficits create alterations in the normal biomechanics of the kinetic chain. The alterations include changes in joint stability; joint instant center of rotation; joint range of motion; forces and application of forces across joints; muscle flexibility; muscle strength and force couple balance across the joint; and alteration in the kinetic chain.

Both types of biomechanical deficits can and should be identified by careful evaluation of the injured athlete prior to initiation of rehabilitation. The evaluation process, which

will be described in some detail in another chapter, evaluates not only the local symptoms but also the distant functional changes that may accompany the clinical findings. The evaluation must be done with knowledge of how the injured anatomic part fits into the normal biomechanical sequencing of the kinetic chain, whether abnormal biomechanics—due to the injury, acquired as part of the injury process, or related to causation of the injury—exist, and how the entire kinetic chain should be rehabilitated.

Rehabilitation of the biomechanical deficits, after they have been identified, depends on how they were caused and where they fit into the kinetic chain. In general, biomechanical deficits that occur distantly in the kinetic chain may be rehabilitated early in the rehabilitation sequence, sometimes while the actual site of pathology is being protected after surgery or other treatment. Deficits that are anatomically or biomechanically more local to the site of clinical symptoms must be rehabilitated when the injured tissues are capable of withstanding the loads. Rehabilitation of hip or trunk inflexibility can be done early in the rehabilitation of rotator cuff injuries, whereas, in the same patient, posterior shoulder inflexibility must be rehabilitated after the acute symptoms and clinical pathology have been normalized. Muscle strength balance and force couple rehabilitation would follow restoration of normal flexibility.

Once the local and kinetic chain deficits have been rehabilitated, emphasis should be placed on sport- and activity-specific progressions before returning to play. Using the muscles, links, and body segments—in the positions and angles, and at the speeds that are encountered in sports or activities—is essential to normal function. This last part of rehabilitation requires knowledge of the mechanical patterns of the sport. For baseball throwing or tennis serving, rotator cuff exercises should be done with the shoulder elevated to about 90 degrees and with very light weights or tubing. This activity will then simulate the arm position and will allow the velocities that will be seen in the normal activity.

In summary, sporting activities require biomechanical kinetic chains to function efficiently. Flaws in the chain, either locally or distantly from the site of clinical symptoms, can alter the chain or can be caused by the pathologic processes that are commonly seen in athletic injuries, especially those due to chronic microtrauma. Evaluation of the injured athlete for local and distant biomechanical alterations allows the establishment of a complete exercise prescription for rehabilitation. This prescription can then be carried out in the context of preparing the athlete for return to the biomechanical demands of the sport or activity.

SUGGESTED READINGS

1. Elliott BC, Marsh T, Blanksby B. A three-dimensional cinematographic analysis of the tennis serve. *Int J Sport Biomech.* 1986;2: 260–271.

2. Kibler WB. Evaluation of sports demands as a diagnostic tool in shoulder disorders. In: Matsen FA, Fu FH, Hawkins RJ, eds. *The Shoulder: A Balance of Mobility and Stability.* Rosemont IL: American Academy of Orthopaedic Surgeons; 1994:379–399.

3. Kibler WB. Biomechanical analysis of the shoulder during throwing activities. *Clin Sports Med.* 1995;14:79–85.

4. Kibler WB, Livingston B, Bruce R. Current concepts in shoulder rehabilitation. *Adv Operative Orthop.* 3:1995;249–300.

5. Nichols TR. A biomechanical perspective on spinal mechanisms of coordinated muscular action: an architectural principle. *Acta Anat.* 1994; 151:1–13.

6. Putnam CA. Sequential motions of body segments in striking and throwing skills: descriptions and explanations. *J Biomech.* 1993;26: 125–135.

7. Spriginig E, Marshall R, Elliott B. A three-dimensional kinematic method for determining the effectiveness of arm segment rotations in producing racquet head speed. *J Biomech.* 1994;27:245–254.

CHAPTER 4

Radiologic Imaging in Rehabilitation

Richard J. Herzog

INTRODUCTION

The foundation of successful rehabilitation rests on an accurate clinical diagnosis. The process to accomplish this goal begins with a complete history and physical examination. If this initial evaluation is not adequate to provide the information needed to explain a patient's symptoms, additional diagnostic testing is usually needed to determine the precise pathoetiology of the dysfunctional condition. The additional data provided by these tests become useful clinical information only when they are integrated with the patient's history, physical exam, and other completed tests. In the past, radiologic imaging studies, e.g., plain films, computed tomography (CT), and radionuclide studies have played a major role in the diagnostic evaluation of patients with musculoskeletal disorders. These studies focused mainly on the detection of osseous abnormalities. With the recent development and implementation of magnetic resonance imaging (MRI), it is now possible to noninvasively evaluate the soft tissue structures of the body, e.g., muscles, tendons, and ligaments, which are the structures most frequently responsible for the majority of symptoms of patients with musculoskeletal dysfunction.

The goal of any imaging study is to accurately define the pathomorphologic changes in a specific tissue, organ, or part of the body. Whenever possible, objective diagnostic criteria should be employed when reporting the findings of an imaging study. Objective categorization of pathologic changes facilitates the interpretation and communication of abnormalities detected on a test, and these same criteria can then be used on follow-up tests to assess the effects of different forms of therapy, e.g., surgical intervention or nonoperative rehabilitation. The reproducibility and reliability of all objective diagnostic criteria must be rigorously evaluated in prospective blinded studies prior to their implementation.[1–4]

With the utilization of different forms of energy, different imaging techniques encode and display different physical properties of tissue. Tissue contrast on plain films and CT is based on the attenuation of X-rays, which is highly dependent on the level of tissue mineralization. Plain films and CT provide excellent delineation of ossified or calcified structures. The most useful application of these modalities has been to evaluate disorders of bone, e.g., fractures, arthritis, and bone destruction by tumor or infection. They are also employed to detect soft-tissue calcification and ossification. Technetium 99m methylene diphosphonate bone scintigraphy predominantly provides information concerning osseous pathology. The localization of the radionuclide activity reflects the metabolic activity of osseous tissue.[5] While radionuclide bone scans may be extremely sensitive to detect pathologic bony conditions, their specificity as to determining the precise etiology of an osseous abnormality is limited.

Magnetic resonance imaging encodes a completely different physical property of tissue compared with studies using an X-ray source or a radioisotope. If a person is placed in a strong extrinsic magnetic field, e.g., in an MR magnet, a small percentage of the mobile hydrogen atoms in the body will become aligned with the magnet's static magnetic field. If a defined radiofrequency energy pulse is then applied to the body, a certain percentage of these aligned atoms will absorb some of this energy and change to a higher energy state. When the extrinsic source of energy is terminated, these energized hydrogen atoms will release this energy back to the environment. The rate of energy release, i.e., the relaxation time, is dependent on the chemical properties of the tissue. An MR image is created by encoding the location of the atoms that undergo this energy transformation. With different MR sequences, it is possible to optimize differences in tissue contrast in different parts of the body. Spatial resolution depends on the MR equipment, including coil design, and the imaging parameters selected by the technologist. Excellent imaging of soft tissue is possible because of the large number of mobile hydrogen ions in their chemical structure. Any structure or material containing mobile hydrogen ions, e.g., water, fat, muscle, blood, or edematous and necrotic tissue, can be evaluated on a standard MRI examination. Tissues that contain few mobile hydrogen ions, e.g., cortical bone, ligaments, and tendons, can still be imaged with MRI if they contain or are in contact with other tissues containing mobile hydrogen ions, e.g., fat or fluid. The standard sequences on an MRI exam to evaluate the musculoskeletal system are the spin-echo and short tau inversion recovery (STIR) sequences. They provide excellent contrast and spatial resolution for the evaluation of normal anatomic structures and pathologic changes within the body (Table 4–1). Spin-echo T1-weighted sequences, i.e., short relaxation time (TR)/short echo time (TE), are optimal to display tissues containing fat or blood. Spin-echo proton density–weighted sequences, i.e., long TR/short TE, also provide excellent anatomic detail. Spin-echo T2-weighted sequences, long TR/long TE, are employed to delineate tissue containing fluid. STIR and fat-suppressed T2-weighted sequences are particularly sensitive to the presence of fluid in both soft tissues or osseous structures. A complete discussion of MRI physics and the different MRI sequences that are currently used can be found in several publications.[6–12] It is necessary to know the contraindications to performing an MRI exam, e.g., patients with cardiac pacemakers, metallic foreign bodies in the eye or spinal canal, cerebral aneurysm clips, infusion pumps, certain vascular stents, and some ocular or cochlear implants.[13]

Ultrasonography (US) is also used to assess soft-tissue disorders of the musculoskeletal system.[14,15] The major advantages of US are its availability, safety, and lower cost compared with MRI. It is limited to the evaluation of tissues that transmit sound waves; therefore, osseous structures or soft tissues shielded by osseous tissue cannot be evaluated. Compared with the other imaging modalities, the efficacy of ultrasound is heavily dependent on the operator of the equipment, but this should not preclude its use in the appropriate clinical situations. Considering its cost and availability, the role of ultrasound may grow as more clinicians become proficient in its application. This is already true in many European countries where ultrasound is heavily utilized in the evaluation of musculoskeletal disorders.[16,17]

As a result of the static nature of most imaging studies, their interpretation is predominantly focused on the detection of structural abnormalities. However, static images are truly a snapshot of the evolution of a pathologic condition, and their value is enhanced if they can elucidate the dynamic pathologic changes occurring in the natural history of a pathologic process. Imaging is a means of assessing the integrity of the components of a functional unit, whether it is a myotendinous junction or a whole knee joint. Whereas each functional unit in the body is unique, their components are similar, e.g., ligaments, tendons, fascia, muscle, cartilage, and bone. By understanding the appearance of normal tissue along with the appearance of the spectrum of pathologic changes affecting these tissues, it is possible to apply this knowledge when imaging any part of the body. This is particularly relevant with the interpretation of MRI examinations because of the wide range of body parts that are assessed. The following sections will focus on the basic types of tissue in the musculoskeletal system and will discuss the most common pathologic conditions afflicting these tissues.

TISSUE COMPOSITION

Prior to the discussion of specific types of tissue, it is important to consider the basic biochemical constituents of tis-

Table 4–1 MR Signal Intensity

	T1-Weighted	*T2-Weighted*	*STIR*
Fat	High	Intermed	Low
Muscle	Intermed	Intermed–Low	Intermed–Low
Hyaline Cartilage	Intermed	Intermed–Low	Intermed–High
Fibrocartilage	Low	Low	Low
Ligaments and Tendons	Low	Low	Low
Cortical Bone	Low	Low	Low
Bulk Water	Intermed	High	High
Granulation Tissue	Intermed	High	High
Fibrous Tissue	Low	Low	Low
Cellular Tumors	Intermed	High	High
Fibrous Tumors	Intermed–Low	Intermed–Low	Intermed–Low

sue and their appearance in health and disease. This is particularly relevant to the understanding of MR images where different imaging sequences are used to enhance tissue contrast, which is directly determined by the chemical composition and organization of the tissue. All tissue in the body is composed of cells and an extracellular matrix. Any tissue containing fat, e.g., bone marrow or subcutaneous tissue, will generate high signal intensity on T1- and proton density–weighted sequences. These sequences will provide excellent anatomic delineation of most normal structures in the musculoskeletal system. Cells usually contain a large amount of fluid. Thus, the more cells in a tissue, whether normal or pathologic, the greater the signal intensity that will be generated on spin-echo T2-weighted or STIR sequences. Extracellular matrix is mainly composed of fluid, proteoglycans, and collagen. As previously discussed, the level of tissue hydration directly affects signal intensity on an MR image. Tissue containing a large component of proteoglycans will demonstrate increased signal intensity on a spin-echo T2-weighted sequence because of the fluid that is imbibed to the proteoglycan. Collagen contains few mobile hydrogen ions and, therefore, generates minimal or no signal on spin-echo or STIR sequences. Thus, any structure that contains a high proportion of collagen, e.g., ligaments, tendons, or fibrous tissue, will generate minimal or no MR signal.

With MRI it is now possible to noninvasively follow the evolution of tissue injury, repair, and remodeling (Table 4–2), as well as changes of tissue aging. Acute injury to vascularized tissue will incite an inflammatory response. There will be an increase in tissue hydration as part of the inflammatory response, which will be detected on spin-echo T2-weighted and STIR sequences as a focus of high signal intensity. With tissue healing, remodeling, and fibrosis, the MR signal intensity on the T2-weighted and STIR sequences decreases due to the increased amount of collagen and the decreased amount of fluid in the tissue. Aging involves changes in both the cellular and extracellular components of tissue.[18] Tissue aging that is accompanied by tissue dessication, e.g., the intervertebral disc, will demonstrate decreased signal intensity on spin-echo T2-weighted sequences. Tissue aging that is accompanied by fatty infiltra-

tion will demonstrate increased signal intensity on spin-echo T1-weighted sequences.

Because the inorganic salts in bone contain few mobile hydrogen ions, any heavily mineralized tissue, e.g., cortical bone, will generate no signal on MR images. The high signal intensity present in cancellous bone on T1-weighted sequences is due to the large amount of fat within the cancellous bone. With any process that replaces this fat, there will be decreased signal intensity on the spin-echo T1-weighted sequence. If the abnormal process contains fluid, e.g., an inflammatory focus or in malignant cells, there will be increased signal intensity in the cancellous bone on spin-echo T2-weighted and STIR sequences. If the process replacing the marrow fat contains fibrous tissue or additional mineralization, there will be an absence of signal intensity on all MR sequences. Soft tissues that become calcified or ossified will also show no signal on MR images.

MUSCLE-TENDON UNIT

The basic function of any muscle in the body is to generate a force by concentric contraction or to resist a load by eccentric contraction. The force of a muscle is transmitted through its tendon to its bony insertion site. To understand the pathophysiology of muscle injuries, it is best to consider the muscle and the tendon as a single functional muscle-tendon unit (MTU). Injury of the MTU may occur at different locations, depending on the nature of the applied force. Whether the force is extrinsically applied, e.g., a direct blow, or intrinsically generated, e.g., by eccentric muscle contraction, will also determine the type and location of fiber failure.

Muscle injuries are one of the most frequent causes of musculoskeletal dysfunction in sports. A direct blow to a muscle may cause a muscle contusion with disruption of muscle fibers. Acute disruption of muscle fibers will incite an inflammatory response associated with soft tissue edema and, frequently, soft tissue hemorrhage and/or hematoma. With the acute pain associated with muscle injury, it may be difficult on the physical exam to determine the precise location and extent of an injury. Prior to the implementation of MRI, radiologic imaging studies were of little value in the evaluation of acute muscle injuries. On plain films, there may be obscuration of the fat planes surrounding an injured muscle secondary to the perimuscular edema. With CT, there may be an alteration of the size or contour of a muscle, but detection of intramuscular hemorrhage or edema is limited. With the excellent soft tissue contrast resolution provided by MRI, it is possible to obtain the following important clinical information related to a muscle injury: (1) the extent of muscle edema and hemorrhage, (2) whether a focal hematoma is present, including its size and location, (3) the degree and extent of the fiber disruption, (4) whether there is complete disruption of the muscle; whether there is associ-

---

Table 4–2 MRI Evaluation of Ligament Injury and Repair

Pathoanatomy	MRI Signal Intensity	
	T1	T2
Hemorrhage or Edema	Intermed to High	High
Granulation Tissue	Intermed	High
Immature Scar	Low to Intermed	Low to High
Mature Scar	Low	Low

ated muscle retraction, (5) whether there is interruption of the overlying fascia and whether there is a muscle herniation, (6) the degree of muscle swelling and the detection of a possible concomitant compartment syndrome, and (7) whether single or multiple muscles are injured. Muscle contusions occur most frequently in the lower extremities, particularly involving the quadriceps mechanism.[19]

On an MRI exam, a muscle contusion is detected by abnormal signal intensity and morphology of the muscle. On spin-echo sequences, normal muscle demonstrates intermediate signal intensity on T1-weighted sequences and intermediate to low signal intensity on T2-weighted sequences. In a contused muscle, the interstitial edema and/or hemorrhage will be detected as high signal intensity on T2-weighted sequences. Because hemorrhage infiltrates through the muscle and mixes with the interstitial edema, it is not possible to separate it from the edematous muscle tissue (Figure 4–1). With a grade 1 contusion, i.e., microstructural fiber failure, there may be slightly increased size of the muscle, and the margins of the muscle may have a feathery appearance due to the extension of interstitial edema into the perimuscular tissue.[20–21] Edematous changes in the adjacent subcutaneous fat are also frequently detected. With a grade 2 muscle contusion, i.e., partial tear, there will be a focus of disrupted muscle fibers in addition to the altered signal intensity from the interstitial edema and hemorrhage (Figure 4–2). A grade 3 muscle contusion will appear similar to a

grade 2 contusion, except there will be complete disruption of the muscle fibers. With a muscle hematoma, there will be a focal accumulation of blood within a muscle. A hematoma demonstrates intermediate or high signal intensity on a T1-weighted sequence, depending on the chemical composition of the hematoma, and high signal intensity on a T2-weighted sequence (Figures 4–3 and 4–4). The sequelae of a muscle contusion may include muscle atrophy, fibrosis, calcification, or ossification.

The role of plain films and CT in the evaluation of these potential complications has focused mainly on the detection of muscle calcification or ossification. Myositis ossificans is a benign ossifying soft tissue mass, typically located within skeletal muscle. A history of prior trauma is present in approximately 50% of the cases, and the episode of trauma is frequently of a minor degree. Plain radiographs show faint calcification within the muscle from two to six weeks after the onset of symptoms and a well-circumscribed osseous mass in approximately six to eight weeks. The lesion will then mature over the next six months and become smaller. In the early stages of the lesion, prior to bony maturation, the margins of the ossified mass may be poorly defined on plain films. If there is a history of only a minor injury or no trauma, the possibility of a soft tissue malignancy, e.g., osteosarcoma, is sometimes explored after obtaining the plain films. If a CT scan is obtained at four to six weeks, it will demonstrate a rim of mineralization surrounding a central area of

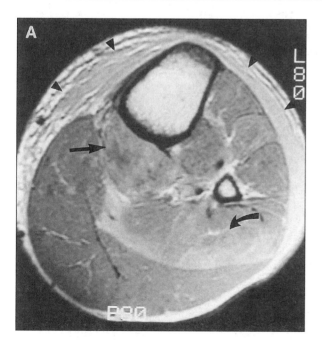
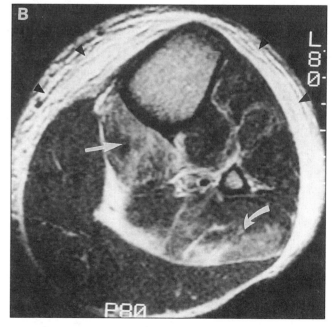

Figure 4–1 Grade 1 muscle contusion secondary to a football injury. On the proton-density (**A**) and T2-weighted (**B**) axial images, there is increased signal intensity in the soleus (*curved arrows*) and the popliteal (*straight arrows*) muscles related to the edema and hemorrhage within the muscle. Edematous changes are also identified in the subcutaneous tissue (*arrowheads*).

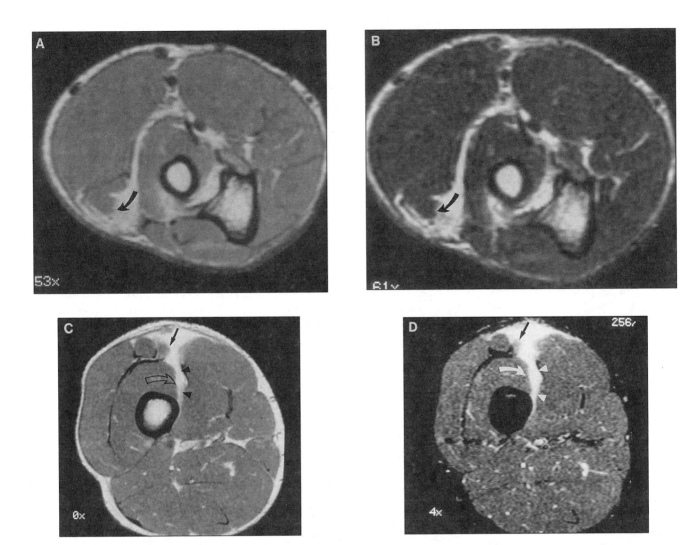

Figure 4–2   Grade 2 muscle contusion secondary to a football injury. On the proton-density (**A**) and T2-weighted (**B**) axial images, there is a tear of the extensor digitorum communis muscle of the forearm, with separation of the muscle from its myotendinous junction (*curved arrows*). In another football injury, on the proton-density (**C**) and T2-weighted (**D**) axial image, there is a tear of the quadriceps muscle involving both the vastus medialis (*straight arrows*) and the vastus intermedius (*curved arrows*) muscles. Hemorrhage/edema (*arrowheads*) extends to the femur.

decreased attenuation. On an MRI examination, the characteristics of myositis ossificans are highly dependent on the age of the lesion. On a T2-weighted sequence, an early lesion usually has poorly defined margins and has inhomogeneous intermediate to high signal intensity within the lesion. Perilesional edema is also identified with an acute lesion. Histologically, an early lesion has a cellular core with an appearance similar to nodular fasciitis. As the lesion matures, it will develop a rim of mature bone.[22] Mature lesions are well defined with inhomogeneous signal intensity similar to fat. The most important finding on all of these imaging modalities is that the areas of ossification are most mature at the periphery of the lesion, and the central core contains

the immature cellular components. This is in contrast to a soft tissue osteosarcoma, which is most mature centrally and immature peripherally. A few months of watchful waiting will demonstrate the normal maturation of myositis ossificans.

Muscle strains are probably the most common type of injury to the MTU. A muscle strain is an acute stretch-induced injury secondary to excessive indirect force generated by eccentric muscular contraction. Muscle strains may occur anywhere in the body, but the most frequent muscles involved are the quadriceps femoris, biceps femoris, semimembranosus, semitendinosus, and the gastrocnemius-soleus complex. Muscles that cross two joints and that have a high proportion

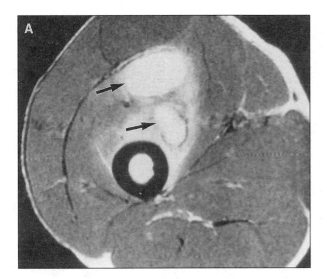
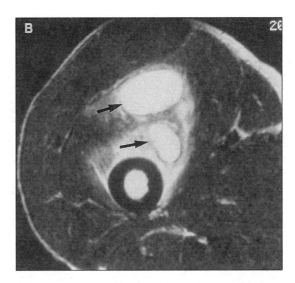

Figure 4–3 Acute hematoma secondary to a cycling injury. On the proton-density (**A**) and T2-weighted (**B**) axial images, there are two focal accumulations of blood in the vastus intermedius muscle (*arrows*). Hemorrhagic/edematous changes are also identified at the muscle-bone interface.

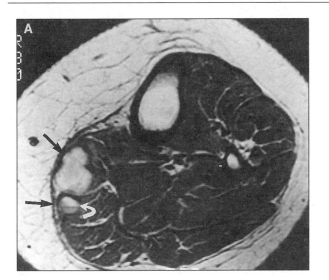
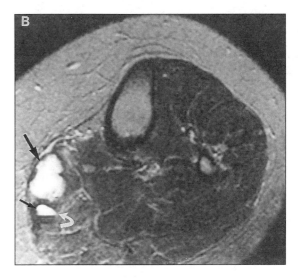

Figure 4–4 Subacute hematoma related to a hiking injury. On the proton-density (**A**) and T2-weighted (**B**) axial images, there are two focal accumulations of fluid representing resolving hematomas (*straight arrows*) in the medial head of the gastrocnemius muscle. There is a fluid-fluid level in the smaller hematoma (*curved arrows*) related to the blood breakdown products.

of fast twitch fibers are more prone to muscle strains. Muscle strains may also involve the muscles stabilizing the hip, shoulder, and the elbow joints. The pain elicited from an acute muscle strain is typically experienced during an athletic activity or immediately at its termination.[23] The pathologic changes in an acutely strained muscle include microtraumatic disruption of the muscle fibers near the myotendinous junction, along with edema and hemorrhage.

The grade of a muscle strain depends on the degree of fiber disruption and the clinical findings.

The appearance of a grade 1 muscle strain with MRI is similar to the findings of a grade 1 muscle contusion. There may be enlargement of the muscle due to interstitial edema and hemorrhage, and on a spin-echo T2-weighted sequence, there will be increased signal intensity within the muscle (Figure 4–5). Muscle strains are frequently located near

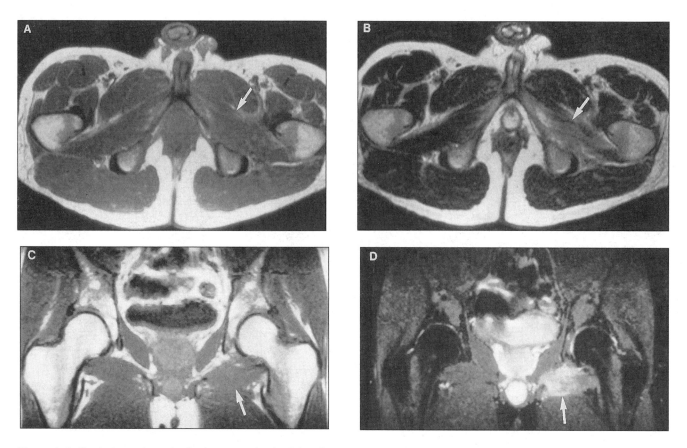

Figure 4–5 Grade 1 muscle strain. On the proton-density (**A**) and T2-weighted (**B**) axial images, there are edematous changes and hypertrophy of the left obturator externus muscle (*arrows*). The edematous changes are not apparent on the T1-weighted coronal image (**C**) (*arrow*) but are easily detected on the STIR coronal image (**D**) (*arrow*).

its myotendinous junction. The tendon of a multipennate muscle extends into the muscle belly; therefore, the symptoms elicited by a strain may be located anywhere within a muscle and not merely at its ends. Magnetic resonance imaging has provided excellent documentation of the extent and location of these injuries (Figure 4–5C, D). Fleckenstein et al.[24] reported on the MRI appearance of the natural history of acute muscle strains. Acutely, the abnormal signal intensity was identified throughout the muscle, but on follow-up studies, the abnormal signal intensity was most prominent in the periphery of the muscle. In one patient, there was persistent abnormal signal intensity within the muscle after complete resolution of symptoms.

A grade 2 muscle strain manifests clinically as muscle pain associated with a loss of strength. Pathologically, there is a macroscopic partial tear of the MTU. On an MRI study, there will be a partial tear of the muscle fibers associated with edema and/or hemorrhage (Figure 4–6). With a grade 3 strain, there is complete disruption of the MTU. Plain films provide little useful information in the evaluation of most

muscle strains. Only if there is a grade 3 strain that results in gross instability or malalignment, e.g., a quadriceps rupture, will plain films be helpful. Computed tomography has also been used to evaluate muscular strain injuries, but it provides less useful clinical information compared with an MRI examination.[25]

While an acute muscle strain elicits pain at the time or immediately following its occurrence, muscle pain and/or dysfunction frequently does not develop until one to two days after the completion of exercise. Delayed-onset muscle soreness (DOMS) is a well-recognized clinical entity in which patients develop muscle pain and stiffness 24–48 hours following an episode of muscular exertion.[26] The pathologic changes with DOMS are similar to those demonstrated with a muscle strain and involve muscles that have performed eccentric contractions.[23] The abnormal signal intensity detected on a T2-weighted or STIR sequence may involve the peripheral muscle fibers or may extend diffusely through the muscle.[26] There have been several reports on the MRI evaluation of DOMS.[24,26,27] The etiology of the in-

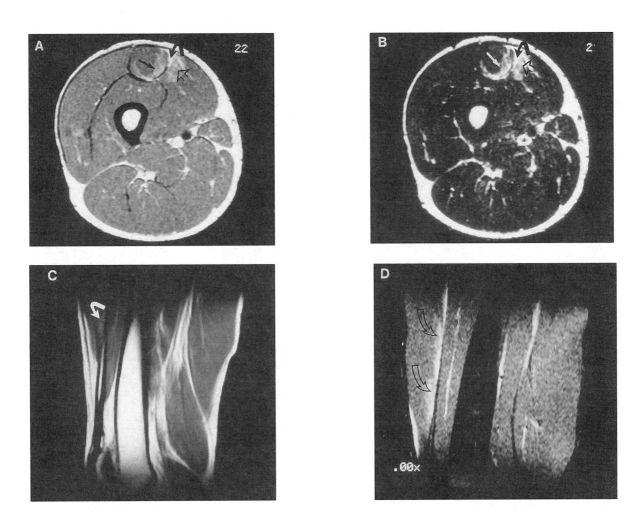

Figure 4–6 Grade 2 muscle strain related to football training. On the proton-density (**A**) and T2-weighted (**B**) axial images, there are edematous changes adjacent to the myotendinous junction of the rectus femoris (*straight arrows*) and vastus medialis (*open arrowheads*) muscles. There is partial separation of the muscles at the myotendinous junction (*curved arrows*). The edematous changes at the myotendinous junction are difficult to detect on the T1-weighted sagittal image (**C**) (*curved arrow*), but are optimally demonstrated on the STIR sagittal image (**D**) (*open curved arrows*).

creased signal intensity within the muscle is probably secondary to an increase in muscle fluid content or a shift of the muscle interstitial fluid from its intracellular to extracellular compartment. In a prospective evaluation of subjects performing exhaustive eccentric and concentric exercises, Shellock et al.[27,28] demonstrated that only muscles performing eccentric contractions demonstrated findings of DOMS. Statistically significant increases in T2 relaxation times indicative of muscle injury peaked from three to ten days after the completion of the exercise. Clinical symptoms of pain and stiffness were present from one to five days after exercise. Abnormalities in some of the muscles were detected up to 75 days after the complete resolution of symptoms. Nurenberg et al.[26] correlated the abnormalities detected on an MRI study to MR-guided muscle biopsies in patients with

DOMS. There was a good correlation between the amount of ultrastructural injury detected on biopsy and the degree of abnormal signal intensity on the MRI exam. An interesting finding was that there was poor correlation between the location of the subjects' experienced pain and the location of the muscle injury detected by biopsy and the MRI. This may explain some of the difficulty in clinically localizing muscle injury, along with the possible limitations of blind muscle biopsies obtained at the site of patients' symptoms.

In addition to the evaluation of acute or delayed muscle injuries, MRI is an ideal imaging modality to follow the evolution of the inflammatory and repair processes within a muscle. With MRI, it is possible to detect any sequelae from an MTU injury, e.g., muscle atrophy or fibrosis.[29] Clinically, it can be extremely difficult to determine when a muscle has completely healed, and with a premature return to athletic activity after injury, an athlete may be predisposed to repeat injury. With MRI, it is possible to detect acute MTU injuries superimposed on subacute or chronic injuries that may have predisposed the patient to reinjury (Figure 4–7).

Magnetic resonance imaging has also been used to study normal muscle physiology, as well as the pathophysiology of muscle overload and injury. The relationship between MR TR and muscle fiber composition has been reported.[30] Longer TRs were detected in fast-twitch fibers compared with slow-twitch fibers. Shellock et al.[27,28] demonstrated that concentric versus eccentric loading of muscles will yield different patterns of altered signal intensity on an MRI exam. Spin-echo T2-weighted sequences were obtained before and

immediately after the performance of concentric or eccentric exercises. Muscles that contracted concentrically had increased signal intensity detected on the MR images compared with nonexercised muscle. Muscles that contracted eccentrically showed little or no change in signal intensity immediately at the termination of the exercise. It was of interest that the actual calculated T2 TRs were significantly increased in both groups of muscles compared with nonexercised muscles, but the T2 TR was significantly longer in the muscles performing concentric contractions, thereby explaining the difference in the appearance of the muscles on the T2-weighted sequence. The exact etiology for the increased signal intensity in the muscles may be related to the nature of the binding of water molecules

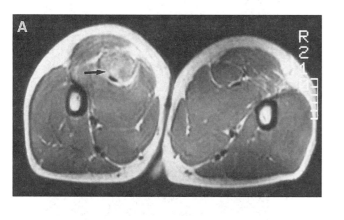

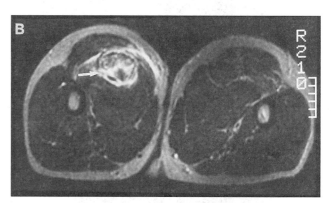

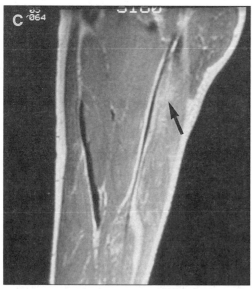

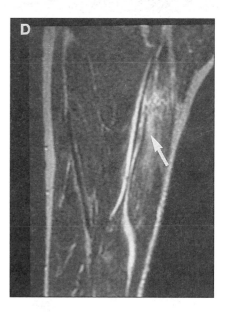

Figure 4–7 Acute grade 1 muscle strain superimposed on a subacute muscle injury in a professional football quarterback. On the proton-density (**A**) and T2-weighted (**B**) axial images (patient positioned prone) and on the proton-density (**C**) and T2-weighted (**D**) sagittal images, there is extensive edema in the semitendinosus muscle. The edematous changes are most prominent at its myotendinous junction (*arrows*). Further distally in the thigh, on the proton-density (**E**) and T2-weighted (**F**) axial images and on the proton-density (**G**) and T2-weighted (**H**) sagittal images, there is a resolving hematoma in the lateral segment of the semitendinosus muscle (*arrows*).

Figure 4–7 continued

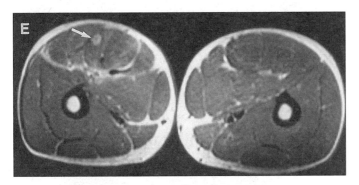

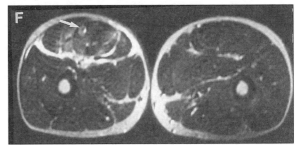

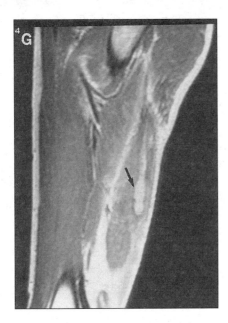

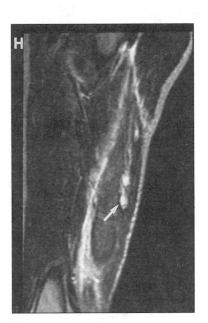

within a muscle.[31] Increased fluid within the muscle secondary to muscle metabolism[32] or increased muscle perfusion[33] related to exercise could also affect the muscle signal intensity.

An additional application of MRI in the evaluation of muscle physiology includes the work performed by Fleckenstein et al.[34] on the assessment of muscle recruitment patterns during exercise. This is particularly relevant to expanding our understanding of the activity of different muscle groups in the kinetic chain. It is now possible to detect which muscles normally act synergistically and to detect which muscles may be overloaded from muscle fatigue or biomechanical imbalance. We recently studied a professional baseball pitcher who was experiencing arm discomfort. After his clinical evaluation, a presumptive diagnosis of a latissimus dorsi strain was reached and rehabilitation started. After he did not improve, an MRI exam was ordered and demonstrated a strain of the lower segment of the subscapularis muscle and only minimal abnormal signal in the latissimus dorsi (Figure 4–8). It is not possible to know whether the subscapularis strain was the etiology of his initial symptoms or whether the strain was related to secondary overload of a synergistic muscle after the injury to the latissimus dorsi.

Another recent application of MRI in the assessment of muscle injury is in the evaluation of patients for the possibility of acute or chronic compartment syndromes (Figure 4–9). An acute compartment syndrome developing after a fracture may be secondary to an accumulation of blood or interstitial edema in a closed muscular compartment. With the application of MRI, Myerson and Manoli[35] detected a hematoma adjacent to a fractured calcaneus, which was the etiology of the patient's posttraumatic compartment syndrome. Acute compartment syndromes most frequently involve the lower extremity, but MRI may be of benefit in demonstrating pathologic changes in any muscle. In a patient with an acute

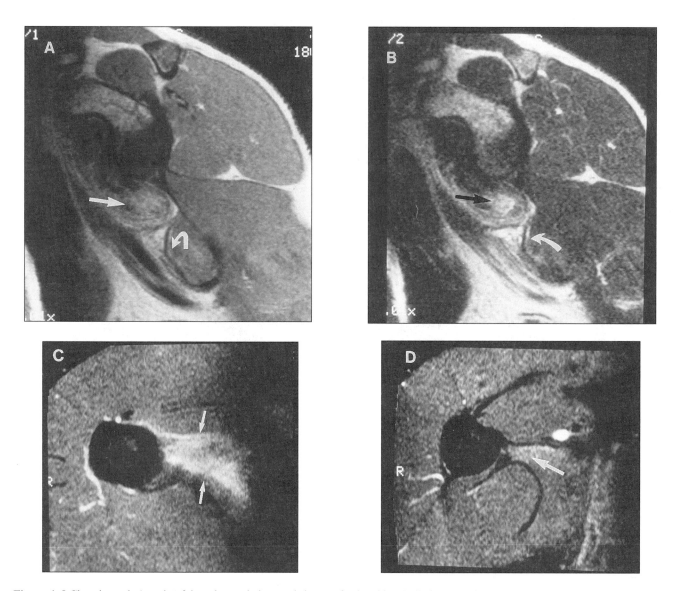

Figure 4–8 Chronic grade 1 strain of the subscapularis muscle in a professional baseball pitcher. On the proton-density (**A**) and T2-weighted (**B**) oblique sagittal images, there are extensive edematous changes in the lower segment of the subscapularis muscle (*straight arrows*) and minimal edematous changes in the latissimus dorsi (*curved arrows*). On the STIR axial image (**C**), there are prominent edematous changes in the subscapularis muscle (*arrows*) extending to its insertion. On the STIR axial image (**D**), there are minimal edematous changes in the latissimus dorsi muscle (*arrow*) at its insertion.

paraspinal lumbar compartment syndrome, an MRI study demonstrated increased signal intensity in the symptomatic paraspinal muscles, which also had abnormal intracompartmental pressures.[36] Resolution of the abnormal signal intensity paralleled the improvement of the patient's symptoms. MRI has also been used in the evaluation of patients with chronic compartment syndromes. Amendola et al.[37] demonstrated that in five patients with a positive clinical history for chronic compartment syndrome and who also had elevated postexercise pressures, four patients demonstrated abnormal MR signal intensity within the muscle. Patients who were

initially thought to have a chronic compartment syndrome but whose pressure measurements were normal also had a normal MRI examination. In a case report of chronic compartment syndrome of the feet, Lokiec et al.[38] demonstrated muscular hypertrophy on an MRI exam after strenuous exercise. There was no pre-exercise MRI exam presented in the report; therefore, it is uncertain whether there was an actual change in muscle morphology with exercise.

Whereas MRI is extremely sensitive in detecting pathologic changes within a muscle due to the accumulation of fluid, it lacks specificity. Any pathologic process that incites

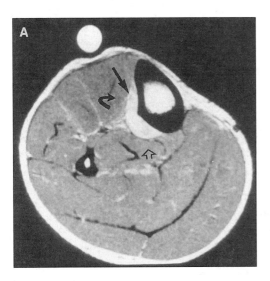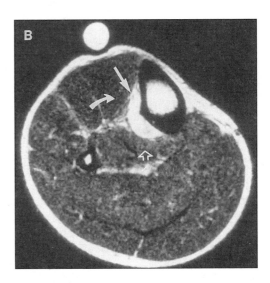

Figure 4–9 Subperiosteal hematoma in an athlete with symptoms of a compartment syndrome. On the proton-density (**A**) and T2-weighted (**B**) axial images, there is a subperiosteal hematoma (*straight arrows*) interposed between the tibia and the anterior (*curved arrows*) and posterior (*open arrows*) tibialis muscles.

an inflammatory response or increases muscle hydration will present with abnormal signal intensity. Other muscular conditions that may present with an appearance similar to muscle injury include metabolic myopathies,[39] dermatomyositis,[40,41] diabetic muscular infarction,[42] vasculitis, viral myositis,[43] sarcoid myopathy,[44] and acute rhabdomyolysis.[45] Even a benign procedure such as an intramuscular injection can be detected on an MRI exam as a focus of abnormal signal intensity in the muscle and perifascial tissue.[46] It is quite apparent that the clinical significance of any abnormal finding on an MRI exam can be determined only by close correlation with a patient's history and physical exam. The value of a negative MRI may also be important in reaching an accurate diagnosis or in directing treatment. An MRI examination was obtained on a group of patients diagnosed with fibromyalgia. There were no abnormalities detected within the muscles or surrounding soft tissues on the MRI study,[47] thereby excluding the possibility of a more ominous process as a cause of the patients' symptomatology.

TENDONS

The function of a tendon is to transmit the force from its muscle of origin to the bone where it inserts. Tendons are stressed by concentric or eccentric muscle contractions, and the highest stress on a tendon is generated with eccentric muscle contractions. Excessive acute or chronic stress on a tendon may precipitate fiber disruption and induce pain. Disruption of a tendon may occur anywhere along its length. Avulsion of a tendon from its bony insertion may or may not be associated with a bony avulsion.[48]

There has been a variety of terms used to describe tendon injuries. To classify tendon injuries, it is necessary to know whether an injury is related to an acute traumatic event or is secondary to chronic overload. The duration of a patient's symptoms must also be considered. An acute injury to a tendon may precipitate fiber failure, i.e., a strain, which is classified as grades 1–3, depending on the degree of fiber disruption. Although the term *tendinitis* is frequently employed when a patient presents with pain related to a tendon or peritendinous tissue, only an injury that acutely precipitates failure of tendon fibers along with disruption of vascularized peritendinous connective tissue can produce an acute inflammatory response in a tendon, i.e., tendinitis.[49] Tendinitis may be acute, subacute, or chronic, depending on the duration of the patient's symptoms. If an acute injury incites an inflammatory response only in the soft tissue surrounding a tendon, e.g., the peritenon or the paratenon, without disruption of the tendon fibers, then the terms *peritendinitis* or *paratendonitis* are the most appropriate to describe a patient's symptomatology.[49,50]

Chronic microtrauma to a tendon, frequently secondary to chronic eccentric overload, may precipitate intrasubstance fiber failure. There is typically no history of an acute injury, and the symptoms have an insidious onset. The chronic pathologic changes identified within the substance of a chronically overloaded tendon include fibrillar degeneration, angiofibroblastic proliferation, fiber necrosis with myxoid and hyaline degeneration, fibrosis, and occasionally chronic inflammation.[51] The term *tendinosis* has been employed to describe these chronic pathologic changes.[49] Tendinosis may represent an abortive healing response of a tendon from chronic overload. It is possible to have changes of acute tendinitis or peritendinitis superimposed on changes of tendinosis.

A normal tendon is composed predominantly of collagen fibers, and it appears as a structure with minimal or no signal intensity on spin-echo or STIR MRI sequences. It is necessary to understand the spectrum of the appearance of normal tendons with MRI prior to attempting to diagnose pathologic changes.[52,53] Certain tendons, e.g., the posterior tibial tendon[54,55] and the rotator cuff[56] will demonstrate increased signal intensity within normal segments of the tendon. This may be related to the orientation of a tendon with respect to the direction of the magnetic field used for MR imaging.

With peritendinitis, pathologically, there will be increased fluid in the peritendinous tissue related to an inflammatory process. This will be detected on an MRI spin-echo T2-weighted or STIR sequence as a focus of high signal intensity surrounding a normal tendon. With tendinosis, a focus of myxoid degeneration or angioblastic proliferation within the substance of a tendon will demonstrate increased signal intensity within the tendon on a spin-echo T1-weighted or STIR sequence. On a T2-weighted sequence, the abnormal signal intensity may persist but typically will not be as bright as it was on the T1-weighted sequence, or the signal intensity within the tendon may become normal. Persistent high signal intensity on a T2-weighted or STIR sequence may be seen if there is inflammatory or degenerative tissue within a tendon. A high-grade partial tear of a tendon provides a mechanism whereby fluid or inflammatory tissue can extend into the substance of a tendon. Short tau inversion sequences have been particularly useful in evaluating tendon disruption. With a STIR sequence, it is also possible to detect pathologic changes within a tendon before the onset or after the resolution of symptoms.

In addition to the abnormal signal intensity identified within inflamed or degenerated tendons, altered morphology is also frequently identified, e.g., hypertrophy or attenuation of a tendon. A grading system of disorders of the posterior tibial tendon has been reported.[54] A hypertrophied tendon containing abnormal signal intensity has been classified as grade 1 degeneration or partial tear; an attenuated tendon containing abnormal signal intensity as grade 2 degeneration or partial tear, and a complete tear of the tendon is classified as grade 3.

Magnetic resonance imaging provides a very sensitive test to detect tendon disorders; unfortunately, it lacks specificity. It is not possible on an MRI study to determine whether a focus of abnormal signal intensity within a tendon is secondary to acute inflammation or to chronic degeneration. If abnormal tendon morphology is also detected, e.g., with an acute partial tendon tear, it may be inferred that some of the abnormal signal intensity is secondary to an acute inflammatory process. However, these acute changes may be superimposed on chronic degenerative changes of a tendon that may not be differentiated on an MRI study. In the assessment of the abnormal signal intensity surrounding a tendon, it is also not possible to determine whether the altered tissue hydration is associated with an inflammatory infiltrate.

Magnetic resonance imaging has had a major impact in the advancement of our understanding of the natural history of tendon failure. With MRI, it is possible to detect subclinical injuries, i.e., pathologic changes in a tendon resulting from chronic microtrauma or aging. These injuries, by definition, do not incite symptoms, but they may predispose a tendon to future dysfunction or failure. When the tendons of patients with an acute complete tendon rupture are studied histologically, changes of chronic tendon degeneration are usually demonstrated adjacent to the area of an acute rupture. Even a great percentage of nonruptured tendons demonstrate pathologic changes of chronic degeneration.[57] These abnormalities can be detected with MRI by the demonstration of abnormal signal intensity or altered morphology of a tendon. These abnormal foci detected on an MRI study are not false-positive findings because they do represent pathologic changes in an asymptomatic tendon. The detection of subclinical tendon degeneration may provide important information with respect to changing training or rehabilitative techniques that may be overloading a tendon.

The location of tendon degeneration and/or tear depends on the etiology of fiber failure. Acute tendon ruptures may occur anywhere in the tendon but are frequently detected at the tendo-osseous junction (Figures 4–10 and 4–11). The nature of the force, the position of the joint at the time of injury, and any predisposing factors that may have weakened the tendon will affect the site of rupture. If failure is secondary to extrinsic impingement, e.g., by a degenerative osseous ridge, the location of tendon failure will occur where the tendon impinges against this extrinsic structure. Chronic overload injuries to a tendon, frequently secondary to eccentric muscle contraction, may cause microstructural damage within the substance of a tendon at a tendon's insertion site, e.g., the quadriceps, patellar, or posterior tibial tendons. Extrinsic impingement or intrinsic overload of a tendon may be amplified if there is also instability of a joint that precipitates external friction or increased tension of a tendon when the MTU is active. With MRI, it is possible to determine the exact location and extent of an injury to a tendon, as well as to define the degree of hypertrophy or attenuation of a tendon. Equally important, an MRI exam provides a comprehensive evaluation of all the peritendinous structures that may impinge a tendon and precipitate failure. Ultrasound has been extensively used in the evaluation of tendon degeneration or tears,[58,59] but US provides little or no information about the status of a tendon when it is located beneath an osseous structure. It also has limited use in defining abnormal osseous structures that may cause extrinsic impingement of a

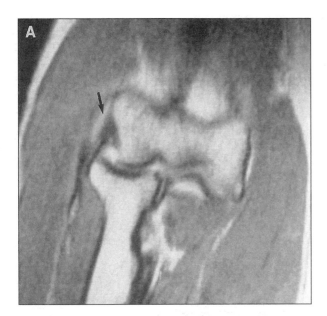 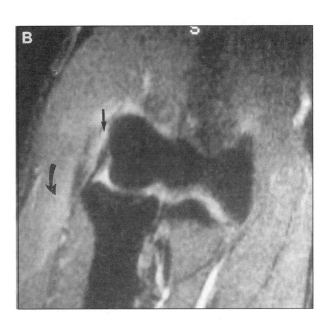

Figure 4–10 Acute grade 1 strain of the extensor carpi radialis brevis tendon. On the T1-weighted (**A**) and STIR (**B**) oblique coronal images, increased signal intensity is identified in the tendon at its insertion site (*straight arrows*). In addition, there are mild edematous changes in the extensor digitorum communis muscle (*curved arrow*).

tendon. Ultrasound is most valuable in the assessment of a superficially located tendon, e.g., the Achilles[60–61] or patellar tendon.

Chronic intrinsic overload of a tendon is a cause of fiber failure and tendon degeneration in a young or middle-aged individual presenting with tendon dysfunction. In patients experiencing debilitating elbow pain, the pain is most commonly located along the lateral side of the elbow. The symptom complex is frequently called *lateral epicondylitis*, even though the pathologic changes are predominantly those of chronic degeneration within the extensor tendons and not in the epicondyle.[51] With MRI, it is possible to noninvasively detect the presence and extent of tendon degeneration (Figure 4–12). Equally important, MRI can detect abnormalities in the peritendinous tissue that may present with symptoms similar to tennis elbow, e.g., entrapment of the posterior interosseous nerve, degenerative arthrosis of the elbow joint, an anconeus or extensor muscle compartment syndrome, lateral ligament insufficiency, or synovitis.[62]

Medial tendinosis of the elbow is not as common as lateral tendon dysfunction. It must be considered as a potential cause of medial elbow pain, particularly in an athlete participating in an activity involving chronic valgus overload to a joint, e.g., baseball pitchers, tennis players, or javelin throwers.[63] Vangsness and Jobe[64] reported on the operative treatment of 35 patients with symptoms of "medial epicondylitis" who had failed conservative care. Approximately 60% of the patients were athletes, and the dominant arm was

involved in 94%. In 20% of the patients, initial plain films demonstrated calcification or spurs adjacent to the medial humeral epicondyle. This is similar to the plain film findings detected adjacent to the lateral humeral epicondyle in patients with tennis elbow. At surgery, visual tears with incomplete healing were identified at the origin of the common flexor tendon. Histologic changes in this tissue included tendon microfragmentation, granulation tissue, calcification, fibrovascular tissue, fibrocartilaginous tissue, inflammatory cells, and necrosis. The value of an MRI study is in determination of the precise location and the extent of tendon pathology prior to debridement or repair.

An MRI exam obtained on a professional quarterback who was experiencing chronic medial elbow pain demonstrated changes of tendinosis at the origin of the common flexor tendon. The athlete continued to play football and, after experiencing increasing severity of pain, a follow-up MRI study demonstrated progression of the tendon tear. Surgical debridement and repair of the tendon were performed, and a postoperative MRI study demonstrated extensive fibrosis of the tendon and peritendinous tissue, and no evidence of tendon disruption. When he resumed athletics, the patient again experienced medial elbow pain, but in a more proximal location compared with his previous symptoms. A repeat MRI exam demonstrated partial disruption of the repaired tendon, along with a new finding of a grade 1 strain of the pronator teres muscle. His pain was located over the region of the abnormal signal intensity in the pronator teres (Figure 4–13).

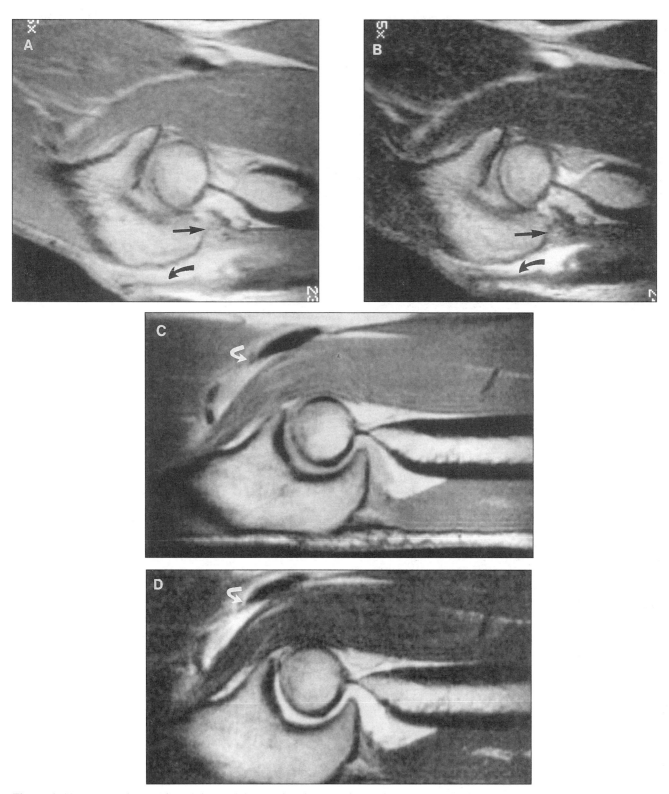

Figure 4–11 Acute grade 3 tendon strain. An injury to the triceps tendon at the tendo-osseous junction secondary to a football injury is identified on the proton-density (**A**) and T2-weighted (**B**) sagittal images with detachment of the triceps tendon (*curved arrows*). The athlete was still able to extend his elbow, due to the intact muscular insertion of the triceps (*straight arrows*). In another athlete, on proton-density (**C**) and T2-weighted (**D**) sagittal images, there is complete disruption of the distal segment of the biceps tendon (*curved arrows*) secondary to a fall.

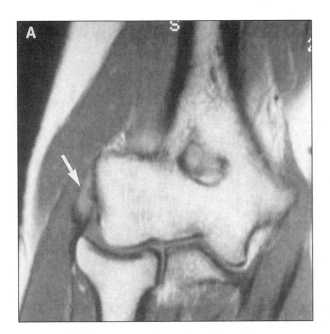 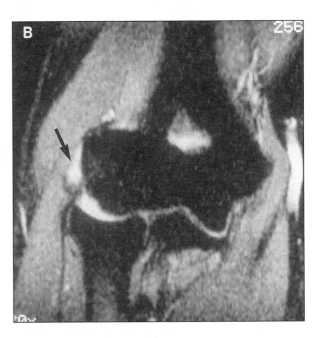

Figure 4–12 Tendinopathy of the extensor carpi radialis brevis tendon in a tennis player. On the T1-weighted (**A**) and STIR (**B**) oblique coronal images, there is a focal area of high signal intensity within the substance of the tendon at its insertion site (*arrows*). There are no edematous changes in the surrounding soft tissue or bone.

This case demonstrates the potential application of MRI to detect an early symptomatic MTU overload injury. With the precise knowledge of which muscle group is injured, rehabilitation may be directed to the exact cause of an athlete's dysfunction. It is also possible to assess the results of therapy with a follow-up MRI study. This may be particularly useful to evaluate the efficacy of different modalities of therapy.

Dysfunction of the Achilles tendon is a frequent cause of debilitating ankle pain in athletes with recurrent episodes of acute pain or persistent chronic pain. There is no tenosynovial sheath surrounding the Achilles tendon; therefore, if acute pain is associated with inflammation in the peritendinous soft tissues, it involves the paratenon or peritenon. Magnetic resonance imaging has proven to be very useful in the evaluation of patients with refractory Achilles pain or acute rupture. Intrasubstance partial tears or degeneration of a tendon are detected as foci of increased signal intensity on spin-echo and STIR sequences due to the increased hydration of the pathologic tissue. Thickening of the tendon is also usually detected. With a partial tear that interrupts the peripheral fibers of the tendon or with a complete tear, focal fiber disruption is identified (Figure 4–14). The MRI exam can be performed with the patient's foot in both dorsiflexion and plantar flexion to assess the size of the gap between the ends of a torn tendon. Weinstabl et al.[65] reported on 28 patients with suspected tendon injury. Of the 13 patients who required operative treatment, all partial and complete tears

detected at surgery were correctly diagnosed on an MRI study. Ultrasonography was also performed on 10 of the 28 patients, and 1 patient with a partial rupture at surgery had a false-negative US. Due to the limited number of patients and the retrospective nature of the data collection, it is not possible to compare the efficacy of MRI versus US in this report.

In several recent reports, US has been useful in the management of patients with chronic painful Achilles tendons by revealing the presence of peritendinitis, tendinosis, and partial or complete tears of the tendon. Martinoli et al.[66] demonstrated the value of high-resolution US in detecting minimal pathologic changes in the structure of tendons in both experimental animals and humans. Kainberger et al.[60] used US to evaluate 73 patients with achillodynia or signs of tendon thickening. Fifty-two of the patients participated in sports, 5 patients had systemic inflammatory diseases, 3 patients had familial hypercholesterolemia, and 13 patients had no known potential etiology for tendon dysfunction. Sonograms were abnormal in 53 patients, and the extent of structural disorders of the tendon could be adequately assessed. Abnormalities included tendon swelling in 45%, abnormal tendon structure in 42%, rupture in 15%, and peritendinous lesions in 47%. Surgical correlation was available for only 18 patients; therefore, it is difficult to determine the accuracy of ultrasonographic findings. Kalebo et al.[61] reported on the diagnostic value of US in the assessment of partial ruptures of the

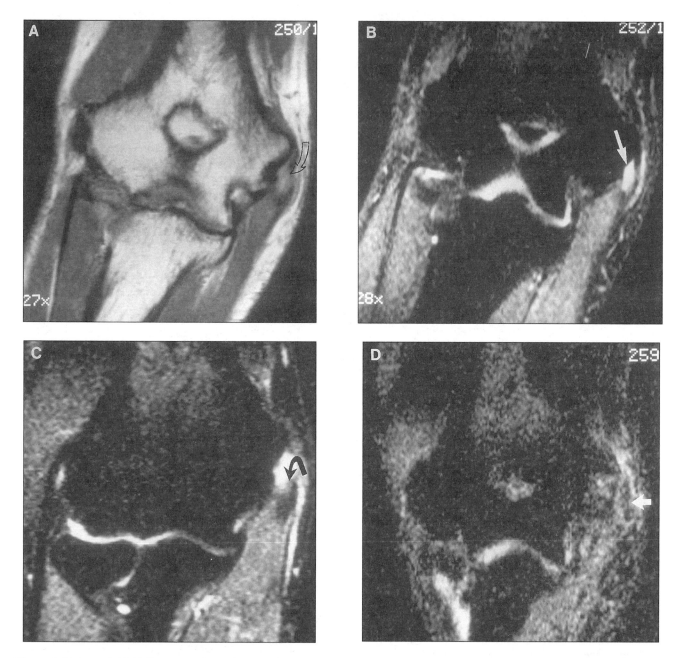

Figure 4–13 On an initial MR exam performed on a professional football quarterback experiencing medial elbow pain, the T1-weighted (**A**) and STIR (**B**) oblique coronal images show a focal area of high signal intensity within the substance of the common flexor tendon at its insertion site (*arrows*). After an exacerbation of his symptoms, a follow-up MRI demonstrated complete detachment of the tendon on the STIR (**C**) oblique coronal image (*curved arrow*). After repair of the tendon, a follow-up MRI (**D**) demonstrated diffuse fibrosis at the surgical site (*arrow*). After the resumption of physical activity, he once again experienced elbow pain, but in a more proximal and anterior location. On a repeat MRI, there was breakdown of the surgical repair (*arrows*) (**E** and **F**), along with a strain of the pronator teres muscle (*arrows*) (**G** and **H**).

Achilles tendon. Of 160 patients with chronic pain of the Achilles tendon evaluated with US, 37 Achilles tendons in 30 patients underwent operative treatment. Surgical findings were compared to the US studies for all of these patients, and histologic examination was also performed on 20 cases. Thirty partial tears were diagnosed by US and were confirmed at surgery. The overall sensitivity for US was 0.94, the specificity was 1.00, and the accuracy was 0.95 in this

Figure 4–13 continued

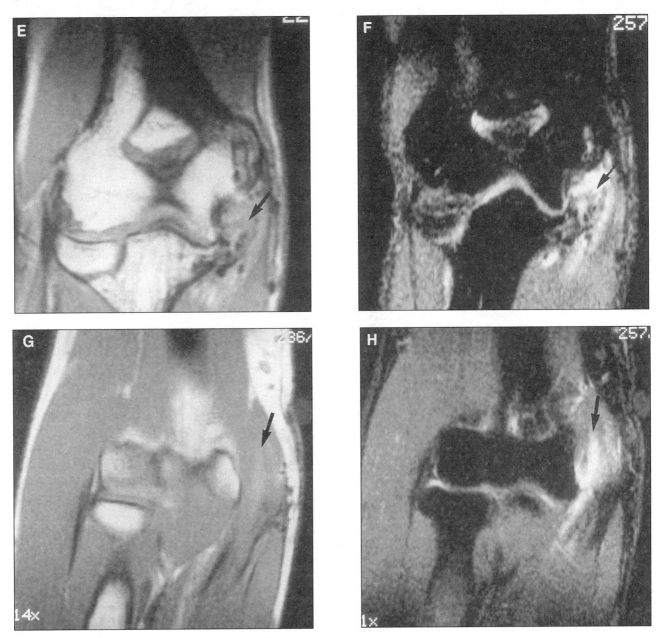

highly selected group of patients. The authors concluded that the advantages of US are its availability, low cost, and real-time imaging capabilities, compared with MRI studies. The authors also stated that MRI is less operator-dependent than is US and renders a better overview of the surrounding tissues, even though no MRI studies were reported for the patients in this report.

Like the Achilles tendon, the patellar tendon is prone to chronic overload injuries.[67] Both US and MRI have been used to evaluate the pathologic changes within the tendon in symptomatic patients. Although pain and dysfunction of the patellar tendon are usually referred to as *patellar tendinitis*, pathologic changes detected within the tendon frequently demonstrate changes of fiber disruption, chronic myxoid degeneration, and focal fibrinoid necrosis.[68] If a patient does not respond to conservative care, an imaging study is frequently ordered to corroborate the presumptive clinical diagnosis and to assist in preoperative planning. With MRI, it is possible to determine the exact location and extent of the pathologic changes within the patellar tendon (Figure

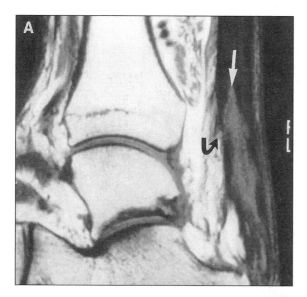
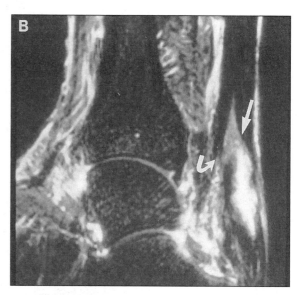

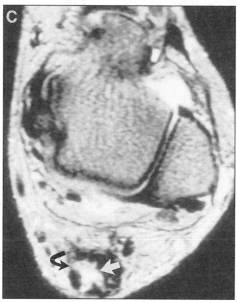

Figure 4–14 Partial tear of the Achilles tendon superimposed on chronic tendon degeneration in a runner. On the T1-weighted (**A**) and STIR (**B**) sagittal images and on the T1-weighted (**C**) axial image, there is diffuse thickening of the tendon, along with a long tubular focus of intratendinous high signal intensity (*straight arrows*). A partial tear of the peripheral margins of the tendon is also identified (*curved arrows*).

4–15).[69] In addition to abnormal signal intensity within a tendon, hypertrophy of a tendon is frequently detected.[70] Patellar "tendinitis" most frequently involves the proximal segment of the tendon, particularly at its insertion into the lower pole of the patella. Magnetic resonance imaging has been utilized to detect partial tears as well as to demonstrate complete tears when they develop.

With MRI, it is not infrequent to detect an enlarged distal segment of the patellar tendon containing bony ossicles secondary to prior Osgood-Schlatter disease.[68] Rosenberg et al.[71] reported on the MRI appearance of acute Osgood-Schlatter disease before and after treatment. In all patients, there was abnormal size of the tendon, along with increased signal intensity within the distal segment of the tendon. A distended infrapatellar bursa was also frequently detected. These abnormalities only partially disappeared on follow-up MRI studies after resolution of symptoms. A CT exam was also performed on these patients; in only 32% of the cases was an ossicle detected in the tendon. In three of seven cases, the ossicle remained ununited to the anterior tibial tubercle

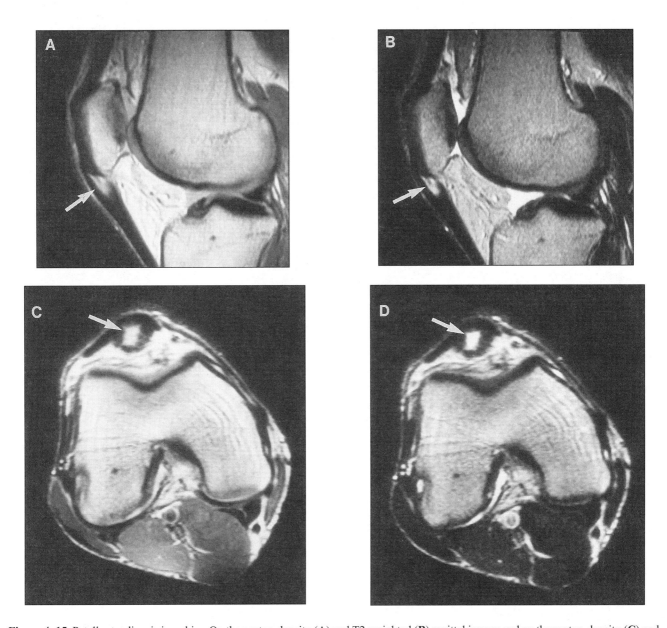

Figure 4–15 Patellar tendinosis in a skier. On the proton-density (**A**) and T2-weighted (**B**) sagittal images and on the proton-density (**C**) and T2-weighted (**D**) axial images, there is a focal area of high signal intensity in the center of the proximal segment of the tendon at its insertion site (*arrows*). At the time of tendon repair, tissue histology revealed chronic degenerative changes within the tendon at this location.

on follow-up studies when the patients were asymptomatic. Marrow edema was also detected in the anterior tibial tuberosity in one third of the cases imaged with MRI. The changes of marrow edema persisted in one third of these cases after the patients became asymptomatic.

Karlsson et al.[72] reported on the US evaluation of partial rupture of the patellar tendon. Eighty-one patients with 91 partial tears of the patellar tendon were classified according to the length of the tear detected with US. Eventually, 27 tendons required an operative procedure, and the surgical findings corroborated the abnormal sonographic findings. Most of the pathologic changes were at the bone-tendon junction at the lower pole of the patella or in the proximal segment of the tendon. The overall need for surgery was greatest in the tendons that had the largest partial tears detected by US. The asymptomatic contralateral patellar tendon was also evaluated in these patients, and in 9 of 71 tendons, small abnormalities in the patellar tendon were also detected. King et al.[73] reported on the use of US and CT in the assessment of lesions of the patellar tendon in 18 patients presenting with infrapatellar pain. Both US and CT showed focal hypertrophy of the patellar tendon in 17 of the 18 patients. The lesions were located in the middle segment of the patellar tendon. These 17 patients subsequently required surgery, and pathologic changes were present in all of the cases. Eight cases detected as cystic on US also had a cystic lesion at the time of surgery. The authors concluded that whereas both CT and US were comparable in lesion detection, US was more accurate in distinguishing between different types of lesions. Davies et al.[74] compared US, CT, and MRI in the evaluation of 16 patients with refractory patellar tendinitis. In 14 cases, US demonstrated hypertrophy of the tendon at its proximal insertion site, and 1 tendon was thickened in its middle segment. Computed tomography was positive in all 16 cases and demonstrated central tendinous expansion at the proximal patellar insertion. With MRI, there was focal thickening of the patellar tendon in all 16 patients. On the MRI study, there was abnormal signal intensity in 14 of the 16 cases. The abnormal signal intensity was present on all of the STIR sequences but on only 57% of the spin-echo T1-weighted images and 64% of the T2-weighted images. In the 15 cases that underwent surgical correction, abnormal tissue was present at the site of the abnormalities detected on the imaging studies. Tendon histology included degenerative changes, perivascular cellular infiltrates, neovascularization, and nodules of granulation tissue. In all three of these studies, a very select group of patients with prominent patellar tendon pathology underwent an operative procedure. It is, therefore, difficult to determine the true accuracy or efficacy of US, MRI, or CT, particularly in the detection of small lesions. If only large lesions are refractory to conservative therapy, the detection of small lesions may not be important, but this will have to be proved with a long-term prospective study.

The rotator cuff is one of the largest tendinous structures in the body and, because of its functional demands, it is prone to degeneration and failure. The two primary mechanisms of injury to the cuff are extrinsic primary impingement and intrinsic chronic overload. The impingement syndrome presents as painful dysfunction of the shoulder, particularly with overhead activities. The pain is precipitated by entrapment or abrasion of the rotator cuff mechanism (i.e., the rotator cuff and the peritendinous soft tissue) under a degenerated acromioclavicular joint or under the coracoacromial arch (i.e., the arch formed by the coracoid process, the coracoacromial ligament, and the acromion). In the supraspinatus outlet, the rotator cuff mechanism may impinge against a thickened coracoacromial ligament, an enthesophyte projecting off the anteroinferior margin of the acromion at the insertion of the coracoclavicular (CA) ligament, or against a curved or hooked acromion. Repetitive abrasion of the rotator cuff mechanism can precipitate bursal inflammation, peritendinous inflammation, or tendon degenera-

tion.[75] Fiber disruption secondary to cuff abrasion will be associated with edema and/or hemorrhage in the cuff and the peritendinous tissues. With MRI, it is possible to precisely define the anatomy of the acromioclavicular (AC) joint and the supraspinatus outlet, and to detect any evidence of a degenerative process affecting these structures (Figure 4–16). It is possible to define the location where the cuff may be impinging against areas of bony proliferation or ligamentous hypertrophy. It is also possible to detect evidence of bursal inflammation. Impingement (to push against) is a physical phenomenon and can be detected by an MRI exam, but diagnosis of impingement syndrome, which is a painful symptom complex secondary to the repetitive abrasion and inflammation of the cuff and/or the peritendinous tissue resulting from impingement, can be made only clinically. With continued injury to a cuff, a focal partial tear or full-thickness tear may develop. If biomechanical imbalance results from a torn rotator cuff or is present secondary to primary shoulder instability, secondary impingement of the cuff may also be present and may elicit symptoms.

Imaging studies of the rotator cuff are frequently obtained after an unsuccessful trial of conservative therapy for rotator cuff impingement or tear. Prior to the development of US and MRI, plain films were the primary diagnostic imaging study to evaluate the shoulder for rotator cuff dysfunction.

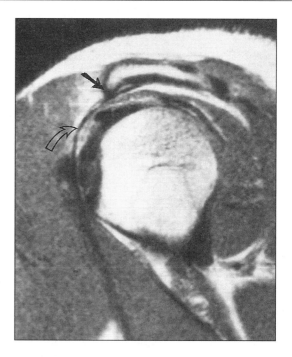

Figure 4–16 Mild impingement of the supraspinatus myotendinous junction by a type III acromion in a tennis player. On the proton density–weighted oblique sagittal image, impingement of the cuff against a hooked acromion is identified (*straight arrow*). There is minimal thickening of the CA ligament (*curved arrow*).

Whereas plain films are helpful in the evaluation of osseous anatomy and pathology, they provide no direct and only limited indirect evidence of rotator cuff pathology. The best indicator for a torn rotator cuff on plain films is when the distance between the humeral head and the acromion is less than 6 mm on an anteroposterior view of the shoulder with the arm in neutral rotation.[76] Unfortunately, this is a very late finding in the natural history of cuff degeneration, and when it is present, there is usually a very large or massive tear of the cuff. The supraspinatus outlet view has recently been implemented to assess the shape of the acromion. Because a plain film is a two-dimensional projection of a three-dimensional structure, it is frequently difficult to determine the true shape of the acromion. Interobserver variability is also a problem with the interpretation of this projection. Special views have also been developed to detect osseous ridges projecting off the anteroinferior margin of the acromion.[77]

The integrity of the rotator cuff can be assessed by arthrography, which is a mildly invasive procedure. After the instillation of contrast into the shoulder joint, full-thickness cuff tears can be detected by the leakage of contrast. The sensitivity of arthrography to detect full-thickness tears measuring over 1 cm is probably over 90%, but the study is less sensitive in detecting small full-thickness tears or partial tears of the articular surface of the cuff. It is insensitive in the detection of partial tears on the bursal side of the cuff, which may result from extrinsic impingement. Arthrography provides little information on the status of the cuff fibers, e.g., evidence of degeneration or attrition, and it provides no information on the assessment of the coracoacromial arch and the supraspinatus outlet. The detection of a full-thickness cuff tear may occur in asymptomatic older patients and in asymptomatic individuals who have undergone a surgical repair of the cuff. Calvert et al.[78] performed arthrography on 20 patients after rotator cuff repair and demonstrated leakage of contrast, indicating a full-thickness cuff tear, in 18 of the patients. Seventeen of the 18 patients were asymptomatic at the time of arthrography.

Ultrasound and MRI are noninvasive tests performed to evaluate the rotator cuff and the surrounding soft-tissue structures. One advantage of US is its capacity to study the cuff with the arm in different positions. This may be particularly useful in the evaluation of patients with shoulder impingement syndrome.[79] There have been several reports on the value of US to detect tears of the rotator cuff.[80–82] Weiner et al.[82] reported on a group of 225 patients who had preoperative sonography and compared the results of US to the surgical findings. The abnormalities detected on the US included partial- and full-thickness cuff tears. The US findings were surgically confirmed in 92% of the cases. Several areas of potential bias may affect the validity of these results. The surgical treatment was generally based on the sonographic classification; therefore, knowledge of the abnormalities de-

tected by US may influence the selection of patients for surgery (work-up bias) and the findings reported at surgery (verification bias). The 225 patients represented a subset from a group of 800 patients who completed US evaluation. With the large number of patients not requiring surgery, it is not possible to determine the overall accuracy of US. Brenneke and Morgan[81] reported on the sonographic evaluation of 120 patients who underwent diagnostic arthroscopy. Compared to the arthroscopic findings, the sensitivity of US for the detection of a full-thickness cuff tear was 95%; for detecting a partial-thickness cuff it was 41%. At arthroscopy, 14 of 20 patients with impingement had a partial-cuff tear and a negative US. The authors concluded that US was an effective modality to detect full-thickness but not partial rotator cuff tears. It is difficult to assess the results of this study, due to its methodological limitations.

Misamore and Woodward[83] reported a prospective study of 32 patients who had degeneration of the rotator cuff and who required surgery. Preoperatively, both US and arthrography were performed. Of the 20 patients who had a full-thickness tear, arthrography detected 100% and US detected 35%. Of the 7 patients with partial-thickness tears, arthrography was accurate in 3, and US was accurate in 2 of the cases. Arthrography was accurate in all 5 patients who did not have a tear, and US was accurate in 3 of the cases. The physicians caring for the patients were not blinded to the results of the imaging studies; therefore, the possibility of bias must be considered. It does appear from the reports in the literature that, in some centers, US provides useful information for a certain subset of patients. The efficacy of US cannot be deduced from these studies in regard to its application as a screening examination for rotator cuff disorders.

Magnetic resonance imaging is the optimal imaging modality to provide a comprehensive evaluation of the shoulder in a patient with shoulder dysfunction. The strengths of MRI are its direct multiplanar capabilities, excellent soft-tissue contrast resolution, and its ability to completely evaluate the osseous architecture of the shoulder girdle. Whereas US has received criticism for its operator dependence, the efficacy of MRI in the assessment of the shoulder is highly dependent on the imaging protocols employed and the expertise of the radiologist interpreting the study. Like all structures in the body, there is a range in the appearance of normal anatomy that must be appreciated.[56,84] The pathoetiology of abnormalities detected on an MRI study can be determined only by precisely comparing the findings on an MRI study to those detected at arthroscopy—an open surgical procedure—or to tissue histology obtained from cadavers.

The appearance of a normal rotator cuff is similar to that of other tendons in the body. With its high collagen content, it demonstrates minimal signal intensity on spin-echo or STIR sequences. There are zones in a cuff that may normally demonstrate intermediate signal intensity on T1-weighted sequences, e.g., the transition point between the supraspinatus and the infraspinatus segments of a cuff. There may also be a segment of increased signal intensity in a cuff if there is lateral extension of muscle fibers into the cuff. It is also possible to detect increased signal in certain segments of a cuff, due to the orientation of a cuff with respect to the direction of the magnetic field of the MR equipment. Whereas all of these variations demonstrate increased signal intensity compared with a normal cuff on spin-echo T1-weighted sequences, on T2-weighted sequences, these areas demonstrate minimal signal intensity, similar to that of normal cuff. Abnormalities of the rotator cuff are detected by altered cuff morphology, along with abnormal signal intensity. Complete assessment of the soft tissues and osseous structures surrounding the cuff is mandatory to achieve a comprehensive evaluation of the shoulder. Imaging of the shoulder in three orthogonal planes should be performed on all patients. The axis of the different scan planes is determined by the orientation of the supraspinatus tendon and the scapula. The coronal sequence is oriented parallel to the long axis of the body of the scapula and the supraspinatus tendon. The sagittal sequence is oriented perpendicular to the coronal sequence. Both the coronal and sagittal sequences are oriented obliquely to the coronal and sagittal planes of the body, due to the normal rotation of the scapula on the chest wall. Therefore, these sequences are referred to as *oblique coronal* or *oblique sagittal* sequences. The axial sequence is oriented perpendicular to the face of the glenoid, and, depending on the degree of scapular rotation, it may be necessary to perform an oblique axial sequence compared with the horizontal plane of the body. Spin-echo T1- and T2-weighted se-

quences are standard for the evaluation of the shoulder, and additional sequences, e.g., gradient-echo or STIR, may be performed to provide supplemental information.

Degeneration and/or intrasubstance tears of the collagenous cuff fibers is detected on an MRI T1-weighted sequence as a focus of increased signal intensity due to increased hydration of the cuff tissue. On a T2-weighted sequence, the abnormal signal intensity may persist or, more commonly, decrease in intensity. The morphology of the cuff may be altered, e.g., attenuated or hypertrophied, and the margins of the cuff may be ill defined but not focally torn. Working with cadavers, Kjellin et al.[85] compared the abnormalities detected in the rotator cuff on an MRI study to histologic findings in the cuff. Areas of the cuff that demonstrated abnormal increased signal intensity on spin-echo proton density–weighted sequences, which did not increase in intensity on T2-weighted sequences, corresponded to areas of eosinophilic, fibrillar, or mucoid degeneration, as well as to areas of fibrosis. Areas of increased signal intensity on a T2-weighted sequence corresponded to areas of severe degeneration and fiber disruption. After analyzing the pathologic changes in the rotator cuff, the authors concluded that these cuff abnormalities detected on the MRI study should be classified as tendinosis or tendinopathy and not tendinitis.

With a partial tear of the rotator cuff, there will be a focal area of fiber disruption on the bursal surface, articular surface, or within the substance of the cuff. With MRI, it is possible to detect partial tears of the cuff surface (Figure 4–17) or intrasubstance cuff tears that do not extend to the surface of the cuff. With a full-thickness cuff tear, there will be complete discontinuity of the cuff fibers. Spin-echo T2-weighted

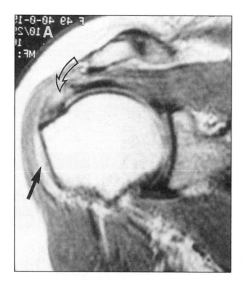 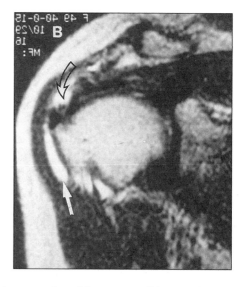

Figure 4–17 Partial tear of the bursal surface of the distal segment of the supraspinatus portion of the rotator cuff in a tennis player. On the proton-density (**A**) and T2-weighted (**B**) oblique sagittal images, there is discontinuity of the superficial fibers of the cuff (*curved arrows*) and fluid in the adjacent subdeltoid bursa (*straight arrows*).

sequences are optimal to diagnose partial- or full-thickness tears by detection of fluid in the cuff defect. In addition to the presence of fluid, Nakagaki et al.[86] detected chondrocyte-like cells in the margin of a torn cuff that may be partially responsible for the high signal intensity identified in a torn cuff. Optimally, to diagnose a full-thickness cuff tear, fluid should be detected extending from the articular to the bursal surface of the cuff, along with fluid present in the adjacent subdeltoid bursa. Unfortunately, this is not always detected with a full-thickness tear, particularly when a tear is chronic and has generated a fibrous reaction in the peritendinous tissue. In these cases, assessment of cuff morphology or detection of cuff retraction may provide the necessary information to reach an accurate diagnosis. With a complete evaluation of a cuff tear in at least two imaging planes, it is possible to accurately measure the size and location of a tear (Figure 4–18). In some reported series, the size of a cuff tear appears to have prognostic significance as to which patients will be

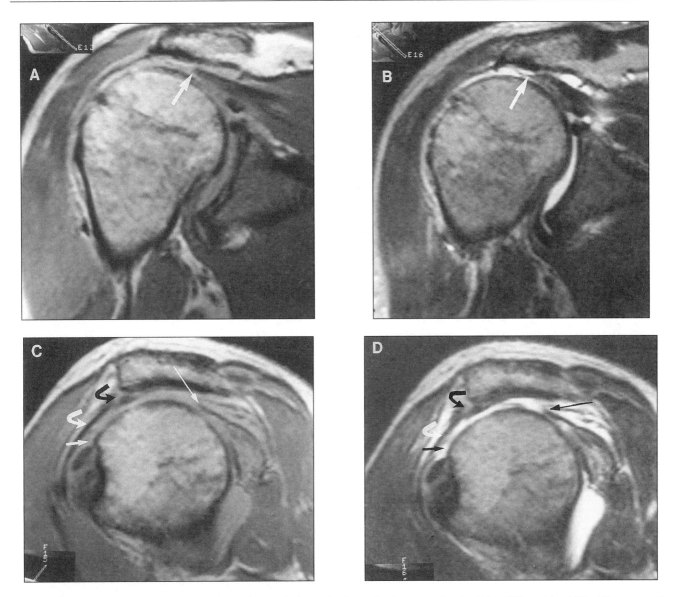

Figure 4–18 Full-thickness tear of the rotator cuff in an elderly tennis player. On the proton-density (**A**) and T2-weighted (**B**) oblique coronal images, there is a full-thickness tear of the rotator cuff. The free margin of the torn cuff is surrounded by fluid, and it is positioned subjacent to the acromion (*arrows*). On the proton-density (**C**) and T2-weighted (**D**) oblique sagittal images, the cuff tear extends from the rotator interval (*short straight arrows*) to the anterior fibers of the infraspinatus segment of the cuff (*long straight arrows*). There is hypertrophy of the CA ligament (*curved white arrow*), along with an enthesophyte projecting off the anteroinferior margin of the acromion at the insertion of the CA ligament (*curved black arrow*).

improved by operative intervention. Full-thickness cuff tears usually first involve the supraspinatus segment of the cuff, posterior to the rotator interval. Isolated full-thickness tears of the subscapularis segment of a cuff may be difficult to detect clinically, but MRI provides an excellent means to detect these tears (Figure 4–19).[87] With MRI, it is also possible to determine the degree of cuff retraction and whether there is associated atrophy of the rotator cuff musculature. The size of recurrent cuff tears also appears to be related to the degree of a patient's dysfunction.[88] The same MRI evaluation performed preoperatively is employed for the postoperative evaluation of the cuff.

Iannotti et al.[89] reported on the efficacy of MRI of the shoulder in the evaluation of 91 patients who required an operative procedure for shoulder dysfunction and for 15 asymptomatic volunteers. In the detection of a complete cuff tear, MRI was 100% sensitive and 95% specific. Tendinitis was defined arthroscopically as an area of hyperemia on the undersurface of the cuff or as thickening of the subacromial bursa. Degeneration or partial tear of the cuff was defined arthroscopically as fraying or fibrillation of the cuff. For the differentiation between cuff tendinitis and degeneration, the sensitivity of MRI was 82%, and the specificity was 85%. In differentiating a normal tendon from one showing signs of impingement, the sensitivity of MRI was 93% and specificity 87%. The authors concluded that high-resolution MRI is an excellent noninvasive tool in the diagnosis of disorders of the rotator cuff mechanism. Both the performance and interpretation of the MRI exams in this study were provided by musculoskeletal radiologists having extensive experience with MRI. There have been several other reports on the high accuracy of MRI in detecting full-thickness cuff tears.[90–93]

The sensitivity of MRI in detecting partial cuff tears is considerably lower than its detection rate for full-thickness tears. In two studies that compared MRI to the findings at arthroscopy, Traughber and Goodwin[91] reported that 4 of 9 partial tears were not detected on an MRI study, and Hodler et al.[90] reported that only 1 of 13 partial tears was detected on an MRI study. They also performed MR arthrography on these patients, and 6 of the partial tears were detected. Both Palmer et al.[94] and Karzel and Snyder[95] have recently reported on the improved detection rate of MR arthrography, compared with standard MRI, to detect partial- and full-thickness rotator cuff tears. Because MR arthrography is a more invasive, costly, and time-consuming examination, compared with a standard MRI study, its efficacy will have to be proved in well-designed prospective studies before it can be recommended.

With the direct multiplanar capabilities of MRI, it is possible to evaluate the condition of any tendon in the body. Yacoe et al.[96] reported on the application of MRI for preoperative assessment of the degree of cellularity in the lesions of patients with Dupuytren's contracture. Magnetic resonance imaging may also be employed to evaluate the position of tendons that may elicit symptoms due to subluxation or dislocation, e.g., the peroneal tendons or the long head of the biceps.[97–98] For patients with peroneal tendon dysfunc-

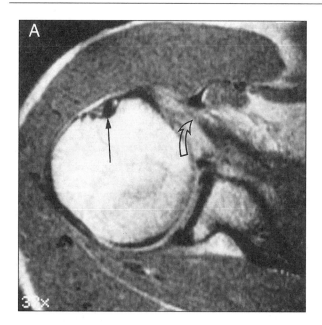 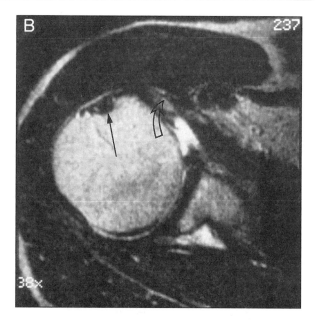

Figure 4–19 Isolated full-thickness tear of the subscapularis segment of the rotator cuff secondary to a ski injury. On the proton-density (**A**) and T2-weighted (**B**) oblique sagittal images, there is a full-thickness tear of the subscapularis tendon (*curved arrows*) but no dislocation of the biceps tendon (*straight arrows*).

tion, it is important to assess the morphology of the posterior surface of the distal fibula. In cases of medial dislocation of the tendon of the long head of the biceps, the integrity of the subscapularis tendon must be determined.

LIGAMENTS

Ligaments are collagenous fibrous structures that act as passive soft-tissue restraints, and their function depends on their morphology and location. Injuries to ligaments are one of the most common injuries incurred in sporting activities. The diagnosis of a ligamentous injury depends on an accurate history and physical exam, sometimes supported by objective tests, e.g., a K-T 1000 exam of the knee. Prior to the implementation of MRI, radiologic imaging studies to detect ligamentous injury focused on plain films to detect evidence of bony avulsion at a ligament's insertion site, stress radiographs to detect abnormal joint alignment[99] or motion, and arthrography[100] to detect evidence of ligament or capsular incompetence. The plain film findings are insensitive to most ligamentous injuries, and positive findings do not elucidate the age of an abnormality. The criteria for normal versus abnormal stress radiography continue to be controversial. The results of stress films are highly dependent on the type of restraint used on the joint when applying stress and the mechanism by which the force is applied. Both tenography and arthrography have also been used to assess ligament integrity, but they are invasive procedures that have only a limited application.

With MRI's excellent soft-tissue resolution and direct multiplanar imaging capabilities, it provides a comprehensive evaluation of normal, degenerated, or torn ligamentous structures. A normal ligament appears on an MRI study as a structure with low signal intensity due to its high collagen content. Ligaments that contain some intrafascicular fat, e.g., the anterior cruciate ligament at its tibial insertion site,[101] may demonstrate higher signal intensity compared with a normal ligament, particularly on a spin-echo T1-weighted sequence. Ligaments are frequently surrounded by fat, which facilitates their evaluation on spin-echo sequences. Optimal imaging planes are needed to assess the integrity of ligaments, and these are performed either perpendicular or parallel to the course of ligamentous structures. Due to the oblique orientation of many ligaments, most imaging planes will be oblique with respect to the standard axes of the body. Accurate interpretation of these oblique planes requires a complete understanding of the three-dimensional orientation of the anatomic structures.

Clinically, ligament sprains have been classified as: a grade 1 injury, microscopic fiber disruption of a ligament associated with no instability and little functional loss; a grade 2 injury, a partial macroscopic tear of a ligament associated with mild to moderate instability; and a grade 3 injury,

a complete tear of a ligament associated with loss of function and/or instability of a joint.[102] Detection of ligamentous injury on an MRI study is dependent on abnormal signal intensity and/or morphology of a ligament. With a grade 1 sprain, there will be increased signal intensity within the ligament on spin-echo and STIR sequences secondary to the increased interstitial fluid in the ligament, e.g., edema or hemorrhage. The ligament may be slightly increased in size, and it may have indistinct margins. With a grade 2 sprain, in addition to the abnormal signal intensity within the ligament, there will be a focal partial discontinuity of a ligament that may contain fluid or inflammatory tissue. Periligamentous edema is usually present secondary to an inflammatory response elicited by a ligament injury. With a grade 3 sprain, complete discontinuity or detachment of a ligament is present, frequently associated with maceration or displacement of the torn ligamentous tissue. Spin-echo T2-weighted sequences are optimal to demonstrate a grade 3 ligamentous sprain.

The most common ligamentous sprain involves the lateral ligamentous complex of the ankle, i.e., the anterior and posterior talofibular ligaments and the calcaneofibular ligament. Plain films are frequently obtained after an acute ankle sprain to evaluate the integrity of the ankle mortise and to detect the presence of a possible avulsion injury. Stress radiography can also be performed to assess the integrity of the ligaments if the physical exam is inconclusive and if this information is needed to guide therapy. The accuracy of MRI in the detection of ankle ligamentous tears has been reported in several studies.[103–106] The use of thin sections and three-dimensional imaging techniques seems to improve the accuracy of an MRI exam. Prior to obtaining an MRI study to assess the ankle ligaments, it is important to determine how the results of an MRI exam will affect clinical care. The information provided by an MRI study may be useful for preoperative planning, but it provides no indication of the degree of joint instability as it is not a functional examination.

Plain film evaluation is also used to detect evidence for injury of the anterior cruciate ligament (ACL). Positive findings include the detection of bony avulsions or osseous impactions. Overall, plain films are extremely insensitive to detecting ACL injuries. The plain film findings, which have a high specificity for ACL tears, e.g., a Segond fracture or gross malalignment of the knee joint, are rarely present with most ACL injuries. Stress radiography[107] may have a role in the assessment of ACL ligamentous dysfunction, but it provides no information on the presence of concomitant knee injuries that may be associated with an ACL tear.

The initial application of MRI in the assessment of ligamentous dysfunction focused on the evaluation of the ACL. In the last few years, there have been many reports documenting the high accuracy of MRI to detect complete tears of the ACL.[108–113] With MRI, it is possible to determine the precise location of an ACL tear, e.g., proximal, midsubstance, or distal (Figure 4–20). Whereas several studies have reported on the value of secondary signs detected in knees with a torn ACL,[114–117] the diagnosis of an ACL tear should be primarily based on the appearance of an ACL on the MRI study.[118] Improvement in the detection of ACL tears is accomplished by imaging the knee in three orthogonal planes.[119] In addition to detecting a torn ACL, it is equally important to determine whether there are any concomitant injuries to the meniscus, cartilage, bone, or other ligaments of the knee, which may affect knee stability. This information is needed when trying to prognosticate the long-term outcome of patients with an ACL injury.[120,121] Oberlander et al.[122] reported a prospective study that assessed the accuracy of the clinical examination of the knee. The diagnostic accu-

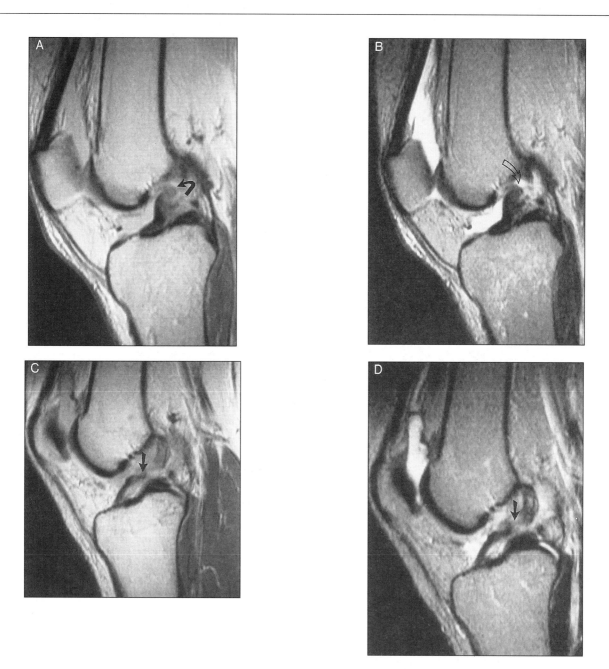

Figure 4–20 Complete tear of the ACL in skiers. On the proton-density (**A**) and T2-weighted (**B**) sagittal images, discontinuity of the proximal segment of the ACL is delineated (*arrow*). There is mild buckling of the distal segment of the ligament. In another skier, on the proton-density (**C**) and T2-weighted (**D**) sagittal images, there is discontinuity of the central third of the ACL (*arrow*).

racy of the clinical exam for intra-articular knee injuries was determined by comparison to arthroscopic findings. An overall correct diagnosis for the clinical exam was present in 56% of the cases, an incomplete diagnosis in 31%, and an incorrect diagnosis in 13%. When a single lesion was present, diagnostic accuracy was 72%, but when more than two abnormalities were present, the accuracy of the clinical exam fell to 30%. Lesions most difficult to diagnose were cartilage fractures, tears of the ACL, and loose bodies. The strength of an MRI exam in the evaluation of an acute or chronically symptomatic knee is its ability not only to assess the integrity of one structure in the knee, e.g., the ACL, but to provide a comprehensive evaluation of the entire knee. This is particularly important in the clinical situation where pain or locking limits the diagnostic capacity of a physical examination.

Complete evaluation of the other ligaments of the knee, e.g., the posterior cruciate ligament,[123–125] the medial collateral ligament,[20,126] and the lateral collateral ligament[126,127] or ligaments of other joints[128] can be achieved with an MRI exam. The same diagnostic criteria applied to ACL tears are applied in the assessment of these ligaments (Figure 4–21). Clinical evaluation of the posterolateral corner of the knee may be difficult,[129] and with MRI, it is possible to detect soft tissue or osseous injuries to this region which may help explain a patient's symptomatology and dysfunction.[130] These include a strain or contusion of the popliteal MTU, an injury and possible avulsion of the biceps femoris MTU, or an im-

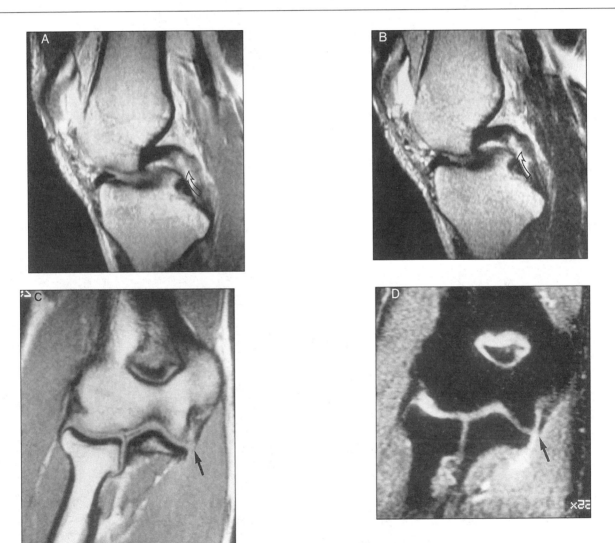

Figure 4–21 Ligamentous injuries in athletes. After a football injury, on the proton-density (**A**) and T2-weighted (**B**) sagittal images, there is a high-grade partial tear of the anterior fibers of the midsegment of the posterior cruciate ligament (*PCL*) (*arrow*). On the T1-weighted (**C**) and STIR (**D**) oblique coronal images, obtained on a baseball player with valgus instability of the elbow, there is a complete tear of the distal fibers of the medial collateral ligament at its ulnar insertion site (*arrow*).

paction injury to the posterosuperior margin of the lateral femoral condyle (Figure 4–22).

In addition to detecting acute ligamentous injuries, it is possible with MRI to assess the degree of ligamentous healing with follow-up studies. I have followed the course of healing of an acute grade 3 medial collateral ligament (MCL) injury in several athletes. On the initial study, diffuse maceration of the ligament was frequently detected and not a focal avulsion of the ligament at its bony insertion site. On the MRI study, the ligament demonstrated diffuse increased signal intensity on the spin-echo and STIR sequences. There was no evidence of normal ligamentous fibers spanning from the femur to the tibia. In addition, prominent thickening of the ligament secondary to the fiber disruption and concomitant edema and hemorrhage was present. On the follow-up MRI studies, the ligament became well defined, thickened, and demonstrated decreased signal intensity compatible with collagenous repair (Figure 4–23). The macerated ligament initially identified probably provides a scaffold for the ingrowth of fibroblastic tissue. The MRI exam provides direct information documenting the structural restoration of a ligament but cannot determine its functional integrity. In the process of healing, a medial collateral ligament is composed of a greater percentage of type III collagen and is weaker than a normal ligament composed of type I collagen. Currently, it is not known whether the MR signal characteristics of type I collagen are different from those of type III collagen. It is interesting that frequently a ligament will appear thickened on an MRI study during its early healing. The increased width of a healing ligament is an important factor in determining its strength.[131] With the final remodeling of the ligament, its signal intensity has a normal appearance, and the ligament is frequently slightly thickened. It is also possible to follow the healing patterns of the posterior and anterior cruciate ligaments. I have identified the healing of partial but not complete tears of both of these ligaments (Figure 4–24). On a follow-up MRI study of patients with posterior cruciate ligament (PCL) injury, the ligament frequently appears normal, but with the few partial ACL tears that have been followed by the author, the ligament has appeared attenuated or lax on follow-up MRI exams.

Magnetic resonance imaging has also been applied in the evaluation of ACL reconstructive surgery. The MRI appearance of both a neoligament composed of gracilis and semitendinosus tendons[132,133] and the patellar tendon[8] have been reported. The neoligaments typically demonstrate increased signal intensity in the first few months after surgery, reflecting the increased hydration and vascularity of the structure. On follow-up MRI studies, there may be a varied appearance of the morphology and the signal intensity of the ligament.

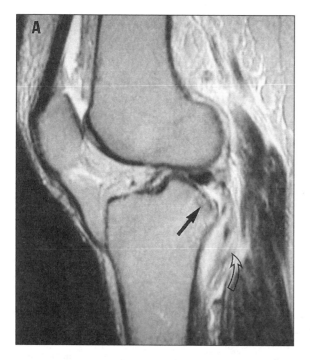
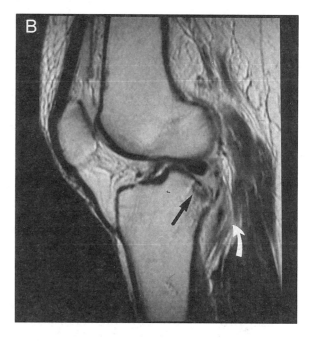

Figure 4–22 Impaction injury of the posterosuperior segment of the tibia in a skier who also sustained a complete ACL tear. On the proton-density (**A**) and T2-weighted (**B**) sagittal images, there is an impaction injury of the posterosuperior segment of the tibia (*straight arrows*). In addition, there are diffuse edematous changes in the popliteus muscle (*curved arrows*).

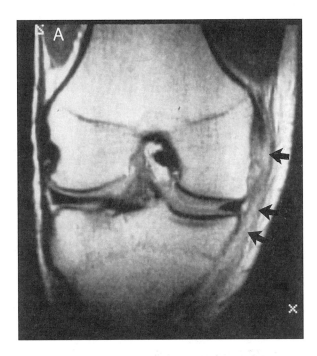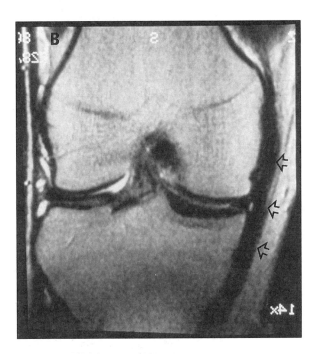

Figure 4–23 Healing of the medial collateral ligament (MCL) after a football injury. After an acute injury, on the proton density–weighted coronal image (**A**), there is diffuse maceration of the MCL (*arrows*). On a follow-up MRI (**B**) obtained approximately 8 months after injury, there is a completely healed, hypertrophied MCL (*arrows*) on the T2-weighted coronal image.

Yamato and Yamagishi[134] reported on the assessment of 15 patients with a clinically stable bone-patellar tendon-bone autograft from three months to three years and three months after reconstructive surgery. In only two patients did the entire ligament appear as a band of low signal intensity. Segmental areas of increased signal intensity were identified on ten studies and nonvisualization of the ligament on three studies. There were no changes in the appearance of the autograft in the patients who had a second MRI study within the first postoperative year. Rak et al.[135] reported on the MRI evaluation of 37 patients with ACL reconstructions using bone-patellar tendon-bone autografts. On 43 of 47 MR examinations, they identified a well-defined ligament with low signal intensity. The correlation between the clinical exam and the MRI was 92% and between the MRI and a second-look arthroscopy was 100%. Howell et al.[136,137] reported on the application of MRI to assist in ACL graft placement and to detect evidence of graft impingement prior to failure. Coupens et al.[138] reported on the follow-up MRI evaluation of the native patellar tendon after it had been used to supply the autograft for ACL reconstruction. They evaluated 20 patients up to 18 months after harvesting the bone-patellar tendon-bone autograft. By 18 months, the signal intensity in the residual patellar tendon appeared normal, but there was a significant increase in the thickness of the tendon on all follow-up studies.

CARTILAGE

Damage to articular cartilage due to an acute traumatic injury or to chronic microtrauma may be an important component in the pathoetiology of joint dysfunction. Prior to the development of MRI, the radiologic detection of cartilage abnormalities on plain films was based on indirect evidence of cartilage damage, e.g., joint space narrowing or secondary osseous degenerative changes. Cartilaginous injury or degeneration can be directly evaluated with arthrography or CT-arthrography. The sensitivity of arthrography is limited, due to the difficulty in evaluating the curved articular surfaces that are present in most joints. The tomographic capability of CT-arthrography improves the detection of cartilaginous lesions[139] but, like standard arthrography, it has limited application and is a relatively invasive procedure.

With the excellent soft-tissue resolution provided by MRI, it was initially hoped that it would be the ideal study for the assessment of cartilage disorders. In addition to excellent contrast resolution, a high degree of spatial resolution is needed to detect cartilage abnormalities, considering that most articular cartilage ranges in thickness from 2 to 3 mm. Because the thickness of the patellar articular cartilage is approximately 5 mm, the initial effort to optimize MRI sequences for the evaluation of articular cartilage has fo-

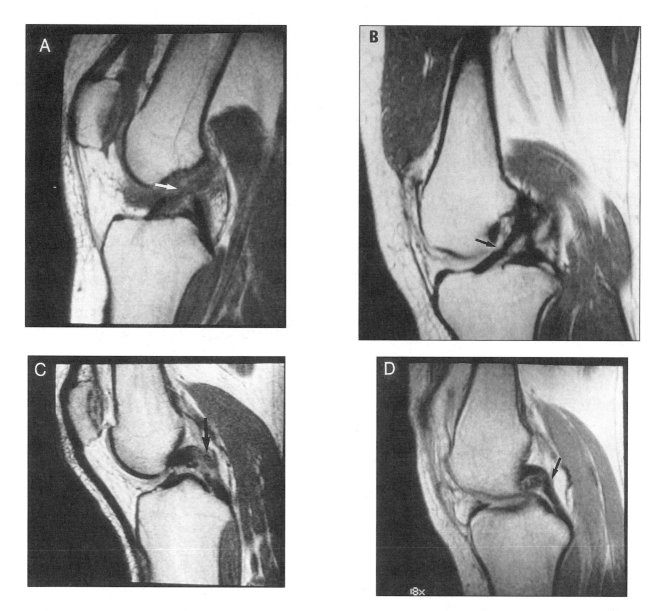

Figure 4–24 Healing of ACL and PCL partial tears. In a skier, on the proton density–weighted sagittal image (**A**), there is a high-grade partial tear of the ACL (*arrow*), which was present at arthroscopy. On a follow-up MRI obtained one year after injury, on the T1-weighted sagittal image (**B**), there is a slightly bowed, completely healed ACL (*arrow*). After a football injury, on the proton density–weighted sagittal image (**C**), there is a high-grade partial tear of the PCL (*arrow*), which appeared normal on a follow-up MRI (**D**) obtained at one year postinjury.

cused on the assessment of normal and abnormal patellar cartilage.

Disorders of patellar articular cartilage are considered a potential source of pain in many patients presenting with knee dysfunction, e.g., young athletes with parapatellar pain syndrome. Therefore, it was hoped that an accurate, noninvasive test to detect these abnormalities would have a significant impact on patient care. Most of the initial investigative work on the efficacy of MRI in the evaluation of patellar

articular cartilage was performed on cadavers. Whereas the results of this work are not necessarily applicable to patients, they at least provide a means to determine the capacity of different imaging sequences to detect cartilage defects or degeneration.[140–143] Hayes et al.[144] evaluated the patellar articular cartilage in 14 cadaveric knees and found that MRI was accurate in detecting moderate and advanced patellar cartilage lesions. Technical factors are extremely important to optimize imaging of articular cartilage.[12] The awareness of chemical shift artifacts is essential for accurate interpretation of cartilage morphology.[145] To compare different imaging protocols, it is necessary to a have a standard objective classification scheme for cartilage abnormalities. Staging of cartilage lesions with the classification system proposed by Shahriaree (grade 0, normal; grade 1, softening; grade 2, blisterlike swelling; grade 3, ulceration or fibrillation not extending to bone; and grade 4, ulceration with exposure of subchondral bone) has been employed in clinical studies.[146] In addition to determining the depth of cartilage lesions, it is also important to determine the size of the abnormality, e.g., less than or greater than 1 cm. With the use of special coils, small fields of view, very thin sections, and special imaging sequences, it is possible with MRI to detect small defects in the articular cartilage in cadaveric specimens. It has become apparent in most studies of articular cartilage that some type of fluid (e.g., a joint effusion, intra-articular saline, or an MRI contrast agent) is needed to accurately assess the appearance of the articular cartilage (Figure 4–25).[147]

Hodler et al.[148] reported on the value of different routine MRI sequences in the detection of focal changes in the articular cartilage of the tibiofemoral joint. Three-millimeter coronal and sagittal anatomic sections were imaged with different pulse sequences, and the MRI studies were compared to the anatomic specimens. Eighty-two defects with a mean diameter of 9.3 mm and a depth of less than 1 mm in 33 cases and greater than 1 mm in 49 cases were evaluated by MRI in a nonblinded fashion. Seventy-two percent of the lesions were detected with a spin-echo T1-weighted sequence, 68% on a T2-weighted sequence, and 66% on a gradient-echo sequence. Twenty-six of the detected lesions had a depth of less than 1 mm and a diameter of 2–20 mm, and 42 of the lesions had a depth greater than 1 mm and a diameter between 1 and 20 mm. Fourteen defects were not detected on the MRI images, even when directly compared to the anatomic sections. Seven of these defects had a depth of less than 1 mm and a diameter between 1 and 15 mm, and the other seven had a depth of greater than 1 mm and a diameter between 1 and 8 mm. In a blinded evaluation of normal and pathologic changes of articular cartilage as part of the same study, there was a sensitivity of 71%, a specificity of 69%, and an accuracy of 70% with MRI in detecting pathologic changes of the cartilage. The authors concluded from this study that the MRI sequences that are routinely used in the analysis of patients with knee dysfunction are limited. Most of the cadaveric studies that report an excellent detection rate in assessment of articular cartilage do not employ the MRI sequences that are currently used for routine knee imaging.

The clinical efficacy of MRI in the detection of chondromalacia of the patella was reported by Conway et al.,[149] who conducted a prospective evaluation of 30 patients with anterior knee pain eventually requiring arthroscopy. Only spin-echo T1-weighted axial and sagittal sequences were used to detect cartilage abnormalities. The authors concluded that MRI was relatively sensitive and had a high predictive value in the detection of grades 3 and 4 chondromalacia lesions, even though no statistical analysis of the data was reported. There was also no discussion concerning the preoperative evaluation of these patients or the criteria employed to determine the indications for arthroscopy. McCauley et al.[146] evaluated the appearance of the articular cartilage of the patella in 52 patients who underwent knee arthroscopy after MRI examination. Twenty-nine of these patients had findings of chondromalacia at arthroscopy, and the remaining 23 patients had normal patellar articular cartilage. The MRI studies were reviewed retrospectively by two radiologists without knowledge of the arthroscopic findings. An MR diagnosis based on focal signal or contour abnormalities detected on an axial spin-echo proton density or T2-weighted sequence had a sensitivity of 86%, a specificity of 74%, and an accuracy of 81%. The sensitivity, specificity, and accuracy to detect chondromalacia was higher in the patients without joint fluid compared to patients with effusions. This finding is at odds with other clinical studies,[147] but the imaging techniques used in the different studies are dissimilar. In the McCauley study, the arthroscopists had knowledge of the MRI reports prior to arthroscopy, which potentially could bias the results. One limitation of the study was the use of 5-mm thick axial sections and a 2.5-mm interslice gap. The authors concluded that thinner sections may improve the accuracy to detect chondromalacia, but this will have to be proven with a prospective blinded study.

Radionuclide imaging has also been used to evaluate the patellofemoral joint in young athletes with knee pain. Dye and Boll[150] studied 167 symptomatic knees with technetium bone scans, and 49% of these knees were determined to have a qualitatively positive bone scan. This was determined by comparing the scans of the symptomatic knees to control scans of asymptomatic knees. At the follow-up evaluation performed at 18 months, 89% of the knees with continued patellar pain had a positive scan, including 10 knees which initially had a negative scan. Arthroscopy or open procedures were performed on 15 patients in this study. Forty-two percent with positive scans had normal patellar cartilage, and 58% had either grade 2 or grade 3 chondromalacia. In this study, it is difficult to determine the precise etiology of a positive bone scan or its efficacy in the evaluation of patellofemoral pain, as there was no independent gold standard used to determine whether these patients had patellofemoral disease. A surgical procedure was performed in only a minority of the cases, and it is uncertain from the study's methodology whether the surgeon was blinded to the findings on the bone scans at the time of surgery.

Speer et al.[147] reported on the value of MRI in the assessment of traumatic articular cartilage injuries. Forty-nine articular cartilage lesions were documented by arthroscopy in

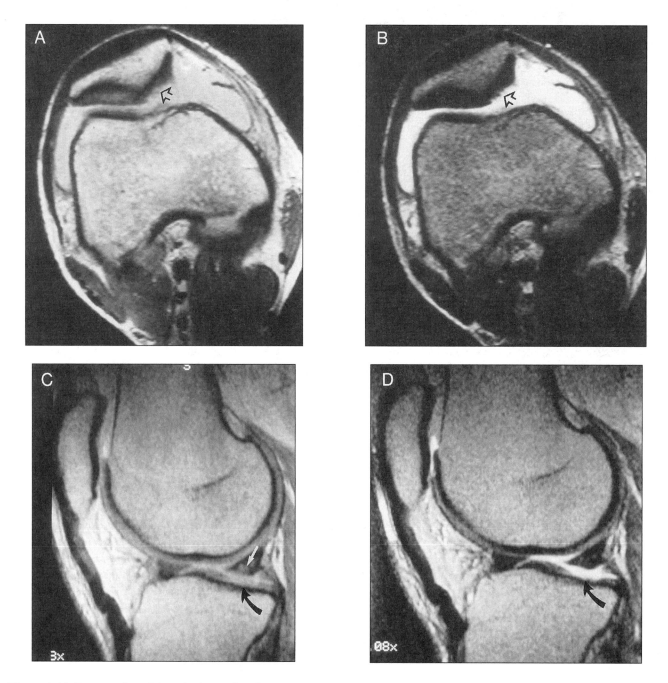

Figure 4–25 Degeneration of the articular cartilage in two runners. On the proton-density (**A**) and T2-weighted (**B**) axial images, there is fibrillation of the articular cartilage (*arrows*) of the medial facet of the patella, best delineated on the T2-weighted image. In another runner, on proton-density (**C**) and T2-weighted (**D**) sagittal images, there is focal denudation of the articular cartilage of the lateral tibial plateau (*curved arrows*), which is detected only on the T2-weighted sequence as a result of the high signal intensity in the joint fluid.

28 knees. The MRI was performed within 4 weeks prior to the arthroscopic procedure. The MRI studies were interpreted twice—once prior to arthroscopy and once after arthroscopy, with the knowledge of the arthroscopic findings. For full-thickness articular cartilage lesions, the pre-

arthroscopic sensitivity of MRI to detect these abnormalities was 41%, and the postarthroscopic sensitivity was 83%. For partial-thickness cartilage lesions, the prearthroscopic sensitivity was 15%, and postarthroscopic sensitivity was 55%. The presence of fluid in the joint facilitated the detection of chondral abnormalities. All lesions were stellate or crater-shaped, and no flap tears were included in the study. Only the full-thickness chondral lesions were associated with bone marrow edema, but no STIR or fat-suppressed T2-weighted sequences were performed. A review of the preoperative clinical charts demonstrated that in 36% of the cases, there was a clinical suspicion of articular cartilage injury. With a high index of suspicion by the radiologist for a chondral injury, the prearthroscopic sensitivity increased to 69%. The authors concluded that the pre- and postarthroscopic sensitivity of MRI was low and that it cannot reliably exclude the presence of an articular cartilage injury. It is of interest that on retrospective analysis, the sensitivity of MRI was 83%, which was much higher than the sensitivity of the clinical evaluation. Few diagnostic tests have a sensitivity of 100% while maintaining an acceptable level of specificity. It is still possible that MRI may provide useful information in the initial clinical assessment of patients with knee pain, particularly if the decision to perform arthroscopy is uncertain. The study did illustrate the importance of experience in detecting cartilage abnormalities with MRI.

Since implementing STIR or fat-suppressed T2-weighted sequences as part of MRI evaluation of the knee, the author has detected many cases that initially appeared to be pure chondral injuries on the spin-echo sequences, but edema in the subjacent cancellous bone was detected on a fat-suppressed sequence (Figure 4–26). This information may be important in determining the healing potential of these lesions. The presence of edema in the cancellous bone probably reflects increased fluid, e.g., edema or hemorrhage, secondary to microfractures of the cancellous trabeculae. Repair of the subchondral bone may influence the healing potential of the overlying cartilage.

By routinely using spin-echo T2-weighted sequences in three orthogonal imaging planes, the author has been able to detect nondisplaced chondral flap tears (Figure 4–27). The presence of fluid in the knee is necessary to detect most chondral lesions, but almost 100% of acutely traumatized knees will contain an adequate amount of fluid to evaluate the articular cartilage. The same principles apply to the MRI assessment of articular cartilage in any large joint in the body. The detection of small chondral lesions in smaller joints such as the elbow has also been successful, as long as there is adequate fluid within the joint.[151]

In addition to the detection and characterization of chondral disorders, MRI has been applied to the evaluation of osteochondral lesions, e.g., osteochondral fractures and osteochondritis dissecans (OCD). Prior to the application of MRI, evaluation of OCD relied on standard X-rays. Routine radiographs are helpful in detecting relatively large lesions of the bone and calcified or ossified loose bodies. The size of the OCD lesion appears to be of prognostic significance in determining which patients may develop osteoarthritis. Twyman

et al.[152] reported on 22 knees with OCD diagnosed before skeletal maturity; these were followed prospectively for an average of 33.6 years. Thirty-two percent had radiographic evidence of moderate or severe osteoarthritis (OA) at follow-up, and 50% had a good or excellent functional result. Osteoarthritis was more likely to occur with a large OCD defect and one that involved the lateral femoral condyle. The osteoarthritic changes were minor in one third of the cases, and only 13.6% had grade 3 changes. One shortcoming of the study was that only one third of the initial patients were contacted for follow-up evaluation. These findings are quite different from those reported by Linden,[153] who followed 76 knees with OCD for an average of 33 years. In the 23 cases of OCD in children detected prior to epiphyseal closure, there were no complications referable to the OCD lesion at follow-up. In the adults who developed OCD after epiphyseal closure, 75% showed evidence of OA. The group of patients who developed OA had an earlier onset of disease when compared to adults with primary OA. The site of the original OCD lesion influenced the pattern of OA. One major limitation in any study relying on plain film evaluation is the relative insensitivity of plain films to detect early changes of OA or to detect other pathologic disorders of the knee, e.g., a torn meniscus, which may precipitate knee dysfunction.

Joint scintigraphy has also been used in the assessment of patients with OCD. Cahill et al.[154] reported a prospective study using radionuclide imaging to investigate conservative treatment of juvenile OCD of the femoral condyle. Over a 10-year period, 92 knees were evaluated, with an average follow-up of 4.2 years. The average age of the patient at detection of an OCD lesion was 12.5 years, and all patients were participants in athletic or exercise programs. Each patient was scanned and reevaluated every two months. Based on specific indications for failure, 50% failed conservative treatment and required surgery. Parameters of location, sex, and scan classification were not statistically significant predictors of eventual outcome. There was a moderate correlation between lesion size and failure of conservative treatment, with larger lesions having a worse prognosis under conservative care.

Clinical staging and management of patients with OCD depend on the mechanical stability of the OCD fragment. At arthroscopy, a stable lesion is attached to the cancellous bone, and the overlying articular cartilage is intact. An unstable lesion may be detached from the underlying bone but the overlying articular cartilage may be intact, i.e., loose in situ. A partially detached lesion is separated from the parent bone, and there is discontinuity of part of the overlying cartilage. A completely detached fragment is detached from the underlying bone, and there is complete discontinuity of the overlying articular cartilage. A completely detached fragment may or may not be displaced from the parent bone. If

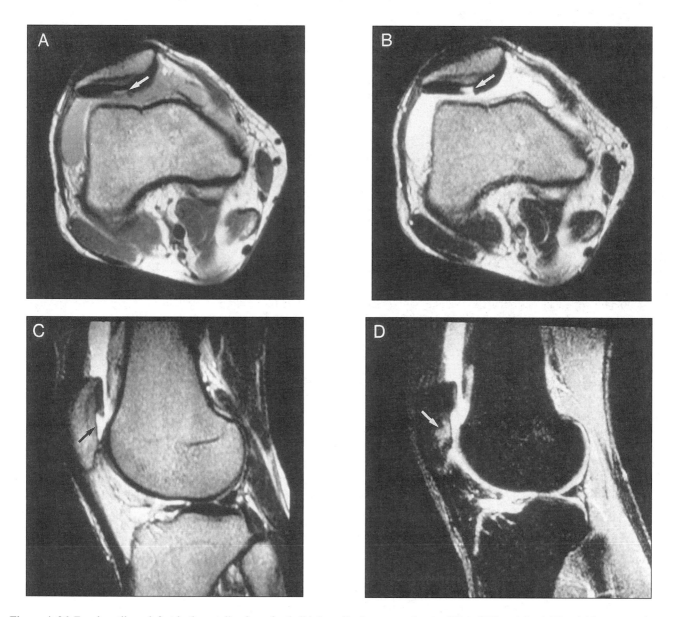

Figure 4–26 Focal cartilage defect in the patella after a football injury. On the proton-density (**A**) and T2-weighted (**B**) axial images, and on the T2-weighted sagittal image (**C**), there is a focal defect in the articular cartilage of the lateral facet of the patella (*arrows*). The defect extends to the subchondral bone plate, which appears normal. Only on the STIR sagittal image (**D**) are the edematous changes in the subjacent cancellous bone appreciated (*arrow*).

early detection of an OCD lesion were possible using a noninvasive test such as MRI, it would provide a means of enhancing our knowledge of the natural history of OCD and, it is hoped, would provide a means to assess the efficacy of different modes of therapy. This cannot be accomplished with plain films because only the ossified component of the lesion can be evaluated.

Mesgarzadeh et al.[155] reported on the evaluation of 21 joints with OCD lesions studied with plain films, MRI, and bone scintigraphy. This was a retrospective study, and all imaging modalities were evaluated without the knowledge of clinical follow-up. Arthroscopy was performed on 13 joints that failed conservative therapy; and loose fragments were detected in 12 of these joints. It was assumed by the authors that the other nine asymptomatic knees were stable because they did not require surgery. On the analysis of the different imaging modalities, the authors reported that the plain film evaluation of the size of the lesions and the amount of surrounding sclerosis was of benefit in predicting a loose fragment. Bone scintigraphy was more sensitive and specific

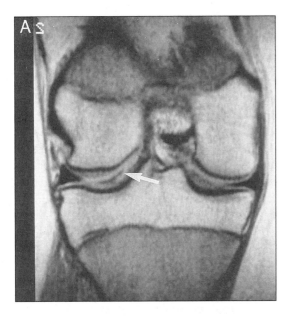 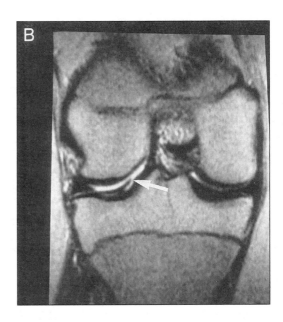

Figure 4–27 Chondral flap tear in a young football player. On the proton-density (**A**) and T2-weighted (**B**) coronal images, there is a flap tear of the articular cartilage of the lateral tibial plateau (*arrows*). It is easier to delineate on the T2-weighted image, due to the high signal intensity of the adjacent joint fluid.

than were plain films for determining the mechanical stability of the OCD fragment. With MRI, the most reliable sign of a loose fragment was the presence of fluid at the interface between the OCD fragment and the parent bone, and this was detected for all loose fragments. Discontinuity of the overlying articular cartilage was diagnosed on MRI for 11 of 12 loose fragments but was detected in only 5 cases at arthroscopy. No discontinuity of the articular cartilage was detected on the MRI studies of the clinically stable cases, but without arthroscopic verification, it is not possible to determine whether there were any false-negative MRI exams. The small number of cases also limited the statistical analysis.

De Smet et al.[156] also reported on the successful application of MRI to detect unstable OCD lesions. A high signal interface between the lesion and the parent bone was considered as evidence for instability, and 14 of 15 lesions with this finding had partially or completely detached OCD fragments at the time of arthroscopy. Patients with a displaced fragment had a large articular defect that was filled with fluid. Similar to the study reported by Mesgarzadeh et al.,[155] this study is limited by its design and small number of patients.

In a recent report by Kramer et al.,[157] 24 cases with OCD were evaluated with MRI prior to arthroscopy. After performing standard spin-echo T1-weighted and gradient-echo sequences, 40 mL of saline and gadolinium-DTPA (Gd-DTPA) were injected intra-articularly, and the same MRI sequences were repeated. A correct diagnosis of the type of OCD present prior to the intra-articular injection of Gd-DTPA was 39.3% for spin-echo T1-weighted sequences and 57.4% for gradient-echo sequences. After the intra-articular injection of Gd-DTPA, the sensitivity of the spin-echo sequence was 92.9%, and the gradient-echo sequence was 100%. One limitation of this study was that a spin-echo T2-weighted sequence was not routinely performed. Prior studies reporting on the efficacy of MRI to evaluate OCD have predominantly relied on T2-weighted sequences to detect the presence of fluid at the OCD–bone interface. While gradient-echo sequences do permit improved spatial resolution, the contrast resolution may be limited, particularly in regions of cancellous bone. Before advocating the application of MR arthrography, which is more invasive and expensive than is a standard MRI exam, its efficacy must be proven in a well-controlled prospective study. Assessment of the efficacy of a standard MRI exam could also be determined as part of this prospective study.

MRI has also been applied to other joints in the body to evaluate OCD lesions.[158,159] De Smet et al.[159] reported on imaging patients with OCD of the talus. In 13 of 14 patients who required surgery, MRI accurately predicted the status of the OCD fragment. The same MRI criteria used in the assessment of OCD in the knee were applied to the talus. The grading system is highly dependent on the results of the spin-echo T2-weighted sequence. Magnetic resonance imaging has also successfully been employed to assess the status of OCD lesions of the elbow. Similar to the evaluation of chondral disorders, the accuracy of predicting the grade of OCD depends on the presence of fluid within the joint.

In addition to the evaluation of hyaline cartilage, one of the initial applications of MRI is in the evaluation of fibrocartilage, e.g., the knee meniscus and the intervertebral disc. The normal knee meniscus is a triangular fibrocartilaginous structure, which generates no signal on an MRI study. Abnormal signal intensity within a meniscus is graded 1, 2, or 3, depending on the shape of the abnormal signal and whether it extends to the articular surface of a meniscus.[27] Grade 1 is a globular focus of increased signal intensity that does not extend to the meniscal articular surface. Grade 2 is a linear focus of increased signal intensity that does not extend to the meniscal articular surface but may extend to the meniscocapsular junction. Grade 3 is any focus of increased abnormal signal intensity that extends to the meniscal articular surface. Several studies have demonstrated the high accuracy of MRI to detect meniscal tears.[108,109,111,125,160,161]

With aging, horizontal meniscal tears are frequently detected in asymptomatic patients,[161] making it more difficult to determine their significance in a symptomatic patient. Flap tears can be a cause of locking of the knee, and on an MRI study, a displaced meniscal fragment may be detected. There have been reports on the evaluation of the meniscus in asymptomatic athletes.[162–164] Reinig et al.[163] reported on asymptomatic football players who demonstrated progression of meniscal degeneration over one season. Shellock et al.[164] evaluated asymptomatic marathon runners and found no increase in meniscal pathology, compared with sedentary persons. Only a limited number of athletes were evaluated in both of these studies. Bodne et al.[165] reported on a prospective blinded investigation of the knee in asymptomatic subjects using MRI. Sixteen percent of the subjects had a meniscal tear. The prevalence of a tear was 13% in subjects under the age of 45 and 36% in subjects over the age of 45.

The diagnosis of a meniscal tear is more difficult in the postoperative knee because of the altered morphology and signal intensity of the meniscus.[166] The study is most valuable if only a small portion of the meniscus has been resected. It is possible to perform an MRI arthrogram with Gd-DPTA to improve the detection rate of postoperative tears, but the MRI study then becomes a relatively invasive and more expensive procedure. In the future, other possible applications of MRI with respect to the meniscus may include kinematic MRI studies to assess meniscal stability and three-dimensional exams to create templates for meniscal implant surgery.

The intervertebral disc is another fibrocartilaginous structure that is prone to degeneration and failure. The chemical composition of the fibrocartilage of the disc is quite different than the meniscus, which accounts for some of the differences in the appearance of the two structures on an MRI study. Whereas the fibrocartilage of the meniscus is composed of type I collagen, the disc is composed of type I collagen in the outer annulus and type II collagen in the inner annulus and nucleus pulposus. The nucleus also contains proteoglycans, which imbibe fluid, resulting in a greater level of hydration of the nucleus, compared with the annulus. The high signal intensity in a disc detected on a spin-echo T2-weighted sequence is located within the nucleus and the inner annular fibers.

For the evaluation of disc degeneration, plain films are of limited value. Decreased disc height, bony sclerosis, gas or calcification within the disc, and end-plate proliferation are associated with disc degeneration, but these findings are of little prognostic value in determining the cause of spinal or radicular pain. Both MRI and CT are excellent studies to detect a disc herniation. The major advantage of MRI is its ability to demonstrate pathoanatomic and chemical changes within the disc prior to disc herniation. It is possible with MRI to detect annular fissures prior to the displacement of nuclear material (Figure 4–28). Magnetic resonance imaging is also the optimal study to follow the natural history of a disc herniation and to determine the degree of disc resorption after it has herniated. There have been several studies that followed patients treated nonoperatively for a disc herniation and documented disc resorption on follow-up MRI or CT exams.[167–170] There have been many excellent papers and texts written about the application of both CT and MRI for the evaluation of discal disorders.[11,171–175] With the increased utilization of MRI, it has become clear that disc herniation and/or degeneration is frequently detected in both symptomatic and asymptomatic individuals; therefore, the significance of these abnormalities can be determined only by precise clinical correlation.

BONE

In the evaluation of acute skeletal trauma, plain films should be the initial radiologic study obtained to detect the presence of an osseous abnormality and to determine the nature and extent of bony disruption. With acute fractures of the skeletal system that involve cortical bone, standard X-rays are usually adequate to assess whether there is an acute cortical injury. Plain films are optimal to determine angulation, rotation, and distraction of the fracture fragments and to evaluate the integrity of the adjacent joints. At least two orthogonal X-ray views, i.e., 90 degrees perpendicular to each other, are required to accurately assess the extent and alignment of a fracture. To optimize the detection of traumatic changes with plain films, it is important that the relevant clinical history is available at the time of plain film interpretation. Berbaum et al.[176] reported on how the knowledge of the location of a patient's symptoms and signs affected the detection rate of fractures. Seven radiologists evaluated a set of 40 radiographs in sessions separated by 4

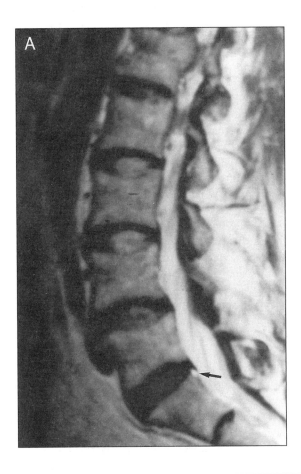

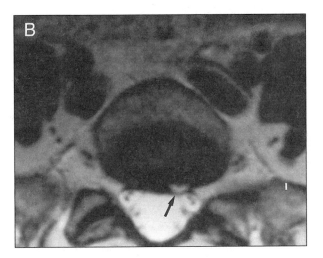

Figure 4–28 Annular fissure in a recreational tennis player experiencing low back pain. On the T2-weighted sagittal (**A**) and axial (**B**) images, there is a small focus of high signal intensity in the outer annular fibers of the posterolateral margin of the L5-S1 disc (*arrows*), which probably represents an annular fissure. There is no posterior protrusion of the disc. Mild to moderate decreased signal intensity of the disc is also present.

months. In half of the cases at each session, the precise location of the patient's symptoms was provided. Analysis of receiver operator characteristic parameters indicated that the clinical information improved the detection rate of fractures. The improvement was based on an improved true-positive rate without an increased false-positive rate.

Several classification systems to describe fractures have been developed to help explain the mechanism of injury and to determine the appropriate form of surgical or nonsurgical care.[177] With simple fractures it is easy to classify a fracture type, e.g., transverse, horizontal, oblique, or impacted, but with more complex fractures, classification becomes more difficult. Few classification systems that are currently utilized to assess fractures have been critically studied to determine intraobserver and interobserver variability utilizing the classification system.[1] Sidor et al.[3] recently reported on the application of the Neer classification system to assess proximal humeral fractures. Fifty fractures of the proximal humerus were evaluated by an orthopedic shoulder specialist, an orthopaedic traumatologist, a skeletal radiologist, and two orthopaedic residents. The X-ray studies included a scapular anteroposterior and lateral view, and an axillary view. These were reviewed by each physician twice, with a six-month in-

terval between interpretations. All five observers agreed on the final classification for 32% of the fractures in the first interpretation and on 30% of the fractures in the second interpretation. Paired comparisons between the five observers, i.e., interobserver variation, showed a mean reliability of approximately 0.5. The mean reproducibility, i.e., intraobserver variability, was 0.66 and ranged from 0.83 for the shoulder specialist to 0.5 for the skeletal radiologist. The purpose of a classification system should be to provide objective information that can be reliably used by the same physician and communicated between physicians. It is obvious that this goal was not achieved with the application of the Neer classification in this series, nor in a similar study reported by Siebenrock et al.[178] Neither study determined the accuracy of the Neer classification by comparing the plain film interpretations to a gold standard, e.g., multiplanar CT.

With complex fractures, plain films are frequently not adequate to determine the nature and extent of the osseous injury. In these cases, CT is the ideal study to perform, after the initial plain film evaluation. With CT, it is possible to determine the precise number and relationship of the different fracture fragments. It also is excellent in determining whether a fracture extends into contiguous joints, information that is critically needed in presurgical planning (Figure 4–29). Several studies have reported on the value of CT in the assessment of shoulder,[179] pelvis, tibial,[180] and calcaneal fractures.

Plain films are also the standard examination to follow fracture healing by detecting the presence and extent of callus formation.[181] Early detection of a delayed union or nonunion is limited with plain films. If there is a clinical concern about the degree of healing, plain films or CT can be performed to determine the extent of fracture healing. Smith et al.[182] reported on the prediction of fracture healing of the tibia by quantitative radionuclide imaging. The test had a sensitivity of 70% and a specificity of 90%. In cases where internal fixation had been applied, the assessment of fracture healing was more difficult, as well as the detection of a nonunion.

Chronic osseous microtrauma may result in fractures of the cortical or cancellous bone if cumulative load exceeds the cell-matrix adaptive capacities. This may occur at the insertion site of tendons into bone, e.g., apophyseal traction injuries,[183] or at sites of mechanical overload related to increased physical activity,[184] e.g., march fractures. Chronic stress fractures are referred to as *fatigue fractures* if they result from excessive load applied to normal bone; or *insufficiency fractures* if they result from the application of physiologic stress to weakened bone.[185,186] Bone normally responds to new functional demands by remodeling, but if the rate of tissue disruption exceeds tissue repair, failure may result. Because the pathologic process involves both bone resorption and healing, the stress fractures that develop will initially have indistinct margins and are difficult to detect with plain films. If a stress fracture involves the cortical bone, periosteal new bone formation may be detected at the fracture site. If the fracture involves the cancellous bone, subtle areas of linear sclerosis may be detected in regions of trabecular compaction or callus formation. It usually takes 5–6 weeks for an X-ray to become positive after the onset of symptoms, and even then, the findings on plain films may be extremely subtle. If the findings on plain films are indeterminate, additional studies, e.g., CT or bone scintigraphy, may be needed to evaluate the bony changes.[187] Computed tomography has proven useful in the assessment of stress fractures of the tarsal navicular[188] and of the pars interarticularis of the spine (Figure 4–30). Computed tomography has also been employed to differentiate between stress fractures and bone tumors, e.g., osteoid osteomas.

As a result of the active bone remodeling at the site of a stress fracture, a bone scan will usually be positive soon after the onset of symptoms, particularly in a young patient. A positive bone scan will occur with any process that increases bone metabolism; therefore, its specificity is limited. In addition, there is limited spatial resolution with a bone scan, and it may be difficult to precisely localize the position of the abnormality and to determine whether adjacent soft tissues or joints are involved by a pathologic process. There also have been case reports of negative bone scans in patients with stress fractures.[189,190]

Magnetic resonance imaging is also extremely sensitive in detecting stress fractures or in any pathologic process that replaces the normal medullary fat in the cancellous bone by edematous tissue or by a cellular infiltrate.[10,191] In both the inflammatory and reparative phases of a fracture, there will be increased fluid and cellular infiltration at the fracture site. These changes will be detected on a spin-echo T1-weighted sequence as a focus of intermediate signal intensity, compared with the high signal of the normal fat and on a T2-weighted or STIR sequence as a focus of high signal intensity. The strength of MRI compared with a bone scan is its excellent spatial resolution, direct multiplanar capabilities, high soft tissue contrast resolution, and the fact that it requires no exposure to ionizing radiation. With an MRI, it is usually possible to precisely localize the position of an abnormality. In cases where other diagnoses are being considered in addition to a stress fracture, e.g., infection or tumor, the utilization of Gd-DTPA can enhance the value of an MRI study. The results of an MRI study are also immediately available after the completion of an exam.

The major drawbacks of MRI compared with bone scans are its higher cost, lower accessibility, and the fact that it is contraindicated for certain patients. One way to curtail MRI costs is to perform only a limited MRI study; this has proven to be extremely valuable in the detection of subtle femoral neck fractures in elderly patients.[192] Deutsch et al.[193] employed a coronal spin-echo T1-weighted sequence in the evaluation of 23 patients in whom there was a high clinical suspicion of fracture and who had normal plain films. A fracture was demonstrated by MRI in 9 of 9 patients who, on follow-up X-rays, had fractures, and the MRI excluded a fracture in 14 of 14 patients without fractures. In the same study, radionuclide scans were positive in 4 of 4 patients with a fracture and equivocal in 1 patient who did not have a fracture. The authors concluded that MRI can provide rapid, cost-effective, and anatomically precise diagnoses of hip fractures in patients with normal or equivocal plain films. Bone scans are also used to detect insufficiency fractures of the femoral neck in older patients,[194] but it may take several days before the scan becomes positive. It also may be difficult with a bone scan to differentiate between a fracture and severe arthritis.

Fractures involving the epiphyseal plate, i.e., growth plate, are usually related to an acute traumatic event but can also result from chronic microtrauma. Plain films are usually adequate to detect epiphyseal plate injuries that also involve the adjacent bone. If a fracture involves only the cartilaginous epiphyseal plate, its acute detection may be difficult. It may take several days before it can be detected on a plain

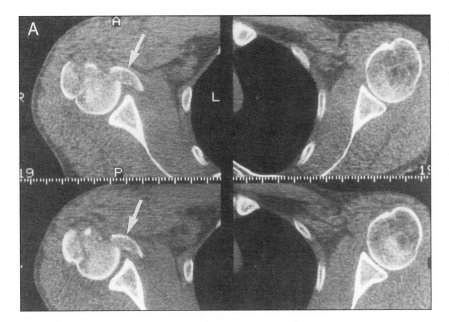

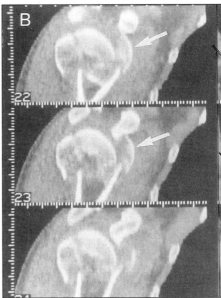

Figure 4–29 Comminuted fracture of the humeral head sustained after a climbing injury. On a multiplanar CT study, on the axial (**A**) and reformatted coronal (**B**) images, there is excellent delineation of the degree of comminution and of the precise location of the fracture fragments. The displaced lesser tuberosity (*arrows*) was difficult to detect on the plain films.

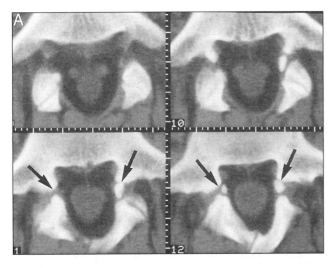

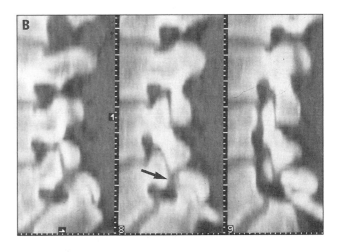

Figure 4–30 Spondylolysis in a young athlete. On a multiplanar CT study, on the axial (**A**) and reformatted sagittal (**B**) images, there is excellent delineation of the defect in the pars interarticularis (*arrows*).

film when the fracture becomes more apparent secondary to osseous resorption or periosteal new bone formation at the fracture site. Magnetic resonance imaging is an excellent modality to evaluate the status of the epiphyseal plate[195] and to detect possible complications of growth plate fractures. Jaramillo et al. [196,197] reported on the appearance of the normal and abnormal growth plate, utilizing MRI. They found that the gradient-echo sequence was optimal to differentiate

between cartilage and bone but suboptimal to spin-echo sequences in evaluating the different zones of the cartilaginous epiphyseal plate. Utilization of MRI was helpful in the evaluation of acute growth plate injuries that had a greater risk of developing future deformity. With vertical injuries to the growth plate, healing will occur by ingrowth of vessels, and deformity may result if a bony bar forms across the plate. This may be difficult to detect with plain X-rays but can be diagnosed with an MRI study. The earlier detection of these abnormalities with MRI will permit earlier resection of a bony bridge. Epiphyseal plate injuries may also occur secondary to chronic overuse injuries. Injury to the proximal humeral epiphyseal plate,[198] olecranon epiphyseal plate,[199] and distal radial epiphyseal plate has been reported in young athletes. The epiphyseal plate injury of the olecranon probably is secondary to traction and shear forces, whereas the injury to the distal radial epiphyseal plate is secondary to chronic compressive overload. Because these are horizontal injuries to the epiphyseal plate, the likelihood of developing a bony bar across the plate is less likely than with an acute traumatic injury. The epiphyseal plate fractures related to chronic microtrauma may lead to disorganization of the plate and to altered patterns of maturation and fusion due to the hyperemia and cartilage injury.

After a direct injury to an extremity, it is fairly common for an individual to experience pain involving an osseous structure but to have a normal plain film. Prior to the application of MRI, the precise etiology of this pain was unclear, and it was uncertain whether it was related to injury of the soft tissue and/or of osseous structures. With the exquisite sensitivity of MRI to detect bone marrow edema, it quickly became apparent that many patients with acute trauma had areas of edematous cancellous bone at the site of an osseous injury.[200–203] The focal areas of bone marrow edema are most likely secondary to trabecular microfractures, i.e., bone contusions or bruises, in the cancellous bone. They may occur secondary to an extrinsic impaction injury or may be secondary to bones impacting against one another as a result of acute instability or malalignment.

One of the first injuries in which bone contusions were frequently detected was in patients with complete tears of the ACL.[204–206] The osseous contusions are typically located in the cancellous bone of the lateral femoral condyle subjacent to the terminal sulcus and in the cancellous bone of the posterosuperior segment of the lateral tibial condyle (Figure 4–31). With complete disruption of the ACL, there may be anterior translation and internal rotation of the tibia with respect to the femur, and if there is an associated valgus force, the posterosuperior segment of the lateral tibial plateau will impact against the lateral femoral condyle.[204] Speer et al.[130] also discussed the possibility of a hyperextension injury, which would impact the anterolateral tibial rim and the lateral meniscus against the femoral condyle, or an injury to the lateral femoral condyle secondary to the reduction and impaction of a displaced tibia against the femoral condyle as potential mechanisms of injury to explain bone contusions.

There are several potential reasons that the detection of these bone contusions is important. Clinically, a patient may have lateral joint line pain, and the possibility of a torn lateral meniscus must be considered as a potential source of this pain. With an MRI exam, it is possible not only to assess the appearance of the meniscus, but also, by demonstrating the presence of a bone contusion, it clarifies the etiology of the pain. The fact that the contusion exists also means that the overlying articular cartilage and/or meniscus also sustained a focal impaction force at the time of the injury (Figure 4–32). Cartilage tears are difficult to detect with MRI, but the presence of a contusion should alert the radiologist to critically evaluate the articular cartilage overlying the region of the contused bone. Vellet et al.[207] reported on a group of 21 patients with acute hemorrhagic knee effusions who underwent MRI study and arthroscopy. Bone contusions adjacent to the subchondral plate were detected with MRI in these patients, but at arthroscopy, the overlying articular cartilage was normal. When these individuals were reevaluated at 6–12 months after the injury with repeat MRI examination, 67% had developed osteochondral abnormalities. It is possible that when these contusions are detected at the time of the initial injury, rehabilitation may be directed to prevent further overload to the articular cartilage. This should be investigated by the appropriate long-term prospective studies.

By the detection of the exact position of bony contusions, it is possible to determine the exact location of the bone subjected to an extrinsic force. This information may help clarify the pathomechanics of different injuries and help to diagnose the precise etiology of knee pain when the history and physical exam is indeterminate. The diagnosis of patel-

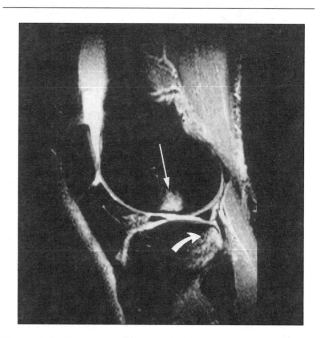

Figure 4–31 Bone contusions associated with a complete ACL tear secondary to a ski injury. On the STIR sagittal image, there are edematous changes in the cancellous bone of the lateral femoral condyle (*straight arrow*) and in the posterosuperior segment of the lateral tibial condyle (*curved arrow*).

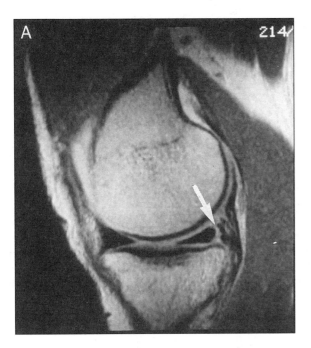 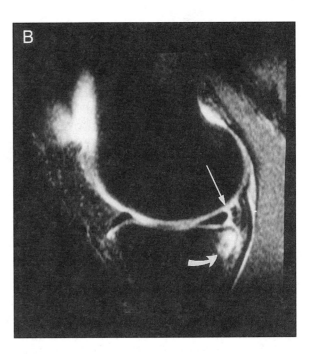

Figure 4–32 Vertical tear of the red zone of the posterior horn of the medial meniscus secondary to a football injury. On the proton density–weighted (**A**) and STIR (**B**) sagittal images, there is a vertical tear in the red zone of the posterior horn of the medial meniscus (*straight arrows*). On the STIR sequence, a focal bone contusion (*curved arrow*) is identified immediately subjacent to the meniscal tear. The detection of a contusion helps to define the direction and location of the applied force.

lar dislocation may be difficult if the patella relocates immediately. A patient may present with parapatellar pain and swelling, and a history of the knee giving out. Magnetic resonance imaging can be particularly helpful in these cases by detecting bone bruises on the anterolateral nonarticular margin of the lateral femoral condyle and in the medial facet of the patella.[208–210] The bony contusions are secondary to impaction of the medial facet of the patella against the lateral femoral condyle when the patella translates medially in the process of relocation. It is also possible to detect injuries of the lateral patellar facet and the lateral facet of the femoral trochlea if they impact against each other as the patella translates laterally. Kirsch et al.[208] reported on the findings of transient lateral patellar dislocation in 26 patients. Partial or complete disruption of the medial patellar retinaculum was detected in 96%, a contusion of the lateral femoral condyle in 81%, osteochondral injuries in 58%, lateral patellar tilt or subluxation in 92%, and a joint effusion in 100%. Patellar dislocation had not been suspected prior to the MRI study in 73% of the patients. Virolainen et al.[209] reported on the application of low field strength MRI in the evaluation of 25 patients with acute lateral patellar dislocation. Twenty-four of these patients also underwent arthroscopy. Bone bruises were detected in 100% of the cases, with a lateral femoral condyle injury in all cases. Osteochondral fragments

detected on plain films and cartilage injury detected at arthroscopy were not identified on the MRI study. This was probably related to the limited spatial resolution of the low-field MR system. In all these studies, the detection of the constellation of abnormalities present with transient lateral patellar dislocation were detected on the axial images. Considering that many of these patients are being imaged for knee dysfunction without the clinical suspicion of transient lateral patellar dislocation, it is mandatory that an axial sequence is part of a standard MRI evaluation for all patients with acute knee dysfunction. From these reports, it appears that the spin-echo[208] and STIR[210] sequences are optimal to detect these abnormalities.

Another important application of MRI in the evaluation of pathologic changes in bone is in the detection of osteonecrosis (ON). STIR and fat-suppressed spin-echo T2-weighted sequences are probably optimal to detect marrow edema. The pathoetiology, e.g., atraumatic or traumatic, and the stage of evolution of ON will determine whether and how it is detected on an MRI study. With an acute traumatic disruption of the vessels supplying the femoral head, which may occur with a displaced femoral neck fracture, it may take up to ten days before there is pathologic evidence of ON[211,212] in the femoral head. Because the femoral head is acutely avascular, cell death will ensue without a secondary inflammatory or reparative response. Atraumatic ON is an evolving process, whether associated with medications, e.g., steroids, or as part of a clinical disorder causing ischemia to the femoral head, e.g., sickle cell or marrow storage diseases. Intermittent ischemia will precipitate microinfarcts with secondary inflammation and repair. The inflammatory and reparative processes are associated with increased fluid in the marrow, which may elevate the marrow pressure due to the constraints of the surrounding bone.[213] It appears that the earliest changes of ON depicted on a routine MRI is the detection of marrow edema, which explains why the study would be negative in detecting ON secondary to acute vascular disruption.[214] The animal studies that have reported early changes on MRI with acute vascular disruption[215,216] may not be applicable to humans because of the differences in the marrow components of the femoral heads in the animal models, compared with humans.[214] It is possible that both dynamic radionuclide and dynamic MRI studies with Gd-DPTA[217] may be able to detect perfusion abnormalities of the femoral head. However, the presence of decreased perfusion does not necessarily mean that ON will develop.

The detection of bone marrow edema on an MRI study is not a specific finding for ON but can be found with other disorders, causing increased marrow hydration, e.g., ischemia,[218] fracture, transient bone marrow edema syndrome,[219,220] infection, or malignancy. Once there is osseous repair and/or replacement of the necrotic trabeculae with new bone, a characteristic "double line" can be detected at the interface between the necrotic and viable bone. On an MRI spin-echo T2-weighted sequence, there will be a zone of high signal intensity secondary to the reparative tissue, surrounded by a zone of low signal intensity representing the repaired thickened trabecular bone. Any area of fibrosis or mineralized tissue will appear on the T2-weighted sequence as a focus of low signal intensity. Contrast-enhanced MRI studies may help differentiate between viable and nonviable marrow at this stage of ON.[221] With progression of ON, fracture and/or collapse of the femoral head can be detected with MRI, but CT is helpful to delineate small areas of cortical disruption or subchondral fractures. The location and extent of the osteonecrotic bone may be of prognostic value in predicting whether the femoral head will collapse[222,223]; therefore, both sagittal and coronal sequences are needed to calculate the extent of ON. Because MRI is noninvasive, it is possible to follow patients who are at high risk for developing ON[224,225] or patients who have undergone core decompression[226,227] to determine the status of their femoral heads. Plain films are insensitive in detecting early ON,[228] and by the time a subchondral fracture or collapse of the femoral head is detected on a plain film, the value of a core decompression may be limited.

In addition to the detection of ON of the hip, MRI is useful in detecting ON of the knee,[229] shoulder, wrist, or ankle.

With the exquisite sensitivity of MRI to detect abnormalities of bone marrow, it was hoped that it could also be applied in assessing patients with reflex sympathetic dystrophy (RSD). Three-phase radionuclide bone scans have a reported 100% sensitivity, 80% specificity, 54% positive predictive value, and 100% negative predictive value for the detection of RSD of the foot.[5] Koch et al.[230] reported on the MRI findings of 17 patients with RSD. Ten of 17 were normal on MRI, 6 of 17 had nonspecific soft tissue changes or bone marrow sclerosis, and 1 of 17 showed changes of abnormal signal intensity. The fact that an MRI is negative with RSD may help elucidate the pathophysiology of RSD. It seems likely that the increased marrow perfusion detected on radionuclide studies may not be associated with concomitant marrow edema. It would be of interest to assess patients at different stages of RSD with both routine MRI and dynamic contrast-enhanced studies to determine whether MRI can provide any useful information in the evaluation or monitoring of patients with RSD.

MUSCULOSKELETAL KINEMATICS

Because symptoms of joint dysfunction are frequently related to a specific motion or position of a joint, diagnostic studies that provide information about a moving structure, e.g., a dynamic electromyogram or fluoroscopy, may help determine the cause of a patient's symptomatology. Abnormal alignment and biomechanics have been implicated in the pathophysiology of patellofemoral dysfunction,[231] shoulder instability and impingement, and ankle and foot disorders. The plain film evaluation of joints to detect evidence for biomechanical dysfunction has focused mainly on measuring various parts of the skeleton and on determining size, shape, position, and angular relationships of different anatomic structures in both symptomatic patients and normal controls. The efficacy of these measurements to differentiate patients with a specific clinical syndrome from the normal patient population can be determined only by a prospective study that includes a gold standard to characterize the disorder under evaluation.

The greatest application of plain film measurements to detect patients with abnormal joint biomechanics has been in the assessment of patients with patellofemoral dysfunction.[232,233] The position and angulation of the patella with respect to the femoral groove can be determined with a variety of radiographic projections, e.g., Merchant, Knutson, and Laurin et al.[234,235] obtained at varying degrees of knee flexion. Patellar height can also be assessed by a variety of measurements, e.g., Insall-Salvati and Blackburne and Peel.[236] Whereas plain film measurements provide some information on osseous morphology and alignment, and appear to have some value in predicting abnormal joint kinematics, they are usually obtained in positions dissimilar from those that precipitate the patient's symptoms of pain or instability. Altered patellar tracking is usually most prominent from 0 to 30 degrees of knee flexion, positions that are difficult to evaluate on standard radiographic views. Equally important is that most plain film studies assess a joint in a static unloaded condition. In addition, standard plain film analysis provides only two-dimensional information.[231] Three-dimensional analysis is possible with plain films, e.g., stereophotogrammetry, but this requires an invasive procedure to implant radio-opaque markers in the anatomic structure being analyzed.

With the application of CT to evaluate the patellofemoral relationship, it is possible to make the same axial measurements as determined on plain films.[237] The major advantage of CT is that these measurements can be performed from full extension to at least 30 degrees of knee flexion, depending on the size of the patient and the size of the CT gantry. In addition, with the cross-sectional evaluation provided by CT, it is possible to identify specific landmarks that facilitate accurate measurements of specific anatomic relationships. Martinez et al.[238] measured the patellar indices on a group of normal patients with their knees positioned at 0, 20, and 45 degrees of knee flexion, with and without quadriceps muscle contraction. In full extension with the quadriceps muscle relaxed, 19 of 20 patients showed the patella centered in the femoral trochlear groove. The tilt and centralization of the patella was unchanged with increased knee flexion with quadriceps muscle contraction. Schutzer et al.[239] reported on the value of CT in the classification of patients with patellofemoral pain and found that dysplasia of the trochlea was most pronounced in patients with a history of patellar dislocation. They studied the knees from full extension to 30 degrees of knee flexion, and 38% of the subluxed patellae were completely reduced by 30 degrees of knee flexion. In an attempt to simulate physiologic conditions of patellofemoral tracking, Stanford et al.[240] evaluated patellofemoral motion with ultrafast CT. The moving knee was imaged from 0 to 90 degrees of flexion. The ultrafast CT views were correlated to Merchant views, and there was a significant correlation in tangent offset, patellar tilt angle, congruence angle, and lateral patellofemoral angles, but no correlation in the measurements of the sulcus angle. The advantage of ultrafast CT over the standard views is that it permits assessment of the dynamic changes with flexing and extending the knee. The major disadvantages with ultrafast CT are the radiation exposure to the patient, the fact that the patient is not erect, and the cost of the study.

The strength of MRI in the assessment of patellofemoral tracking is that, in contrast to CT, it does not require radiation exposure, and the parapatellar soft tissues, along with the patellar and trochlear articular cartilage, can be evaluated with MRI. The evolution of kinematic MRI evaluation of the patellofemoral joint was similar to the evolution with CT. The first studies provided information on the static relationships of the patella to the femur at different degrees of knee flexion.[241] Passive evaluation of the patellofemoral joint involves acquiring a series of axial MR images with a patient's knee passively positioned at different degrees of flexion or extension. A cinematic movie, to simulate knee motion, can be created by combining the series of static axial images. Using this technique, Shellock et al.[242] evaluated both normal subjects and patients with symptomatic patellofemoral disorders. Normal patellofemoral tracking was observed in all asymptomatic patients and in 7% of the symptomatic knees. In 26% of symptomatic knees, there was lateral subluxation of the patella, 41% medial subluxation, 8% excessive lateral pressure syndrome, 7% lateral to medial subluxation, and in 1% a patellar dislocation. In the patients who had undergone prior surgery on the patellofemoral joint, 87% had abnormal patellar tracking. The evaluation of the joint kinematics was based on subjective observations. To test interobserver and intraobserver precision and accuracy, some type of objective criteria will be needed if the effectiveness of kinematic studies is to be determined.

Reports on the value of passive versus active MRI kinematic evaluation of the patellofemoral joint have been reported.[243–245] With active evaluation, the axial MR images are obtained at fixed time intervals while the patient is actively flexing or extending the knee. The patient may be prone or supine during the study, depending on the equipment being utilized for the study. Brossmann et al.[244] reported on motion-triggered cinematic MRI in 13 patients with known patellar maltracking and in 15 controls. In both the patient group and the control group, there were significant differences in the patellofemoral tracking comparing the passive to the active studies. The comparison between the patient group and the control group was statistically different on active but not passive studies. The authors concluded that active MRI evaluation with quadriceps muscle contraction was essential for the diagnosis of patellofemoral tracking disorders. There were several limitations in the methodology of this study. At the time of the interpretation of the different studies, the observers were not blinded as to the status of the patients. There was also no assessment of interobserver or intraobserver variability.

Shellock et al.[245] also reported on passive and active kinematic MR imaging of the patellofemoral joint in 16 symptomatic joints and in 10 controls. The appearance of normal and abnormal patellar tracking was similar with the two techniques. The main advantage of the active study was a shorter examination time and the ability to assess the appearance of the activated muscle. Only subjective impressions of patellar position and tracking were recorded. Shellock et al.[246] have also reported on the development and application of "loaded" kinematic MR imaging of the patellofemoral joint. The technique is similar to an active study but, in addition, the positioning device incorporates a mechanism that has an adjustable resistance applied to the patellofemoral joint in the sagittal plane. The patient is studied in the prone position, and the movement against resistance primarily loads the quadriceps muscle. A force of 30 ft-lb/sec is applied during the active movement. Twenty-three symptomatic joints were studied with both the active loaded and unloaded techniques, and blinded qualitative assessment of patellofemoral tracking was recorded. With the unloaded technique, seven joints were normal, nine had lateral subluxation, three had lateral tilt, and four had medial subluxation. With the loaded technique, one was normal, thirteen had lateral subluxation, four had lateral tilt, and five had medial subluxation. Comparing the initially abnormal appearance of the knees on an unloaded study to their appearance on a loaded study demonstrated that the severity of the tracking abnormality was similar in nine cases and greater with loading in seven cases. Five control subjects were also studied, and they demonstrated normal patellar tracking with both techniques. It is uncertain whether the control studies were interpreted blindly and/or intermixed with the studies performed on the symptomatic knees. The authors concluded that active loaded kinematic MR imaging facilitated the detection of patellofemoral tracking abnormalities.

One of the greatest shortcomings in all of these studies assessing patellofemoral tracking in symptomatic patients is that the precise etiology of the patient's pain is uncertain. There is no proof, e.g., positive arthroscopy or successful surgical correction of patellar malalignment, that the patella or patellar mechanism is the source of the patient's pain. There are also no long-term studies reassessing the patients' symptomatology or function. These studies also have been performed in the recumbent position, which does not simulate the loaded conditions that precipitate a patient's dysfunction. There has been a report by Stein et al.[247] on the fluoroscopic assessment of the patella during walking. This technique has the advantage of examining the patient in an erect position, but it is uncertain from this preliminary study whether the information provided by this study is accurate or reproducible. It also requires radiation exposure to the patient.

Kinematic MR imaging of other joints in the body, e.g., shoulder, elbow, and hip,[248] is also possible. Most of these studies use a positioning device to passively position the extremity and create a cine movie by combining a set of static images. These studies are subject to the same criticisms as already discussed concerning the MRI evaluation of the knee. Until a joint can be evaluated in the same position and performing the same function that precipitates a patient's symptoms, the value of kinematic studies will be limited.

CONCLUSION

Musculoskeletal dysfunction occurs when the capacity of the cell–matrix complex to adapt to biomechanical force is exceeded. Whether this is an acute or chronic process will determine the nature of an injury and the secondary tissue response, e.g., inflammation or degeneration. By understanding the initial mechanism of injury and the spectrum of tissue reaction to structural failure, it is possible to predict the manifestations of a myriad of musculoskeletal disorders on any type of imaging study. Each study, e.g., plain films, CT, MRI, and radionuclide imaging, encodes a different physical property of tissue; therefore, each study should be used in specific clinical situations. Redundant studies must be eliminated if the costs of health care are to be controlled. Prospective controlled studies that compare the various imaging modalities to determine their cost-effectiveness must be performed. It is also possible that certain imaging studies may decrease medical costs by eliminating more expensive diagnostic procedures, e.g., arthroscopy.[249]

An imaging study should be ordered only when the results will directly affect patient management. This implies that the physician has a specific working diagnosis beyond the general categories of "derangement" or "dysfunction." The data from an imaging study can be transformed into useful clinical information only when correlated to the patient's history, physical exam, and any completed diagnostic test. Magnetic resonance imaging has already had a major impact on the diagnosis and treatment of musculoskeletal disorders, but its efficacy could be significantly enhanced with a closer working relationship among the physicians caring for patients with musculoskeletal disorders. With the sharing of knowledge, it will be possible to optimize diagnostic studies to address specific clinical problems, thereby having a greater impact on patient care.

REFERENCES

1. Burstein AH. Fracture classification systems: do they work and are they useful? *J Bone Joint Surgery Am.* 1993;75:1743–1744. Editorial.

2. Scott WW, Lethbridge-Cejku M, Reichle R, Wigley FM, Tobin JD, Hochbert MC. Reliability of grading scales for individual radiographic features of osteoarthritis of the knee: the Baltimore longitudinal study of aging atlas of knee osteoarthritis. *Invest Radiol.* 1993;28:497–501.

3. Sidor ML, Zuckerman JD, Lyon T, Koval K, Cuomo F, Schoenberg N. The Nee classification system for proximal humeral fractures: an as-

sessment of interobserver reliability and intraobserver reproducibility. *J Bone Joint Surg Am.* 1993;75:1745–1750.

4. Wright JG, Feinstein AR. Improving the reliability of orthopaedic measurements. *J Bone Joint Surg Br.* 1992;74:287–291.

5. Holder LE, Cole LA, Myerson MS. Reflex sympathetic dystrophy in the foot: clinical and scintigraphic criteria. *Radiology.* 1992;184: 531–535.

6. Bushong SC. Magnetic resonance imaging: physical and biological principles. St Louis: Mosby, 1988; 382.

7. Crues JV. Technical considerations. In: Mink JH, Reicher MA, Crues JV, Deutsch AL, eds. *Magnetic Resonance Imaging of the Knee.* 2nd ed. New York: Raven Press; 1993:1.

8. Fleckenstein JL, Archer BT, Barker BA, Vaughan JT, Parkey RW, Peshock R. Fast short-tau inversion-recovery MR imaging. *Radiology.* 1991;179:499–504.

9. Mirowitz SA. Fast scanning and fat-suppression MR imaging of musculoskeletal disorders. *AJR.* 1993;161:1147–1157.

10. Mirowitz SA, Apicella P, Reinus WR, Hammerman AM. MR imaging of bone marrow lesions: relative conspicuousness on T1-weighted, fat-suppressed T2-weighted, and STIR images. *AJR.* 1994;162:215–221.

11. Modic MT, Masaryk TJ, Ross JS. *Magnetic Imaging of the Spine.* Chicago: Year Book Medical Publishers, 1989.

12. Yao L, Lee JK. Avulsion of the posteromedial tibial plateau by the semimembranosus tendon: diagnosis with MR imaging. *Radiology.* 1989;172:513–514.

13. Shellock FG. MRI biological effects, safety, and patient management. In: Mink JH, Reicher MA, Crues JV, Deutsch AL, eds. *Magnetic Resonance Imaging of the Knee.* 2nd ed. New York: Raven Press; 1993:25.

14. Kaplan PA, Matamoros A, Anderson JC. Sonography of the musculoskeletal system. *AJR.* 1990;155:237–245.

15. Harcke HT, Grissom LE, Finkelstein MS. Evaluation of the musculoskeletal system with sonography. *AJR.* 1988;150:1253–1261.

16. Aspelin P, Ekberg O, Thorsson O, Wilhelmsson M, Westlin N. Ultrasound examination of soft tissue injury of the lower limb in athletes. *Am J Sports Med.* 1992;20:601–603.

17. O'Keeffe D, Mamtora H. Ultrasound in clinical orthopaedics. *J Bone Joint Surg Br.* 1992;74:488–494.

18. Buckwalter JA, Woo Sly, Goldberg VM, et al. Current concepts review: soft-tissue aging and musculoskeletal function. *J Bone Joint Surg Am.* 1993;75:1533–1548.

19. Ryan JB, Wheeler JH, Hopkinson WJ, Arciero RA, Kolakowski KR. Quadriceps contusions. *Am J Sports Med.* 1991;19:299–304.

20. Deutsch AL, Mink JH. Articular disorders of the knee. *Magn Reson Imaging.* 1989;1(3):43–56.

21. Mink JH. Muscle injuries. In: Mink JH, Reicher MA, Crues JV, Deutsch AL, eds. *Magnetic Resonance Imaging of the Knee.* 2nd ed. New York: Raven Press, 1993:401.

22. Kransdorf MJ, Meis JM, Jelinek JS. Myositis ossificans: MR appearance with radiologic-pathologic correlation. *AJR.* 1991;157:1243–1248.

23. Noonnan TJ, Garrett WF. Injuries at the myotendinous junction. *Clin Sports Med.* 1992;11:738–806.

24. Fleckenstein JL, Weatherall PT, Parkey RW, Payne JA, Peshock RM. Sports-related muscle injuries: evaluation with MR imaging. *Radiology.* 1989;172:793–798.

25. Speer KP, Lohnes J, Garrett WE. Radiographic imaging of muscle strain injury. *Am J Sports Med.* 1993;21:89–96.

26. Nurenberg P, Giddings CJ, Stray-Gundersen J, Fleckenstein JL, Gonyea WJ, Peshock RM. MR imaging-guided muscle biopsy for correlation of increased signal intensity with ultrastructural change and delayed-onset muscle soreness after exercise. *Radiology.* 1992;184:865–869.

27. Shellock FG, Fukunaga T, Mink JH, Edgerton VR. Exertional muscle injury: evaluation of concentric versus eccentric actions with serial MR imaging. *Radiology.* 1991;179:659–664.

28. Shellock FG, Fukunaga T, Mink JH, Edgerton VR. Acute effects of exercise on MR imaging of skeletal muscle: concentric vs eccentric actions. *AJR.* 1991;156:765–768.

29. Greco A, McNamara MT, Escher MB, Trifilio G, Parienti J. Spin-echo and STIR MR imaging of sports-related muscle injuries at 1.5 T. *J Comput Assist Tomogr.* 1991;15: 994–999.

30. Kuno Sy, Katsuta S, Inouye T, Matsumoto K, Akisada M. Relationship between MR relaxation time and muscle fiber composition. *Radiology.* 1988;169:567–568.

31. Polak JF, Jolesz FA, Adams DF. NMR of skeletal muscle differences in relaxation parameters related to extracellular/intracellular fluid spaces. *Invest Radiol.* 1998;23:107–112.

32. Fleckenstein JL, Haller RG, Bertocci LA, Parkey RW, Peshock RM. Glycogenolysis, not perfusion, is the critical mediator of exercise-induced muscle modifications on MR images. *Radiology.* 1992; 183:25–27.

33. de Kerviler E, Leroy-Willig A, Jehenson P, Duboc D, Eymard B, Syrota A. Exercise-induced muscle modifications: study of healthy subjects and patients with metabolic myopathies with MR imaging and P-31 spectroscopy. *Radiology.* 1991;181:259–264.

34. Fleckenstein JL, Watumull D, Bertocci LA, Parkey RW, Peshock RM. Finger-specific flexor recruitment in humans: depiction by exercise-enhanced MRI. *Am Physiol Soc.* 1992;5:1974–1977.

35. Myerson M, Manoli A. Compartment syndromes of the foot after calcaneal fractures. *Clin Orthop.* 1993;290:142–150.

36. DiFazio FA, Barth RA, Frymoyer JW. Acute lumbar paraspinal compartment syndrome. *J Bone Joint Surg Am.* 1991;73:1101–1103.

37. Amendola A, Rorabeck CH, Vellett FD, Vezina W, Rutt B, Nott L. The use of magnetic resonance imaging in exertional compartment syndromes. *Am J Sports Med.* 1990;18:29–34.

38. Lokiec F, Siev-Ner I, Pritsch M. Chronic compartment syndrome of both feet. *J Bone Joint Surg Br.* 1991;73:178–179.

39. Jehenson P, Leroy-Willig A, de Kerviler E, Duboc D, Syrota A. MR imaging as a potential diagnostic test for metabolic myopathies: importance of variations in the T2 of muscle with exercise. *AJR.* 1993;161:347–351.

40. Hernandez RJ, Sullivan DB, Chenevert TL, Keim DR. MR imaging in children with dermatomyositis: musculoskeletal findings and correlation with clinical and laboratory findings. *AJR.* 1993;161:359–366.

41. Park JH, Vansant JP, Kumar NG, et al. Dermatomyositis: correlative MR imaging and P-31 MR spectroscopy for quantitative characterization of inflammatory disease. *Radiology.* 1990;177:473–479.

42. Nunez-Hoyo M, Gradner CL, Motta AO, Ashmead JW. Case report—skeletal muscle infarction in diabetes: MR findings. *J Comput Assist Tomogr.* 1993;17:986–988.

43. Hernandez RJ, Keim DR, Chenevert TL, Sullivan DB, Aisen AM. Fat-suppressed MR imaging of myositis. *Radiology.* 1992;182:217–219.

44. Kurashima K, Shimizu H, Ogawa H. MR and CT in the evaluation of sarcoid myopathy. *J Comput Assist Tomogr.* 1991;15:1004–1007.

45. Shintani S, Shiigai T. Repeat MRI in acute rhabdomyolysis: correlation with clinicopathological findings. *J Comput Assist Tomogr.* 1993;17:786–791.

46. Resendes M, Helms CA, Fritz RC, Genant H. MR appearance of intramuscular injections. *AJR.* 1992;158:1293–1294.

47. Kravis MMM, Munk PL, McCain GA, Vellet AD, Levin MF. MR imaging of muscle and tender points in fibromyalgia. *JMRI.* 1993;3:669–670.

48. Rao L, Lee JK. Occult intraosseous fracture: detection with MR imaging. *Radiology.* 1988;167:749–751.

49. Leadbetter WB. Cell-matrix response in tendon injury. In: Renstrom AFH, Leadbetter WB, eds. *Clinics in Sports Medicine: Tendinitis 1 Basic Concepts.* W.B. Saunders, 1992:533.

50. Puddu G, Ippolito E, Postacchini F. A classification of Achilles tendon disease. *Am J Sports Med.* 1976;4:145–150.

51. Regan W, Wold LE, Coonrad R. Morrey BF. Microscopic histopathology of chronic refractory lateral epicondylitis. *Am J Sports Med.* 1992;20:746–749.

52. Kaplan PA, Bryans KC, Davick JP, Otte M, Stinson WW, Dussault RG. MR imaging of the normal shoulder: variants and pitfalls. *Radiology.* 1992;184:519–524.

53. Zeiss J, Saddemi SR, Ebraheim NA. MR imaging of the quadriceps tendon: normal layered configuration and its importance in cases of tendon rupture. *AJR.* 1992;159:1031–1034.

54. Schweitzer ME, Caccese R, Karasick D, Wapner KL, Mitchell DG. Posterior tibial tendon tears: utility of secondary signs for MR imaging diagnosis. *Radiology.* 1993;188:655–659.

55. Erickson SJ, Cox JH, Hyde JS, Carrera GF, Strandt JA, Estkowski RTR. Effect of tendon orientation on MR imaging signal intensity: a manifestation of the "magic angle" phenomenon. *Radiology.* 1991;181:389–392.

56. Mirowitz SA. Normal rotator cuff: MR imaging with conventional and fat-suppression techniques. *Radiology.* 1991;180:735–740.

57. Kannus P, Jozsa L. Histopathological changes preceding spontaneous rupture of a tendon: a controlled study of 891 patients. *J Bone Joint Surg Am.* 1991;73:1507–1525.

58. Kalebo P, Karlsson J, Sward L, Peterson L. Ultrasonography of chronic tendon injuries in the groin. *Am J Sports Med.* 1992;20:634–639.

59. Middleton WD, Reinus WR, Totty WG, Melson CL, Murphy WA. Ultrasonographic evaluation of the rotator cuff and biceps tendon. *J Bone Joint Surg Am.* 1986;68:440–450.

60. Kainberger FM, Engel A, Barton P, Huebsch P, Neuhold A, Salomonowitz E. Injury of the Achilles tendon: diagnosis with sonography. *AJR.* 1990;155:1031–1036.

61. Kalebo P, Allenmark C, Peterson L, Sward L. Diagnostic value of ultrasonography in partial ruptures of the Achilles tendon. *Am J Sports Med.* 1992;20:378–381.

62. Morrey BC. Reoperation for failed surgical treatment of refractory lateral epicondylitis. *J Shoulder Elbow Surg.* 1992;1:47–55.

63. Coonrad RW. *Tendonopathies at the Elbow.* AAOS Instructional Course Lectures. 1991;40:25–32.

64. Vangsness CT, Jobe FW. Surgical treatment of medial epicondylitis. *J Bone Joint Surg Br.* 1991;73:409–411.

65. Weinstabl R, Stiskal M, Neuhold A, Aamlid B, Hertz H. Classifying calcaneal tendon injury according to MRI findings. *J Bone Joint Surg Br.* 1991;73:683–685.

66. Martinoli C, Derchi LE, Pastorino C, Bertolotto M, Silvestri E. Analysis of echotexture of tendons with US. *Radiology.* 1993;186:839–843.

67. Ferretti A, Ippolito E, Mariani P, Puddu G. Jumper's knee. *Am J Sports Med.* 1983;11:58–62.

68. Bodne D, Quinn SF, Murray WT, et al. Magnetic resonance images of chronic patellar tendinitis. *Skeletal Radiol.* 1988;17:24–28.

69. Scranton PE, Farrar EL. Mucoid degeneration of the patellar ligament in athletes. *J Bone Joint Surg Am.* 1992;74:435–437.

70. El-Khoury GY, Wira RL, Berbaum KS, Pope TL, Monu JUV. MR imaging of patellar tendinitis. *Radiology.* 1992;184:849–854.

71. Rosenberg ZS, Kawelblum M, Cheung YY, Beltran J, Lehman WB, Grant AD. Osgood-Schlatter lesion: fracture or tendinitis? Scintigraphic, CT, and MR imaging features. *Radiology.* 1992;185:853–858.

72. Karlsson J, Kalebo P, Goksor LA, Thomee R, Sward L. Partial rupture of the patellar ligament. *Am J Sports Med.* 1992;20:390–395.

73. King JB, Perry DJ, Mourad K, Kumar SJ. Lesions of the patellar ligament. *J Bone Joint Surg Br.* 1990;72:46–48.

74. Davies SG, Baudouin CJ, King JB, Perry JD. Ultrasound, computed tomography and magnetic resonance imaging in patellar tendinitis. *Clin Radiol.* 1991;43:52–56.

75. Seeger LL, Gold RH, Bassett LW, Ellman H. Shoulder impingement syndrome: MR findings in 53 shoulders. *AJR.* 1988;150:343–347.

76. Weiner DS, Macnab I. Superior migration of the humeral head: a radiological aid in the diagnosis of tears of the rotator cuff. *J Bone Joint Surg Br.* 1970;52:524–527.

77. Ono K, Yamamuro T, Rockwood CA. Use of a thirty-degree caudal tilt radiograph in the shoulder impingement syndrome. *J Shoulder Elbow Surg.* 1992;246–252.

78. Calvert PT, Packer NP, Stoker DJ, Bayley JIL, Kessel L. Arthrography of the shoulder after operative repair of the torn rotator cuff. *J Bone Joint Surgery Br.* 1986;68:147–150.

79. Farin PU, Jaroma H, Harju A, Soimakallio S. Shoulder impingement syndrome: sonographic evaluation. *Radiology.* 1990;176:845–849.

80. Mack LA, Gannon MK, Kilcoyne RF, Matsen FA. Sonographic evaluation of the rotator cuff: accuracy in patients without prior surgery. *Clin Orthop.* 1988;234:21–27.

81. Brenneke SL, Morgan CJ. Evaluation of ultrasonography as a diagnostic technique in the assessment of rotator cuff tendon tears. *Am J Sports Med.* 1989;20:287–288.

82. Wiener SN, Seitz WH. Sonography of the shoulder in patients with tears of the rotator cuff: accuracy and value for selecting surgical options. *AJR.* 1993;160:103–107.

83. Misamore GW, Woodward C. Evaluation of degenerative lesions of the rotator cuff: a comparison of arthrography and ultrasonography. *J Bone Joint Surg Am.* 1991;73:704–706.

84. Neumann CH, Holt RG, Steinbach LS, Jahnke AH, Petersen SA. MR imaging the shoulder: appearance of the supraspinatus tendon in asymptomatic volunteers. *AJR.* 1992;158:1281–1287.

85. Kjellin I, Ho CP, Cervilla V. Alterations in the supraspinatus tendon at MR imaging: correlation with histopathologic findings in cadavers. *Radiology.* 1991;181:837–841.

86. Nakagaki K, Ozaki J, Tomita Y, Tamai S. Magnetic resonance imaging of rotator cuff tearing and degenerative tendon changes: correlation with histologic. *J Shoulder Elbow Surg.* 1993;2:156–164.

87. Gerber C, Krushell RJ. Isolated rupture of the tendon of the subscapularis muscle: clinical features in 16 cases. *J Bone Joint Surg Br.* 1991;73:389–394.

88. Harryman DT, Mack LA, Wang KY, et al. Repairs of the rotator cuff: correlation of functional results with integrity of the cuff. *J Bone Joint Surg Am.* 1991;73:1982–1989.

89. Iannotti JP, Zlatkin MB, Esterhai JL, Kressel HY, Dalinka MK, Spindler KP. Magnetic resonance imaging of the shoulder. *Magn Reson Imaging.* 1991;73:17–29.

90. Hodler J, Kursunoglu-Brahme S, Snyder SJ, et al. Rotator cuff disease: assessment with MR arthrography versus standard MR imaging in 36 patients with arthroscopic confirmation. *Radiology.* 1992;182:431–436.

91. Traughber PD, Goodwin TE. Shoulder MRI: arthroscopic correlation with emphasis on partial tears. *J Comput Assist Tomogr.* 1992;16:129–133.

92. Rafii M, Firooznia H, Sherman O, et al. Rotator cuff lesions: signal patterns at MR imaging. *Radiology.* 1990;177:817–823.

93. Farley TE, Neumann CH, Steinbach LS, Jahnke AJ, Petersen SS. Full-thickness tears of the rotator cuff of the shoulder: diagnosis with MR imaging. *AJR.* 1992;158:347–351.

94. Palmer WE, Brown JH, Rosenthal DI. Rotator cuff: evaluation with fat-suppressed MR arthrograph. *Radiology.* 1993;188:683–687.

95. Karzel RP, Snyder SJ. Magnetic resonance arthrography of the shoulder. *Clin Sports Med.* 1993;12:123–136.

96. Yacoe ME, Bergman AG, Ladd AL, Hellman BH. Dupuytren's contracture: MR imaging findings and correlation between MR signal intensity and cellularity of lesions. *AJR.* 1993;160:813–817.

97. Cervilla V, Schweitzer ME, Ho C, Motta A, Kerr R, Resnick D. Medial dislocation of the biceps brachii tendon: appearance at MR imaging. *Radiology.* 1991;180:523–526.

98. Chan TW, Dalinka MK, Kneeland JB, Chervot A. Biceps tendon dislocation: evaluation with MR imaging. *Radiology.* 1991;179:649–652.

99. Faciszewski T, Burks RT, Manaster BJ. Subtle injuries of the lisfranc joint. *J Bone Joint Surg Am.* 1990;72:1519–1522.

100. Raatikainen T, Putkonen M, Puranen J. Arthrography, clinical examination, and stress radiograph in the diagnosis of acute injury to the lateral ligaments of the ankle. *Am J Sports Med.* 1992;20:2–12.

101. Hodler J, Haghighi P, Trudell D, Resnick D. The cruciate ligaments of the knee: correlative between MR appearance and gross and histologic findings in cadaveric specimens. *AJR.* 1992;159:357–360.

102. Kannus P, Renstrom P. Current concepts review: treatment for acute tears of the lateral ligaments of the ankle. *J Bone Joint Surg Am.* 1991;73:305–312.

103. Schneck CD, Mesgarzadeh M, Bonakdarpour A. MR imaging of the most commonly injured ankle ligaments, Part II: ligament injuries. *Radiology.* 1992;184:507–512.

104. Rijke AM, Goitz HT, McCue FC, Dee PM. Magnetic resonance imaging of injury to the lateral ankle ligaments. *Am J Sports Med.* 1993;21:528–534.

105. Verhaven EFC, Shahabpour M, Handelberg FWJ, Vaes PHEG, Opdecam PJE. The accuracy of three-dimensional magnetic resonance imaging in the diagnosis of ruptures of the lateral ligaments of the ankle. *Am J Sports Med.* 1991;19:583–587.

106. Cardone BW, Erickson SJ, Den Hartog BD, Carrera GF. MRI of injury to the lateral collateral ligamentous complex of the ankle. *J Comput Assist Tomogr.* 1993;17:102–107.

107. Franklin JL, Rosenberg TD, Paulos LE, France EP. Radiographic assessment of instability of the knee due to rupture of the anterior cruciate ligament: a quadriceps-contraction technique. *J Bone Joint Surg Am.* 1991;73:365–372.

108. Glashow JL, Katz R, Schneider M, Scott WN. Double-blind assessment of the value of magnetic resonance imaging in the diagnosis of anterior cruciate and meniscal lesions. *J Bone Joint Surg Am.* 1989;71:113–119.

109. Jackson DW, Jennings LD, Maywood RM, Beger PE. Magnetic resonance imaging of the knee. *Am J Sports Med.* 1988;16:29–38.

110. Lee JK, Yao L, Phelps CT, Wirth CR, Czajka J, Lozman. Anterior cruciate ligament tears: MR imaging compared with arthroscopy and clinical tests. *Radiology.* 1988;166:861–864.

111. Mink JH, Levy T, Crues JV. Tears of the anterior cruciate ligament and menisci of the knee: MR imaging evaluation. *Radiology.* 1988;167:769–774.

112. Vahey TN, Broome DR, Kayes KJ, Shelbourne KD. Acute and chronic tears of the anterior cruciate ligament: differential features at MRI imaging. *Radiology.* 1991;181:251–253.

113. Remer EM, Fitzgerald SW, Friedman H, Rogers LF, Hendrix RW, Schafer MF. Anterior cruciate ligament injury: MR imaging diagnosis and patterns of injury. *Radiographics.* 1991;12:901–915.

114. Vahey TN, Hunt JE, Shelbourne KD. Anterior translocation of the tibia at MR imaging: a secondary sign of anterior cruciate ligament tear. *Radiology.* 1993;187:817–819.

115. Cobby MJ, Schweitzer ME, Resnick D. The deep lateral femoral notch: an indirect sign of a torn anterior cruciate ligament. *Radiology.* 1992;184:855–858.

116. Stallenberg B, Gevenois PA, Sintzoff SA, Matos C, Andrianne Y, Struyven J. Fracture of the posterior aspect of the lateral tibial plateau: radiographic sign of anterior cruciate ligament tear. *Radiology.* 1993;187:821–825.

117. McCauley TR, Moses M, Kier R, Lynch JK, Barton JW, Jokl P. MR diagnosis of tears of anterior cruciate ligament of the knee: importance of ancillary findings. *AJR.* 1994;162:115–119.

118. Tung GA, Davis LM, Wiggins ME, Fadale PD. Tears of the anterior cruciate ligament: primary and secondary signs at MR imaging. *Radiology.* 1993;188:661–667.

119. Fitzgerald SW, Remer EM, Friedman H, Rogers LF. MR evaluation of the anterior cruciate ligament: value of supplementing sagittal images with coronal and axial images. *AJR.* 1993;160:1233–1237.

120. Sommerlath K, Lysholm J, Gillquist J. The long-term course after treatment of acute anterior cruciate ligament ruptures : a 9 to 16 year follow-up. *Am J Sports Med.* 1991;19:156–162.

121. O'Brien WR. Degenerative arthritis of the knee following anterior cruciate ligament injury: role of the meniscus. *Sports Med Arthroscopy Rev.* 1994;1:114–118.

122. Oberlander MA, Shalvoy RM, Hughston JC. The accuracy of the clinical knee examination documented by arthroscopy: a prospective study. *Am J Sports Med.* 1993;21:773–778.

123. Grover JS, Bassett LW, Gross ML, Seeger LL, Finerman GAM. Posterior cruciate ligament: MR imaging. *Radiology.* 1990;174:527–530.

124. Gross ML, Grover JS, Bassett LW, Seeger LL, Finerman GAM. Magnetic resonance imaging of the posterior cruciate ligament. *Am J Sports Med.* 1992;20:732–737.

125. Fischer SP, Fox JM, De Pizzo W, Friedman MJ, Snyder SJ, Ferkel RD. Accuracy of diagnoses from magnetic resonance imaging of the knee. *J Bone Joint Surg Am.* 1991;73:2–10.

126. Mink JH. The cruciate and collateral ligaments. In: Mink JH, Reicher MA, Crues JV, Deutsch AL, eds. *Magnetic Resonance Imaging of the Knee.* 2nd ed. New York: Raven Press, 1993:141.

127. Weber WN, Neumann CH, Barakos JA, Petersen SA, Steinbach LS, Genant HK. Lateral tibial rim (segond) fractures: MR imaging characteristics. *Radiology.* 1991;180:731–734.

128. Spaeth HJ, Abrams RA, Bock GW, et al. Gamekeeper thumb: differentiation of nondisplaced and displaced tears of the ulnar collateral ligament with MR imaging. *Radiology.* 1993;188:553–556.

129. Noyes FR, Cummings JF, Grood ES, Walz-Hasselfeld, Wroble RR. The diagnosis of knee motion limits, subluxations, and ligament injury. *Am J Sports Med.* 1991;19:163–171.

130. Speer KP, Spritzer CE, Bassett FH, Feagin JA, Garrett WE. Osseous injury associated with acute tears of the anterior cruciate ligament. *Am J Sports Med.* 1992;20:382–389.

131. Fu FH, Harner CD, Johnson DL, Miller MD, Woo SLY. Biomechanics of knee ligaments. *J Bone Joint Surg Am.* 1993;75:1716–1727.

132. Cheung Y, Magee TH, Rosenberg ZS, Rose DJ. MRI of anterior cruciate ligament reconstruction. *J Comput Assist Tomogr.* 1992;16:134–137.

133. Howell SM, Clark JA, Blasier RD. Serial magnetic resonance imaging of hamstring anterior cruciate ligament autografts during the first year of implantation: a preliminary study. *Am J Sports Med.* 1991;19:42–47.

134. Yamato M, Yamagishi T. MRI of patellar tendon anterior cruciate ligament autografts. *J Comput Assist Tomogr.* 1992;16:604–607.

135. Rak KM, Gillogly SD, Schaefer RA, Yakes WF, Liljedahl RR. Anterior cruciate ligament reconstruction: evaluation with MR imaging. *Radiology.* 1991;178:553–556.

136. Howell SM, Berns GS, Farley TE. Unimpinged and impinged anterior cruciate ligament grafts: MR signal intensity measurements. *Radiology.* 1991;179:639–643.

137. Howell SM, Clark JA, Farley TE. A rationale for predicting anterior cruciate grant impingement by the intercondylar roof: a magnetic resonance imaging study. *Am J Sports Med.* 1991;19:276–28.

138. Coupens SD, Yates CK, Sheldon C, Ward C. Magnetic resonance imaging evaluation of the patellar tendon after use of its central one-third for anterior cruciate ligament reconstruction. *Am J Sports Med.* 1992; 20:332–335.

139. Hodge JC, Ghelman B, O'Brien SJ, Wickiewicz TL. Synovial plicae and chondromalacia patellae: correlation of results of CT arthrography with results of arthroscopy. *Radiology.* 1993;186: 827–831.

140. Recht MP, Kramer J, Marcelis S, et al. Abnormalities of articular cartilage in the knee: analysis of available MR techniques. *Radiology.* 1993;187:473–478.

141. Paul PK, Jasani MK, Sebok D, Rakhit A, Dunton AW, Douglas FL. Variation in MR signal intensity across normal human knee cartilage. *JMRI.* 1993;3:569–574.

142. Tervonen O, Dietz MJ, Carmichael SW, Ehman RL. MR imaging of knee hyaline cartilage: evaluation of two- and three-dimensional sequences. *JMRI.* 1993;3:663–668.

143. Chandnani VP, Ho C, Chu P, Trudell D, Resnick D. Knee hyaline cartilage evaluated with MR imaging: a cadaveric study involving multiple imaging sequences and intraarticular injection of gadolinium and saline solution. *Radiology.* 1991;178:557–561.

144. Hayes CW, Sawyer RW, Conway WF. Patellar cartilage lesions: in vitro detection and staging with MR imaging and pathologic correlation. *Radiology.* 1990;176:479–483.

145. Hayes CW, Conway WF. Evaluation of articular cartilage radiographic and cross-sectional imaging techniques. *Radiographics.* 1992;12:409–428.

146. McCauley TR, Kier R, Lynch KJ, Jokl P. Chondromalacia patellae: diagnosis with MR imaging. *AJR.* 1992;158:101–105.

147. Speer KP, Spritzer CE, Goldner JL, Garrett WE. Magnetic resonance imaging of traumatic knee articular cartilage injuries. *Am J Sports Med.* 1991;19:396–402.

148. Hodler J, Berthiaume MF, Schweitzer ME, Resnick D. Knee joint hyaline cartilage defects: a comparative study of MR and anatomic sections. *J Comput Assist Tomogr.* 1992;16:597–603.

149. Conway WF, Hayes CW, Loughran T, et al. Cross-sectional imaging of the patellofemoral joint and surrounding structures. *Radiographics.* 1991;11:195–217.

150. Dye SF, Boll DA. Radionuclide imaging of the patellofemoral joint in young adults with anterior knee pain. *Orthop Clin North Am.* 1986;17:249–262.

151. Herzog RJ. Magnetic resonance imaging of the elbow. *Magn Reson Q.* 1993; 3:188–210.

152. Twyman RS, Desai K, Aichroth PM. Osteochondritis dissecans of the knee. *J Bone Joint Surg Br.* 1991;73:461–464.

153. Linden B. Osteochondritis dissecans of the femoral condyles: a long-term follow-up study. *J Bone Joint Surg Am.* 1977;59:769–776.

154. Cahill BR, Phillips MR, Navarro R. The results of conservative management of juvenile osteochondritis dissecans using joint scintigraphy. *Am J Sports Med.* 1989;17:601–606.

155. Mesgarzadeh M, Sapega AA, Bonakdarpour A, et al. Osteochondritis dissecans: analysis of mechanical stability with radiography, scintingraphy, and MR imaging. *Radiology.* 1987;165:775–780.

156. De Smet AA, Fisher DR, Graf BK, Lange RH. Osteochondritis dissecans of the knee: value of MR imaging in determining lesion stability and the presence of articular cartilage defects. *AJR.* 1990;155:549–553.

157. Kramer J, Stiglbauer R, Engel A, Prayer L, Imhof H. MR contrast arthrography (MRA) in osteochondrosis dissecans. *J Comput Assist Tomogr.* 1992;16:254–260.

158. Nelson DW, DiPaola J, Colville M, Schmidgall J. Osteochondritis dissecans of the talus and knee: prospective comparison of MR and arthroscopic classifications. *J Comput Assist Tomogr.* 1990;14: 804–808.

159. De Smet AA, Fisher D, Burnstein MI, Graf BK, Lange RH. Value of MR imaging in staging osteochondral lesions of the talus (osteochondritis dissecans): results in 14 patients. *AJR.* 1990;154:555–558.

160. Boeree NR, Watkinson AF, Ackroyd CE, et al. Magnetic resonance imaging of meniscal and cruciate injuries of the knee. *J Bone Joint Surg Br.* 1991;73:452–457.

161. Kornick J, Trefelner E, McCarthy S, et al. Meniscal abnormalities in the asymptomatic population at MR imaging. *Radiology.* 1990; 177:463–465.

162. Brunner MC, Flower SP, Evancho AM, Allman FL, Apple DF, Fajman WA. MRI of the athletic knee findings in asymptomatic professional basketball and collegiate football players. *Invest Radiol.* 1989;24:72–75.

163. Reinig JW, McDevitt ER, Ove PN. Progression of meniscal degenerative changes in college football players: evaluation with MR imaging. *Radiology.* 1991;181:255–257.

164. Shellock FG, Deutsch AL, Mink JH, Kerr R. Do asymptomatic marathon runners have an increased prevalence of meniscal abnormalities? An MR study of the knee in 23 volunteers. *AJR.* 1991;157:1239–1241.

165. Bodne SD, David DO, Dina TS, et al. A prospective and blinded investigation of magnetic resonance imaging of the knee. *Clin Orthop.* 1992;282:177–185.

166. Deutsch AL, Mink JH. The postoperative knee. In: Mink JH, Reicher MA, Crues JV, Deutsch AL, eds. *Magnetic Resonance Imaging of the Knee.* 2nd ed. New York: Raven Press, 1993;237.

167. Saal JA, Saal JS, Herzog RJ. The natural history of lumbar intervertebral disc extrusions treated nonoperatively. *Spine.* 1990;15:683–686.

168. Bozzao A, Gallucci M, Masciocchi C, Aprile I, Barile A, Passariello R. Lumbar disk herniation: MR imaging assessment of natural history in patients treated without surgery. *Radiology.* 1992;185:135–141.

169. Delauche-Cavallier MC, Budet C, Laredo JD, et al. Lumbar disc herniation: computed tomography scan changes after conservation treatment of nerve root compression. *Spine.* 1992;17:927–933.

170. Maigne JY, Rime B, Deligne B. Computed tomographic follow-up study of forty-eight cases of nonoperatively treated lumbar intervertebral disc herniation. *Spine.* 1992;17:1071–1074.

171. Modic MT, Masaryk T, Boumphrey F, et al. Lumbar herniated disk disease and canal stenosis: prospective evaluation by surface coil MR, CT and myelography. *AJR.* 1986;147:757–765.

172. Modic MT, Masaryk TJ, Ross JS, Carter JR. Imaging of degenerative disk disease. *Radiology.* 1988;168:177–186.

173. Modic MT, Steinberg PM, Ross JS, et al. Degenerative disk disease: assessment of changes in vertebral body marrow with MR imaging. *Radiology.* 1988;166:193–199.

174. Glenn WV Jr, Rothman SLG, Rhodes ML, Kerber CW. An overview of lumbar computed tomography/multiplanar reformations: what are its elements and how do they fit together? In: Post MJD, ed. *Computed Tomography of the Spine.* Baltimore: Williams & Wilkins, 1984; 135–154.

175. Masaryk TJ, Ross JS, Modic MT, Boumphrey F, Bohlman H, Wilber G. High-resolution MR imaging of sequestered lumbar intervertebral disks. *AJR.* 1988;150:115–162.

176. Berbaum KS, El-Khoury GY, Franken EA, Kathol M, Montgomery WJ, Hesson W. Impact of clinical history on fracture detection with radiography. *Radiology.* 1988;168:507–511.

177. Young JWR, Resnik CS. Fracture of the pelvis: current concepts of classification. *AJR.* 1990;155:1169–1175.

178. Siebenrock KA, Gerber C. The reproducibility of classification of fractures of the proximal end of the humerus. *J Bone Joint Surg Am.* 1993;75:1751–1715.

179. Kilcoyne RF, Shuman WP, Matsen FA, Moris M, Rockwood CA. The Neer classification of displaced proximal humeral fractures: spectrum of findings on plain radiographs and CT scans. *AJR.* 1990;154:1029–1033.

180. Dias JJ, Stirling AJ, Finlay DBL, Gregg PJ. Computerised axial tomography for tibial plateau fractures. *J Bone Joint Surgery Br.* 1987;69:84–88.

181. Rogers LF, Hendrix RW. Radiography of fracture healing. *Curr Imaging.* 1990;2:194–200.

182. Smith MA, Jones EA, Strachan RK, et al. Prediction of fracture healing in the tibia by quantitative radionuclide imaging. *J Bone Joint Surg Br.* 1987;69:441–447.

183. Lombardo SJ, Retting AC, Kerlan RK. Radiographic abnormalities of the iliac apophysis in adolescent athletes. *J Bone Joint Surg Am.* 1983;65:444–446.

184. Eisele SA, Sammarco GJ. Fatigue fractures of the foot and ankle in the athlete. *J Bone Joint Surg Am.* 1993;75:290–298.

185. Daffner RH, Pavlov H. Stress fractures: current concepts. *AJR.* 1992;159:245–252.

186. Kathol MH, El-Khoury GY, Moore TE, Marsh JL. Calcaneal insufficiency avulsion fractures in patients with diabetes mellitus. *Radiology.* 1991;180:725–772.

187. Satku K, Kumar VP, Chacha PB. Stress fractures around the knee in elderly patients: a cause of acute pain in the knee. *J Bone Joint Surg Am.* 1990;72:918–922.

188. Kiss ZS, Khan KM, Fuller PJ. Stress fractures of the tarsal navicular bone: CT findings in 55 cases. *AJR.* 1993;160:111–115.

189. Keene JS, Lash EG. Negative bone scan in a femoral neck stress fracture: a case report. *Am J Sports Med.* 1992;20:234–236.

190. Sterling JC, Webb RF, Meyers MC, Calvo RD. False negative bone scan in a female runner. *Med Sci Sports Exerc.* 1993;25:179–185.

191. Hosten N, Schorner W, Neumann K, Huhn D, Felix R. MR imaging of bone marrow—review of the literature and possible indications for contrast-enhanced studies. *Adv MRI Contrast.* 1993;1:84–98.

192. Rizzo PF, Gould ES, Lyden JP, Asnis SE. Diagnosis of occult fractures about the hip: magnetic resonance imaging compared with bone-scanning. *J Bone Joint Surg Am.* 1993;75:395–401.

193. Deutsch AL, Mink JH, Waxman AD. Occult fractures of the proximal femur: MR imaging. *Radiology.* 1989;170:113–116.

194. Tountas AA. Insufficiency stress fractures of the femoral neck in elderly women. *Clin Orthop.* 1993;292:202–209.

195. Harcke HT, Synder M, Caro PA, Bowen JR. Growth plate of the normal knee: evaluation with MR imaging. *Radiology.* 1992;183:119–123.

196. Jaramillo D, Hoffer FA. Cartilaginous epiphysis and growth plate: normal and abnormal MR imaging findings. *AJR.* 1992;158:1105–1110.

197. Jaramillo D, Hoffer FA, Shapiro F, Rand F. MR imaging of fractures of the growth plate. *AJR.* 1990;155:1261–1265.

198. Dotter WE. Little leaguer's shoulder: a fracture of the proximal epiphyseal cartilage of the humerus due to baseball pitching. *Guthrie Clin Bull.* 1953;23:68–72.

199. Maffulli N, Chan D, Aldridge MJ. Overuse injuries of the olecranon in young gymnasts. *J Bone Joint Surg Br.* 1992;74:305–308.

200. Yao L, Sinha S, Seeger LL. MR imaging of joints: analytic optimization of GRE techniques at 1.5T. *AJR.* 1992;158:339–345.

201. Lee JK, Yao L. Occult intraosseous fracture: magnetic resonance appearance versus age of injury. *Am J Sports Med.* 1989;17:620–623.

202. Mink JH, Deutsch AL. Occult cartilage and bone injuries of the knee: detection, classification, and assessment with MR imaging. *Radiology.* 1989;170:823–829.

203. Lynch TCP, Crues JV, Morgan FW, Sheehan WE, Harter LP, Ryu R. Bone abnormalities of the knee: prevalence and significance at MR imaging. *Radiology.* 1989;171:761–766.

204. Murphy BJ, Smith RL, Uribe JW, Janecki CJ, Hechtman SK, Mangasarian RA. Bone signal abnormalities in the posterolateral tibia and lateral femoral condyle in complete tears of the anterior cruciate ligament: a specific sign? *Radiology.* 1992;182:221–224.

205. Spindler KP, Schils JP, Bergfeld JA, et al. Prospective study of osseous, articular, and meniscal lesions in recent anterior cruciate ligament tears by magnetic resonance imaging and arthroscopy. *Am J Sports Med.* 1993;21:551–557.

206. Kaplan PA, Walker CW, Kilcoyne RF, Brown DE, Tusek D, Dussault RG. Occult fracture patterns of the knee associated with anterior cruciate ligament tears: assessment with MR imaging. *Radiology.* 1992;183:835–838.

207. Vellet AD, Marks PH, Fowler PJ, Munro TG. Occult posttraumatic osteochondral lesions of the knee: prevalence, classification, and short-term sequelae evaluated with MR imaging. *Radiology.* 1991;178:271–276.

208. Kirsch MD, Fitzgerald SW, Friedman H, Rogers LF. Transient lateral patellar dislocation: diagnosis with MR imaging. *AJR.* 1993;161:109–113.

209. Virolainen H, Visuri T, Kuusela T. Acute dislocation of the patella: MR findings. *Radiology.* 1993;189:243–246.

210. Lance E, Deutsch AL, Mink JH. Prior lateral patellar dislocation MR imaging findings. *Radiology.* 1993;189:905–907.

211. Catto M. Histological study of avascular necrosis of the femoral head after transcervical fracture. *J Bone Joint Surg Br.* 1965;47:749–776.

212. Catto M. The histological appearances of late segmental collapse of the femoral head after transcervical fracture. *J Bone Joint Surg Br.* 1965;47:777.

213. Kiaer T, Pedersen NW, Kristensen KD, Starklint H. Intra-osseous pressure and oxygen tension in avascular necrosis and osteoarthritis of the hip. *J Bone Joint Surg Br.* 1990;72:1023–1030.

214. Asnis SE, Gould ES, Bansal M, Rizzo PF, Bullough PG. Magnetic resonance imaging of the hip after displaced femoral neck fractures. *Clin Orthop.* 1994;298:191–198.

215. Brody AS, Strong M, Babikian G, Sweet DE, Seidel FG, Kuhn JP. Avascular necrosis: early MR imaging and histologic findings in a canine model. *AJR.* 1991;157:341–345.

216. Ruland LJ, Wang GJ, Teates CD, Gay S, Rijke A. A comparison of magnetic resonance imaging to bone scintigraphy in early traumatic ischemia of the femoral head. *Clin Orthop.* 1992;285:30–34.

217. Nadel SN, Debatin JF, Richardson WJ. Detection of acute avascular necrosis of the femoral head in dogs: dynamic contrast-enhanced MR imaging vs spin-echo and STIR sequences. *AJR.* 1992;159:1255–1261.

218. Vande Berg B, Malghem J, Labaisse MA, Michaux JL, Maldague B. Apparent focal bone marrow ischemia in patients with marrow disorders: MR studies. *J Comput Assist Tomogr.* 1993;17:792–797.

219. Hayes CW, Conway WF, Daniel WW. MR imaging of bone marrow edema pattern: transient osteoporosis, transient bone marrow edema syndrome, or osteonecrosis. *Radiographics.* 1993;13:1001–1011.

220. Vande Berg BE, Malghem JJ, Labaisse MA, Noel HM, Maldague B. MR imaging of avascular necrosis and transient marrow edema of the femoral head. *Radiographics.* 1993;13:501–520.

221. Vande Berg B, Malghem J, Labaisse MA, Noel H, Maldague B. Avascular necrosis of the hip: comparison of contrast-enhanced and nonenhanced MR imaging with histologic correlation work in progress. *Radiology.* 1992;182:445–450.

222. Ohzono K, Saito M, Takaoka K, et al. Natural history of nontraumatic avascular necrosis of the femoral head. *J Bone Joint Surg Br.* 1991;73:68–72.

223. Takatori Y, Kokubo T, Ninomiya S, Nakamura S, Morimoto S, Kusaba I. Avascular necrosis of the femoral head: natural history and magnetic resonance imaging. *J Bone Joint Surg Br.* 1993;75:217–221.

224. Genez BM, Wilson MR, Houk RW, et al. Early osteonecrosis of the femoral head: detection in high-risk patients with MR imaging. *Radiology.* 1988;168:521.

225. Tervonen O, Mueller DM, Matteson EL, Velossa JA, Ginsburg WW, Ehman RL. Clinically occult avascular necrosis of the hip: prevalence in an asymptomatic population at risk. *Radiology.* 1992;182:845–847.

226. Hofmann S, Engel A, Neuhold A, Leder K, Kramer J, Plenk H. Bone-marrow edema syndrome and transient osteoporosis of the hip: an MRI-controlled study of treatment by core decompression. *J Bone Joint Surg Br.* 1993;75:210–216.

227. Neuhold A, Hofmann S, Engel A, et al. Bone marrow edema of the hip: MR findings after core decompression. *J Comput Assist Tomogr.* 1992;16:951–955.

228. Turner DA, Templeton AC, Selzer PM, Rosenberg AG, Petasnick JP. Femoral capital osteonecrosis: MR findings of diffuse marrow abnormalities without focal lesions. *Radiology.* 1989;171:135–140.

229. Bjokengren AG, Airowaih A, Lindstrand A, Wingstrand H, Thorngren KG, Pettersson H. Spontaneous osteonecrosis of the knee: value of MR imaging in determining prognosis. *AJR.* 1990;154:331–336.

230. Koch E, Hofer HO, Sialer G, Marincek B, von Schulthess GK. Failure of MR imaging to detect reflex sympathetic dystrophy of the extremities. *AJR.* 1991;156:113–115.

231. Grabiner MD, Koh TJ, Draganich LF. Neuromechanics of the patellofemoral joint: clinical review. *Med Sci Sports Exerc.* 1994;26:10–21.

232. Kujala UM, Osterman K, Kormano M, Nelimarka O, Hurme M, Taimela S. Patellofemoral relationships in recurrent patellar dislocation. *J Bone Joint Surg Br.* 1989;71:788–792.

233. Merchant AC, Mercer RL, Jacobsen RH, Cool CR. Roentgenographic analysis of patellofemoral congruence. *J Bone Joint Surg Am.* 1974;56:1391–1396.

234. Laurin CA, Levesque HP, Dussault R, Labelle H, Peides JP. The abnormal lateral patellofemoral angle. *J Bone Joint Surg Am.* 1978;60:55–60.

235. Minkoff J, Fein L. The role of radiography in the evaluation and treatment of common anarthrotic disorders of the patellofemoral joint. *Clin Sports Med.* 1989;8:203–260.

236. Aglietti P, Insall JN, Cerulli G. Patellar pain and incongruence: measurements of incongruence. *Clin Orthop.* 1983;176:217–224.

237. Reikeras O, Hoiseth A. Patellofemoral relationships in normal subjects determined by computed tomography. *Skeletal Radiol.* 1990;19:591–592.

238. Martinez S, Korobkin M, Fondren FB, Hedlund LW, Goldner JL. Computed tomography of the normal patellofemoral joint. *Invest Radiol.* 1983;18:249–253.

239. Schutzer SF, Ramsby GR, Fulkerson JP. Computed tomographic classification of patellofemoral pain patients. *Orthop Clin North Am.* 1986;17:235–248.

240. Stanford W, Phelan J, Kathol MH, et al. Patellofemoral joint motion: evaluation by ultrafast computed tomography. *Skeletal Radiol.* 1988;17:487–492.

241. Kujala UM, Osterman K, Kormano M, Komu M, Schlenzka D. Patellar motion analyzed by magnetic resonance imaging. *Acta Orthop Scand.* 1989;60:13–16.

242. Shellock FG, Mink JH, Deutsch AL, Fox JM. Patellar tracking abnormalities: clinical experience with kinematic MR imaging in 130 patients. *Radiology.* 1989;172:799–804.

243. Brossmann J, Muhle C, Bull CC, et al. Evaluation of patellar tracking in patients with suspected patellar malalignment: cine MR imaging vs. arthroscopy. *AJR.* 1994;162:361–367.

244. Brossmann J, Muhle C, Schroder C, et al. Patellar tracking patterns during active and passive knee extension: evaluation with motion-triggered cine MR imaging. *Radiology.* 1993;187:205–212.

245. Shellock FG, Mink JH, Deutsch AL, Foo TK. Kinematic MR imaging of the patellofemoral joint: comparison of passive positioning and active movement techniques. *Radiology.* 1992;184:574–577.

246. Shellock FG, Mink JH, Deutsch AL, Foo TK, Sullenberge P. Patellofemoral joint: identification of abnormalities with active-movement, "unloaded" versus "loaded" kinematic MR imaging techniques. *Radiology.* 1993;188:575–578.

247. Stein LA, Endicott AN, Sampalis JS, Kaplow MA, Patel MD, Mitchell NS. Motion of the patella during walking: a video digital-fluoroscopic study in healthy volunteers. *AJR.* 1993;161:617–620.

248. Minami M, Yoshikawa K, Matsuoka Y, Itai Y, Kokubo T, Iio Masahiro. MR study of normal joint function using a low field strength system. *J Comput Assist Tomogr.* 1991;15:1017–1023.

249. Ruwe PA, McCarthy S. Cost-effectiveness of magnetic resonance imaging. In: Mink JH, Reicher MA, Crues JV, Deutsch AL, eds. *Magnetic Resonance Imaging of the Knee.* 2nd ed. New York: Raven Press, 1993:463.

CHAPTER 5

Medication Use in Sports Rehabilitation

Daniel J. Mazanec

INTRODUCTION

Medications, particularly antiinflammatory drugs, are frequently included in the treatment approach to both acute and chronic sports injuries. The objectives of drug therapy in the sports injury setting include relief of pain, suppression of inflammation, and reduction in muscle spasm. The ultimate goal is enhancement of tissue healing and facilitation of the rehabilitation process. Adequate analgesia may allow earlier mobilization after injury and resumption of activity. In chronic overuse injuries, however, analgesics to permit continued activity despite symptoms may be inappropriate. Reduction in inflammatory reaction immediately after injury may also reduce symptoms and enable earlier mobilization. That suppression of the inflammatory response may have adverse consequences on tissue repair is at least a theoretical concern. Many injuries are complicated by secondary muscle spasm, which further increases pain and may interfere with rehabilitation efforts. Relief of spasm by local modalities, better analgesia, or centrally acting muscle relaxants may be appropriate in such circumstances.

The following groups of medications have been used in the treatment of sports injuries:

- pure analgesics
- nonsteroidal antiinflammatory drugs (NSAIDs)
- muscle relaxants
- corticosteroids
  - systemic
  - intra-articular
  - intraspinal
- tricyclic antidepressants (TCAs)

Despite the scarcity of well-designed clinical trials supporting a role for these groups of medications in acute or chronic sports injury, many of these agents are widely used in the medical management of the injured athlete.

Drug therapy plays an adjunctive role in the comprehensive management of sports injuries. Thorough working knowledge of the principles of effective rehabilitation of the particular injury is fundamental to optimal medication use. Obviously, a clear appreciation of the clinical pharmacology of the agents themselves is mandatory. In addition, an understanding of the pathophysiology of acute soft tissue injury and healing provides the scientific basis for effective drug therapy.

PATHOPHYSIOLOGY OF SOFT TISSUE INJURY

The mechanism of most acute athletic injuries is either muscle or ligament stretch or tear—overload of the musculotendinous unit—or direct contusion. The histopathology of the acute lesion provides some justification for the use of antiinflammatory drug therapy. The evolution of the micropathology with healing suggests appropriate timing of antiinflammatory therapy. Based on pathologic study, three stages have been described in the progression from acute injury to healing.[1] The first phase, lasting up to 72 hours, is characterized by an acute inflammatory response. The cellular infiltrate is comprised primarily of polymorphonuclear cells, which release inflammatory and immunomodulating chemical mediators, including prostaglandins, kinins, and histamine. The complement system is activated and fibrinolysis occurs. During the second phase, repair begins with removal of cellular debris by macrophages, vascular regeneration, and collagen fiber synthesis. Fibroblasts and macrophages dominate the cellular infiltrate at this stage. During the final phase of remodeling, tensile strength of the injured tissue improves as collagen matures and is oriented for maximal strength in the direction of forces imposed during the rehabilitation process.

Medications may affect all stages of this process. Early treatment with antiinflammatory drugs (phase 1) is intended to reduce pain and swelling by suppressing the acute inflammatory reaction. This may allow earlier mobilization of the injury and speed restoration of function. The possibility that long-term antiinflammatory drug therapy may interfere with the repair process (phase 2) is a theoretical concern.[2] Clearly, the inflammatory response is not entirely pathologic and plays a pivotal role in clearing cellular debris and fibrin clot. Furthermore, elements of the inflammatory cascade directly enhance repair. Prostaglandins of the F series, for example, may play a role by enhancing collagen formation.[3] Finally, relief of pain and muscle spasm during the long rehabilitation process (phase 3) by local modalities or systemic drug therapy facilitates mobilization, i.e., stretching and strengthening of the injured tissue.

Chronic musculotendinous injuries in distance runners are typically the result of cumulative trauma related to repetitive overuse. The pathophysiology of these injuries is probably more complex but resembles the acute lesion with an inflammatory cell component and healing by fibrosis.[4] The role of drug therapy in these conditions is not well studied. If analgesic or antiinflammatory therapy is used to permit the athlete to continue performing despite symptoms, the potential for additional cumulative injury is increased.

PURE ANALGESICS

Beyond the relief of acute pain, the ultimate objective of analgesic therapy in sports injury is facilitation of rehabilitation and more rapid return to full function. Analgesics may be divided into centrally acting (opioid) and peripherally acting (nonopioid) groups:

Nonopioid, peripherally acting analgesics
- acetaminophen
- NSAIDs

Opioid, centrally acting analgesics
- propoxyphene
- codeine
- dihydrocodeine
- pentazocine
- oxycodone
- hydrocodone

Nonopioid analgesics are effective for mild to moderate pain. Centrally acting agents are reserved for severe pain or pain unresponsive to peripherally acting agents.[5] Addition of a centrally acting drug to a nonopioid analgesic is an effective strategy in this situation.[6]

Acetaminophen is primarily analgesic without clinically significant antiinflammatory action. It is effective in mild to moderate pain, with analgesia comparable to that of NSAIDs. Toxicity at doses less than 4 g daily is rare. Higher doses, particularly in association with substantial alcohol intake, may be associated with hepatic dysfunction.[7] Unlike most NSAIDs, acetaminophen does not interfere with prostaglandin synthesis. Serious prostaglandin-related toxicity, including gastric ulceration, perforation, or bleeding, does not occur during therapy with acetaminophen.

Opioid analgesics act primarily by binding with opiate receptors in the central nervous system (CNS). Opioids are indicated for relief of acute, moderate to severe pain. Long-term use may be associated with tolerance, toxicity, addiction, and illicit use and is not appropriate in sports rehabilitation.[8,9] Studies comparing opioid and nonopioid analgesics in sports injuries are scarce and flawed. In a study of 50 college athletes, diflunisal, a peripherally acting nonnarcotic nonsteroidal antiinflammatory drug, was as effective as was acetaminophen with codeine in the treatment of mild to moderate pain due to sprains and strains.[10] Naproxen, another NSAID, was superior to propoxyphene in relief of pain in a short-term study of 98 patients with a mix of "soft-tissue disorders."[11] That opioid or nonopioid analgesic therapy affects longer-term outcomes, such as accelerating rehabilitation resulting in earlier return to full activity, has not been demonstrated.

NONSTEROIDAL ANTIINFLAMMATORY DRUGS

An ever-expanding array of NSAIDs (Exhibit 5–1) is widely used in clinical management of musculoskeletal pain and injury. More than 100 million prescriptions for the various NSAIDs are written in the United States annually, and worldwide sales exceed 1 billion dollars.[12,13] Relief of pain and inflammation is the most common rationale for NSAID therapy in sports injury. Despite frequent use, important questions remain regarding the role of NSAIDs in management of soft tissue injury:

1. Does treatment with an antiinflammatory drug (rather than with a nonopioid or opioid pure analgesic) result in improved short-term or long-term outcome of sports injury treatment? This issue has important clinical implications as nonopioid pure analgesics such as acetaminophen are clearly less toxic than are NSAIDs.
2. Does treatment with an NSAID slow or delay healing by interfering with inflammation helpful in the repair process? The answer to this question may depend on how soon after injury NSAID therapy is initiated and the duration of drug therapy.
3. Are certain NSAIDs preferred in treatment of sports injury? Drug-specific differences in toxicity and compliance, rather than efficacy, may direct the choice of agent.[14]

All NSAIDs are analgesic, antipyretic, and antiinflammatory. Most NSAIDs are highly protein bound, primarily to

Exhibit 5–1 Available Nonsteroidal Antiiflammatory Drugs

Salicylates
    Acetylated
        Aspirin
    Nonacetylated
        Choline Magnesium Trisalicylate
        Diflunisal
        Magnesium salicylate
        Salsalate
        Sodium salicylate

Acetic Acids
    Diclofenac
    Indomethacin
    Tolmetin
    Sulindac
    Etodolac

Proprionic Acids
    Ibuprofen
    Naproxen
    Fenoprofen
    Oxaprozin
    Ketoprofen
    Flurbiprofen

Fenamic Acids
    Mefenamic acid
    Meclofenamic acid

Enolic Acids
    Phenylbutazone
    Piroxicam

albumin. Potential for interaction with other highly bound drugs including oral anticoagulants, Dilantin, or oral hypoglycemics, is a theoretical concern.[12] In general, NSAIDs are metabolized in the liver to inactive drug. Renal excretion represents a minor mode of excretion of active drug. Clearance of NSAIDs is slower in older patients, who demonstrate significant increases in drug half-life.[15]

The hypothesis that NSAID antiinflammatory effect is a consequence of inhibition of cyclooxygenase activity and, therefore, prostaglandin synthesis, was first proposed in 1971.[16] It is now clear that at least some NSAIDs influence the inflammatory process in other, non–prostaglandin-dependent ways, including direct effects on neutrophil function, interference with cell-cell binding, and suppression of enzymatic activity.[12,17,18] Inhibition of prostaglandin synthesis is, however, the primary mechanism of NSAID toxicity.

No significant differences in efficacy have been demonstrated among currently available NSAIDs in numerous clinical trials.[12,19] Considerable variability in efficacy and toxicity is observed from patient to patient, however, even

within the same chemical class of NSAIDs. Similar patients express marked variation in preference for various NSAIDs.[20,21] Because of the similar efficacy and significant variability in response to a particular agent, choice of NSAID is empiric. Rather than efficacy, initial drug choice may be based on physician preference, cost, the patient's prior experience with various NSAIDs, duration of effect of the particular NSAID (half-life), drug formulation (liquid vs. capsule), and perhaps perceived or theoretical differences in potential toxicity. For example, nonacetylated salicylates as weak prostaglandin synthesis inhibitors may be selected in certain subgroups of patients in whom prostaglandin-mediated renal or gastrointestinal (GI) toxicity is a major concern. An adequate trial of any NSAID is two to three weeks. In view of the individual variation in response to these drugs, it is reasonable to try a series of NSAIDs, if indicated, in a single patient, looking for the best response and least toxicity.

Most adverse effects of NSAID therapy occur as a result of drug interference with prostaglandin synthesis. However, several rare but serious problems related to NSAID therapy, including clinical hepatitis and agranulocytosis or aplastic anemia, are idiosyncratic and of less clear etiology. In sports medicine, the relatively short duration of NSAID therapy effectively limits the risk of prostaglandin-mediated toxicity.

Gastrointestinal side effects occur in approximately 25% of NSAID users, though silent endoscopically demonstrated lesions occur in as many as 60%.[22,23] The term *NSAID gastropathy* has been applied to the spectrum of NSAID-induced GI lesions, which range from simple erythema through erosion, ulceration, and ulcer complications of perforation and bleeding.[23,24] Recently, NSAID-induced colitis, presumably also related to prostaglandin synthesis inhibition, has been described.[25] The relative risk of serious GI disease or complications (ulcer, bleeding, death) has been reported to range from 1.4 to 10.5 in NSAID users.[26] Risk factors for NSAID gastropathy probably include age greater than 60 years, history of prior ulcer disease, concomitant corticosteroid therapy, and higher-dose NSAID therapy.[27–29] Recognition of NSAID gastropathy is complicated by the poor correlation between symptoms and endoscopic findings. The absence of dyspeptic symptoms does not exclude the possibility of NSAID-induced ulcer disease.[30,31] Though all NSAIDs have been associated with gastropathy, nonacetylated salicylates may be less likely to adversely affect the GI tract. Nonacetylated salicylates are approximately 100 times less effective than is aspirin as inhibitors of prostaglandin synthesis.[14] Misoprostol, an analog of prostaglandin E_1, when coadministered with an NSAID, significantly reduces the likelihood of endoscopically demonstrable ulceration.[23,32] Whether or not misoprostol decreases the risk of ulcer complication—bleeding or perforation—is less clear. About 25% of patients taking misoprostol develop diarrhea. Misoprostol also increases uterine contractility and can precipitate abortion. Routine clinical use of prophylactic misoprostol in all NSAID users is not indicated. H_2 blockers such as cimetidine and ranitidine have not been shown to reduce the likelihood of gastric ulcer.[23]

A wide spectrum of renal syndromes may occur in patients taking NSAIDs.[33,34] The most common is sodium retention, largely an effect of prostaglandin synthesis inhibition, manifested as peripheral edema in up to 25% of patients taking a particular agent. Much less common, but potentially more serious, is reversible acute renal failure, also a result of cyclooxygenase inhibition. Individuals at risk for this complication are dependent on renal prostaglandin production for maintenance of renal function, including patients with congestive heart failure, intrinsic renal disease, cirrhosis and ascites, increasing age, and atherosclerotic cardiovascular disease. Athletes such as long-distance runners in sports predisposing to dehydration may be at increased risk for this problem as well. Diuretic therapy amplifies the risk of NSAID-induced acute renal failure. Rare renal syndromes also associated with NSAID therapy include papillary necrosis, interstitial nephritis (most commonly associated with fenoprofen), and hyporeninemic hypoaldosteronism. Sulindac and nonacetylated salicylates are probably associated with a lesser incidence of renal toxicity than are other NSAIDs.[14,35,36]

Several important drug interactions may occur with NSAID therapy. Agents that are strong inhibitors of prostaglandin synthesis attenuate the effect of diuretics, beta blockers, and angiotensin-converting enzyme inhibitors on control of blood pressure.[14,37] In hypertensive patients requiring antiinflammatory drug therapy, nonacetylated salicylates are preferred. Lithium clearance is reduced by NSAIDs, mandating careful monitoring of lithium levels in such patients when an NSAID is prescribed. Interaction with other highly protein-bound drugs has already been described. Other NSAID side effects include elevation of liver enzymes in up to 3% of patients, changes in cognitive function, headache, and impaired platelet aggregation.[14,38]

The studies exploring the role of NSAIDs in sports medicine have recently been critically reviewed.[13,39] Many of the more than 50 studies are significantly flawed. Only 36% have placebo controls, and only 66% are randomized. Only 7% of 44 studies examined met the following criteria: are randomized, have placebo controls, allow physical therapy, and control time between injury and treatment.[13] Most are short term (one week or less) in duration and do not assess longer-term outcomes. Despite these limitations, several conclusions about the role of NSAIDs in the management of sports injuries can be drawn from review of the better clinical trials.[40–45] NSAIDs are effective analgesics and superior to placebo within the first week following injury. Some clinical signs of inflammatory activity—swelling and tenderness—are more rapidly reduced with NSAID therapy within the 7 to 14 days following injury. NSAID-treated patients returned to activity earlier than did placebo-treated patients in some studies, though by 14 days following injury, most athletes were significantly improved, irrespective of drug therapy. Side effects from NSAIDs were uncommon in patients treated in these short-term trials.

The short-term clinical trials described above do not address two additional concerns that have been raised regarding NSAID therapy in the athlete. The first of these is whether NSAIDs delay healing by interfering with the inflammatory process and its role in clearing cellular debris and initiating neovascularization and fibrosis. Two recent studies in animal models of muscle strain have demonstrated histologic evidence that NSAID therapy delays degradation of damaged tissue and slows muscle regeneration.[46,47] However, functional parameters of contractile and tensile strength were not significantly different from controls at 7 to 14 days following treatment. This finding is consistent with the fact that the cells most important in healing of injured tissue—macrophages and fibroblasts—are largely unaffected by NSAIDs.[48] A second concern is whether NSAIDs adversely affect proteoglycan metabolism in articular cartilage.[49,50] Various NSAIDs have been demonstrated to affect proteoglycan synthesis in vitro. The clinical significance of these observations in the injured athlete is unknown.

In sum, NSAIDs provide effective analgesia and perhaps clinical antiinflammatory benefit when administered early after injury. NSAID therapy can facilitate early active rehabilitation. Short-term use is not associated with any clinically detectable delay in healing or any significant toxicity in most patients. Optimal duration of treatment has not been effectively studied. No agent has been shown to be preferred on the basis of efficacy or toxicity in these patients.

MUSCLE RELAXANTS

Muscle relaxants are frequently prescribed in addition to NSAIDs or other analgesic agents in acute musculoskeletal injury (Exhibit 5–2). Though structurally unrelated, these agents share common pharmacologic properties. They are all centrally acting drugs that alter polysynaptic supraspinal and spinal pathways, which modulate stretch reflexes.[51] In addition, all available agents produce nonspecific sedation, which may also account for muscle relaxation.

Review of the studies assessing the efficacy of muscle relaxants in the treatment of acute musculoskeletal disorders suggests that these agents are more effective than placebo in relief of symptoms.[52] However, in studies comparing muscle relaxant therapy with pure analgesics, no significant difference in outcomes has been demonstrated. Interpretation of these studies is complicated by the diversity of the injuries included, the difficulty in objective documentation of muscle

Exhibit 5–2 Centrally Acting Oral Skeletal Muscle Relaxants

cyclobenzaprine
chlorzoxazone
carisoprodol
diazepam
baclofen
methocarbamol
orphenadrine

spasm, the vague outcome parameters, and the frequent uncontrolled use of physical therapy. Further, because the natural history of untreated soft tissue musculoskeletal injury is generally favorable, all patients (including placebo-treated) are significantly better in one or two weeks. Most studies do not specifically address sports-related musculoskeletal trauma or pain. Studies comparing two or more muscle relaxants have failed to demonstrate superiority of any single agent over another.[53–55]

Muscle relaxants are commonly administered with analgesics or NSAIDs, sometimes in the form of a single combination product. In a prospective trial comparing cyclobenzaprine, 5 mg twice daily; diflunisal, 500 mg twice daily; combined therapy with both drugs; and placebo in treatment of acute back spasms, combined therapy was superior at day 4, but no differences were demonstrated at 2, 7, or 10 days.[56] Almost all patients recovered within 7 to 10 days, irrespective of therapy. Studies of other combinations support a modest short-term advantage to combination therapy over single-agent treatment alone.[57–59]

The most common adverse effect of muscle relaxants is sedation, though other CNS toxicity, including headache, dizziness, nausea, and vomiting, has been described. Sedation may facilitate treatment early after the injury by enhancing compliance with recommendations for rest. Cyclobenzaprine may cause dryness of the mouth.

In sum, muscle relaxants have a limited, short-term role in the early management of musculoskeletal injuries. They should be coadministered with an analgesic or NSAID. There is no evidence to support long-term use in sports injury care. Alternative, nonpharmacologic modalities to reduce posttraumatic muscle spasm, such as manipulation, myofascial release techniques, ultrasound, or hot packs, may be as effective as systemic agents, though a prospective comparative trial has not been performed.

CORTICOSTEROIDS

Glucocorticoids have been used orally, intra-articularly, periarticularly, intramuscularly, and intraspinally in the treatment of musculoskeletal pain. In sports injury, as with NSAIDs, the rationale for steroid use is relief of the early inflammatory response, including pain and swelling, facilitating early active movement and rehabilitation. Corticosteroids are both antiinflammatory and immunosuppressive. Perhaps the most important immediate affect on inflammation is reduction in leukocyte migration to the injured site.[51] Other potential antiinflammatory effects of steroids include inhibition of prostaglandin synthesis, lymphocytopenia, and impairment of macrophage functions, including phagocytosis.[51,60]

Adverse consequences of systemic corticosteroids are well known. Intraspinal, intra-articular, or periarticular injections are, in general, associated with less systemic absorption and less risk of systemic effects such as suppression of the hypothalamic-pituitary-adrenal axis, glucose intolerance, osteoporosis, avascular necrosis, myopathy, and posterior subcapsular cataracts. The risk of these serious complications of steroid therapy is related to the dose and duration of treatment. Short-term use (7–10 days) of even high-dose (30–40 mg prednisone or equivalent) corticosteroids has not been associated with major adverse effects. Long-acting injectable preparations of glucocorticoids, such as triamcinolone hexacetonide and tertiary butyl acetate esters, are locally effective, with little systemic absorption.[61]

Two serious potential adverse reactions to injected corticosteroids are most feared: infection and tendon or ligamentous rupture.[61,62] With aseptic technique, infection is extremely rare (.005% in a large series of intraarticular injections).[63] Tendon rupture following injection of an inflamed tendon sheath is also uncommon. Tensile strength of a tendon may be reduced transiently by as much as 40% following injection.[62] Other adverse reactions to injected corticosteroids include atrophy of overlying skin and soft tissue at the injection site and (with intra-articular injections) a postinjection "flare" related to corticosteroid crystal-induced synovitis. Multiple intra-articular injections may accelerate degenerative changes in the joint. This problem may be related to direct effect of steroid on articular cartilage, as well as overuse of a damaged joint. Intraarticular injections should probably be limited to three or four per year in any weight-bearing joint.

Of even greater concern than with nonsteroidal antiinflammatory therapy in sports injury is the possibility that corticosteroids might suppress components of the inflammatory response important in the healing process. In particular, steroid inhibition of macrophage function might slow removal of cellular debris and interfere with collagen (scar) formation. Limiting the duration of steroid therapy reduces the possibility of this complication.

Corticosteroids should be considered in treatment of acute musculoskeletal injury when NSAIDs are contraindicated or have been ineffective. Clinical trials comparing steroids, NSAIDs, and analgesics in sports trauma are lacking, and treatment is empirical. Comparisons of oral and injected steroids in musculoskeletal trauma in terms of efficacy and toxicity have not been made. There is controversy regarding the efficacy of both intraspinal steroids and facet joint injections.[64–67] These techniques are intended for short-term symptom control so that the patient can participate in active rehabilitation. The decision to use intraspinal versus oral steroids is economic as well as clinical. Intraspinal steroids are clearly more costly and are probably less likely to cause side effects. Studies comparing efficacy of these two modalities have not been done.

ANTIDEPRESSANTS

Tricyclic antidepressants are widely used in the management of chronic pain. Chronic musculoskeletal pain, as well as headache, facial pain, and diabetic neuropathy, has been demonstrated to respond to some degree to treatment with these agents.[68–71] Originally, it was believed that the therapeutic effect of TCAs was related to their antidepressant properties, which, by improving mood, enhanced the efficacy of coadministered analgesics. Analgesic efficacy of TCAs at doses below those needed to achieve psychotropic effects and improvement in pain without demonstrable change in depression suggests that another mechanism of action for pain relief is operative. TCAs block presynaptic reuptake of monamine neurotransmitters such as serotonin, increasing their action at the postsynaptic receptor site. This is believed to affect pain modulation. Sedating antidepressants may also modulate pain perception by augmenting non-REM, phase 4 sleep, a mechanism believed to contribute to the efficacy of TCAs in patients with fibromyalgia.[72,73]

Side effects vary in frequency and intensity according to the specific drug, and there is significant patient variability. Excess daytime sedation, dry mouth, difficulty with visual accommodation, urinary retention, constipation, weight gain, and orthostatic hypotension are adverse effects associated with TCA therapy.

The efficacy of TCAs in the treatment of chronic musculoskeletal pain is reasonably well established.[74–76] Effects are modest in such patients, and significant changes in functional status beyond analgesia have not been demonstrated. It is unclear from these trials and others whether improvement is related to analgesia, antidepressant effects, or even improvement in sleep. No studies have evaluated the effect of TCA therapy in acute pain syndromes.

Clearly, TCAs do not have a role in the management of acute sports injury. However, in patients with more chronic musculoskeletal pain, antidepressant therapy may be useful. TCAs should definitely be considered when pain, depression, or sleep disturbance coexist. Therapy should begin with low bedtime dosing and should be titrated upward slowly, depending on patient response. Endpoints include improvement in restorative sleep, reduction in pain, improvement in mood, and improvement in ability to participate in reconditioning and rehabilitative activities. Antidepressants can be administered as adjuncts to other analgesics, such as NSAIDs.

REFERENCES

1. Kellet J. Acute soft tissue injuries—a review of the literature. *Med Sci Sports Exer.* 1986;18:489–500.

2. Almekinders LC. Anti-inflammatory treatment of muscular injuries in sports. *Sports Med.* 1993;15:139–145.

3. Calabrese LH, Rooney TW. The use of nonsteroidal anti-inflammatory drugs in sports. *Physician Sports Med.* 1986;14:89–97.

4. Warhol MJ, Siegel AJ, Evans WJ, Silverman LM. Skeletal muscle injury and repair in marathon runners after completion. *Am J Pathol.* 1985;118:331–339.

5. Acute Pain Management Guideline Panel. *Acute Pain Management: Operative or Medical Procedures and Trauma. Clinical Practice Guideline.* AHCPR Pub. No. 92-00332. Rockville, MD: Agency for Health Care Policy and Human Research, Public Health Service, U.S. Dept. of Health and Human Services. February 1992.

6. Kantor TG. Control of pain by nonsteroidal antiinflammatory drugs. *Med Clin North Am.* 1982;66:1053–1059.

7. Hyman SE, Cassem NH. Current topics in medicine: pain. In: Rubensein E, Federman DD, eds. *Scientific American Medicine.* New York: Scientific American; 1989;2:1–17.

8. Portenoy RK. Chronic opioid therapy in nonmalignant pain. *J Pain Symptom Manage.* 1990;5:46–61.

9. Savage SR. Addiction in the treatment of pain: significance, recognition and management. *J Pain Symptom Manage.* 1993;8:265–278.

10. Indelicato PA. Comparison of diflunisal and acetaminophen with codeine in the treatment of mild to moderate pain due to strains and sprains. *Clin Ther.* 1986;8:269–274.

11. Abbott CJA, Bouchier-Hayes TAI, Hunt HA. A comparison of the efficacy of naproxen sodium and a paracetamol/dextropropoxyphene combination in the treatment of soft-tissue disorders. *Br J Sports Med.* 1980;14:213–218.

12. Brooks PM, Day RO. Nonsteroidal antiinflammatory drugs—differences and similarities. *N Engl J Med.* 1991;324:1716–1725.

13. Weiler JM. Medical modifiers of sports injury. The use of nonsteroidal anti-inflammatory drugs (NSAIDs) in sports soft-tissue injury. *Clin Sports Med.* 1992;11:625–644.

14. Furst DE. Are there differences among nonsteroidal antiinflammatory drugs? Comparing acetylated salicylates, and nonacetylated nonsteroidal antiinflammatory drugs. *Arthritis Rheum.* 1994;37:1–9.

15. Mazanec DJ. Conservative treatment of rheumatic disorders in the elderly. *Geriatrics.* 1991;46:41–45.

16. Vane JR. Inhibition of prostaglandin synthesis as a mechanism of action for aspirin-like drugs. *Nature.* 1971;231:232–235.

17. Goodwin JS, Ceuppens JL, Rodriquez MA. Effect of non-steroidal anti-inflammatory agents on immunologic function in patients with rheumatoid arthritis. *JAMA*. 1983;25:2485–2488.

18. Abramson SB, Weissman G. The mechanisms of action of nonsteroidal antiinflammatory drugs. *Arthritis Rheum*. 1989;32:1–9.

19. Huskisson EC. How to choose a non-steroidal antiinflammatory drug. *Clin Rheum Dis*. 1984;10:313–323.

20. Huskisson EC, Woolf DL, Balme HW, Scott J, Franklyn S. Four new antiinflammatory drugs: responses and variations. *Br Med J*. 1976; 1:1048–1049.

21. Scott DL, Roden S, Marshall T, Kendall MJ. Variations in response to nonsteroidal antiinflammatory drugs. *Br J Clin Pharmacol*. 1982; 14:691–694.

22. Greene JM, Winickoff RN. Cost-conscious prescribing of nonsteroidal anti-inflammatory drugs for adults with arthritis. *Arch Intern Med*. 1992;152:1995–2002.

23. Loeb DS, Ahlquist DA, Talley NJ. Management of gastro-duodenopathy associated with use of nonsteroidal anti-inflammatory drugs. *Mayo Clin Proc*. 1992;67:354–364.

24. Roth SH, Bennett RE. Nonsteroidal anti-inflammatory drug gastropathy. Recognition and response. *Arch Intern Med*. 1987;147:2093–2100.

25. Gibson GR, Whitacre EB, Ricotti CA. Colitis induced by nonsteroidal anti-inflammatory drugs. Report of four cases and review of the literature. *Arch Intern Med*. 1992;152:625–632.

26. Soll AH, Weinstein WM, Kurata J, McCarty D. NSAIDs and peptic ulcer disease. *Ann Intern Med*. 1991;114:307–319.

27. Fries JF, Williams CA, Bloch DA, Michel BA. NSAID-associated gastropathy: incidence and risk factor models. *Am J Med*. 1991;91:213–221.

28. Carson JL, Strom BL, Soper KA, West SL, Morse ML. The association of nonsteroidal anti-inflammatory drugs with upper gastrointestinal tract bleeding. *Arch Intern Med*. 1987;147:85–88.

29. Griffin MR, Ray WA, Schaffner W. Nonsteroidal anti-inflammatory drug use and death from peptic ulcer in elderly persons. *Ann Intern Med*. 1988;109:359–363.

30. Larkai EN, Smith JL, Lidsky MD, Graham DY. Gastroduodenal mucosa and dyspeptic symptoms in arthritic patients during chronic nonsteroidal anti-inflammatory drug use. *Am J Gastroenterol*. 1987; 82:1153–1158.

31. Pounder R. Silent peptic ulceration: deadly silence or golden silence? *Gastroenterology*. 1989;96:626–631.

32. Walt RP. Misoprostol for the treatment of peptic ulcer and anti-inflammatory drug-induced gastroduodenal ulceration. *N Engl J Med*. 1992;327:1575–1580.

33. Clive DM, Stoff JS. Renal syndromes associated with nonsteroidal antiinflammatory drugs. *N Engl J Med*. 1984;310:563–572.

34. Blackshear JL, Napier JS, Davidman M, Stillman NT. Renal complications of nonsteroidal antiinflammatory drugs: identification and monitoring of those at risk. *Semin Arthritis Rheum*. 1985;14:163–175.

35. Ciabattoni G, Cinotti GA, Pierucci A, et al. Effects of sulindac and ibuprofen in patients with chronic glomerular disease. *N Engl J Med*. 1984;310:279–283.

36. Roberts DG, Gerber JG, Barnes JS, Zerbe GO, Nies AS. Sulindac is not renal sparing in man. *Clin Pharmacol Ther*. 1985;38:258–265.

37. Cinquergrani MP, Liang C. Indomethacin attenuates the hypotensive action of hydralazine. *Clin Pharmacol Ther*. 1986;39:564–570.

38. Hoppman RA, Peden JG, Ober SK. Central nervous system side effects of nonsteroidal anti-inflammatory drugs. *Arch Intern Med*. 1991; 151:1309–1313.

39. Almekinders LC. The efficacy of nonsteroidal anti-inflammatory drugs in the treatment of ligament injuries. *Sports Med*. 1990;9:137–142.

40. Huskisson EC, Berry H, Street FC, Medhurst HE. Indomethacin for soft-tissue injuries. A double-blind study in football players. *Rheumatol Rehabil*. 1973;12:159–160.

41. van Marion WF. Indomethacin in the treatment of soft tissue lesions. *J Int Med Res*. 1973;1:151–158.

42. McLatchie GR, Allister C, Hamilton G, McGregor H, Colquhuon I, Pickvance NJ. Variable schedules of ibuprofen for ankle sprains. *Br J Sports Med*. 1985;19:203–206.

43. Hutson MA. A double-blind study comparing ibuprofen 1800 mg or 2400 mg daily and placebo in sports injuries. *J Int Med Res*. 1986;14:142–146.

44. Fredberg U, Hansen PA, Skinhoj A. Ibuprofen in the treatment of acute ankle joint injuries. A double-blind study. *Am J Sports Med*. 1989; 17:564–566.

45. Lereim P, Gabor I. Piroxicam and naproxen in acute sports injuries. *Am J Med*. 1988;84(suppl5A):45–49.

46. Almekinders LC, Gilbert JA. Healing of experimental muscle strains and the effects of nonsteroidal antiinflammatory medication. *Am J Sports Med*. 1986;14:303–308.

47. Obremsky WT, Seaber AV, Ribbeck BM, Garrett WE. Biomechanical and histologic assessment of a controlled muscle strain injury treated with piroxicam. *Am J Sports Med*. 1994;22:558–561.

48. Abramson S. Mechanism of action of nonsteroidal anti-inflammatory drugs and therapeutic considerations. *Bull Hosp Jt Dis Orthop Inst*. 1990;50:107–115.

49. Palmoski MJ, Brandt KD. Effect of salicylate on proteoglycan metabolism in normal canine articular cartilage in vitro. *Arthritis Rheum*. 1979;22:746–754.

50. Palmoski MJ, Brandt KD. Effects of some nonsteroidal antiinflammatory drugs on proteoglycan metabolism and organization in canine articular cartilage. *Arthritis Rheum*. 1980;23:1010–1020.

51. Robinson JP, Brown PB. Medications in low back pain. *Phys Med Rehabil Clin North Am*. 1991;2:97–126.

52. Elenbaas JK. Centrally acting oral skeletal muscle relaxants. *Am J Hosp Pharm*. 1980;37:1313–1323.

53. Stern FH. A controlled comparison of three muscle relaxant agents. *Clin Med*. 1964;71:367–372.

54. Brown BR, Womble J. Cyclobenzaprine in intractable pain syndromes with muscle spasm. *JAMA*. 1978;240:1151–1152.

55. Basmajian JV. Cyclobenzaprine hydrochloride effect on skeletal muscle spasm in the lumbar region and neck: two double blind controlled clinical and laboratory studies. *Arch Phys Med Rehabil*. 1978;59:58–63.

56. Basmajian JV. Acute back pain and spasm. A controlled multicenter trial of combined analgesic and antispasm agents. *Spine*. 1989;14:438–439.

57. Tisdale SA, Ervin DK. Controlled clinical trial of Robaxisal. *Curr Ther Res Clin Exp*. 1978;23:166–172.

58. Walker JM. Value of an acetaminophen-chlorzoxazone combination (Parafon Forte) in the treatment of acute musculoskeletal disorders. *Curr Ther Res Clin Exp*. 1973;15:248–252.

59. Borenstein DG, Lacks S, Wiesel SW. Cyclobenzaprine and naproxen versus naproxen alone in the treatment of acute low back pain and muscle spasm. *Clin Ther*. 1990;12:125–132.

60. Robinson DR. Prostaglandins and the mechanism of action of anti-inflammatory drugs. *Am J Med*. 1983;26:26–31.

61. Gatter RA. Arthrocentesis technique and intrasynovial therapy. In: McCarty DJ, Koopman WJ, eds. *Arthritis and Allied Conditions. A*

Textbook of Rheumatology. Philadelphia: Lea & Febiger; 1993:711–720.

62. Fitzgerald RH. Intrasynovial injection of steroids. *Mayo Clin Proc*. 1976;51:655–659.

63. Hollander JL, Jessar RA, Brown EM Jr. Intra-synovial corticosteroid therapy: a decade of use. *Bull Rheum Dis*. 1961;11:239–240.

64. Dilke TFW, Burry HC, Grahame R. Extradural corticosteroid injection in management of lumbar nerve root compression. *Br Med J*. 1973;2:635–637.

65. Yates DW. A comparison of the types of epidural injection commonly used in the treatment of low back pain and sciatica. *Rheum Rehabil*. 1978;17:181–186.

66. Cuckler JM, Bernini PA, Wiesel SW, Booth RE, Rothman RH, Pickens GT. The use of epidural steroids in treatment of lumbar radicular pain. *J Bone Joint Surg*. 1985;67A:63–66.

67. Carette S, Marcoux S, Truchon R, et al. A controlled trial of corticosteroid injections into facet joints for chronic low back pain. *N Engl J Med*. 1991;325:1002–1007.

68. France RD, Houpt JL, Ellinwood EH. Therapeutic effects of antidepressants in chronic pain. *Gen Hosp Psychiatry*. 1984;6:55–63.

69. Jenkins DG, Ebbutt AF, Evans CD. Tofranil in the treatment of low back pain. *J Int Med Res*. 1976;4(supp):28–40.

70. Rosenblatt RM, Reich J, Dehring D. Tricyclic antidepressants in treatment of depression and chronic pain: analysis of the supporting evidence. *Anesth Analg*. 1984;63:1025–1032.

71. Getto CJ, Sorkness CA, Howell T. Antidepressants and chronic nonmalignant pain: a review. *J Pain Symptom Manage*. 1987;2:9–18.

72. Bennett RM, Gatter RA, Campbell SM, Andrews RP, Clark SR, Scarola JA. A comparison of cyclobenzaprine and placebo in the management of fibrositis. *Arthritis Rheum*. 1988;31:1535–1542.

73. Carette S, Bell MJ, Reynolds WJ, et al. Comparison of amitriptyline, cyclobenzaprine, and placebo in the treatment of fibromyalgia. *Arthritis Rheum*. 1994;37:32–40.

74. Ward NG, Bloom VL, Friedel RO. The effectiveness of tricyclic antidepressants in the treatment of coexisting pain and depression. *Pain*. 1979;7:331–341.

75. Ward NG. Tricyclic antidepressants for chronic low back pain. Mechanisms of action and predictors of response. *Spine*. 1986;11:661–665.

76. Zitman FG, Linssen ACG, Edelborek PM, Steynen TM. Low-dose amitriptyline in chronic pain: the gain is modest. *Pain*. 1990;42:35–42.

CHAPTER 6

The Effective Use of Rehabilitation Modalities

Joel M. Press and Beven Pace Livingston

INTRODUCTION

The number of therapeutic modalities used in the rehabilitation environment is increasing. Such modalities include forms of heat, cold, electricity, light, water, and any mechanical means that promote healing. These modalities help in minimizing time lost due to injury, which is a major goal of patients and rehabilitation professionals. Unfortunately, in rehabilitation practice, many of the modalities are often applied without an understanding of the principles that relate to a particular modality, such as when it is indicated and contraindicated, and how it should be properly used. When used by the rehabilitation professional as part of a comprehensive rehabilitation program and when the subjective and unique responses of each patient are abided by, modalities can be very helpful.

In this chapter, the therapeutic and physical principles, therapeutic responses, and clinical applications, as well as the cautions and contraindications of these various modalities will be discussed.

HEAT MODALITIES

Superficial Heating

Heat may be transferred to body tissue using conduction, convection, or conversion. Conduction and convection are forms of superficial heat.

Hydrocollator packs transfer heat using conduction. These packs are heated in steel containers with water temperatures between 65 and 90 degrees Centigrade.[1] They maintain heat for about 30 minutes, and treatment sessions usually last 20–30 minutes. Other convection modes include hot water bottles, electric heating pads, and chemical packs, but these have the disadvantage of limited temperature control.

Whirlpools and Hubbard tanks transfer heat using convection. The body part or the entire body is submerged in heated water. Due to increased risk of elevating the patient's core body temperature, the water temperature for Hubbard tanks rarely exceeds 40 degrees Centigrade for total body immersion.

Cautions/Contraindications

Before deciding to use heat as a therapeutic modality, it is important to assess the patient's sensitivity to temperature, pain, and circulation status. Patients with circulatory impairment or arterial disease should not be treated with superficial heat as they are at a high risk for tissue burns.[2]

Also, patients with body areas prone to increased bleeding should not be treated with superficial heating agents. These patients include those with hemophilia and individuals experiencing an acute stage of inflammation.

Finally, superficial heat should not be used in areas of decreased sensation or on those individuals who suffer heat sensitivity or heat illness. Exhibit 6–1 summarizes these contraindications.

Misuses

The most common misuse of heat occurs when deciding whether to use heat or cold, superficial or deep heat, and moist or dry heat.

Factors to be considered include: (1) stage of injury; (2) area of the body to be treated; (3) medical status; and (4) patient preference. Cold is preferred during acute stages of inflammation. In contrast, heat may be better tolerated psychologically by individuals with pain or muscle spasm. Temperature elevation increases collagen extensibility and decreases joint stiffness, so heat is a better choice.

The decision to use superficial or deep heat depends on the location and degree of temperature elevation. Many individuals claim moist heat is more penetrating than dry heat. Few clinical studies have examined this question, however.

Exhibit 6–1 General Contraindications to Therapeutic Heat

- Not to be used when the individual is unable to safely report sensation of pain
- Not to be used over anesthetic regions
- Not to be used in individuals with bleeding tendencies
- Not to be used over areas with diminished circulation due to inability for adequate blood flow to meet demands of increased metabolism
- Not to be used in the acute stages of inflammation or trauma

Shortwave and Microwave Diathermy

Diathermy, or deep-heating modalities, use conversion to heat deeper body tissues.

Cautions/Contraindications

Special consideration should be given to the use of diathermy as a deep-heating modality because it is difficult to treat localized body areas and because the dosage is subjective. The applicator for both shortwave and microwave diathermy should *never* come in contact with the skin. If a deep aching sensation is reported by the patient during treatment, overheating may be indicated. It is important that the operator pay attention when using this modality so that the patient's pain tolerance is not exceeded. The absolute contraindications are similar to those of other thermomodalities and are listed in Exhibit 6–2.

Misuses

Diathermy as a modality has become fairly obsolete with the advent of ultrasound as a form of deep-heating modality.[3]

CRYOTHERAPY

Using cold for therapeutic treatment results in vasoconstriction with vasodilation following reflexively, decreased local metabolism, and minimized enzymatic activity and oxygen demand.[1,4] Cold treatments are used for pain control and for decreasing muscle spasticity and guarding.[1,4] Because cold increases connective tissue stiffness and muscle viscosity, it diminishes flexibility. Cryotherapy is usually applied during the first 48 hours of acute musculoskeletal injuries to decrease the inflammatory response.

Cold Bath/Whirlpools

This method of cryotherapy is preferred for cooling the feet, ankles, hands, arms, and elbows, typically during cryo-

Exhibit 6–2 Contraindications and Precautions for the Use of Shortwave and Microwave Diathermy

- Not to be used over mental implants, jewelry, or when IUDs are present
- Not to be applied over the pelvis during pregnancy or menstruation
- Not to be used with cardiac pacemakers, due to potential for electrical interference
- Not to be used over the eyes
- Not to be used over open wounds, moist dressings, or areas of increased perspiration, due to selective heating effects
- Not to be used over epiphyseal growth plates in children
- Not to be used over the gonads
- Not to be used over an area of infection due to potential spread
- To be used with caution in the obese individual, due to selective heating of the subcutaneous fat

kinetics. While the optimum temperature is not known, the recommended temperature is between 33 and 59 degrees Fahrenheit.[5]

Cold Machines

Various appliances exist in the marketplace that have reservoirs for holding ice and water; the chilled fluid is circulated through pads that are applied to the body. These appliances provide cold and compression and are used postoperatively or for acute injuries.

Cautions/Contraindications

Cryotherapy, like other modalities, is not without problems. However, fear of misusing it by rehabilitation professionals causes treatment sessions to be too conservative, and, as a result, patients do not receive the full treatment benefit.[5] Rehabilitation professionals fear inducing frostbite from direct application of ice packs and or gel-packs to the skin. Most of the current cryotherapy techniques are probably not cold enough to cause tissue damage unless they are used continuously for one hour or more or combined with pressure.[2,5,6] Gel-packs, however, are an exception because they are much colder. There should be an inverse relationship between the intensity of cold and the duration of exposure.[5]

Another problem with cold application is nerve palsy or neuropraxia. Drez[7] reported a case of nerve palsy using cryotherapy in 1981. He postulated that it was due to ice application in close proximity to a superficial nerve. Knight[5] did a follow-up study and concluded that it was the pressure that resulted in the decreased blood flow (ischemia) to the nerve. Knight estimated that this problem occurs in less than .001% of instances in which cold packs are used.

Cold hypersensitivity is another contraindication to cold therapy. Clinicians should be especially careful when using cryotherapy to treat a person who suffers from cold hypersensitivity; the patient should make the choice about whether to use it or not. Individuals who suffer from vasospastic disorders such as Raynaud's disease should *never* be treated with cryotherapy, as it could result in ischemic necrosis. Exhibit 6–3 presents the cautions and contraindications for cryotherapy.

Misuses

Some standard recommendations about the use of cryotherapy are probably misleading. One recommendation is to limit ice application to 20 minutes, which will not provide adequate time to cool the injured tissue for most injuries. Another is the rule never to apply ice directly to the skin. In most cases, this results in less than optimal cooling. Care should be taken when using commercial gel-packs, as they are sometimes many degrees below freezing and should not be applied over superficial nerves. Finally, some individuals advise avoiding compression when applying ice. Actually, it is imperative to combine cold and compression in the immediate care of musculoskeletal injuries.

ELECTROTHERAPY

Therapeutic electricity has been used to treat musculoskeletal problems for a long time. Electrical devices can put out alternating current (AC), as in most household appliances, or direct current (DC), as in a generator or battery.

Direct current can be continuous or intermittent. It can also have different wave forms, frequencies, durations, and amplitudes; adjustments in these parameters affect the quality, type, and form of electrical stimulation received.

Muscle and nerve have different responses to electrical stimulation. For instance, nerve stimulation needs a current that rises quickly to maximum intensity, and high frequencies and short durations are used. Muscle, however, can be stimulated with very slowly rising currents.

Many different electrotherapeutic modalities, such as galvanic stimulation and iontophoresis, are available for treating sport injuries. Their uses vary widely among physical therapists and athletic trainers, and many times they are based on anecdotal and empirical support rather than scientific research. The efficacy of these modalities has been the topic of considerable debate in the rehabilitation community. Yet a role exists for these electrotherapeutic modalities in rehabilitation. A summary of the different electrotherapeutic modalities and their general indications is shown in Exhibits 6–4 and 6–5.

Exhibit 6–4 Forms of Therapeutic Electricity

- Galvanic stimulation (direct current)
- Faradic stimulation (alternating current)
- Iontophoresis
- Electrical muscle stimulation
- Transcutaneous electrical nerve stimulation
- Interferential current
- Neuroprobe™
- Electro-Accuscope™

Exhibit 6–5 General Indications for Therapeutic Electricity

- Decrease muscle atrophy due to immobilization or partial denervation
- Decrease muscle spasm and guarding
- Promote tissue healing
- Increase local blood flow
- Decrease edema
- Decrease pain
- Drive ions into the skin and subcutaneous tissue
- Promote muscle relaxation

Exhibit 6–3 Contraindications to Cryotherapy

- Cold hypersensitivity

    Raynaud's phenomenon

    Cold urticaria

    Cryoglobulinemia

    Paroxysmal cold hemoglobinuria

- Circulatory compromise
- Anesthetic skin
- Cardiovascular/respiratory disease

Cautions/Contraindications

Electrotherapeutic modalities should be applied using solid clinical judgment. Two contraindications to the use of electrical stimulation have been clearly stated by the Food and Drug Administration.[8] Transcutaneous electric nerve stimulation (TENS) and neuromuscular electric stimulation (NMES) should not be used for patients with a synchronous cardiac pacemaker. In addition, they should not be applied over the carotid sinus because stimulation of the vasovagal reflex could result in hypotensive response or cardiac arrest.

Because the effect of electrical stimulation on fetal development and health has not been defined, the use of NMES on the abdominal or lumbar region of a patient who is pregnant is not recommended.

Another area of concern is the placement of electrodes over or close to an incision site or recent scar, as this could impair healing. Scar tissue has a higher impedance, which could result in skin irritation or in an electrochemical burn. Any form of electricity should be avoided near an area of acute injury if there is active bleeding to prevent worsening the hemorrhage. In any area where there is a sensory deficit of the skin, electrical stimulation should be avoided to prevent local burns.

Further cautions should be taken when arterial disease, deep vein thrombosis, local infection, or malignant tumor are present. All the contraindications are listed in Exhibit 6–6.

Misuses

Improper electrode placement is a common problem in the use of electrotherapeutic modalities. Electrode placement over significant adipose tissue can significantly impede cur-

---

Exhibit 6–6 Contraindications to Electrical Stimulation of Muscle or Nerve

- Anesthetic areas
- Incompletely healed wounds
- Areas where metal is imbedded close to the skin
- Active bleeding
- Cardiac pacemakers
- Pregnancy
- The carotid sinus
- Sensitive mucous membranes
- The eyes

---

rent flow and prevent effective treatment.[8] Skin irritation may be caused by improper electrode-skin interface. Thermal burns can occur if the current density is too high beneath or between electrodes. Smaller electrodes have higher current density. To decrease the possibility of skin irritation or burn, the clinician should use a larger electrode, uniform contact with a conducting medium, and an interelectrode distance at least equal to the size of the electrodes.[9]

ULTRASOUND

Ultrasound involves sound waves classified within the acoustic spectrum above 20,000 Hz (cycles per second). The production of heat is due to high-frequency alternating electric current (0.8–1.0 MHz), which is converted via a crystal transducer to acoustic vibrations. Energy transfer occurs as the crystal undergoes changes in shape when voltage is applied, creating vibrations that pass through the tissue being treated.

Cautions/Contraindications

Ultrasound is generally considered to be safe. Many of the harmful effects of ultrasound are associated with dosages beyond the recommended therapeutic ranges.

Because the harm would exceed the benefit, ultrasound is contraindicated for use over the uterus during pregnancy; over the eyes, due to possible cataract production; in thrombophlebitic conditions; and in peripheral vascular disease or loss of sensation as the thermal response might not be apparent.[2,10]

Use of ultrasound on immature epiphyses is also not recommended. There have been conflicting reports about this in the medical literature. Vaughen and Bender[11] found no effect on the closure time or integrity in rabbits. De Forest and associates[12] reported increased chondroblast activity that resulted in widening, slipping, and fracture of the tibial epiphysis in rabbits at doses of 5–10 W. The literature suggests that therapeutic ranges may be safe, but the benefits to the patient must outweigh the risks.

Ultrasound should not be used over the brain and spine, due to the increased possibility of cavitation in fluid-filled cavities and vascular compromise in the cord and meninges.[10] Ultrasound should not be used over the reproductive organs, pacemakers, the heart, in acute inflammation or infection, or over malignancies (Exhibit 6–7).

Misuses

Some common problems exist with the therapeutic use of ultrasound. One frequent mistake often made by rehabilitation professionals is in treating too large an area. Also, it is

Exhibit 6–7 Contraindications to Ultrasound Use

- Acute injury

- Not to be used over fluid-filled cavities due to risk of cavitation

    Eye

    Heart

    Uterus

    Testes

- Avoid over epiphyseal growth plates or healing fractures

- Avoid over joint replacements with methyl methacrylate

- Avoid in the presence of an acute herniated disc with radiculopathic findings

---

important to know the crystal size versus the sound head size. This information is usually given in the machine specifications under "Effective Radiating Area" (ERA). The treatment area should not exceed two times the ERA.[13]

Other common errors are made when inappropriate treatment time is selected with preset intensities. Many have thought that the longer the treatment time and the higher the intensity, the greater the temperature increase. However, this is variable and depends on the frequency of the ultrasound unit. Draper et al[13] demonstrated in their study that to achieve the tissue temperature rise of 4 degrees Centigrade, a marked increase in intensity and treatment time (1 MHz at 1.5 W/cm^2=13 min, 3 MHz at 1.5 W/cm^2=4.5 min) was required.

Another widespread misconception has to do with the depth of the target tissue. It is thought that the higher the intensity, the deeper the penetration. Actually, this is a function of the frequency of the ultrasound beam. Typically, 1 MHz ultrasound is used to heat tissues 2.5–5.0 cm deep, and 3 MHz ultrasound is used to heat tissues less than 2.5 cm.[14]

Other errors include ignoring the stretch window, icing prior to treatment, using unresearched coupling agents, and moving the sound head too fast. Care must be taken when using ultrasound for treating an acute injury. Deep heating of an acutely injured tissue, such as an acutely herniated disc, can increase the inflammatory response and exacerbate the problem, and is contraindicated.

It is recommended that the patient stretch prior to treatment and up to 2–3 minutes afterward to maximize the heating effect. Icing before treatment only creates greater skin temperature difference to overcome. The clinician should move the sound head as slowly as possible without causing the patient pain (approximately 4 cm/sec). Burning the patient may be due to a poor beam nonuniformity ratio (BMR), which can create hot spots.

TRACTION

This technique uses a distractive force on a particular body part to stretch soft tissues and to separate joint surfaces or bone fragments. Traction was popularized in the 1950s as a treatment for lumbar disc lesions.

Cautions/Contraindications

The contraindications to treating with traction include patients with spinal tumors, bone disease, infection, osteoporosis, and rheumatoid arthritis. Additionally, cervical segmental instability or acute ligamentous injury are conditions in which traction would not be indicated as it may perpetuate the instability or cause further strain (Exhibit 6–8).

Misuses

With traction, the most common misuse during treatment occurs during patient setup, which includes the positioning of the patient, the amount of weight or force of pull, duration and frequency of treatment, and continuous versus intermittent traction.

Body position has been reported to have a large impact on traction results. Generally, the neutral spine position of the lumbar spine allows for the largest intervertebral foramen opening and is usually the position of choice. Saunder[15] recommends the prone position as the position of choice in disc protrusions as it allows the easy application of other modalities and is an easier way to assess the amount of spinous process separation. When applying traction in the supine position, the hip position was found to affect vertebral separation. As the degree of hip flexion increased from 0 to 90 degrees, traction produced greater posterior intervertebral separation.[16] When positioning patients for cervical traction,

---

Exhibit 6–8 Contraindications to the Use of Traction

- Spinal neoplasms or metastasis

- Segmental instability

- Spinal infections

- Acute ligamentous injuries

- Osteoporosis

- Rheumatoid arthritis

---

it is very important to place the patient's neck in the proper position (20–30 degrees of flexion) to impart the proper pull along the cervical spine.[1]

The amount of force necessary when performing lumbar traction should be at least one-fourth of the patient's body weight to overcome the friction of the patient on a table. Traction imparts little movement on the lumbar spine without large forces, usually in the range of a patient's body weight. These high forces pose no danger to the lumbar spine components unless they exceed 440 pounds.[17] However, there is a tendency for lumbar traction to cause the nucleus pulposus to imbibe fluid, to increase pressure in the disc, and to increase patients' symptoms. Less force should be used on the initial treatments and it should be determined whether there are any negative effects. It makes sense that the forces necessary to impact movement in the

cervical spine are much less, approximately 20–50 pounds. Greater separation is expected in younger patients than in older ones, and in the lower cervical segments versus the upper.[17]

Duration of treatment times is only partially research-based. When treating disc-related symptoms, duration should start at 10 minutes. If this is successful, treatment time should remain at that length. However, if it is only partially successful or not successful at all, treatment time should be increased up to 30 minutes.[1]

Finally, good results have been reported with both continuous and intermittent traction. Continuous traction should be used to relieve muscle spasm or disc pressure. Intermittent traction is more easily tolerated and creates a massage effect, which can be helpful for a patient who is new to treatment with traction.

REFERENCES

1. Prentice W. *Therapeutic Modalities in Sports Medicine.* 2nd ed. St. Louis, MO: Mosby–Year Book; 1990.

2. Michlovitz S, ed. *Thermal Agents in Rehabilitation.* Philadelphia: FA Davis; 1990.

3. American Academy of Orthopaedic Surgeons. *Athletic Training and Sports Medicine.* 2nd ed. Park Ridge, IL: American Academy of Orthopaedic Surgeons; 1991.

4. Lehman JF. *Therapeutic Heat and Cold.* 3rd ed. Baltimore: Williams & Wilkins; 1982.

5. Knight K. *Cryotherapy in Sport Injury Management.* Champaign, IL: Human Kinetics; 1995.

6. Meeusen R, Lievens P. The use of cryotherapy in sports injuries. *Sports Med.* 1986;3:398–414.

7. Drez D, Faust DC, Evans IP. Cryotherapy and nerve palsy. *Am J Sports Med.* 1981;9:256–257.

8. Gersh MR. *Electrotherapy in Rehabilitation.* Philadelphia: FA Davis; 1992.

9. Balmaseda MT, et al. Burns in functional electrical stimulation: two case reports. *Arch Phys Med Rehabil.* 1987;68:452.

10. Leadbetter W, Buckwalter J, Gordon S, eds. *Sports-Induced Inflammation.* Park Ridge, IL: American Academy of Orthopaedic Surgeons; 1990.

11. Vaughen JL, Bender LF. Effects of ultrasound on growing bone. *Arch Phys Med Rehabil.* 1959;40:158–160.

12. De Forest RE, Herrick JF, Janes JM, et al. Effects of ultrasound on growing bone: an experimental study. *Arch Phys Med Rehabil.* 1953;34:21–30.

13. Draper DO, Castel JC, Castel D. Rate of temperature increase in human muscle during 1-MHz and 3-MHz continuous ultrasound. *JOSPT.* 1995;22:142–150.

14. Gann N. Ultrasound: current concepts. *Clin Manage.* 1991;11(4):64–69.

15. Saunder HD. Use of spinal traction in the treatment of neck and back conditions. *Clin Orthop.* 1983;179:31–38.

16. Reilly J, et al. Pelvic femoral position on vertebral separation produced by lumbar traction. *Phys Ther.* 1979;59:282–286.

17. Mathews JA. The effects of spinal traction. *Physiotherapy.* 1972; 58:64–66.

SELECTED READINGS

Bruckner P, Khan K. *Clinical Sports Medicine.* Sydney, Australia: McGraw-Hill; 1993.

Dreyfuss P, Stratton S. The Low-energy laser, electro-acuscope, and neuroprobe. *Phys Sports Med.* 1993;21(8):47–57.

Lake DA. Neuromuscular electrical stimulation: An overview and its application in the treatment of sports injuries. *Sports Med.* 1992;13:320–326.

Snyder-Mackler L, Robinson A. *Clinical Electrophysiology: Electrotherapy and Electrophysiology.* Baltimore: Williams & Wilkins; 1989.

CHAPTER 7

Flexibility Training

Joel S. Saal

INTRODUCTION

Stretching has become a popular prelude to most athletic events. Flexibility training is widely accepted as an essential part of any conditioning program and has been promoted as a means of avoiding injury and improving performance.[1–15] A considerable sport experience and theoretical basis support the importance of adequate flexibility in all athletes.[6,9,16–22] Flexibility training is a two-edged sword, however, as it is not without risk, having the potential to cause significant injury if performed incorrectly.[14, 21–23] It must be approached within a program outlined for the specific needs of the individual athlete's body and sport.

The nature of flexibility is complex, with an interplay of connective tissue biophysics, the neurophysiology of motor control, and human joint kinematics. A flexibility training program should be approached with a view toward the full complement of tissues that must be stretched. Although flexibility clearly plays a role in sports injury and performance,[1,2,4,6,8,12–15, 20,22, 24–37] there is conjecture regarding optimal stretching methods, indications, and measurement. Whereas a great deal of information is available in basic science, the clinical literature is less precise. There is, however, an adequate basis for necessitating flexibility training and for establishing criteria for safe and effective stretching programs.

DEFINITION

For the purposes of this chapter, *flexibility* is defined as "the total achievable excursion (within limits of pain) of a body part through its potential range of motion." This includes the range of motion not only of the major joint involved, but also of all contiguous joints and soft tissues. For example, shoulder girdle flexibility includes glenohumeral,

scapulothoracic, sternoclavicular, acromioclavicular, sternocostal, and costochondral motion, as well as soft tissues of the anterior chest wall (including intercostal musculature). It also includes the periscapular and intrinsic shoulder musculature, and the above-mentioned joints' capsules and attendant ligamentous support.

It is important to clearly establish the differences between flexibility and joint laxity. *Flexibility* refers to extensibility of periarticular tissues to allow normal or physiologic motion of a joint or limb. *Laxity* refers to the stability of a joint, which is dependent on its supporting structures (ligaments, capsule, and bony continuity). Excessive laxity could result from chronic injury or congenital hyperelasticity (eg, Ehlers-Danlos syndrome) of stabilizing capsular structures with the presence of positive instability maneuvers (eg, anterior drawer in knee or ankle, talar tilt, etc.). In general and for the purpose of this chapter, the term *flexibility* refers to the degree of normal motion and *laxity* to the degree of abnormal motion of a given joint.

Adequate flexibility implies an ideal state of length and elasticity of the structures crossing joints and affecting single or multiple joint motion (such as the hamstring muscle crossing the hip and knee joints). The goal of a flexibility training program is to develop adequate flexibility without causing injury or excessive joint laxity. To accomplish this, the program must consider the axis and potential range of motion of the joints involved. This potential range includes all planes of motion of a given joint (within physiologic limits of boundary tissues). Flexibility training includes stretching and mobilization. The term *stretching* is used to define an activity that applies a deforming force along the rotational or translational planes of motion of a joint. It should be performed along the lines of geometry of the joint and within the planes of stability of the joint. Theoretically, joint capsular structures, as well as nonarticular structures, have a basic requirement to maintain optimal elasticity. In the injured athlete, this may assume an even greater significance. A combination of these activities is necessary for complete flexibility training.

DETERMINANTS OF BODY FLEXIBILITY

The determinants of normal joint mobility include both static and dynamic factors. Among the static factors are the type and state of collagen subunits in the tissue, types of intervening tissue (i.e., ligament, tendon, muscle, loose connective tissues), presence or absence of inflammation, and, within limits, the temperature of the tissue. The dynamic factors include voluntary muscle control variables, the length-tension "thermostat" of the musculotendinous unit, and the presence or absence of painful or other inhibitory factors associated with injury. Each of these will be discussed individually in the context of its contribution to flexibility and normal joint mobility.

The muscle-tendon unit is probably the most important target site of flexibility training. It is the basic functional effector unit of motion and must withstand forces greater than body weight delivered over a small area. It is also the major site of injury related to lack of flexibility.[2–4,20,28,38] The muscle-tendon unit includes the full length of the muscle and its supporting tissue, the full length of the tendon and tendon-bone junction, as well as the musculotendinous junction. Specific studies of the forces delivered to these structures separately have not been performed, and precisely which structures are lengthened with each given stretching maneuver is not known. There is conjecture about the relative contribution of various individual tissues, the most widely accepted view being that the greatest role is played by muscle, followed by loose (areolar) connective tissue, then dense connective tissue (ligament and tendon).[39–46] Each of these tissues has the capacity to lengthen in response to an applied force, as is shown with in vivo and in vitro animal studies.[40,42,47–53]

Although muscle differs structurally from the other components of the stretch, there is evidence that its mechanical behavior is in part due to its connective tissue components,[39,43] with some qualification as to what degree this behavior exists in intact muscle under conditions of physiologic loading. Sapega et al[43] argues that muscle behaves primarily in this manner. However, in the awake and alert state, muscle is not relaxed enough or electrically silent at all levels to behave purely in this manner. This is evident in the effectiveness of physiologic maneuvers aimed at neural inhibition for facilitating stretch.[29,54–57] Additionally, the bending stiffness of the trunk is greater in the alert than in the anesthetized state, presumably because of dynamic muscle factors (static contraction), rather than material stiffness.[58] Hill[59,60] theorized that muscles' elastic properties are due to

an elastic component in parallel to the contractile component.

Of the tissues involved in a stretch, muscle probably has the largest capacity for percent lengthening.[11,45,46,61] One study demonstrated a ratio of 95:5% for muscle:tendon length change.[45] However, the capacity of a given tissue for absolute lengthening is not necessarily equivalent to the importance of that tissue in a stretching program. In this regard, tendon may have the greatest significance. Despite its limited capacity for lengthening (2–3% of its length, compared with approximately 20% for muscle),[45–47,62,63] tendon must withstand repeated stresses that require it to be maintained at its optimal length and elasticity. Similarly, fibrous joint capsules supply a significant percentage of overall stiffness of a joint[61] and, therefore, have a minimum requirement for an applied stretching force.

IMPORTANCE OF FLEXIBILITY

The inability to clearly define injuries by a "gold standard" diagnostic test has made it difficult to draw definitive conclusions regarding the relevance of any of the interventions used in daily practice on all levels of sports medicine. Although it has been demonstrated that the application of flexibility programs can prevent muscle injuries,[6,20,24,64] it has been difficult to document the full extent of the observed empirical benefit of flexibility on injury prevention (further divided into categories of major knee injuries, tendinitis, and muscle tears), performance enhancement, and rehabilitation of sports surgeries.

The relationship between degree of flexibility and the occurrence of major knee injuries (ligament disruption, internal derangement) has received a great deal of attention in the literature. The results, however, are far from conclusive. Nicholas[64] demonstrated a correlation between five tests of laxity/flexibility and the occurrence of third-degree muscle strains and major knee injuries in a group of professional football players. There was an increased relative incidence of knee injuries in players with increased joint laxity and an increased incidence of muscle tears in players with poor flexibility. There was no clear separation between flexibility and laxity, however, and subsequent attempts by other authors gave conflicting results. Subsequent studies[32,65,66] found a wide variation in subjective assessment of joint laxity between different trained examiners, with results contrary to those of Nicholas. Numerous clinical studies to date (both prospective cohort studies and retrospective cross-sectional studies) display a general agreement that the major predictive factor for joint injury was a previous joint injury or the presence of excessive joint laxity, and not necessarily inadequate flexibility.[6,9,20,22,38,65,66] A prospective study of a flexibility program in soccer players showed a correlation of improved range of motion and a decrease in muscle tears.[6]

Additionally, this study revealed poorer flexibility in hip range of motion in soccer players than in age-matched controls. A more recent review of all studies of soccer injuries[38] suggested an important role for flexibility in the prevention of injury, especially in older players. Muscle strain and tendinitis are more common in older and less flexible soccer players, and up to 11% of all injuries are related to poor flexibility.[6,38]

There are major injuries incurred as a direct result or indirect result of inadequate flexibility that were not evaluated by any of these studies. There is detailed biomechanical evidence to show that the lower extremity flexibility is needed for prevention of lumbar spine injuries.[67,68] Indeed, there is report of increased frequency of spondylolysis/spondylolisthesis in kindreds with severe hamstring inflexibility.[69] In a given individual with a history of back injury, flexibility plays a vital role in reducing further stresses on the spine. Khalil[70] has shown that flexibility may help reduce pain complaints and improve function in patients with chronic low back pain. Adequate cervical spine mobility and flexibility in both uninjured and injured athletes is important to allow for the normal function of this very complex structure. However, no systematic evaluation of the role of flexibility in spine injury prevention in athletes has been performed. An anthropometric analysis of adolescents with and without back pain found a significant association of lower extremity inflexibility and back symptoms.[71] In the industrial setting, Cady[72] found an inverse relationship between the degree of flexibility and the incidence of back injuries and Workers' Compensation costs in a cohort study of firefighters placed on a fitness program. Considering the high incidence of spine injury and related complaints that exist at all levels of organized football, this is an area that requires investigation.

Again, it is important to distinguish between flexibility and laxity in reference to cervical spine injuries in football. Adequate soft tissue flexibility and intervertebral joint mobility do not imply lack of muscular strength or stability. Improved flexibility allows for a better dynamic stability, which is critical for the prevention of cervical spine injury. In this setting, the presence of adequate flexibility in no way militates against adequate stability.

There are areas of inflexibility common to a large percentage of athletes that contribute to excessive forces at the intervertebral joints, the knee, and the ankle. The iliopsoas and anterior hip soft tissues are frequently overlooked and directly contribute to excessive torque at the intervertebral disk if their inflexibility does not allow for full excursion at hip extension. This requires greater pelvic rotation in both the transverse and the sagittal planes, transferring increased forces across the lower lumbar disk spaces.[67,68] The position of pelvic tilt is also important in improving hamstring muscle flexibility. Patients who performed a hamstring stretch with an anterior pelvic tilt as opposed to a posterior pelvic tilt showed greater improvement in hamstring flexibility regardless of stretching method.[73] The hip rotators have a similar role in indirect injury prevention. The flexibility of the iliotibial band has implications in patellar tracking problems.[5,74] The sternoclavicular and costoclavicular joints, in combination with the anterior chest and chest wall soft tissues, are important for adequate rotation at the level of thoracic spine, in maintenance of thoracic and cervicothoracic posture, and in the prevention of untoward traction on neurovascular structures in the thoracic outlet. This is an area without a quantifiable measure of range of motion or a controlled evaluation of injury prevention.

In the setting of injury, flexibility takes on an even more crucial role in the function of the athlete. Where strength has been lost or pain limits force production, the resistance offered by soft tissues can lead to abnormal movement patterns. The abnormal excursions of joints allow for further adaptive shortening of soft tissues as well as excessive forces on joints, thereby establishing a vicious circle. This is especially common in the spine and shoulder girdle. Restoration of adequate flexibility on a regional basis, along with specific strength and movement training, is the cornerstone of physical rehabilitation. There are, however, situations in which withholding stretching is in order. Craib and associates[75] showed that subelite distance runners who were less flexible in ankle dorsiflexion and standing hip rotation had a more economical gait, as measured by submaximal volume of oxygen utilization ($\dot{V}o_2$). They speculated that inflexibility in certain areas of the musculoskeletal system may enhance running economy in this group of subelite runners by increasing storage and return of elastic energy and minimizing the need for muscle-stabilizing activity. Joint instability should not be treated by mobilization and aggressive stretching. A hypermobile structure requires stabilization, not mobilization. This is an issue commonly faced in spine and shoulder rehabilitation. In the presence of anterior instability of the shoulder, stretching the posterior capsule while allowing for adaptive shortening of the anterior capsule is the program of choice. Conversely, a frozen or severely hypomobile joint requires mobilization (for a capsular stretch), as well as stretch of extra-articular structures. In general, these principles govern the major use of flexibility within rehabilitation of sports and other musculoskeletal injuries.

There appears to be less controversy regarding the importance of inflexibility of soft tissue (i.e., muscle and tendon) in the pathogenesis of tendinitis than in the etiology of major joint injury. It is considered by many researchers to play a causative role in Achilles tendinitis. However, the mechanism of its role is not clear. Although biomechanical properties of tendon have been shown to involve a change in fiber pattern following application of stretching force in vitro, the in vivo event is not certain.[75] The sites of tendinitis have been demonstrated to coincide with areas of relatively lower blood flow than in neighboring portions of tendon.[4,76] There are no data to prove that flexibility training alters that blood flow per se. As previously mentioned, the relative change in length with an applied stretching force for tendon is much smaller than for muscle. Although common stretching maneuvers may deliver some force to the tendon itself, the majority of deformation probably occurs in the muscle bellies.[11,27,45,46] The force generated at the tendon insertion increases in a nonlinear manner as the elasticity of intervening tissues along the lever arm of force decrease.[2-4] However, the symptomatic improvements noted with flexibility programs in the treatment of tendinitis may be due largely to a change in muscle function, rather than simply to a change in the biomechanical profile of the tendon substance. Janda and associates[77] have shown that tight and inflexible muscles can act like an effusion and have an inhibitory effect on antagonist muscle groups. This inhibitory effect occurs through the afferent proprioceptive arc, and preparticipation stretching might decrease facilitation of muscle spindle afferents and assist the facilitation of Golgi tendon organs. Despite the mechanical uncertainties, flexibility training appears to be valuable in the treatment and prevention of many sites of tendinitis.

Despite interest on the part of many experts, there exists little experimental documentation of enhancement of sports performance by improved flexibility. A program of sprint training combined with flexibility training failed to show a significant improvement in running speed, compared with sprint training alone.[65] There is, however, a physiologic basis upon which speed, strength, and agility may be improved with ideal flexibility. The performance of fine and repetitive motor control requires a delicately balanced sensitivity of proprioception ("muscle-tendon memory"), as transmitted through a complex arrangement of receptors in series and in parallel within the muscle and connective tissue architecture. Owing to the plastic nature of collagen-based connective tissue, a regularly applied stretching force will affect the fiber array of collagen and thereby determine the mechanical properties of the musculotendinous or ligament-bone unit. Similarly, the arrangement of tension control receptors and effectors within muscle would also be directly affected by an applied stretching force. In the author's opinion, an ideal state of flexibility in the individual would heighten the sensory feedback mechanism to the athlete's advantage of increased proprioceptive accuracy and sensitivity.

Some variables in performance—such as grace, ease of movement, fluidity, and style—are difficult to measure in a quantitative or isolated manner. These play specific performance roles in dance, gymnastics, and ice and figure skating, but they are becoming more influential in an overall sense of ability in sports such as basketball, football, and soccer.[27] The feedback system of joint proprioceptor and pressure sensors, and the interplay of musculotendinous receptors of stretch (Golgi tendon, intrafusal) underlie this aspect of performance.

It should be noted that delayed muscular soreness may be altered by a flexibility program. Although the etiology of this troublesome condition is controversial and probably multifactorial, there is some evidence that it can be prevented and treated by static stretching.[28,78] Enhancement of the force of muscle contraction has been demonstrated in prestretched muscle, with an increase relative to the degree of prestretch.[2,3,44,79-82] Training methods based on elastic stretch followed by immediate contraction have been developed to capitalize on this observed effect. Although Cavagna et al[81] demonstrated that the greater amount of work performed could not be accounted for purely on the basis of the elastic property of muscle, this type of activity places a greater stress on the elastic component. A study of the effect of intense flexibility training on the function profile of knee extensors revealed no change in maximum force of contraction, but significant improvement was seen in speed of repetitive isometric contractions, relaxation time, and stride frequency on treadmill running.[11] The optimization of muscle performance by improvement in flexibility, therefore, has a theoretical basis.

BIOPHYSICAL ASPECTS OF FLEXIBILITY

The manner in which muscle and connective tissue respond to stretching is a direct reflection of their structure and chemistry. Although they differ in their overall structure, there are similarities that allow each of these tissue types to respond to stretching with a permanent (lasting, but not irreversible) elongation. Muscle is arranged on a cellular level as overlapping filaments of actin-myosin, with a varying number of tropomyosin cross-bridges (Figure 7–1). These are enclosed within the sarcolemma (muscle cell membrane) delineating individual myofibrils. The myofibrils are arranged in parallel and in series within a sequence of connective tissue layers (endomysium, perimysium, then epimysium) to form the whole muscle. Within an individual myofibril, the contractile units are divided into sarcomeres (Figure 7–1).

Connective tissue is composed largely of collagen fibers, which are made up of individual fibrils composed of an overlapping arrangement of tropocollagen subunits (Figure 7–2). The collagen fibers are combined with a smaller number of elastin fibers, woven as a mesh within a matrix ground substance composed of varying amounts of proteoglycans and numbers of fibroblasts. The collagen fibers are found in a wavy, longitudinal arrangement in ligament and in a more parallel arrangement in tendon. In areolar connective tissue (loose connective tissue that surrounds other structures such as organs or tendons and muscle), the fibers are oriented in a more random fashion, resulting in slightly different physical

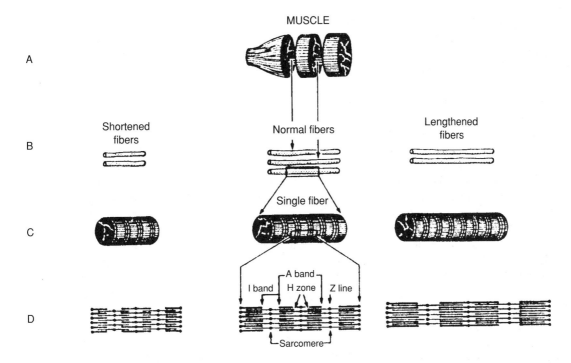

Figure 7–1 The structure of normal muscle (*center*) and the relative changes that occur when a muscle undergoes changes due to shortened position (*left*) or lengthened position (*right*). **A**, Skeletal muscle composed of single fibers (cells). **B**, Single fibers. **C**, Single fiber enlarged to show myofibrils; note decreased and increased sarcomere numbers in the shortened and lengthened fibers, respectively. **D**, Myofibril enlarged to show contractile proteins of the sarcomere (actin and myosin myofilaments); note increased and decreased sarcomere length in the shortened and lengthened fibers, respectively. Both neurophysiologic (alteration in sarcomere length) and structural (change in sarcomere number) adaptations are presented. *Source:* Reprinted from *Physical Therapy,* Grossman, M., Sahrmann, S., and Rose, S. Experimental Evidence and Clinical Implications, 1982, Vol. 62, pp. 1799–1808, with permission of the APTA.

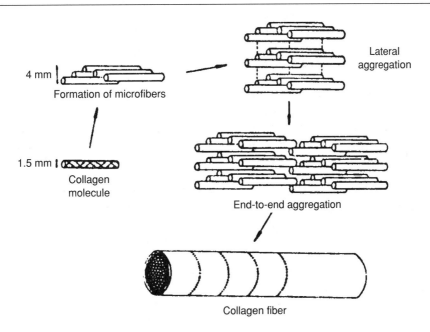

Figure 7–2 Formation of the five-membered microfibril and its potential for lateral and end-to-end aggregation to form fibers. *Source:* Reprinted with permission from M.E. Nimni, Collagen: Structure, Function, and Metabolism in Normal and Fibrotic Tissue, *Seminars in Arthritis and Rheumatism,* Vol. 13, pp. 1–86, © 1983, W.B. Saunders.

properties (i.e., increased deformation with low-level force). There are specific subtypes of collagen, categorized according to the specific tissue, with differing physical properties. In general, tendon and ligament are composed of Type 1 collagen. There are a few specialized structures, such as ligamentum flavum and ligamentum nuchae, that contain a greater amount of elastic tissue.

Connective tissues are, for the most part, sparsely cellular in their mature state. They are, however, metabolically active tissues, relying on the continued synthesis of specialized matrix substances (proteoglycans) and collagen turnover for the maintenance of their specific function. There is, to some degree, a natural order to connective tissue; it has an inherent tensile force and will naturally shorten to the shape in which it is maintained if not subjected to an outside deforming force on a regular basis.[42,83–85] This occurs through the continuous remodeling of collagen, the turnover of collagen molecules, and the production and removal of the proteoglycan matrix.[17,18,84,85] This entire process is accelerated in the presence of wound healing (the entire spectrum of injury).[63,83,84,86,87]

The viscoelastic properties (exhibiting features of both fluid and solid nature) of connective tissue and the contractile-elastic properties of muscle determine their response to stretching. Muscle and connective tissue (tendon and connective tissues surrounding muscle) are aligned in series along the axis of an applied stretch. Muscle has been described mechanically as composed of contractile and elastic elements[59] arranged in parallel.[88] Huxley and Simons[88] demonstrated this feature to be secondary to the cross-bridges of actin and myosin. As mentioned earlier, muscle can respond to an applied force with permanent elongation. Animal studies have demonstrated that this is due to an increase in the number of sarcomeres. Additionally, this affects the contractile nature of the muscle, with an increase in its peak tension at a longer resting length.[52,53,89–91] Muscle at rest has a constant tendency to shorten, based on its contractile element. Animal studies have shown that this results in permanent shortening, most likely due to a reduction in the number of sarcomeres.[52,53,91]

Similarly, connective tissue will adapt its structure based upon the forces to which it is subjected. Both tendon and ligament have been demonstrated to respond to regularly applied force (exercise versus immobilization) with increased strength:weight ratios.[16,18,19,30,83,84,92,93] The improved strength is due to both increased proteoglycan content and collagen cross-links.[30,83,84,92,93] The organization of fibers is related to the amount of applied forces, with a more random organization of fibers in the absence of outside force. Both the strength and elasticity of tendon and ligament are reduced in this state.[2,3,50,83] Connective tissues respond to stretch in a viscoelastic manner.[48,50,94,95] This describes characteristics of reversible (elastic) and plastic (nonreversible) deformation.

These properties have been extensively studied in tendon, in both animal and ex vivo human studies.

In the laboratory, when tendon is subjected to a tensile force, its response is depicted graphically by a stress force (force per unit area) strain (percent length change/original length). As shown in Figure 7–3, this is not a linear function. There is a greater deformation at low loads, followed by a rapid increase in stress until rapid deformation occurs (rupture). The initial change is related to the gradual elongation of elastic fibers, along with the straightening of the wavy arrangement of collagen fibers. This is followed by rupture of smaller collagen fibers with disruption of cross-links. The shape of this curve can be altered by prestretching the tendon. The stiffness of the tendon varies inversely with its length. Therefore, a tendon of greater length will show greater flexibility.[3] Within the initial part of the curve, the deformation is time-dependent, a feature known as *creep* (percent length change/time at constant applied force). A low load applied for a prolonged time will produce a greater length change than will a large force applied rapidly.[3,42,48,94,95] The amount of force required is also influenced by temperature, local blood flow, and nutritional state.[41,42,51] On this basis, it can be concluded that a stretching program should include the regular application of forces in a gradual and prolonged manner, with an adequate tissue temperature. Because the presence of inflammation will also affect the response, attention to the injury must be appropriately maintained.

MUSCLE FACTORS

Whole muscle is a heterogeneous structure, with components of varying flexibility. Following the external to internal organization, each muscle contains an outer connective tissue sheath (epimysium), inner connective tissue sheaths surrounding fiber groups (perimysium), individual fibers (endomysium), and the sarcolemma (membrane that delineates individual fibers). These cells, known as *extrafusal fibers*, are innervated by alpha-motoneurons. These are the contractile elements, and they determine the power of the muscle. In parallel with these fibers are the intrafusal fibers (muscle spindles). They are innervated by gamma-motoneurons and, although given a contractile function, they serve the purpose of length/tension control for the muscle as a whole (Figure 7–4).[62,96] Their length and tension are determined by the input of the gamma-motoneuron, whose activity, in turn, is influenced by numerous factors, including suprasegmental input via descending cerebellar and cortical tracts, segmental input through direct sources (muscle tension and force development via the segmental innervation by alpha-motoneuron), and indirect sources (overlap of cutaneous afferents and receptors of multiple types). In this manner, there can be multiple simultaneous inputs to the determi-

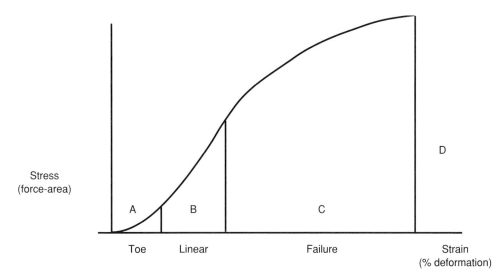

Figure 7–3 Representative stress/strain deformation curve for tendon. **A**, toe; **B**, linear formation; **C**, failure (individual fibrils); **D**, rupture. *Source:* Reprinted with permission from D. Stromberg and C. Weiderheilmn, Viscoelastic Description of a Collagenous Tissue in Simple Elongation, *Journal of Applied Physiology,* Vol. 26, pp. 857–862, © 1969, The American Physiological Society.

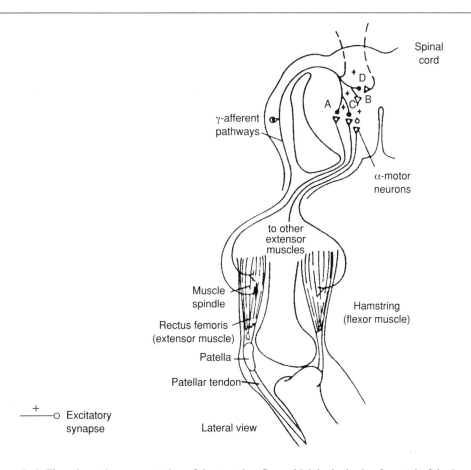

Figure 7–4 The schematic representation of the stretch reflex, which is the basis of control of the length/tension ratio. Alpha-motoneuron innervates extrafusal muscle fibers. Gamma-motoneuron innervates intrafusal muscle fibers (muscle spindles), with both suprasegmental and segmental input via IA afferent fibers. *Source*: Reprinted with permission from Brooks and Fahey: *Exercise Physiology: Human Bioenergetics and Its Applications,* © 1984, The McGraw-Hill Companies.

nation of muscle length and tension. Additionally, there are receptors in the musculotendinous unit (Golgi tendon organ) that operate in a fail-safe manner (all or none) at the point of critical stresses to the structure, delivering inhibitory input and preventing further muscle contraction (thus allowing lengthening and facilitating relaxation). This has been referred to by some[15,26] as the *inverse stretch reflex*. The intrafusal fibers operate on a continuous basis, adjusting length via speed and force considerations (a more slowly applied stretch elicits less response from the muscle spindles).[62,96] When the muscle spindle is stretched, it sends impulses to the spinal cord, which reflectively causes the muscle to contract. If the stretch is maintained (longer than six seconds) the Golgi tendon organ will fire, causing relaxation.[22,62,96] This has direct implications for slow, prolonged stretching and for specific adaptations of stretching techniques. The resetting of the length/tension base line in muscle may be achieved by applying a stretch in this manner.

The length- and tension-setting physiology is the basis for the use of neuromuscular facilitation techniques. These techniques were first developed as a means of increasing strength in paralyzed limbs but soon gained an increasing utility in the treatment of spastic extremities and, subsequently, in neurally intact limbs. The reflex loops described above, in combination with the Sherrington law of reciprocal inhibition (antagonist muscle group), have resulted in numerous stretching techniques with varying degrees of direct neurophysiologic rationale. The cellular and extracellular electrophysiology of the basis of these methods has been investigated by numerous researchers.[4,26,29,54–57,62,97–104] Although these methods have been demonstrated to be effective in increasing flexibility, there is conflicting evidence regarding the specific basis for the observed effect.[56] In Moore and Hutton's study[56] of female gymnasts, electromyographic (EMG) activity during stretch was greater, as were mobility gains in the proprioceptive neuromuscular facilitation (PNF) group. There is evidence that a preceding muscle contraction will cause a lingering after-discharge that results in persistent muscle activation.[56,98,101,105] Whereas this may play a facilitating role in enhancing muscle strength and contraction efficiency, it should have the opposite effect on flexibility characteristics. It appears likely that the observed benefits are due to neural factors, although the interaction of excitatory and inhibitory activity is apparently more complex than the model drawn up to this point, with the inability to measure the specific "message" within the electric signal.

It is apparent that the precise discrete in vivo physiologic event that occurs during stretching is not known. While animal studies have demonstrated that muscle, tendon, and loose connective tissue will change physical and mechanical properties with prolonged immobilization at different lengths, the correlate to human "tightness" and inflexibil-

ity (in the absence of immobilization-induced contracture) is not clear. Athletic flexibility training is performed for much shorter time periods than those employed in the aforementioned studies. It is not known whether absolute length changes (secondary to protein synthesis) are involved at all in vivo. The dynamic factors affecting muscle length (i.e., muscle spindle, gamma loop, and Golgi tendon organ) clearly play a role in the flexibility changes observed with the use of stretching programs. The changes in hamstring flexibility noted immediately after the institution of a stretching program are too rapid to be accounted for on the basis of change in the number of sarcomeres or alteration in protein synthesis alone. The tremendous stiffness of tendon compared with muscle makes it unlikely that tendon length change plays any role in this phenomenon. It is unclear whether the improved flexibility occurs secondary to alteration in actin-myosin cross-bridges, tension by neural factors. The relative contribution of each of these components is controversial. In the initial phases of training, neural factors probably play the major role in the observed flexibility changes. After prolonged periods of flexibility training, changes in sarcomere number may play a role in reaching the new steady-state muscle length.

FLEXIBILITY MEASUREMENT/OBJECTIVE ASSESSMENT

The measurement of flexibility is a complex task that is difficult to standardize. Measurement of joint range of motion and assessment of flexibility are not necessarily equivalent, but in a practical sense they are usually considered as such. There is a good standardization of method and normal ranges are recorded for static goniometric recording of single joints.[41,106,107] The equipment (goniometer) is a protractor designed for easy application to joints. Its use is relatively simple, producing quantitative results with good inter- and intraobserver reproducibility.[106] Limitations include static measurements only, single joints at a given time, and difficulty in application to certain joints (e.g., sternoclavicular and costoclavicular). To ease the application to whole body parts, Leighton designed the flexometer, which consists of a weighted circular dial with a needle enclosed, which can be strapped to the body part. Its reliability is good but not quite so high as that of the standard goniometer.[108] The electrogoniometer designed by Karpovich et al[109] substitutes a potentiometer for a protractor. Its advantage is the ability to record range of dynamic motion with fair accuracy, somewhat less than that for static measurements. Few specific joints, however, can be measured with this device.

The measurement of trunk flexibility has special limitations and inherent difficulties. The standard goniometer is not appropriate for measuring trunk motion in the sagittal plane and is entirely inadequate in the coronal and rotational planes.[33,107] To this end, the Schober test (originally designed for spinal range of flexion and extension in patients with ankylosing spondylitis) was modified by Moll and Wright[102] as a method of reproducible and semiquantitative compound spine movements. Two marks are made along the ends of the lumbar spine, and the tape-measured distance between them is determined in flexion, neutral, and extension. Lack of a normal standard makes interpretation between the ends of a range difficult to interpret clinically. Similarly, the inclinometer method was designed by Loebl.[110] An evaluation of the difference between these methods and simple "fingertip-to-floor" measurement for inter- and intraexaminer variability[111] demonstrated good reliability for the Moll and Schober tests only. "Eyeball" measurements have variability up to 30%.[33] Other methods with good reliability but requiring the use of special equipment or X-rays are available but have obvious drawbacks. At this point, it appears that for a reproducible, quantitative assessment of lumbar spine motion, these tests are recommended. Disadvantages include their inapplicability to the cervical or thoracic spine and their limitation to measurement of compound motion only (the entire thoracolumbar spine). None of these methods can assess articular mobility in the translational or rotational planes. Furthermore, they cannot measure flexibility of nonarticulating soft tissue (fascia, chest wall tissue) or of joints that have motion patterns less well defined by external landmarks (i.e., intercostal, thoracic, rib/spine articulations, abdominal wall).

METHODS OF STRETCHING

Stretching techniques have evolved over the recent years to include numerous options for improving flexibility. Although each method has its share of faithful supporters, the distinct superiority of one method has not been demonstrated.[3,14,15,26,29,54,55,62,76,99,100,112–115] There are indications for the relative superiority of a given method in individual clinical situations. Prevention of injury (as in general warm-up), treatment of specific joint injury, flexibility needs in the presence of pain, and muscle spasm require modification of the basic method. The objectives of a flexibility program must be established with a perspective on the specific needs of the athlete. To obtain and maintain a level of flexibility is the general rule. Progressive daily gains in range of motion are unnecessary once a basic level has been achieved. The postures utilized are designed to optimize stretch on the target tissue while minimizing stress on vulnerable structures (most notably the spine and knees). The stretching options available can be divided into the following categories: ballistic, static, passive, and neuromuscular facilitation. Additionally, each of these methods can be combined with modalities.

Ballistic Stretching

Ballistic stretching employs the rapid application of force in a repeated manner in a bouncing, throwing, or jerking maneuver. This method was the standard in the last decade but is no longer recommended. The rapid increase in force can cause injury and is less efficient than are other available methods.[15,22,26,42,116]

Passive Stretching

Passive stretching is performed with a partner applying a stretch to a relaxed extremity. This method has limited usefulness because of the increased risk of injury. There must be excellent communication between the partners, with slow and sensitive application of force. Gymnasts, dancers, football kickers, and soccer players have used this method for hamstring and adductor stretching, and swimmers have used it for anterior shoulder and chest wall stretching. This method is commonly employed in the training room and physical therapy department, and is safest when used in this context.

Static Stretching

Static stretching is the easiest and probably the safest method and is recommended for preparticipation flexibility exercise in combination with a warmup. A steady force is applied for a period of 15–60 seconds. The duration of the applied stretch has been recently suggested to be equally effective at 15 seconds compared with 45–60 seconds.[111] This is the basis of yoga-type stretching and was advocated by deVries.[113] More recent studies suggest that 30–60 seconds of stretching was more effective at increasing flexibility of the hamstring muscles (as determined by increased range of motion of knee extension) than was 15 seconds of stretching or no stretching. In addition, no significant difference existed between stretching for 30 seconds and for one minute, indicating that 30 seconds of stretching was as effective as the longer duration of one minute. The added advantage of decreased muscular soreness after exercise is a factor supporting the use of static stretching methods.[28,117] Yoga-type stretching can be very effective, although specific cautions are necessary. These methods have been tested over centuries, but they carry a definite risk of injury if performed incorrectly or in the presence of certain injuries (specific joint instabilities, degenerative disk disease—especially cervical—or in association with instability).

Neuromuscular Facilitation

Neuromuscular facilitation techniques have been demonstrated in numerous studies to be effective methods for stretch.[14,26,29,54,56,57] Most of these methods require an experienced partner (usually a physical therapist or trainer). Hold-relax and contract-relax (with or without agonist contraction) are the activities most frequently employed. In the experienced and attentive athlete, the contract-relax activity with added agonist contraction can be a very effective and safe method. For hamstring stretch, the hamstring is isometrically contracted for five seconds, while a gentle submaximal hip flexor contraction is maintained.[56] The author recommends this method for quadriceps, hamstring, and gastrocnemius/soleus/Achilles complex. A cross-training effect has been demonstrated with PNF techniques on hip flexibility.[55] This has a direct implication for flexibility training in the contralateral immobilized leg of the injured athlete.

In addition to manipulation of the neuromuscular system to enhance flexibility, the thermal characteristics of connective tissue can be exploited to improve flexibility programs in certain circumstances. Warmup exercises[22,36,95,118] or conduction heating methods prior to stretching take advantage of the viscoelastic nature of collagen with increased temperature within the physiologic range. Warmup prior to stretch[118] or instead of stretch[36] failed to increase the level of flexibility except in ankle dorsiflexion, which showed significant gains beyond stretching alone. The ease of stretch and prevention of injuries was not studied, however, and this is an equally important consideration. Therefore, the author recommends 5–10 minutes of warmup activity prior to stretching. This could be in the form of light jogging, fast walking, or stationary bike work.

Cold application has been used following flexibility training exercises to take advantage of the thermal characteristics of connective tissue.[43] Once plastic deformation has occurred, lowering the temperature can theoretically prolong the length changes. This has not been proved to be effective except in the setting of treatment of injury. In this setting, muscle spasm and painful inhibition of joint and limb range of movement can be suppressed by cold application in the form of ice massage, cold immersion, or ice packs (time period for use varies with each of these methods).[42,55] The use of a vapocoolant spray has been demonstrated to be of no significant benefit for flexibility gains in the absence of treatment of the injury.[119] However, in the setting of injury where muscle spasm is a factor, this can be a very effective modality (myofascial syndromes).[42,62] Stimulation of cutaneous afferents with the coolant spray can effect muscle relaxation on a physiologic basis similar to the PNF techniques.

Whereas there are data to suggest improved static or passive stretching when combined with ultrasound,[120] there are few data at this time to support its routine use in the absence of injury or fixed joint contracture. The ideal flexibility program should, therefore, include a combination of stretching and mobilizing techniques ("stretching" across the long axis of the joint and "mobilizing" along the translational and rotational axes). A combination of passive, static, and PNF techniques should be utilized, with specific target sites and motions for each sport. Within each sport, there will be variation of needs according to individual flexibility profiles. The program should be designed with these factors in mind and should be performed routinely: in off-season three times per week and daily during the regular season. Gains in flexibility have been shown to be superior in athletes with a postactivity program.[121] Therefore, pre- and post-competition routines should be established. The "after" routine can be more specific and abbreviated, focusing on muscle groups most stressfully involved in the athletic event. Because the short-term effect of stretching diminishes significantly after 90 minutes, the program should be exercised within this time frame.[31] It should be performed for at least 15–20 minutes, as this appears to be the minimum time period for achieving adequate gains in temperature and extensibility.[22,122] The author recommends five repetitions for each motion with each extremity. The duration of "hold" on static stretches should be *15–30 seconds* with the initial stretch, to *30–60 seconds* on the last repetition. Stretches of longer duration have not been demonstrated to have increased effectiveness.[50,123] Self-mobilization exercises at the segmental level of the thoracic and lumbar spine are recommended for most athletes who require upper body rotation and load bearing. Finally, stretching and mobilization techniques should be exercised with careful attention to form to stay within the "window" of safety and effectiveness.

SUMMARY

Flexibility is a characteristic of musculoskeletal function that is more than simple joint range of motion. Flexibility training invokes a complex interaction of biophysical and neurophysiologic factors. A variety of tissue types are involved in stretching maneuvers, but the exact target site or discrete physiologic event is not completely known. Whereas the majority of attention has been focused upon the musculotendinous unit, a complete flexibility training program should also include maneuvers aimed at improvement of joint capsule and pericapsular tissue flexibility. In the setting of athletic injury rehabilitation, especially with attendant weakness (either from pain or neurally induced), this becomes an important issue. Though flexibility training is widely employed for the prevention and treatment of overuse injuries, the mechanism of its action in this setting is not well understood. Although adaptive shortening of connective tissue can occur, whether actual tissue length changes or neurally mediated relaxation play major roles in flexibility gains is not known. At the present time, there is enough epidemiologic evidence to support the routine use of flexibility training programs in most sports. No single stretching method has been shown to be singularly superior, but the evidence implies that PNF methods can achieve the greatest overall flexibility gains. Programs should include a variety of methods and must be designed with consideration of the abilities and specific needs of the athlete. Constant awareness to avoid spinal or peripheral joint injury is imperative. The major evidence regarding the influence of flexibility training on injury prevention and treatment, as well as alteration of sports performances, is theoretical. In the absence of controlled studies with large groups of subjects, this theoretical basis will have to be relied on to guide the use of flexibility training in the near future.

REFERENCES

1. Cohen DB, Mont MA, Campbell KK, Vogelstein BN, Loewy JW. Upper extremity physical factors affecting tennis serve velocity. *Am J Sports Med.* 1994;22:746–750.

2. Curwin S, Stanish W. *Tendinitis: Its Etiology and Treatment.* Lexington, MA: DC Heath & Company, 1984.

3. Curwin S, Stanish W. Tendinitis: its etiology and treatment. In: Butler D, Grood E, Noyes F, Zernicke R, eds. Biomechanics of ligaments and tendons. *Exerc Sport Sci Rev.* 1978;6:125–182.

4. D'Ambrosia R, Drez D. Prevention and treatment of running injuries. In: Stanish W, ed. *Neurophysiology of Stretching.* Thorofare, NJ: Charles Slack, 1982.

5. Doucette SA, Goble EM. The effect of exercise on patellar tracking in lateral patellar compression syndrome. *Am J Sports Med.* 1992;20:434–440.

6. Ekstrand J, Gillquist J. The avoidability of soccer injuries. *Int J Sports Med.* 1983;4:124–128.

7. Fleisg G, Andrews J, Dillman C, Escamilla R. Kinetics of baseball pitching with implication about injury mechanisms. *Am J Sports Med.* 1995;23:233–239.

8. Glick J. Muscle strains: prevention and treatment. *Physician Sports Med.* 1980;6:73–77.

9. Gordon N, Moolman J, Van Rensburg J, et al. The South African Defense Force Physical Training Programme. *S Afr Med J.* 1986;69:483–490.

10. Hilyer J, Brown K, Sirles A, Peoples L. A flexibility intervention to reduce the incidence and severity of joint injuries among municipal firefighters. *J Occup Med.* 1990;32:631–637.

11. Hortbagyi T, Faludi J, Merkely B. Effects of intense "stretching"-flexibility training on the mechanical profile of the knee extensors and on the range of motion of the hip joint. *Int J Sport Med.* 1985;6:317–321.

12. Johnson J, Sim F, Scott S. Musculoskeletal injuries in competitive swimmers. *Mayo Clin Proc.* 1987;62:289–304.

13. Millar A. An early stretching routine for calf muscle strains. *Med Sci Sports Exerc.* 1976;8:39–42.

14. Sady S, Wortman M, Blanke D. Flexibility training: ballistic, static or proprioceptive neuromuscular facilitation. *Arch Phys Med Rehabil.* 1982;63:261–263.

15. Surburg P. Flexibility exercises re-examined. *Athlet Train.* Spring 1983;37040.

16. Akeson W, Amiel D, Abel M, et al. Effects of immobilization on joints. *Clin Orthop.* 1987;219:28–37.

17. Amiel D, Akeson W, Harwood F, Mechanic G. The effect of immobilization on the types of collagen synthesized in periarticular connective tissue. *Connect Tissue Res.* 1980;8:27–32.

18. Amiel D, Woo S, Harwood F, Akeson W. The effect of immobilization on collagen turnover in connective tissue: a biochemical-biomechanical correlation. *Acta Orthop Scand.* 1982;53:325–332.

19. Booth F. Physiologic and biochemical effects of immobilization on muscle. *Clin Orthop.* 1987;219:15–20.

20. Ekstrand J, Gillquist J. The frequencies of muscle tightness and injuries in soccer players. *Am J Sports Med.* 1982;10:75–78.

21. Schultz P. Flexibility: day of the static stretch. *Physician Sports Med.* 1979;7:109–117.

22. Shellock F, Prentice W. Warming up and stretching for improved physical performance and prevention of sports-related injuries. *Sports Med.* 1985;2:267–278.

23. Shyne K, Dominguez R. To stretch or not to stretch? *Physician Sports Med.* 1982;10:137–140.

24. Agre J. Hamstring injuries: proposed etiological factors, prevention, and treatment. *Sports Med.* 1985;2:21–33.

25. Anderson B. *Stretching.* Bolinas, CA: Shelter Publications; 1980.

26. Beaulieu J. Developing a stretching program. *Physician Sports Med.* 1981;9:59–69.

27. Corbin C. Flexibility. *Clin Sports Med.* 1984;3:101–117.

28. deVries H. Prevention of muscular distress after exercise. *Res Q.* 1960;32:177–185.

29. Knott M, Voss D. Proprioceptive neuromuscular facilitation: patterns and techniques. New York: 1956. As cited in Basmajian J: *Therapeutic Exercise.* 3rd ed. Baltimore: Williams & Wilkins, 1978.

30. Laros G, Tipton C, Cooper R. Influence of physical activity on ligament insertions in the knees of dogs. *J Bone Joint Surg Am.* 1971;53:275–286.

31. Moller M, Ekstrand J, Oberg B, Gillquist J. Duration of stretching effect on range of motion in lower extremities. *Arch Phys Med Rehabil.* 1985;66:171–173.

32. Moretz J, Walters R, Smith L. Flexibility as a predictor of knee injuries in college football players. *Physician Sports Med.* 1982;10:93–97.

33. Nelson M, Allen P, Clamp SE, Dombal FT. Reliability and reproducibility of clinical findings in low back pain. *Spine.* 1979;4:97–101.

34. Sammarco G. Diagnosis and treatment in dancers. *Clin Orthop.* 1984;187:176–187.

35. Smith CA. The warm-up procedure: to stretch or not to stretch. A brief review. *J Orthop Sports Phys Ther.* 1994;19:12–17.

36. Wiktorsson-Moller M, Oberg M, Ekstrand J, Gillquist J. Effects of warming up, massage, and stretching on range of motion and muscle strength in the lower extremity. *Am J Sports Med.* 1983;11:249–252.

37. Wooden M. Preseason screening of the lumbar spine. *J Orthop Sports Phys Ther.* 1981;3:6–10.

38. Keller C, Noyes F, Buchner R. Sports traumatology series: the medical aspects of soccer injury epidemiology. *Am J Sports Med.* 1987;15:230–237.

39. Casella C. Tensile force in total striated muscle, isolated fiber sarcolemma. *Acta Physiol Scand.* 1950;21:380–401.

40. Harkness R. Mechanical properties of collagenous tissue. In: Gould BS, ed. *Treatise on Collagen.* New York: Academic Press, 1968;2(A): 247–310.

41. Kottke F, Stillwell K, Lehmann JF. *Krusen's Handbook of Physical Medicine and Rehabilitation.* 3rd ed. Philadelphia: WB Saunders Company; 1982.

42. Kottke F, Pauley D, Ptak R. The rationale for prolonged stretching for correction of shortening of connective tissue. *Arch Phys Med Rehabil.* 1966;47:345–352.

43. Sapega A, Quedenfeld T, Moyer R, Butler R. Biophysical factors in range-of-motion exercise. *Physician Sports Med.* 1981;9:57–65.

44. Steben R, Steben A. The validity of the stretch shortening cycle in selected jumping events. *J Sports Med.* 1981;21:28–37.

45. Stolov W, Weilepp T, Riddell W. Passive length-tension relationship and hydroxyproline content of chronically denervated skeletal muscle. *Arch Phys Med Rehabil.* 1970;51:517–525.

46. Stolov W, Weillepp T. Passive length-tension relationship of intact muscle, epimysium, and tendon in normal and denervated gastrocnemius of the rat. *Arch Phys Med Rehabil.* 1966;47:612–620.

47. Gossman M, Sahrmann S, Rose S. Experimental evidence and clinical implications. *Phys Ther.* 1982;62:1799–1808.

48. Haute R, Little R. A constitutive equation for collagen fibers. *J Biomech.* 1972;5:423–430.

49. Jenkins R, Little R. A constitutive equation for parallel-fibered elastic tissue.

50. LaBan M. Collagen tissue: implications of its response to stress in vitro. *Arch Phys Med Rehabil.* 1962;43:461–466.

51. Lehmann J, Masock A, et al. Effect of therapeutic temperature on tendon extensibility. *Arch Phys Med Rehabil.* 1970;51:481–487.

52. Tabary JC, Tabary C, Tardieu C, et al. Physiological and structural changes in the cat's soleus muscle due to immobilization at different lengths by plaster casts. *J Physiol (Lond).* 1972;224:231–244.

53. Tardieu C, Tarbary J, Tardieu G, et al. Adaptation of sarcomere numbers to the length imposed on muscle. In: Gubba F, Marechal G, Takacs O, eds. *Mechanism of Muscle Adaptation to Functional Requirements.* Tarrytown, NY: Pergamon, 1981.

54. Kabat H. Studies of neuromuscular dysfunction: the role of central facilitation in restoration of motor function in paralysis. *Arch Phys Med Rehabil.* 1952;33:523.

55. Markos P. Ipsilateral and contralateral effects of proprioceptive neuromuscular facilitation techniques on hip motion and electromyographic activity. *Phys Ther.* 1979;59:366–373.

56. Moore M, Hutton R. Electromyographic investigation of muscle stretching techniques. *Med Sci Sports Exerc.* 1980;12:322–329.

57. Surbug P. Neuromuscular facilitation techniques in sports medicine. *Physician Sports Med.* 1981;9:115–127.

58. Scholten P, Veldhuizen A. The bending stiffness of the trunk. *Spine.* 1986;11:463–467.

59. Hill AV. The heat of shortening and the dynamic constraints of muscle. *Proc R Soc Lond.* 1938;126(B):136–195.

60. Hill A. The mechanics of active muscle. *Proc R Soc Lond.* 1938;141(B):136–195.

61. Johns R, Wright V. Relative importance of various tissues in joint stiffness. *J Appl Physiol.* 1962;17:824–828.

62. Downey J, Darling R. *Physiological Basis of Rehabilitation Medicine.* Philadelphia: WB Saunders Company, 1971.

63. Zarins B. Soft tissue repair: biomechanical aspects. *Int J Sports Med.* 1982;3:9–11.

64. Nicholas J. Injuries to knee ligaments: relationship to looseness and tightness in football players. *JAMA.* 1970;212:2236–2239.

65. Godshall R. The predictability of athletic injuries: an eight-year study. *J Sports Med.* 1975;3:50–54.

66. Kalenak A, Morehouse C. Knee stability and knee ligament injuries. *JAMA.* 1975;234:1143–1145.

67. Farfan H, Gracovetsky S. The mechanism of the lumbar spine. *Spine.* 1989;6:249–262.

68. Farfan H, Gracovetsky S. The optimum spine. *Spine.* 1986;11:543–573.

69. Phalen GS, Dickson JA. Spondylolisthesis and tight hamstrings. *J Bone Joint Surg Am.* 1961;43:505–512.

70. Khalil T, Asfour S, Martinez L, Waly S, Rosomoff R, Rosomoff H. Stretching in rehabilitation of low-back pain patients. *Spine.* 1992;17:311–317.

71. Fairbank J, Pynsent P. Influence of anthropometric factors and joint laxity in the incidence of adolescent back pain. *Spine.* 1984;9:461–464.

72. Cady L, Thomas P, Karwasky R. Program for increasing health and physical fitness of firefighters. *J Occup Med.* 1985;27:110–114.

73. Sullivan MK, Dejulia JJ, Worrell TW. Effect of pelvic position and stretching method on hamstring muscle flexibility. *Med Sci Sports Exerc.* 1992;24:1383–1389.

74. Puniello MS. Iliotibial band tightness and medical patellar glide in patients with patellofemoral dysfunction. *J Orthop Sports Phys Ther.* 1993;17:144–148.

75. Craib MW, Mithcell VA, Fields KB, Cooper TR, Hopewell R, Morgan DW. The association between flexibility and running economy sub-elite male distance runners. *Med Sci Sports Exerc.* 1996;28: 737–743.

76. MacNab I, Rathbun M. The microvascular pattern of the rotator cuff. *J Bone Joint Surg Br.* 1970;52.

77. Janda DH, Wojtys EM, Hankin FM, et al. A three phase analysis of the prevention of recreational softball injuries. *Am J Sports Med.* 1990;18:632.

78. deVries H. Electromyographic observations of effects of static stretching upon muscular distress. *Res Q.* 1960;32:468–479.

79. Bosco C, Komi P. Potentiation of the mechanical behavior of the human skeletal muscle through prestretching. *Acta Physiol Scand.* 1979;106:467–472.

80. Bosco C, Tihani J, Komi P, et al. Store and recoil of elastic energy in slow and fast types of human skeletal muscles. *Acta Physiol Scand.* 1982;116:343–349.

81. Cavagna G, Saibene F, Margaria R. Effects of negative work on the amount of positive work performed by an isolated muscle. *J Appl Physiol.* 1965;20:157–158.

82. Cavagna G, Dusman B, Margaria R. Positive work done by a previously stretched muscle. *J Appl Physiol.* 1968;24:21–32.

83. Nimni ME. Collagen: structure, function, and metabolism in normal and fibrotic tissue. *Semin Arthritis Rheum.* 1983;13:1–86.

84. Noyes F, Torvik P, Hyde W, DeLucas J. Biomechanics of ligament failure: an analysis of immobilization, exercise, and reconditioning effects in primates. *J Bone Joint Surg Am.* 1974;56:1406–1418.

85. Peacock EE. Some biomechanical and biophysical aspects of joint stiffness: role of collagen synthesis as opposed to altered molecular bonding. *Ann Surg.* 1986;164:1–12.

86. Klein L, Dawson J, Heiple K. Turnover of collagen in the adult rat after denervation. *J Bone Joint Surg Am.* 1977;59:1065–1067.

87. Young A, Stokes M, Illes J. Effects of joint pathology on muscle. *Clin Orthop.* 1987;219:21–27.

88. Huxley A, Simmons R. Mechanical properties of the cross-bridges of frog striated muscle. *J Physiol Lond.* 1971;218:59P–60P.

89. Goldspink D. The influence of immobilization and stretch on protein turnover of rat skeletal muscle. *J Physiol.* 1977;264:267–282.

90. Goldspink G, Williams PE. The nature of the increased passive resistance in muscle following immobilization of the mouse soleus muscle. *J Physiol (Lond).* 1979;289:55–58.

91. Williams PE, Goldspink G. Changes in sarcomere length and physiological properties in immobilized muscle. *J Anat.* 1978;127:459–468.

92. Tipton C, James S, Mergner W, Tcheng T. Influence of exercise of strength of medial collateral knee ligaments of dogs. *Am J Physiol.* 1970;218:894–902.

93. Woo S, Ritter M, Amiel D, et al. The biomechanical and biochemical properties of swine tendons: long-term effects of exercise on the digital extensors. *Connect Tissue Res.* 1981;7:177–183.

94. Stromberg D, Weiderheilm C. Viscoelastic description of a collagenous tissue in simple elongation. *J Appl Physiol.* 1969;26:857–862.

95. Warren C, Lehmann J, Koblanski J. Heat and stretch procedures: an evaluation using rat tail tendon. *Arch Phys Med Rehabil.* 1976;57:122–126.

96. Basmajian J. *Therapeutic Exercise.* 3rd ed. Baltimore: Williams & Wilkins, 1978.

97. Tanigawa M. Comparison of the hold-relax procedure and passive mobilization on increasing muscle length. *Phys Ther.* 1972;52:725–735.

98. Hagbarth K, Vallbo A. Discharge characteristics of human muscle afferents during muscle stretch and contraction. *Exp Neurol.* 1968;22:674–694.

99. Hartley-O'Brien. Six mobilization exercises for active range of hip flexion. *Res Q Exerc Sport.* 1991;51:625–635.

100. Holt L, Travis T, Okita T. Comparative study of three stretching techniques. *Percept Mot Skills.* 1970;31:611–616.

101. Hutton R, Smith J, Eldred E. Persisting changes in sensory and motor activity of a muscle following its reflex activation. *Pflugers Arch.* 1975;353:327–336.

102. Moll J, Wright V. Normal range of spinal mobility: a clinical study. *Ann Rheum Dis.* 1976;30:381–386.

103. Smith J, Hutton R, Eldred E. Postcontraction changes in sensitivity of muscle afferents to static and dynamic stretch. *Brain Res.* 1974;78:192–202.

104. Wilkerson G. Developing flexibility by overcoming the stretch reflex. *Physician Sports Med.* 1981;9:189–191.

105. Devanandan M, Eccles R, Yokota T. Muscle stretch and the presynaptic inhibition of the group 1a pathway to motorneurons. *J Physiol.* 1965;179:430–441.

106. Ekstrand J, Wiktorsson M, Oberg B, Gillquist J. Lower extremity goniometric measurements: a study to determine their reliability. *Arch Phys Med Rehabil.* 1982;63:171–175.

107. Polley H, Hunder G. *Physical Examination of the Joints.* 2nd ed. Philadelphia: WB Saunders Company, 1978.

108. Harris M. Flexibility. *Phys Ther.* 1968;49:591–601.

109. Karpovich PV, et al. Electrogoniometer: a new device for study of joints in action. *Fed Proc.* 1959;18:79.

110. Loeble W. Measurement of spinal posture and range of spinal movement. *Ann Phys Med.* 1967;9:104–111.

111. Medeiros J, Madding SW. Effect of duration of passive stretch on hip abduction range of motion. *J Orthop Sports Phys Ther.* 1987;8:409–411.

112. Cornelius WL, Ebrahim K, Watson J, Hill DW. The effects of cold application and modified PNF stretching techniques on hip joint flexibility in college males. *Res Q Exerc Sports.* 1992;63:311–314.

113. deVries H. Evaluation of static stretching procedures for improvement of flexibility. *Res Q.* 1962;33:222–229.

114. Gajdosik R, LeVeau B, Bohannon R. Effects of ankle dorsiflexion on active and passive unilateral straight leg raising. *Phys Ther.* 1985;65:1478–1482.

115. Madding S, Wong J, Hallum A, Medeiros J. Effect of duration of passive stretch on hip abduction range of motion. *J Orthop Sports Phys Ther.* 1987;8:409–416.

116. Wallin D, Ekblom B, Grahn R, Nordenborg T. Improvement of muscle flexibility: a comparison of two techniques. *Am J Sports Med.* 1985;13:263–268.

117. deVries H. Quantitative electromyographic investigation of the spasm theory of muscle pain. *Am J Sports Med.* 1966;45:119–134.

118. East J, Smith F, Burry L. Evaluation of warm-up for improvement in flexibility. *Am J Sports Med.* 1986;14:316–319.

119. Newton R. Effects of vapocoolants on passive hip flexion in healthy subjects. *Phys Ther.* 1985;65:1034–1036.

120. Wessling K, DeVane D, Hylton C. Effects of static stretch versus static stretch and ultrasound combined on triceps surae muscle extensibility in healthy women. *Phys Ther.* 1987;67:674–678.

121. Moller M, Oberg B, Gillquist J. Stretching exercise and soccer: effect of stretching on range of motion in the lower extremity in connection with soccer training. *Int J Sports Med.* 1985;6:50–52.

122. Bohannon R. Effect of repeated eight-minute muscle loading on the angle of straight-leg raising. *Phys Ther.* 1984;64:491–497.

123. Bandy WD, Irion JM. The effect of time on static stretch of the flexibility of the hamstring muscles. *Phys Ther.* 1994;74:845–850.

CHAPTER 8

Functional Reconditioning

Jeffrey Chandler

INTRODUCTION

The importance of conditioning for athletes is becoming increasingly apparent as athletes in all sports continue to improve in speed and size, and to set new performance records in a variety of sporting activities. Injured athletes will undoubtedly experience some loss of conditioning, depending on the amount of time lost from participation or conditioning. When a significant injury does occur, the athlete will generally undergo an intense rehabilitation program, generally directed at the specific joint or location of the injury. This chapter will describe the process of reconditioning, which consists of progressive, sport-specific, functional exercises designed to ensure that the injured athlete is returned to competition in a state of optimal conditioning.

Conditioning is important to athletes in a number of ways, including injury prevention and performance enhancement. Conditioning is thought by many[1-4] to be important for the prevention of musculoskeletal injuries. When conditioning exercises are ceased, as may occur after an injury, detraining will occur.

Rehabilitation is generally carried out by a physical therapist or athletic trainer. During the acute phase of an injury, it is the responsibility of this person to see that the athlete avoids any activity that may cause further injury, to begin rehabilitation at the appropriate time, and to determine, with appropriate guidance of the physician, when soft tissues have healed and when normal strength and range of motion have been attained. Once this occurs, the athlete should begin a functional reconditioning program to prepare for a return to participation.

In some instances, athletes are allowed to return to play after a significant injury when the strength and range of motion measurements return to preinjury levels or to a level comparable to the contralateral limb. However, it must be considered that the athlete was injured at that particular level of strength and range of motion. Therefore, comparisons to sport-specific normative data may also be used as a goal for return to play. If normal strength and range of motion are the only criteria used for return to play, the athlete's chance of reinjury may be high. Of course, other factors play a role in the chance of reinjury, such as altered biomechanics that cannot be restored surgically and psychological factors that may alter the athlete's style of play. These factors aside, many sports require highly complex movement patterns that must be incorporated into the traditional rehabilitation program[5] if the athlete is to return to full participation.

The purpose of functional reconditioning is to "bridge the gap" between rehabilitation and the return to play. It can be performed by a knowledgeable physical therapist, athletic trainer, certified strength and conditioning specialist, or coach. Most importantly, it should be directed by someone who understands the rehabilitation process, the concept of soft tissue healing, the demands of the sport on the musculoskeletal system, the musculoskeletal deficits of the individual athlete, and the principles of sound exercise program design, including the appropriate frequency, intensity, and duration of the exercises, and the concepts of specificity, recovery, and gradual progression.

GENERAL RECONDITIONING

Many athletes go through rigorous weight-training programs to improve performance in a particular sport. By including a progressive weight training program in the reconditioning programs, it can be ensured that the athlete can perform at least at the preinjury level. Athletes are at times allowed to return to play when they reach 90% of the strength in the uninjured extremity. As a long-term goal, strength in the injured extremity should be increased to preinjury levels and perhaps even higher to minimize the chance of reinjury.

Conditioning for general athletic fitness (Exhibit 8–1) may include such exercises as the squat, bench press, power clean, dead lift, or other large muscle-mass exercises. Other activities can be used, such as exercises with body weight, with a medicine ball to work on muscular endurance, or with machines to work on specific muscle groups. The abdominal muscle group is one of the most important, yet it is often omitted from exercises in a rehabilitative conditioning program for athletes. The trunk and abdomen are critical in the efficient transfer of forces from the lower body to the upper body, and exercises to strengthen these muscles (i.e., abdominal crunches, side crunches, Figure 8–1) can be performed in spite of most injuries to the extremities. Whereas injury-specific flexibility exercises are likely performed in rehabilitation, general athletic flexibility may be neglected. The reconditioning period is the time to restore general athletic flexibility. Aerobic fitness, as well, may be neglected in the rehabilitation phase. It is possible that an injury does not allow the athlete the ability to perform adequate levels of aerobic exercise. The reconditioning phase of training is the time to evaluate and restore aerobic conditioning necessary for a particular sport.

SPORT-SPECIFIC RECONDITIONING

Once athletes have attained the prior level of general athletic fitness, they can progress to sport-specific functional activities. Athletic fitness, speed, power, quickness, balance, and agility are important in most sports. In fact, these factors may be of major importance to separate great athletes from good athletes. Sport-specific reconditioning exercises should include a variety of movements at a variety of speeds and intensities. By gradually introducing these exercises dur-

ing the reconditioning process, the athlete can most likely be safely returned to full participation in their sport or activity, perhaps in some cases at a higher functional level than when they were injured.

Many exercises may be helpful in improving lower body power, including the squat (Figure 8–2), the power clean, lunges (Figure 8–3), jumping drills (Figure 8–4), bounding, and box jumping. Single leg squats can be especially important for athletes, particularly in sports requiring many changes of direction, which are generally performed on a single leg. Vertical jumping drills can be with body weight

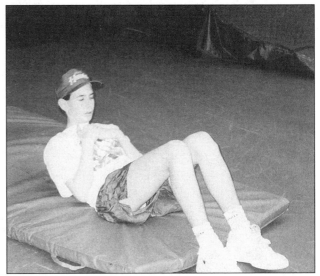

A

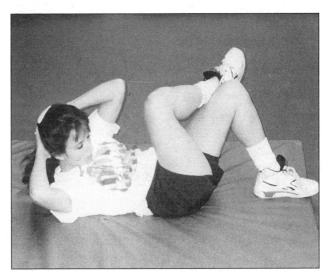

B

Figure 8–1 Abdominal exercises can generally be performed in spite of an injury to an extremity. Even so, they are often neglected as part of a rehabilitation and reconditioning program.

Exhibit 8–1 Exercises for Reconditioning: Begin with Building a General Athletic Fitness Base

Exercises for general strength
- Medicine ball
- Body weight
- Dumbbell free weight
- Barbell free weight
- Machines

Exercises for flexibility
- Total body flexibility
- Individual needs

Exercises for building the aerobic base

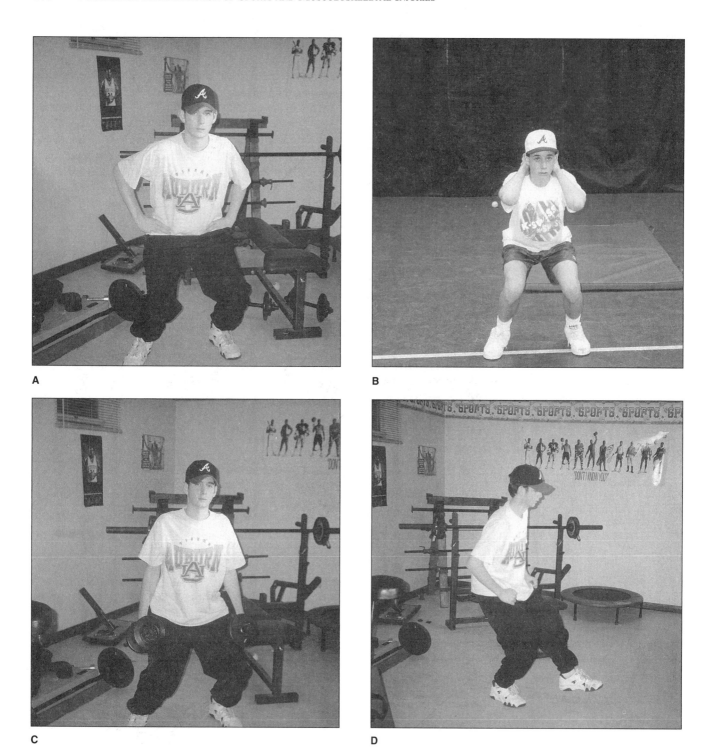

Figure 8–2 The squat exercise is important to performance in most sports. In addition to barbell squats, squats can be performed with body weight (**A**), medicine balls (**B**), dumbbells (**C**), and on a single leg (**D**).

or with resistance, such as having the athlete hold dumbbells during the activity. Box jumps should be added to the program as a final progression, and only in athletes with an adequate strength base. Because many of these drills are plyometric in nature, they must be introduced slowly and cautiously as a part of the functional rehabilitation program. Plyometric exercises involve the stretch-shortening cycle, where a muscle is eccentrically stretched and immediately

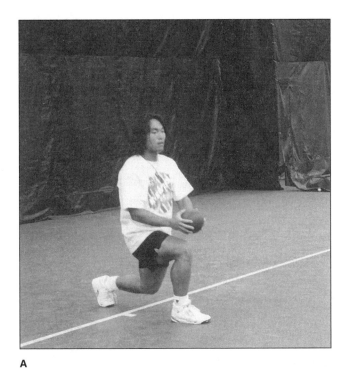

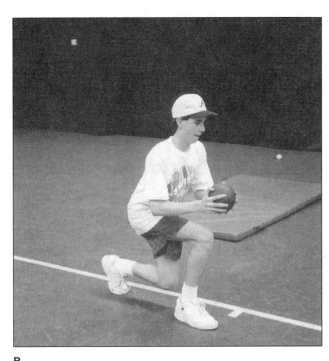

A   **B**

Figure 8–3 Lunges are important to strengthen the hips and legs in a single leg position. Lunges can be performed straight ahead, with a side step (**A**), or with a crossover step (**B**).

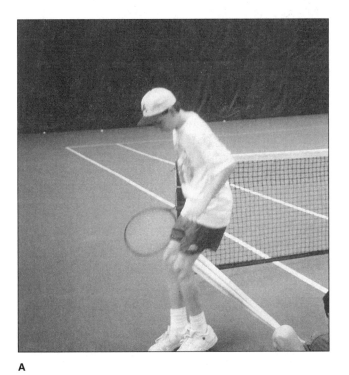

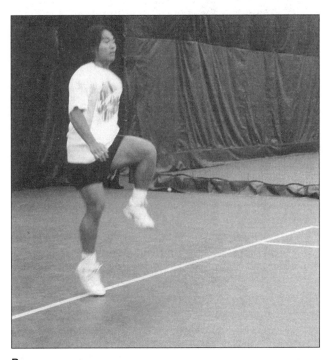

A   **B**

Figure 8–4 Jumping drills can be performed over an elastic cord (**A**) or on a single leg (**B**).

performs a concentric contraction. This improves power output by utilizing the stored elastic energy in a stretched muscle.

For throwing and striking sports, such as baseball and tennis, functional abdominal strengthening exercises can be incorporated in the reconditioning program at the appropriate time. Medicine ball rotational exercises (Figure 8–5) can be effective to increase rotational trunk strength, promote muscle strength balance, and facilitate the transfer of ground reaction forces from the lower extremities. As a progression of this drill, the athlete can perform the drill with a sport-specific implement, such as a tennis racquet (Figure 8–6).

In rehabilitation, even relatively low-intensity plyometric exercises should not be performed until all soft tissue has healed, and the athlete is back to near normal strength and range of motion. Even in the healthy athlete, it has been recommended that the athlete be able to perform a squat with a resistance of two times body weight before undergoing a plyometric exercise routine. It is possible, however, to begin with a low-intensity plyometric routine with less lower body strength. Some experts fear that plyometric exercises will cause injury—or reinjury, in the case of an injured athlete. It must be realized, however, that plyometrics include some activities that are generally considered safe, such as jumping rope. The intensity of a plyometric program should be moni-

tored carefully by recording such variables as the number of single leg-foot contacts, the number of double leg-foot contacts, and the height of a box or bench. The total number of foot contacts should be increased by no more than 10% per week. Due to the intensity of this type of workout, the athlete should not exceed two to three sessions per week. With practice and consistency, these drills can be very beneficial as a component of a reconditioning program designed to bring athletes back to a high level of performance while minimizing the risk of reinjury.

Quickness can be improved in the upper body by using hand slap drills (Figure 8–7), punching bag drills, and balls made to bounce in unpredictable directions. Because the upper body is non–weight-bearing in most sports, these drills can begin early—within certain guidelines—during the reconditioning phase. Quickness for the lower body can be improved using a number of quick foot drills, including ladder drills, the hexagon drill, the five-dot drill, the cross drill, and others. In these drills, athletes are pushed to move their feet as fast as possible while minimizing contact time with the ground. The footwork ladder (Speed City, Portland, Oregon) is an excellent tool for all areas of athletic fitness, including foot quickness. As discussed later, a wide variety of footwork patterns can be trained using the footwork ladder.

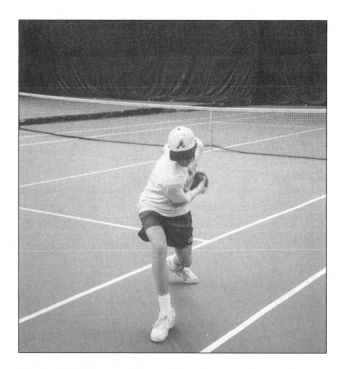

Figure 8–5 Sport-specific trunk rotation exercises can be performed with a medicine ball. These drills are particularly important in throwing and striking sports.

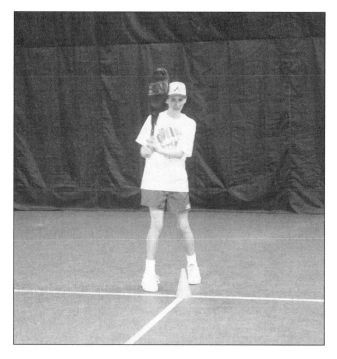

Figure 8–6 Progressing to trunk rotation exercises with a sports implement is a logical progression of a sport-specific reconditioning program.

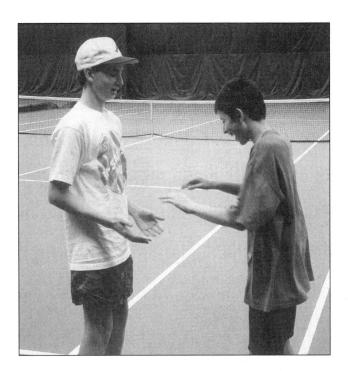

Figure 8–7 Hand slap drills can be used for upper body speed and quickness.

Balance and agility are important to many sports. It may be possible to improve parameters such as balance and agility by training the nervous system. In the case of injury and reconditioning, the goal should be to return balance and agility to preinjury levels of performance and perhaps beyond. Footwork drills, including ladder and cone drills, can improve balance and agility. Single leg drills, including strengthening exercises such as single leg squats and lunges, as well as single leg movement drills such as the hexagon and five-dot drill can improve balance. These drills are particularly important in the case of a lower extremity injury. Single leg exercises are particularly important in sports such as tennis and soccer, where the athlete changes direction often by stopping and pushing off of a single leg.

Speed—the ability to move rapidly from one point to another—is mostly dependent on stride frequency and stride length. Stride frequency is a function of neural drive, causing the muscles to contract as rapidly as possible, which should be a part of the reconditioning process. Generally, an athlete will plateau rapidly with respect to stride frequency, and further gains in speed must be a result of increasing stride length. Stride length can be improved with a number of exercises, including ladder drills, cone drills, form sprints, and changing footwork sprints. With the footwork ladder or cones, the stride length can be gradually increased by increasing the distance between cones or the number of boxes skipped.

For speed improvement, horizontal movement must be maximized, and vertical movement minimized. Athletes must be encouraged to maintain speed and momentum during the exercises. With changing footwork sprints, the athlete is performing one footwork pattern and is required to rapidly change to a second footwork pattern. The first step is critically important to athletes in many sports. The length may be shortened for some athletes after an injury due to inadequate range of motion.

The intensity of training, as well as the length of both the work and rest intervals between sets or exercises, is important to maximize performance and to minimize the chance of reinjury. Injured athletes should have progressed through the soft tissue healing phase before beginning many of these exercises. Initially, the length of time the athlete performs the drill may be limited by fatigue or inability to perform the activity. As the athlete becomes better conditioned, work sets can last from 3 seconds to 1–2 minutes. Athletes should progress from low-intensity exercises to intensities that match those of their specific sport; this is also the case with work/rest intervals.

SPECIFIC DRILLS FOR IMPROVING ATHLETIC FITNESS

Certainly, there are many drills that can be used to improve speed, coordination, balance, power, explosiveness, and other related characteristics of athletic fitness (Exhibit 8–2). The following is certainly not an exhaustive list of drills for improving athletic fitness. All of these drills can be modified to be used at various points in rehabilitation, reconditioning, and conditioning programs for a variety of sports and for athletes of all ages.

Line Drill

The line drill (Figure 8–8) uses a single line, which can be the line on a tennis court, a basketball court line, a piece of tape on the floor, or a line drawn with chalk. The basic movements for the line drill include (1) double leg front to back (jumping forward and backward over the line as quickly as possible), (2) single leg front to back, (3) stagger step front to back (with one foot in front of the line and one foot behind the line, alternating jumping forward with one foot and backward with the second foot at the same time), (4) double leg side to side, (5) single leg side to side, and (6) straddle with crossover (standing with one foot on each side of the line, crossing the feet so one leg is in front with the legs crossed, then back to the straddle position, then with the same leg behind the other leg, then back to the straddle position). The drills can vary in length from a few seconds to a few minutes. Athletes can move consecutively from one drill to the next without rest, once they have become conditioned to the exer-

Exhibit 8–2 Exercises for Reconditioning Progressing to Sport-Specific Athletic Fitness

Exercises for power
- Vertical jumps
- Bounding
- Barrier jumps
- Heel to butt, knee to chest, single and double
- Bounding ladder drills
- Medicine ball drills for trunk rotation, flexion, and extension

Exercises for hand and foot quickness
- Hand slap drills
- Crazy ball
- Punching bag
- Hexagon
- Five-dot drills
- Line jumps
- Quick foot ladder drills
- Cone drills

Exercises for balance and agility
- Ladder drills
- Shuffle drills
- Cone drills
- Single leg drills

Exercises for speed
- Ladder drills
- Form sprints
- Resisted/assisted sprints
- Changing foot pattern sprints

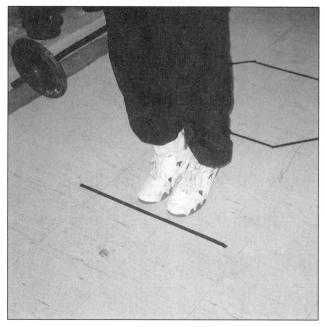

A

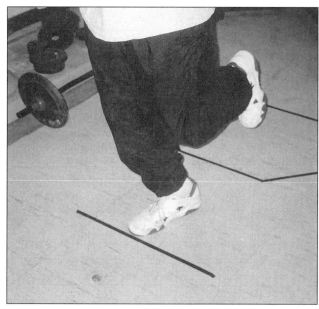

B

Figure 8–8 The line drill can be used with a variety of movement patterns.

cise. While performing single leg drills, athletes may need to switch between the right and left leg every few seconds until they become conditioned to the exercise. To make the drill harder, roll up a towel from the bathroom (or use some other type of soft barrier) and jump over the towel instead of a line. A variety of work/rest intervals should be utilized, progressing to the work/rest intervals and intensities specific to a particular sport.

Five-Dot Drill

For the five-dot drill (Figure 8–9), five dots are placed on the floor, four dots in a 2 × 3 foot rectangle, and one dot in the center. The dots can be a bit closer for young players and beginners, or a bit larger for experienced athletes. The basic movements in the five-dot drill are (1) front to back (or together apart, one foot on each dot on the narrow end of the rectangle, the athlete jumps and lands with the feet together on the middle dot, apart on the next two dots, then backward

and together to the middle dot, then backward to the original starting position), (2) two feet together (in a "skiing motion," two feet stay together and hit each dot going forward, then backward to the starting dot), (3) right leg only (same as two feet together except on one leg), (4) left leg only, (5) turnaround (the athlete starts with the feet apart on two dots,

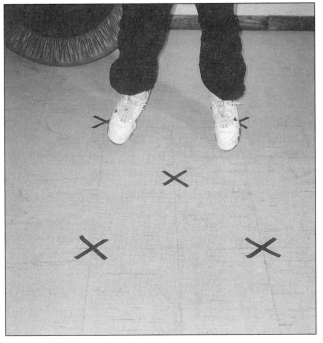

A

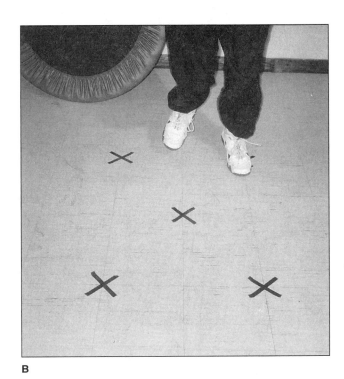

B

Figure 8–9   The five-dot drill can be used to improve foot speed, quickness, balance, and agility.

jumps to the middle dot for both feet, then the end dots with one foot on each dot; the athlete then jumps in the air, turning the body 180 degrees to face in the opposite direction with one foot on each dot; the athlete then jumps to the middle dot, the end dot, and continues to turn around on each end of the drill).

Hexagon Drill

The hexagon (Figure 8–10) consists of generally a 24-inch-sided hexagon drawn with chalk or tape on the floor. The hexagon can be smaller for smaller athletes or beginners. The hexagon drill was first used as a training drill for

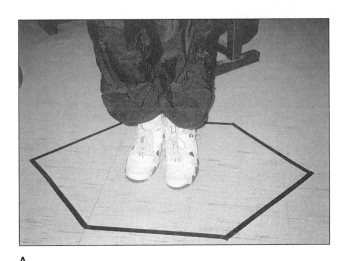

A

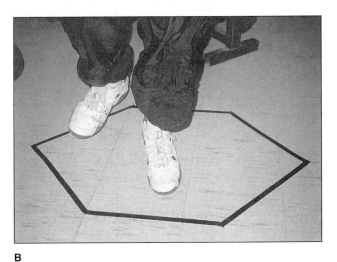

B

Figure 8–10   The hexagon drill is another drill that can be used in a variety of ways to improve athletic fitness.

skiers, keeping both feet together and jumping in and out of the hexagon. Variations include two feet clockwise, two feet counter-clockwise, one foot clockwise, and one foot counter-clockwise. Time intervals can vary, and athletes can switch directions or feet during the drill.

Ladder Drills

The footwork ladder (Figure 8–11) is a versatile tool that can be used in a variety of ways to train a variety of footwork patterns. Athletes can work on foot speed, quickness, balance, and agility by using such drills as alternating two feet in one box, alternating one foot in each box, skipping one box, jumping through boxes on one foot and two feet, and quick feet drills that can be referred to as *in-in-out* and *front-to-back*. To perform in-in-out, the athlete is moving forward through the ladder, both feet go in one box alternately, then one foot to the right, followed by each foot alternately going in to the next box. The proper teaching cadence is "in-in-right, in-in-left." Front-to-back is a similar

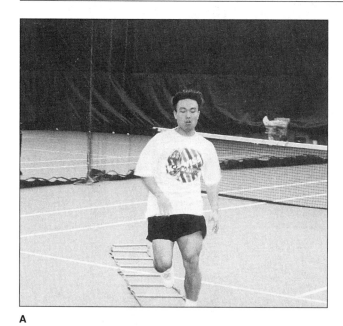

A

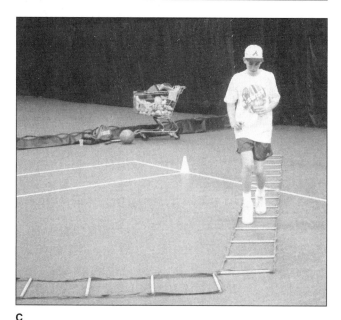

C

B

Figure 8–11 Ladder drills can be used in a wide variety of ways to improve footwork and explosiveness.

drill, except the athlete is moving sideways through the ladder. One foot touches in front of the ladder, followed by two feet alternately touching inside the box, then one foot touches behind the ladder, followed by both feet alternately touching in the next box. For side-to-side drills using the ladder, be sure the athlete moves both to the right and to the left.

The ladder drill can be used to train for speed, power, and explosiveness by using tall cones to jump over on both feet and on one foot, by skipping an increasing number of boxes to increase stride length (Figure 8–11B), and by using the ladder to perform bounding drills. The footwork ladder can also incorporate a 90-degree bend (Figure 8–11C) for the athlete to work on changes of direction.

Cross Drill

To perform the cross drill, use chalk to draw a large cross on the floor (Figure 8–12). Number the boxes as shown in Figure 8–13. Perform the drill as follows: (a) double leg clockwise (1, 2, 3, 4), (b) double leg counterclockwise (4, 3, 2, 1), (c) right foot clockwise, (d) left foot clockwise, (e) right foot counter-clockwise, (f) left foot counterclockwise, (g) double leg with "X pattern" (2, 3, 4, 1), and (e) single leg with "X pattern." Again, the length of each set will average from 5 to 15 seconds, with some longer sets as the athlete improves, and some shorter sets to work on power. Drills can be performed consecutively to increase the

difficulty, and towels can be used instead of lines to make the athlete jump higher in the air.

Flexibility, although not discussed in detail, is extremely important in the reconditioning program. Most general flexibility exercises can be maintained during the rehabilitation phase after injury (Figure 8–14). Specific flexibility exercises related to a particular injury will likely continue during the reconditioning phase. Also of interest relative to flexibility is the linked chain concept of movement and transfer of ground reaction forces. Inflexibilities may occur in body segments not directly linked to the injury. Research on inflexibilities common to a particular sport can point to musculoskeletal areas of high risk. A thorough evaluation of the athlete measuring flexibility throughout the linked chain, particularly those areas at high risk of injury, is important to the reconditioning process.

SUMMARY

Reconditioning is a critical component of the complete rehabilitation process. It should begin with a general conditioning phase, where the athlete builds a strength, flexibility, and aerobic base. In specific sports, functional rehabilitation begins at low intensity but should build to high intensity as the athlete approaches unrestricted return to play. With a gradual and functional return to activity using a wide variety of movement patterns, the athlete will be best prepared to perform at the highest possible level with a decreased risk of injury.

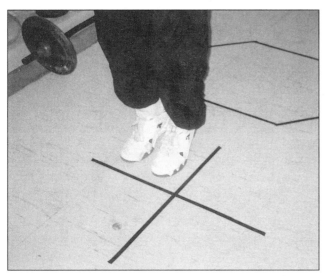

A

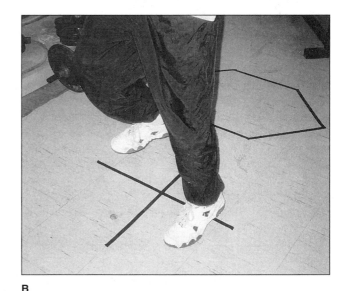

B

Figure 8–12 The cross drill can also be used as one of a variety of exercises to improve athletic fitness.

13A. Numbered quadrants for the cross drill

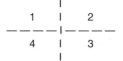

13B. Arrangement of dots for the five-dot drill

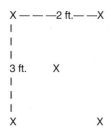

13C. Instructions for drawing a hexagon for the hexagon drill

_____

24-inch sides
120-degree angles

_____

Figure 8–13 Instructions for marking a court or floor for the hexagon, cross, and five-dot drills.

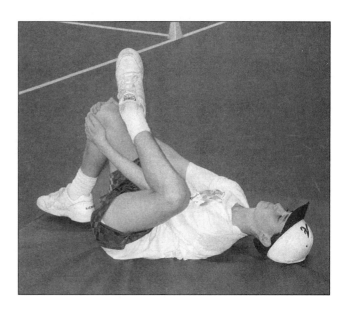

Figure 8–14 Flexibility, including general flexibility, flexibility specific to an injury, or flexibility specific to a particular sport, is important to prevent injury and improve or maintain performance levels.

REFERENCES

1. Kibler WB, Chandler TJ, Uhl TL, et al. A musculoskeletal approach to the preparticipation physical examination. Preventing injury and improving performance. *Am J Sports Med.* 1989;17:525–531.

2. Fleck SJ, Falkel JE. Value of resistance training for the reduction of sports injuries. *Sports Med.* 1986;3:61–68.

3. Chandler TJ, Kibler WB. The role of muscular strength in injury prevention. In: Renstrom PAFH, ed. *The Encyclopedia of Sports Medicine, Sports Injuries, Basic Principles of Prevention and Care.* Oxford, England: Blackwell Scientific Publications. 1992;252–261.

4. Chandler TJ. Exercise training for tennis. Lehman R, ed. *Clin Sports Med.* 1995.

5. Lephart SM, Henry TJ. Functional rehabilitation for the upper and lower extremity. *Orthop Clin North Am.* 1995;26:579–572.

6. Kibler WB. *The Sport Preparticipation Fitness Examination.* Champaign, IL: Human Kinetics, 1990.

CHAPTER 9

Aquatic Strategies for Athletic Rehabilitation

Robert P. Wilder, Andrew J. Cole, and Bruce E. Becker

INTRODUCTION

The use of the aquatic environment for rehabilitating sports injuries is rapidly increasing because the physiologic and biodynamic properties of water allow an athlete's injury to be rehabilitated rapidly and safely. Aquatic rehabilitation techniques allow earlier and more aggressive intervention that helps maximize physiologic function and recovery from injury.

Nearly all of the biologic effects of immersion are related to the fundamental principles of hydrodynamics. These include buoyancy, hydrostatic pressure, viscosity, refraction, specific heat, thermal conductivity, and temperature. Understanding these principles and their effects on the body's systems during immersion allows the astute clinician to prescribe safe, comprehensive, and effective rehabilitation programs. This chapter will review the fundamental principles of hydrodynamics and will apply these principles to the development of aquatic spine stabilization and aqua running programs.

PRINCIPLES OF HYDROTHERAPY[1]

Buoyancy

A body submerged in water is supported by a counterforce that supports the submerged object against the downward pull of gravity. The submerged body seems to lose weight equal to the weight of the water displaced, thus resulting in less stress and pressure on bone, muscle, and connective tissue. When patients are vertically immersed up to their necks, gravitational forces are reduced about 90%.[2] Buoyancy also allows for depth-dependent graded reduction of gravitational forces. Thus, by exercising in progressively shallower water, the athlete is reintroduced to weight-bearing exercise in a gradual, progressive fashion.

The center of buoyancy is located in the pleural cavity in supine patients. This center is distinct from the center of gravity, which is located at the level of the second sacral segment or anterosuperior iliac spine. In water, the more caudal the center of gravity, the greater degree of spine extension required to keep a supine patient afloat, i.e., to put the center of buoyancy in an optimal position to balance downward forces at the center of gravity. This has obvious implications for managing athletes with spine pain and should be assessed for each patient prior to beginning an aquatic exercise program.

Hydrostatic Pressure

Hydrostatic pressure is the pressure exerted by water on a submerged body. It is proportional to depth and equal in all directions. Hydrostatic pressure appears to increase the venous return to the heart and to effect changes in renal blood flow and sinus pressure; it may also assist resolution of edema related to musculoskeletal injuries.

Viscosity

Viscosity is defined as "the frictional resistance presented to a body moving through a fluid." This resistance is proportional to the effort exerted and allows the aquatic environment to be used as a useful strengthening medium. Because water is more viscous than air, the resistance it offers can also assist in increasing proprioceptive and kinesthetic awareness.

Refraction

Refraction results from the deflection of light as it passes from air into water. A visual distortion of submerged objects occurs when viewed from above the water. Refraction can affect visual feedback; therefore, appropriate guidance should be given when acquiring new skills and coordinated movements.

Specific Heat and Thermal Conductivity

Specific heat is the amount of heat needed to raise the temperature of a substance by 1 degree Centigrade. The specific heat of water is much greater than that of air (0.001–1); therefore, the rate of heat loss to water at moderate temperatures is much greater than the rate of heat loss to air at the same temperature. Additionally, water is an efficient conductor of heat, transferring heat 25 times faster than air. Thus, the risk of heat illness commonly associated with exercise is minimized in the aquatic environment.

Temperature

The aquatic environment allows regulation of the temperature during exercise. A pool temperature 80–86 degrees Fahrenheit (28–30 degrees Centigrade) appears to be an ideal range for exercise. In this range, the metabolic heat generated during exercise is easily transferred to the water without additional energy loss due to cold-water stress, thus avoiding impaired performance.[3,4] In the authors' experience, competitive athletes typically prefer a slightly cooler environment.

BIOLOGIC AND PHYSIOLOGIC EFFECTS OF IMMERSION[5]

Aquatic immersion has profound biologic effects, extending across essentially all homeostatic systems. These effects are both immediate and delayed, and allow water to be used with therapeutic efficacy in a great variety of rehabilitative problems. An understanding of these aquatic principles is beneficial in the management of patients with musculoskeletal and neurologic problems, cardiopulmonary pathology, and other medical concerns, both alone and in combination.

Circulatory System

Water exerts pressure upon the immersed body. Because the pressure exerted is greater than venous pressure, blood is displaced upward, first into the thighs, then into the abdominal cavity vessels, and finally into the great vessels of the chest cavity and into the heart. Venous return is enhanced by the shift of blood from the periphery to trunk vessels to thorax to heart. Central venous pressure begins to rise with immersion to the xiphoid and increases until the body is completely immersed. Right atrial pressure increases by 14–18 mm Hg with immersion to the neck going from about

−2 mm Hg to −4 mm Hg to about +14 to +17 mm Hg.[6,7] The transmural pressure gradient of the right atrium increases by 13 mm Hg, going from 2 to 15 mm Hg. Extra systoles may result, especially early into immersion.[6]

Pulmonary blood flow increases with increased central blood volume and pressure. Mean pulmonary artery wedge pressure increases from 5 mm Hg on land to 22 mm Hg immersed to the neck.[6] Most of the increased pulmonary blood volume is distributed in the larger vessels of the pulmonary vascular bed, and only a small percentage (5% or less) at the capillary level. This is validated by the fact that the diffusion capacity of the lungs changes very little.

Central blood volume increases by 0.7 L.[6] This represents a 60% increase in central volume, with one-third of this volume taken up by the heart and the remainder by the great vessels of the lungs. Cardiac volume increases 27–30% with immersion to the neck.[7] However, the heart is not a static receptacle. The healthy cardiac response to increased volume (stretch) is to increase force of contraction. As the myocardium stretches, an improved actin-myosin filament relationship is produced, enhancing the myocardial efficiency.[8] This has been researched for nearly 70 years and is commonly referred to as Starling's Law. Stroke volume increases as a result of this increased stretch. Whereas normal resting stroke volume is about 71 mL/beat, the additional 25 mL from immersion totals about 100 mL, which is close to the exercise maximum for a sedentary individual on land.[9] Mean stroke volume increases by 35%, on average, with immersion to the neck.[6] There is both an increase in end-diastolic volume and a decrease in end-systolic volume.[8]

In land-based studies, stroke volume is a major determinant of the rise in cardiac output seen in training; maximum heart rate response ranges remain relatively fixed.[8] In an untrained individual, maximum heart rate is commonly approximated by subtracting the individual's age from a pulse rate of 220 bpm. There is little change in the maximum heart rate achieved by the elite conditioned athlete; that is to say, the upper limit in an untrained individual is only 10–15% less than that of a trained one. As heart rate increases beyond an optimal point, cardiac output begins to decrease, due to shortening of diastole, which reduces time for ventricular filling, as well as for coronary blood flow in the left ventricle circulatory tree.[8] Maximum stroke volume is reached at 40–50% of maximum O_2 consumption, which equals a heart rate of 110–120 bpm on land. This is generally accepted as the rate at which aerobic training begins to occur.[9]

During immersion, as cardiac filling and stroke volume increase with increase in depth from symphysis to xiphoid, the heart rate typically drops.[10] This drop is variable, the amount of decrease depending on water temperature. Typically, at average pool temperatures, the rate lowers by 12–15%.[7] There is a significant relationship between water temperature and heart rate. At 25 degrees Centigrade, heart rate drops approximately 10 bpm,[11] whereas at higher temperatures, the rate drop is less than 15%. In warm water, the rate may drop little, if at all.[12] At very high temperatures, the rate may even rise slightly. The reduction variability is related to decreased peripheral resistance at higher temperatures and increased vagal effects. A proposed diving response may be involved as well in colder temperatures.

Water-based exercise has often been said to be less effective than land-based exercise for improving cardiovascular fitness.[8,9] Yet, during exercise, maximal myocardial oxygen consumption efficiency occurs with stroke volume increase because heart rate rise is less efficient.[8,9] Stated another way, the most efficient way for the heart to deliver more blood is to increase stroke volume, as heart rate increase places greater demands on the myocardium. Energy is wasted at the onset of myocardial contraction, when the heart is contracting but moving no volume, and at the end point of contraction when the heart is moving little volume and the myocardium is maximally contracted. The optimal length/tension relationship develops with increased stroke volume. Thus, as cardiovascular conditioning occurs, cardiac output increases are achieved with smaller increases in heart rate but greater stroke volumes.

Two recent studies by McMurray et al.[13] and by N. Tanaka and C. Tei (unpublished data, 1994) have validated the aquatic environment for cardiovascular rehabilitation following infarct and ischemic cardiomyopathy. In both studies, the investigators took the bold step of actively rehabilitating cardiac-diseased patients in an aquatic environment. Tanaka and Tei found that a single immersion in a very hot water (41 degrees Centigrade) bath dropped both pulmonary wedge pressure and right atrial pressure by nearly 30%. Over a period of one month, therapy patients showed nearly a 30% rise in ejection fraction, significantly improving by one, and sometimes two, New York Heart Association classifications.

Cardiac output is the product of stroke volume multiplied by pulse rate per unit of time. The heart as an organ is meant to pump blood; therefore, the measure of its performance is the amount of blood pumped per unit of time. Submersion to the neck increases cardiac output by 32%.[6] Output increases by about 1500 mL/min, of which 50% is directed to increased muscle blood flow.[14] Normal cardiac output is approximately 5 L/min in a resting individual. Maximum output in a conditioned athlete is about 40 L/min, which is equivalent to 205 mL/beat × 195 bpm. Maximum output at exercise for a sedentary individual on land is approximately 20 L/min, equivalent to 105 mL/beat × 195 bpm.[9] Because immersion to the neck produces a cardiac stroke volume of about 100 mL/beat, a resting pulse of 86 bpm produces a cardiac output of 8.6 L/min and is already producing cardiac exercise. Therefore, the concept that water exercise is not aerobically efficient is a myth—it may be an ideal cardiovascular conditioning medium. Unfortunately, there has been little direct research data on water exercise–produced cardiac output, only on oxygen consumption, a useful but derivative relationship to cardiovascular workload.

It is possible to measure the resistance of the left ventricle. Resistance is derived from the formula

$$P_{sa} - P_{ra}/Q$$

where P_{sa} = mean arterial pressure, P_{ra} = mean right atrial pressure, and Q = cardiac output. During immersion to the neck, systemic vascular resistance decreases by 30%.[6] Decreased sympathetic vasoconstriction produces this decrease, peripheral venous tone diminishing by 30%[15] from 17 mm Hg to 12 mm Hg. Total peripheral resistance lowers during the first hour of immersion and persists for a time thereafter. This drop is related to temperature, with higher temperatures producing greater drops. This decreases end diastolic pressures. Systolic pressures increase with increasing workload, but appear to be approximately 20% less in water than on land.[13]

In 1989, Gleim and Nicholas[16] found that oxygen consumption ($\dot{V}_{O_2}$) during water treadmill walking was three times greater at a given speed (53 m/min) in water than on land. Thus, looking at the reverse effect, during water walking and running, only one-half to one-third the speed was required to achieve the same metabolic intensity as on land.[11] It is important to note that the relationship of heart rate to $\dot{V}_{O_2}$ parallels the relationship extent on land-based exercise, although water heart rate averages 10 beat/min less, for reasons discussed earlier.[11] Consequently, metabolic intensity in water can be predicted as it is on land by monitoring the heart rate.

Pulmonary System

The pulmonary system is profoundly affected by immersion of the body to the level of the thorax, partly due to the blood shifting into the chest cavity and partly due to compression of the chest wall itself by water. The combined effect is to alter pulmonary function, increase the work of breathing, and change respiratory dynamics.

An overview of pulmonary physiology helps us understand the changes involved. When an individual is at rest and breathing comfortably, the normal excursion of air during inspiration and expiration is called *tidal volume*. At the end point of nonforced expiration, there is still a volume of air left in the lungs that can be expelled with increased effort. This volume is called *expiratory reserve volume* (ERV). Even when this volume has been expelled, there is air left in the lungs that cannot be voluntarily expelled. This remainder is called *residual volume* (RV). The combination of ERV and RV is called *functional residual capacity* (FRC). It is thought that this volume of residual air is a buffer for blood oxygen and carbon dioxide saturation levels, preventing extreme fluctuation. At the end of comfortable inspiration, there is still room for more air to be inhaled. This is called *inspiratory reserve volume* (IRV). As one exercises and increases the need for more oxygen, tidal volume increases, reducing both ERV and IRV. The combination of IRV and ERV with tidal volume is called *vital capacity* (VC) and represents a laboratory measurement of the maximum amount of air that can be inhaled and subsequently exhaled. Vital capacity varies widely with stature, gender, and individual variation. A low VC per body mass reduces the amount of oxygen available for metabolism, whereas a large VC to body mass ratio increases aerobic potential.

Functional residual capacity reduces to about 54% of the normal value with immersion to the xiphoid.[17] Most of this loss is due to reduction in ERV, which decreases by 75% at this level of immersion.[18] Expired reserve volume is reduced to 11% of VC, equal to breathing at a negative pressure of −20.5 cm H_2O.[17] There is some loss of RV, which drops by 15%.[18] Vital capacity decreases about 6–9% when neck submersion is compared to controls submerged to the xiphoid.[17,18] About 50–60% of this VC reduction is due to increased thoracic blood volume, and 40–50% is due to hydrostatic forces counteracting the inspiratory musculature.[17,18] Pressure on the rib cage shrinks rib cage circumference by about 10% during submersion.[17] Vital capacity does appear to fluctuate somewhat with temperature, decreasing with cooler-water immersion (25 degrees Centigrade) and increasing slightly in warm-water immersion (40 degrees Centigrade).[19]

The ability of the alveolar membrane to exchange gases is called *diffusion capacity*. Diffusion capacity reduces slightly, as does partial pressure of oxygen (Po_2) as the lung beds become distended with blood shifted from the extremities and abdomen. Total intrapulmonary pressure shifts to the right by 16 cm H_2O.[18] This causes airway resistance to the movement of air to increase by 58% or more, resulting from reduced lung volume.[17] Expiratory flow rates are reduced, increasing the time to move air into and out of the lungs. Chest wall compliance is reduced to the pressure of water on the chest wall, increasing pleural pressure from −1 to +1 mm Hg.[6]

The combined effect of all these changes is to increase the total work of breathing. The total work of breathing for a tidal volume of 1 L increases by 60% during submersion to the neck. This effort increases by approximately 4,000 g-cm, 75% of which is attributable to increase in elastic work (redistribution of blood from the thorax), and the rest to dynamic work (hydrostatic force upon the thorax).[18] Thus, for an athlete used to land-based conditioning exercises, a program of water-based exercise results in a significant workload challenge to the respiratory apparatus. This challenge can raise the efficiency of the respiratory system if the time spent in water conditioning is sufficient to achieve respiratory apparatus strength gains.

Musculoskeletal System

There are significant effects from water immersion upon the musculoskeletal system as well, resulting from compression due to immersion and reflex regulation of blood vessel tone. Resting muscle blood flow has been found to increase from a dry base line of 1.8 mL/min/100 g tissue to 4.1 mL/min/100 g tissue with neck immersion. Xenon clearance in the tibialis anterior during immersion to the heart increases 130% above dry land clearance.[14] Thus, oxygen delivery is significantly increased during immersion, as is the removal of muscle metabolic waste products. To resist blood pooling during dry conditions, sympathetic vasoconstriction tightens the resistance vessels of skeletal muscle. Immersion pressure removes the biologic need for vasoconstriction, thus increasing muscle blood flow. Hydrostatic forces add an additional circulatory drive. Because half-inch water depth equals 1 mm Hg, immersion to only 36 inches of depth causes a pressure head exceeding average diastolic pressure and acts to drive out edema, muscle lactate, and other metabolic end products.

Renal System

Aquatic immersion affects renal blood flow and the renal regulatory systems in many ways. The flow of blood to the kidneys increases immediately upon immersion. This causes an increase in creatinine clearance initially upon immersion.[15] Renal sympathetic nerve activity decreases due to left atrial distension, which increases renal tubular sodium transport.[15] Sodium excretion increases tenfold in sodium-replete subjects, and sodium excretion is accompanied by free water, creating part of the diuretic effect of immersion. This increase is time-dependent. Sodium excretion also increases as a function of depth,[15] due to the shifting of circulating central blood volume. Release of a humeral natriuretic factor occurs through distension of the atria, and the peptide produced—atriopeptigen—has both natriuretic and diuretic activity. Atriopeptigen relaxes vascular smooth muscle and inhibits production of aldosterone, and it appears to persist for a period of time following immersion. Potassium excretion also increases with immersion.[8]

Renal function is largely regulated by the hormones renin, aldosterone, and antidiuretic hormone. All these hormones are greatly affected by immersion. Aldosterone controls sodium reabsorption in the distal renal tubule, and its suppression accounts for most of the sodium loss with immersion. Suppression begins upon immersion, reaches maximum at 120 min, but is 60% of maximum at 1 hour of immersion time. Aldosterone production is reduced by

80% of control at 30 min of immersion time, 60% of control at 1 hour, and 35% of control at 3 hours. Antidiuretic hormone release is significantly suppressed with immersion by 50% or more and is the other major contributor to diuresis.[15]

Renin stimulates angiotensin, which, in turn, stimulates aldosterone release. Renin activity reduces by 20% of control at 30 min of immersion, 38% at 1 hour, and reduction maximizes at 62% of control at 3 hours' immersion. Plasma renin activity is reduced by 33–50% at 2 hours of immersion to the neck.[15] The combination of these renal and sympathetic nervous system effects is to lower blood pressure in the immersed individual with sustained immersion and to create a period of lowered pressure for a time thereafter.

Central and Peripheral Nervous System

There are many effects that have been anecdotally noted throughout centuries of use of aquatic environments for health maintenance and restoration but that are difficult to study. Predominant among these are the relaxation effect of water immersion and the effect that water immersion has on pain perception. Skin sensor nerve endings are all affected, including temperature, touch, and pressure receptors. Sensory overflow has been suggested as the mechanism by which pain is less well perceived when the affected body part is immersed in water. Pain modulation is consequently affected with a rise in pain threshold, which increases with temperature and water turbulence, producing the therapeutic effect long known with agitated spa immersion.

A relaxation effect is produced by a central process not well understood, likely multifactorial, and likely produced within the reticular activating system deep within the brain. Mood state has been found to improve following dry-land exercise but has not been studied in an aquatic environment. Similarly, anxiety and depression are reduced following dry-land exercise, but research to test these effects following aquatic exercise has not been done. Plasma catecholamines are known to increase during exercise and to decrease following exercise, and the rise decreases with training effect, which may account for some of these psychologic changes.[20]

Weight Control Issues

Water exercise seems to have a fat-sparing quality, as similar exercise intensities and durations do not produce similar body fat decreases.[21,22] It has been noted that elite aquatic distance athletes do not lower their body fat percentages to the same extent that elite track distance athletes do, corroborating this research. Nonetheless, aquatic exercise programs may be highly beneficial in the restoration of fitness in obese patients because of the protective effects against heavy joint loading achieved in the aquatic environment. The ability to achieve an aerobic exercise level long enough to produce a conditioning effect may be difficult in this population on dry land. A program initiating in water and transitioning to land as tolerance builds may be the most effective method of achieving both conditioning and weight loss.

Summary

There are many physiologic effects produced by the immersion of the human body in water. The cardiac effects produced through immersion are profound and probably very salutary, for both the healthy and the rehabilitating heart. Prominent among these effects are the increase in stroke volume and cardiac output resulting from immersion.

The effects of immersion on the respiratory apparatus and the pulmonary system have been found to increase respiratory effort and work. Therefore, a program of regular aquatic exercise should produce a significant training effect and increase pulmonary functioning.

The effects on the circulatory system and the autonomic nervous system, as well as the compressive effect of water pressure, dramatically alter muscle blood flow, increasing both O_2 delivery and metabolic waste product removal. These effects are salutary on both healing and normal exercising muscle and ligament structures.

The aquatic environment produces renal system changes that promote removal of metabolic waste products and produce diuresis, lower blood pressure, and assist the body in regulation of sodium and potassium. These effects persist longer than the period of immersion and may have general applicability in the management of some forms of hypertension. Moreover, they happen in a medium that produces an increase in relaxation and in pain threshold. These pain effects are significant for the rehabilitative practitioner and may facilitate program adherence and consistency.

AQUATIC STRATEGIES FOR LUMBAR STABILIZATION IN ATHLETES

Although many athletes with spine pain have been told by their physicians to swim for rehabilitation and aerobic cross-training, the role that the aquatic environment can play in spine rehabilitation has been further developed. The unique properties of water make it an ideal medium for rehabilitating athletic spinal injuries. A variety of methods may be used to integrate a water-based program into a comprehensive spine rehabilitation program.

Aquatic activity is the most prevalent participation sport in the United States and is an extremely popular form of exercise for recreation, competition, and rehabilitation.[23] Current estimates reveal that there are over 26,000 people involved with United States Masters Swimming and over

2,000 centers using aquatic techniques for rehabilitative purposes (United States Masters Swimming and YMCA of America, personal communication, 1993). The rising popularity of aquatic activities has resulted in ever-increasing numbers of spine and associated musculoskeletal injuries.

Land exercise, swimming, or an inappropriate aquatic rehabilitation program can cause a new spine injury or exacerbate a preexisting spine disorder, but a properly designed aquatic program can help rehabilitate an athlete with a spine injury. Aquatic stabilization techniques and swimming programs may be used in conjunction with an aggressive, comprehensive land-based spine stabilization program or as the sole rehabilitative tool[24] (also, R.E. Eagleston, personal communication, 1991). Swimming skills alone do not determine whether or not an athlete's spine injury can be rehabilitated in the water, because swim stroke proficiency does not correlate with successful treatment outcomes (M.L. Moschetti, personal communication, 1992).

Diagnosis and Treatment

The work-up and diagnosis of spine pain require a thorough understanding of anatomy, physiology, and activity-specific functional biomechanics. After eliciting a careful history, with close attention to the specific mechanism of injury, a thorough yet directed musculoskeletal and neurologic examination of the injured structure and its contiguous supporting elements is performed. A functional evaluation is conducted in which the patient reproduces any painful motion. Finally, appropriate ancillary testing is ordered, and the correct final diagnosis is confirmed.

Because the rehabilitation specialist has a thorough understanding of anatomy and stroke-specific functional biomechanics, he or she is able to develop a thorough treatment plan, including a complete rehabilitation program. The rehabilitation program must address the primary injury, whether spinal or peripheral joint, as well as any secondary sites of dysfunction.[25–28]

The rehabilitation specialist recognizes the functional relationship between the spine and peripheral joints. This "motion cascade" relationship was originally described by Cole et al.[25,29] Peripheral joint dysfunction can set off a cascading series of motion changes throughout the spinal axis. In particular, the cervicothoracic and thoracolumbar transition zones are most commonly affected because they are the junction between the more mobile and less mobile sections of the spine.[30]

When prescribing a rehabilitation plan, the rehabilitation specialist also must be aware that physiologic and psychologic needs vary among different patient populations. For example, highly competitive athletes require alternative training regimens during their rehabilitation programs to maintain peak flexibility, strength, and aerobic conditioning. Recreational performers may be more *flexible* in this regard.

The competitive athlete requires a specific training schedule and goals to compete effectively during this particular athletic season. On the other hand, a weekend athlete's needs usually are not as rigorous. Specific patient goals are met by tailoring the work-up and rehabilitation program to the level of athletic demand. Finally, changes in training routines and sports-specific mechanics require close cooperation among the physician, patient, therapist, and coach.[31]

Rehabilitation Programs

The aquatic rehabilitation programs that will be reviewed are based on the techniques of land-based dynamic spinal stabilization.[32,33] Dynamic land-based stabilization training is a specific type of therapeutic exercise that can help athletes gain dynamic control of segmental spine forces, eliminate repetitive injury to their motion segments (i.e., discs, zygapophyseal joints, and related structures), encourage healing of injured motion segments, and possibly alter the degenerative process. The underlying premise is that motion segments and their supporting soft tissues react to minimize applied stresses and thereby reduce risk of injury. The goals of aquatic stabilization exercise and swimming programs incorporate these elements but take into account the unique properties of water so that the risk of a spine injury is minimized. In particular, aquatic stabilization programs help develop an athlete's flexibility, strength, and body mechanics so that smooth transition to aquatic stabilization swimming programs or other spine-stabilized sports activities may occur. Aquatic stabilization swimming programs can, in addition, help the competitive swimming athlete further develop good swimming spine mechanics by minimizing segmental trunk motion and shear forces, reinforcing lumbar control, encouraging hip, knee, and ankle propulsion, developing head and neck stability, and establishing arm control and strength.[24,34–38] A review of the incorporation of stabilization principles in stroke technique will therefore also be reviewed.

Aquatic Spine Stabilization Techniques

The same principles of land spine stabilization are applicable to aquatic programs. Certain exercises, however, that can be performed on land cannot be reproduced in water, and vice versa. Aquatic programs can be designed for those athletes unable to train on land or for those whose land training has plateaued. Aquatic stabilization programs were first described by Richard Eagleston in 1989.[38]

The advantages aquatic spine programs offer are directly related to the intrinsic properties of water, including buoyancy, resistance, viscosity, hydrostatic pressure, temperature, turbulence, and refraction. The details regarding these properties have been described previously. Graded elimination of gravitational forces through buoyancy allows an athlete to train with decreased yet variable axial loads and shear forces. In essence, water increases the safety margin of an athlete's postural error by decreasing the compressive and shear forces on the spine. The velocity of motion can be controlled better by water resistance, viscosity, buoyancy, and training device use. Buoyancy increases the available range of training positions. The psychologic outlook of aquatic athletes, in particular, can be enhanced because rehabilitation occurs in their competitive environment. Many believe that a certain degree of pain attenuation takes place in the water because of the "sensory overload" generated by hydrostatic pressure, temperature, and turbulence.

Cole et al have developed a set of eight core aquatic stabilization exercises with four levels of difficulty that provide graded training of stabilization skills[24,35-37,39-42] (also A.J. Cole, M.L. Moschetti, and R.E. Eagleston, unpublished data, 1994). Programs must be customized to meet the needs of each athlete's unique spine pathology, related musculoskeletal dysfunctions, and comfort with the aquatic environment. The authors use a modification of the Brennan Scale of Perceived Exertion in the aquatic environment (utilizing numerical and simple verbal descriptors only) because it is simple and reproducible (Table 9–1). Although originally designed exclusively for deep-water running, the Brennan Scale and its verbal descriptors are easily adapted to aquatic stabilization programs.[43,44] Once mastered, a more advanced program is provided. Eventually, if an athlete would like to incorporate a swimming program, a series of transitional aquatic stabilization exercises are initiated to help establish a spine-stabilized swimming style that minimizes the risk of further spine injury and helps maximize swimming performance.

THE EIGHT CORE AQUATIC STABILIZATION EXERCISES: DISCOGENIC PAIN

Wall Sit

Wall sit develops isometric strength, primarily in the quadriceps and hamstring groups. Abdominal muscles are trained to hold the appropriate neutral spine posture.

- Level I (Figure 9–1): The athlete is supported by the pool wall in the vertical position with hips and knees in 90-degree flexion. This position is held for one minute.
- Level II: The position described in Level I is held for two minutes.
- Level III: The position described in Level I is held for three minutes.
- Level IV: The position described in Level I is held for five minutes.

Modified Superman

Modified superman trains ipsilateral hip flexors, extensors, and contralateral gluteus medius, as well as isometric strength in abdominal and paraspinal stabilizers.

- Level I (Figure 9–2): The athlete stands facing the pool wall in the vertical position, holding on to the edge of the pool with both hands. Movement is unilateral, one lower extremity at a time, with the knee flexed to 45 degrees. The hip is actively extended to 20 degrees and then returned to the neutral position. This movement pattern is continued for 60 seconds at modified Brennan Scale Level 1.
- Level II: Level II is performed exactly as in Level I, except that the knee is maintained in full extension, and

Table 9–1 Brennan Scale of Perceived Exertion

Level	RPE
1	Very Light
2	Light
3	Somewhat hard
4	Hard
5	Very Hard

Courtesy of Houston International Running Center, Houston, Texas.

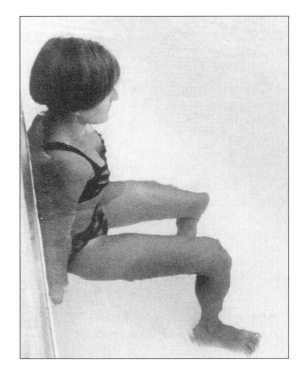

Figure 9–1 Wall sit, level I. Courtesy of Aquatechnics Consulting Group, Inc., Aptos, California.

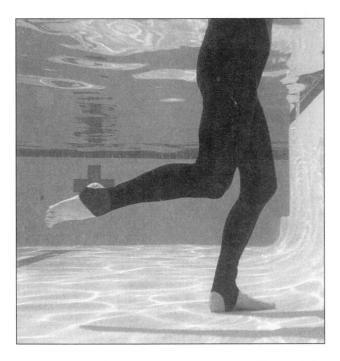

Figure 9–2 Modified superman, level I. Courtesy of Aquatechnics Consulting Group, Inc., Aptos, California.

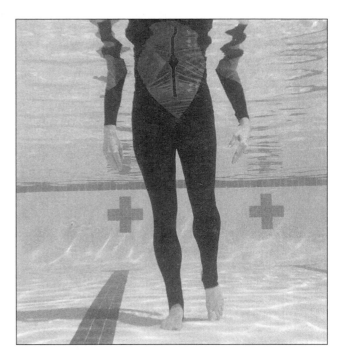

Figure 9–3 Water walking forward, Level I. Courtesy of Aquatechnics Consulting Group, Inc., Aptos, California.

the movement pattern is continued for two minutes at modified Brennan Scale Level 1.5.

- Level III: Level III is performed exactly as in Level II except that a 3-pound ankle cuff is applied to each ankle. This movement pattern is continued for two minutes at modified Brennan Scale Level 1.5.
- Level IV: Level IV is performed exactly as in Level III except that the pattern is continued for three to five minutes at modified Brennan Scale Level 2.

Water Walking Forward

Water walking forward (Figure 9–3) isometrically strengthens the abdominal muscle groups and those groups involved in maintaining proper posture. Isotonic strengthening occurs in those muscles dynamically involved in gait. Please see below for a description of the functional progression for this exercise.

Water Walking Backward

Water walking backward provides a strengthening pattern similar to water walking forward, but with greater emphasis on isometric paraspinal muscle conditioning.

- Level I (Figure 9–4): The athlete begins in the vertical standing position, unsupported, with the water depth at the xiphoid level. Elbows are kept extended with the

arm fully supinated and palm open. The patient water walks for three minutes at modified Brennan Scale Level 1.

- Level II: Level II provides for an incrementally greater challenge for all muscle groups described in Level I. The arms are abducted to 45 degrees, and hand mitts are used. The athlete walks for five minutes at modified Brennan Scale Level 1.5.
- Level III: Level III further enhances resistive training. Hand paddles are used, and the athlete walks for 10 minutes at modified Brennan Scale Level 2.
- Level IV: The athlete walks forward and backward with water shoes or 3-lb ankle weights applied to the ankles, or both. A piece of Plexiglas (36 in × 24 in) or a kickboard held vertically beneath the surface of the water is used to further increase the resistance. This exercise is performed for 10 minutes at a velocity of modified Brennan Scale Level 3.

Supine Sculling

Supine sculling simultaneously initiates strengthening in both upper- and lower-extremity muscle groups. Posterior and anterior muscle groups of the lower extremities, gluteals, shoulder complex, and paraspinals are incrementally challenged.

- Level I (Figure 9–5): The athlete wears a flotation jacket for support of the torso and a flotation collar for

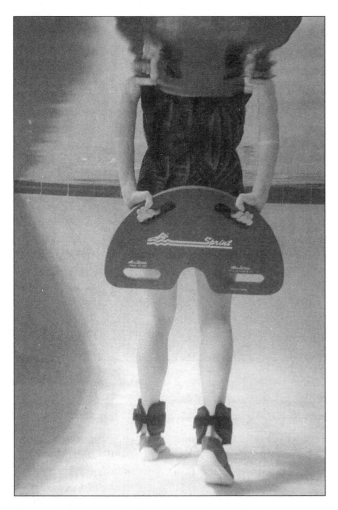

Figure 9–4 Water walking backward, Level I. Courtesy of Aquatechnics Consulting Group, Inc., Aptos, California.

the neck while being maintained in a supine, supported position by the therapist. Upper extremities, arms, and hands simultaneously perform a sculling figure 8 movement at the hip, while the lower extremities initiate a flutter kick. This exercise is performed for one minute at modified Brennan Scale Level 1.

- Level II: A flotation belt is substituted for the flotation jacket, and the cervical flotation support is maintained. The therapist supervises but does not support the athlete. Arms are abducted to 40 degrees, and the flutter is increased in intensity. This exercise is performed for three minutes at modified Brennan Scale Level 2.
- Level III: Hand mitts and short fins are added. The flotation belt continues to be used while the cervical support device is eliminated. This exercise pattern is performed for five minutes at modified Brennan Scale Level 2.
- Level IV: The flotation device is eliminated. Short-blade fins and hand mitts are used. Sculling and kicking are performed for 30 seconds with 15 seconds of rest. The exercise is performed at modified Brennan Scale Level 3; 12 sets are performed.

Wall Crunch

Wall crunch exercises train muscles activated in the wall sit and additionally challenge contralateral gluteals, ipsilateral hip flexors, rotational abdominals, and paraspinals.

- Level I (Figure 9–6): Standing with the spine against the pool wall, unilateral hip flexion to 90 degrees with the knee at 90-degree flexion occurs. This position is then isometrically resisted by the unilateral hand, and this

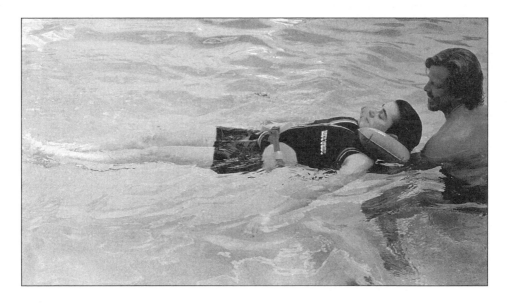

Figure 9–5 Supine sculling, Level I. Courtesy of Aquatechnics Consulting Group, Inc., Aptos, California.

isometric contraction is held for five seconds. Ten repetitions at modified Brennan Scale Level 2 are performed.

- Level II: Standing with the spine against the pool and the arms hooked over the pool ledge, simultaneous bilateral hip flexion to 90 degrees with the knees at 90-degree flexion occurs. This position is held for 10 seconds; 10 repetitions at modified Brennan Scale Level 2 are performed.
- Level III: Standing with the spine against the pool and the arms hooked over the pool ledge, simultaneous bilateral hip flexion to 90 degrees with the knees at full extension occurs. Three-pound ankle weights are applied to the ankle. This position is held for 10 seconds. Twenty repetitions at modified Brennan Scale Level 2 are performed.
- Level IV: This level is performed the same as Level III; however, there is no isometric hold. The motion is continuous for three minutes at modified Brennan Scale Level 3.

Quadruped

Quadruped is performed in the prone position, using a snorkel and mask to avoid the struggle for air while arm and leg mechanics are trained. Athletes who are unfamiliar with the proper use of the snorkel and mask may be taught by the therapist in one-on-one instruction in shallow water. All skills must be performed comfortably by the athlete prior to proceeding. Correct recovery from prone position to vertical standing must be performed. The therapist should not leave the athlete unattended while using any equipment in the therapy pool. Quadruped Level I activities (legs only) challenge lumbar spine stabilizer groups isometrically and lower extremity hip flexors and extensors isotonically. Level I quadruped activities (arms only) challenge lumbar spine stabilizer groups isometrically and upper extremity shoulder groups that reproduce flexion and extension isotonically.

- Level I (Figure 9–7): Begin with the athlete in a semisupported prone position with a flotation belt at the hip level. The therapist supports the legs and hips. The athlete moves both arms simultaneously with the elbows extended from 0 degrees to 180 degrees forward flexion. This motion is performed for one minute at 50% of maximum velocity. Next, the therapist supports the arms and instructs the patient simultaneously to move the legs from 0 degrees hip position to 90 degrees hip and knee flexed position. This motion is performed for one minute at modified Brennan Scale Level 2.
- Level II: The flotation device is removed, and the therapist supports only the athlete's hips. Alternating arm

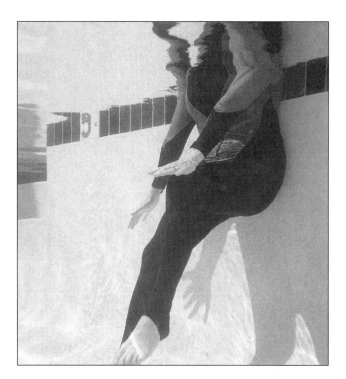

Figure 9–6 Wall crunch, Level I. Courtesy of Aquatechnics Consulting Group, Inc., Aptos, California.

movements are performed in a pattern similar to Level I for three minutes at modified Brennan Scale Level 2. The legs are then trained in an alternating pattern through the same range of motion as in Level I. This occurs for three minutes at modified Brennan Scale Level 2.

- Level III: Level III increases the training intensity by requiring greater independence during activity. All therapist support is removed, but a flotation vest is used. Simultaneous, alternating upper- and lower-extremity patterns as described in Level II occur for three minutes at modified Brennan Scale Level 2.5.
- Level IV: Weights are added to both ankles and wrists for an additional challenge, and a flotation is placed only at the waist to prevent the athlete from sinking. The movement pattern is similar to Level III but continues for five minutes at modified Brennan Scale 3. Once the athlete can perform quadruped, the log roll swim (an exercise transitioning to spine stabilized swimming) is introduced.

Log Roll Swim

The log roll swim teaches the appropriate spine movement, thus eliminating segmental rotation through the spinal axis. The athlete is supported at the hip with a small flotation

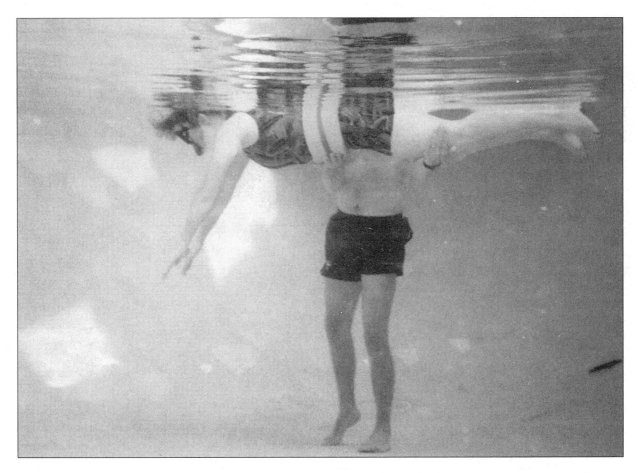

Figure 9–7 Quadruped, Level I. Courtesy of Aquatechnics Consulting Group, Inc., Aptos, California.

belt. A snorkel and mask are used to eliminate the struggle for air. It should be noted that the therapist may tape the lumbar spine with strapping tape to give proprioceptive cues and to avoid segmental spine movement.

- Level I (Figure 9–8): The therapist instructs the athlete to prone float with the knees flexed to 25 degrees and the arms at 0-degrees flexion. The cervical spine should be maintained at approximately 20 degrees of flexion. Proper breathing and relaxation are emphasized; upper-extremity movement of the entire shoulder complex begins with small rotatory movement of the lower arms under the chest, as if the athlete is rototilling water. The hips are maintained at 25-degree flexion. Small flexion/extension knee movements are initiated simultaneously with small rotary arm movements. Both of these movements cause propulsion. A lateral rocking movement is taught so that the athlete logrolls as a single unit in the water. This logroll motion minimizes the amount of segmental stress placed across each motion segment in the lumbar spine. The exercise pattern is performed for five minutes at modified Brennan Scale Level 2. Lateral flexion and rotation must be avoided.

- Level II: Level II begins with the upper extremity performing a scooping movement under the body. The arm is lifted in an arc for recovery above the head, just like the freestyle stroke, and the hand enters the water to repeat the cycle. The logroll pattern must be maintained. Once the upper body motion is correctly performed, Level I kicking is added. This exercise pattern is continued for five minutes at modified Brennan Scale Level 2.

- Level III: The Level II exercise is continued, except that the arm motion advances to that of normal freestyle, and kicking from the hip and not the knee is initiated. This pattern is continued for five minutes at modified Brennan Scale Level 2.

- Level IV: Level IV is performed similarly to Level III, except that the flotation belt is eliminated, and short-blade fins are used. This pattern continues for 10 minutes at modified Brennan Scale Level 2. At this point,

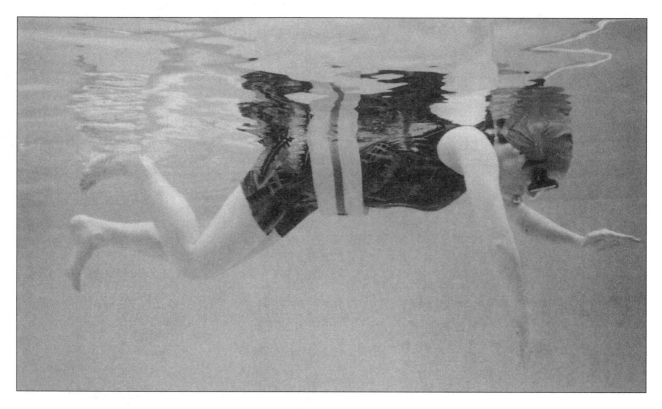

Figure 9–8 Log roll swim, Level I. Courtesy of Aquatechnics Consulting Group, Inc., Aptos, California.

the athlete sequentially can eliminate the mask and snorkel, as well as fins, and can begin a spine-stabilized swimming program.

SPINE-STABILIZED SWIMMING PROGRAMS FOR THE SWIMMING ATHLETE

Once stabilization skills have progressed to the point that a return to swimming is possible, a thorough analysis of stroke technique and its effect on spine motion is critical.[45] The following brief overview will focus on lumbar spine injury and will indicate the role that the cervical spine plays in the mechanics of lumbar aquatic motion. Stroke mechanics analysis, like gait analysis, should be done in an ordered, sequential manner so that all deficits and the relationships among them are carefully and fully scrutinized. We typically begin the analysis from the head and work distally.[24,25,33–36,39–41,45]

Prone Swimming

In prone swimming, the head should be midline. Breathing should occur by turning the head, i.e., rotating the head along the axial plane. There should be no craning, i.e., exces-

sive suboccipital cervical extension (OA) and rotation (AA), or cervical extension and rotation (C2–7) (Figure 9–9). Body roll also contributes to proper breathing mechanics and is essential to minimize dysfunctional cervical positioning and subsequent pain. The cervical spine should be kept in the neutral position along the sagittal plane because excessive extension causes the legs and torso to drop in the water, while excessive flexion can cause a struggle for air. Upper body arm position is evaluated by stroke phase. Freestyle is broken into three phases. The entry phase includes both hand entry and hand submersion ("ride"). The pull phase incorporates insweep, outsweep, and finish components. The recovery phase includes exit and arm swing. There are several stroke defects that can cause poor lumbar mechanics. If the arm abducts beyond 180 degrees, lateral lumbar flexion and rotation are produced (Figure 9–10). During the pull phase, decreased body rotation can cause lateral lumbar flexion and rotation that stress the lumbar motion segments, particularly the annular fibers surrounding the nucleus pulposus. Inadequate triceps strength during the finish phase results in low arm recovery, which, in turn, generates secondary lateral flexion and rotation through the lumbar spine. During recovery, inadequate body roll causes the neck to crane, which results in a struggle for air and accompanying lateral flexion and rotation through the lumbar spine.

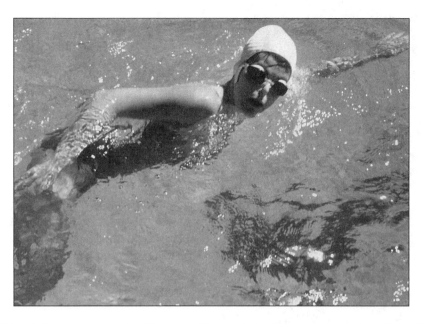

Figure 9–9 Cervical position during prone swimming. Courtesy of Aquatechnics Consulting Group, Inc., Aptos, California.

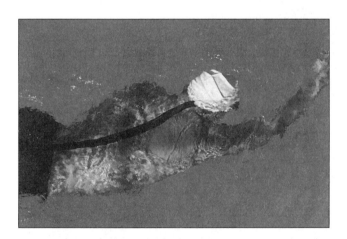

Figure 9–10 Stroke defects during prone swimming. Courtesy of Aquatechnics Consulting Group, Inc., Aptos, California.

Trunk motion is monitored closely for any primary or secondary lumbar flexion, both sagittal and coronal, or for axial rotation. If not corrected by simple changes in stroke mechanics, additional proprioceptive cues can be provided by taping the lumbar spine region. The tape pulls on the skin each time the lumbar spine moves in a segmental manner, ie, when the athlete generates excessive lumbar rotation or lateral lumbar flexion (Figure 9–11).

Flip turns are discouraged. Instead, stabilized turns are employed, in which the athlete initially comes to a vertical position before turning. This vertical position allows the athlete the opportunity to stabilize the spine in preparation for changing direction. Eventually, a horizontal spin is incorporated into the turn, and the vertical position is eliminated. Flip turns may then be resumed.

Supine Swimming

The supine position, starting with a simple kicking program with arms at the side, is best because adequate stabilization can be maintained easily. The use of fins often is suggested to improve propulsion. While supine, extension of the cervical spine will induce lumbar extension. On the other hand, cervical flexion will cause the patient to "sit" in the water, with lowered leg position and decreased propulsion. Extreme cervical extension or flexion is to be avoided in favor of a more neutral, stabilized cervical posture.

Problems with stroke technique usually can be solved with simple changes in stroke mechanics or by the addition of adaptive equipment. For example, a struggle for air can be resolved by the addition of a mask and snorkel. Trunk position can be improved by using the taping technique already mentioned. Poor propulsion can be remedied with an appropriate choice of fins. Hand paddles can provide better kinesthetic awareness of hand and arm position.

FUNDAMENTALS OF AQUA RUNNING FOR ATHLETIC REHABILITATION

Deep-water exercise is currently being incorporated into the treatment and conditioning programs of a number of our

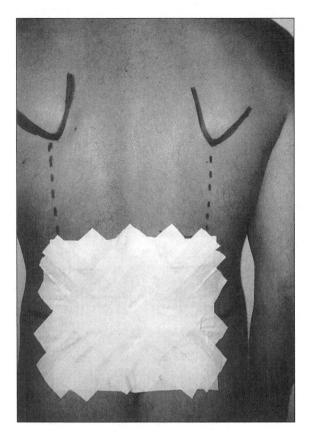

Figure 9–11 Taping techniques to control lumbar segmental motion. Courtesy of Aquatechnics Consulting Group, Inc., Aptos, California.

rehabilitation populations. This is especially true in the field of sports medicine where aqua running serves as an effective form of cardiovascular conditioning for the injured athlete, as well as for others who desire a low-impact aerobic workout. Aqua running, or deep-water running, consists of simulated running in the deep end of a pool, aided by a flotation device (vest or belt) that maintains the head above water. The form of running in the water is patterned as closely as possible after the pattern used on land. The participant may be held in one location by a tether cord—essentially running in place—or may actually run through the water the width of the pool. The tether may serve to increase resistance, as well as to facilitate monitoring of exercise by a physician, therapist, or coach. No contact is made with the bottom of the pool, thus eliminating impact. The elimination of weight-bearing makes this an ideal method for rehabilitating or conditioning the injured athlete, particularly those with foot, ankle, or knee injuries, for whom running on land is contraindicated. An understanding of proper technique, physiologic responses, and methods of exercise prescription will assist practitioners in incorporating aqua running into the rehabilitation and training programs of their athletes.

Biomechanics of Aqua Running

The form of running in water is patterned as closely as possible after that form used on land. For the runner or any athlete whose sport requires running, aqua running represents a biomechanically specific means of conditioning during a rehabilitation program or when supplementing regular training. This has special importance as the effects of training include improvement in cardiac and pulmonary performance, as well as improvement in those muscle groups being used that undergo enzyme changes, capillary density changes, etc. The elimination of weight-bearing and the addition of resistance change the relative contribution of each muscle group, as compared with land-based running. Every effort is made, therefore, to reproduce the running form used on land and to ensure the incorporation of those muscle groups that are used in land-based running. The following guidelines will assist in maintaining proper form during aqua running[43]:

1. The water line should be at the shoulder level. The mouth should be comfortably out of the water without having to tilt the head back. The head should be looking ahead, not down.
2. The body should assume a position slightly forward of the vertical, with the spine maintained in a neutral position.
3. Arm motion is identical to that used on land with primary motion at the shoulder. Hip flexion should reach approximately 60–80 degrees. As the hip is being flexed, the leg is extended at the knee (from the flexed position). When end hip flexion is reached, the lower leg should be perpendicular to the horizontal. The hip and knee are then extended together, the knee reaching full extension when the hip is in neutral (0 degrees of flexion). As the hip is extended, the leg is flexed at the knee. The cycle then repeats itself. The foot undergoes dorsiflexion and plantarflexion at the ankle throughout the cycle. The ankle is in a position of dorsiflexion when the hip is in neutral and the leg is extended at the knee. Plantarflexion is assumed as the hip is extended and the leg is flexed. Dorsiflexion is reassumed as the hip is flexed and the leg is extended. Underwater viewing has shown us that inversion and eversion will accompany dorsiflexion and plantarflexion as it does with land-based running.

The authors' experience at the Tom Landry Sports Medicine and Research Center and the Houston International Running Center has shown that a greater physiologic response in terms of maximum oxygen uptake and heart rate can be obtained by strict adherence to proper technique. The use of a flotation device is important for maintenance of proper technique.

Exercise Response to Aqua Running

Significant differences exist in metabolic response between aqua running and land-based running. In spite of these differences, however, aqua running has been shown to elicit sufficient cardiovascular response to result in a training effect, thus supporting anecdotal evidence of its usefulness in the rehabilitation of the athlete. The American College of Sports Medicine Guidelines for Exercise Prescription state that to obtain a training effect, one must exercise at an intensity level between 40% and 85% of maximum Vo_2 or 55–90% of maximum heart rate, maintaining this level for 15–60 minutes, 3–5 times per week.[46] Studies have demonstrated that aqua running elicits responses well within these suggested ranges.

Maximal Physiologic Responses

Several studies have compared maximal physiologic responses to aqua running and land-based running.[44,47–51] Important measures of response to exercise of maximal intensity include maximum oxygen uptake ($\dot{V}o_2$max) and maximal heart rate. $\dot{V}o_2$max values during supported deep-water running (with a flotation device) have ranged from 83% to 89% of those values obtained during land-based running; heart rates during deepwater running have ranged from 80% to 95% of those values obtained during land-based running, well within those ranges necessary to obtain a training effect.

Submaximal Physiologic Responses

Important relationships have also been noted during deep-water running at submaximal intensities.[44,49,50–54] It appears that for a given level of perceived exertion, heart rates and oxygen uptake levels tend to be lower during deep-water running than during treadmill running. Examining the relationship between heart rate and $\dot{V}o_2$ during submaximal graded exercise, Svedenhag and Seger[49] reported lower heart rates during deepwater running than during treadmill running at any given level of oxygen uptake. A similar relationship between heart rate and $\dot{V}o_2$ was noted by Navia[50] at higher workloads. These results suggest that an aerobic training effect may occur at lower heart rates during deep-water running than during treadmill running.

Long-Term Training Effects

Four studies have reported on the long-term training effects of a deepwater exercise program. Michaud et al[55] reported on ten subjects who underwent an eight-week training program of aqua running and showed improvements in maximal oxygen uptake during both water-based and land-based graded exercise testing (19.6% and 10.7%, respectively), thus demonstrating a training effect as well as a crossover effect to land-based exercise.

Eyestone et al[56] demonstrated that deep-water running was comparable to land-based running and cycling for preserving levels of fitness during a six-week training period at maintenance duration (20–30 min) and frequency (3–5 times/week). Although a small decrease in $\dot{V}o_2$max was noted for each group, this was much less than the 16%–17% loss previously reported during a six-week rest period.

Wilber et al[57] demonstrated no significant differences in treadmill $\dot{V}o_2$max, ventilatory threshold, running economy, and blood lactate at $\dot{V}o_2$max following six weeks of training in two groups, one training on land, the other training exclusively in water. Additionally, glucose and norepinephrine levels were similar between the two groups. Of note, both groups improved treadmill $\dot{V}o_2$max levels. Bushman et al[58] found no significant differences in simulated 5-km run time, submaximal and maximal oxygen consumption, or lactate threshold following four weeks of deep-water training in recreationally competitive distance runners.

Several possible explanations exist for the differences in metabolic response to deep-water running and land-based running.[44] Differences in muscle use and activation patterns contribute to these differences in exercise response. Furthermore, owing to the elimination of weight-bearing and the addition of resistance, less work is likely to be performed by the larger muscle groups of the lower extremities, and a comparatively increased proportion of work is done by the upper extremities than during land-based exercise. This may contribute to the lower maximal oxygen uptakes recorded during deep-water running. Lower perfusion pressures in the legs during immersion with resultant decreases in total muscle blood flow have also been proposed to influence a high anaerobic metabolism during deep-water running.[49]

Hydrostatic pressure is postulated to assist cardiac performance by promoting venous return; thus, the heart does not have to beat as fast to maintain cardiac output. This may contribute to the lower heart rates observed during both submaximal and maximal deep-water running. Temperature has also been demonstrated to have an effect on heart rate during exercise, with higher temperatures correlating with higher heart rates.

Familiarity with this form of exercise also appears to be an important factor in maximizing physiologic response to deep-water running when measured at a particular level of perceived exertion. Our experience at the Tom Landry Sports Medicine and Research Center and the Houston International Running Center has indicated that strict adherence to proper form and technique ensures higher physiologic responses, as measured by $\dot{V}o_2$ and heart rate.

Exercise Prescription for Aqua Running

Three methods are used for grading aqua running exercise intensity: heart rate, rating of perceived exertion, and cadence. Workout programs are typically designed to reproduce the work the athlete would do on land and to incorporate both long runs as well as interval/speed training.

Heart Rate

A high correlation exists between heart rate and oxygen uptake. The American College of Sports Medicine guidelines recommend that for a training effect, one must exercise at a level between 55% and 90% of the maximum heart rate (the target heart rate range).[46] The maximum heart rate can be estimated (220 minus age) or can be based on heart rate levels attained during exercise of maximum effort. Although heart rate levels in the water tend to be lower than those attained on land, it is possible to approach land-based values by adherence to proper technique. Heart rate can be monitored by a waterproof heart monitor or can be periodically monitored by palpation.

Rating of Perceived Exertion

Rating of perceived exertion refers to a subjective grading of how hard the athlete feels he or she is working.[59,60] Thus, if the athlete is jogging, perceived exertion is rated low. Sprinting would be rated with a high level of perceived exertion. The most commonly used scale of perceived exertion is the Borg Scale, a 16-point scale with verbal descriptors ranging from very, very light to very, very hard. We have been using the Brennan Scale, a five-point scale designed exclusively for aqua running with verbal descriptors ranging from very light to very hard (see Table 9–1).[43] We further instruct our athletes that Level 1 (very light) corresponds to a light jog or recovery run, Level 2 (light) to a long steady run, Level 3 (somewhat hard) to 5 to 10-km road race pace, Level 4 (hard) to 400 to 800-m track speed, and Level 5 (very hard) to sprinting (100 to 200-m speed). The Brennan Scale facilitates the incorporation of both speed and distance work

into workouts in a manner easily understood by both coach and athlete. A sample workout protocol is presented (Table 9–2).

Cadence

Wilder et al demonstrated a very high correlation between cadence and heart rate with intraindividual correlations averaging 0.98.[61] The authors treat competitive athletes who undergo a graded exercise test of aqua running following a standard protocol (Table 9–3). Cadence is controlled through the use of an auditory metronome. By recording heart rate responses to varying levels of cadence, we can anticipate an expected physiologic response to a particular cadence level. We can then design workouts using timed intervals at particular cadence levels.

The heart rate response is used primarily during long runs—prolonged periods of exercise at a specified rate (the target rate). Ratings of perceived exertion and cadence are most often used for interval sessions. Rating of perceived exertion is most useful in group settings, whereas cadence is most appropriate for individual sessions.

Maintaining conditioning is a challenge for the injured athlete. Aqua running provides an effective means to continue training during rehabilitation. Aqua running may then be incorporated into a regular training program, providing a low-stress form of additional cardiovascular exercise.

SUMMARY

The rehabilitation of the injured athlete employs a multidisciplinary approach to promote injury healing as well as maintenance of fitness. The aquatic environment offers an additional tool to assist in this rehabilitation, and its use should especially be considered with those athletes for whom exercise on land is difficult or contraindicated.

Table 9–2 Sample Workout Protocol

Total Workout Time and Workout No.	No. of Repetitions	×	Duration of Repetitions (min)	@	Exertion	Level	(Recovery Periods)
(37:00) 1	5	×	2:00	@	RPE	SH	(:30)
	8	×	1:00	@	RPE	H	(:30)
	5	×	2:00	@	RPE	SH	(:30)

In this case, the workout protocol (#1) would call for five repetitions of two minutes' duration each at a perceived exertion level of somewhat hard (SH), followed by eight repetitions of one minute's duration each at a perceived exertion level of hard (H), followed by five repetitions of two minutes' duration each at a perceived exertion level of somewhat hard, with a 30-second recovery period consisting of easy jogging after each interval, for a total workout time of 37 minutes. RPE, rating of perceived exertion.

Courtesy of Houston International Running Center, Houston, Texas.

Table 9–3 Houston International Running Center Data Collection Sheet: Wilder Graded Exercise Test for Aqua Running

Name: Date:
Predicted 90% Max Heart Rate:

Stage	End Point	Heart Rate	Cadence	RPE	Comments
W	4:00	48			
1	6:00	66			
2	8:00	69			
3	10:00	72			
4	12:00	76			
5	14:00	80			
6	16:00	84			
7	18:00	88			
8	20:00	92			
9	22:00	96			
10	24:00	100			
11	26:00	104			
Post	27:00	48			
	28:00	48			
	29:00	48			

W, warm-up phase; RPE, rating of perceived exertion; Post, postexercise values during cool down

Courtesy of Houston International Running Center, Houston, Texas.

REFERENCES

1. Edlich R, Towler M, Goitz R, Wilder R, et al. Bioengineering principles of hydrotherapy. *J Burn Care Rehabil.* 1987;8:580–584.

2. Harrison R, Bulstrode S. Percentage weight bearing during partial immersion in the hydrotherapy pool. *Physiother Pract.* 1987;3:60–63.

3. Nadel E, Holmer I, Bergh U, et al. Energy exchanges of swimming man. *J Appl Physiol.* 1974;36:465–471.

4. Astrand P, Rodahl K. Applied sports physiology. In: Astrand P, Rodahl K, eds. *Textbook of Work Physiology: Physiological Bases of Exercise.* 2nd ed. New York: McGraw-Hill Book Co; 1986:654–657.

5. Becker BE. The biologic aspects of hydrotherapy. *J Back Musculoskel Rehabil.* 1994;4:255–264.

6. Arborelius M, Balldin UI, Lilja B, Lundgren CE. Hemodynamic changes in man during immersion with the head above water. *Aerospace Med.* 1972;43:593–599.

7. Risch WD, Koubenec HJ, Beckmann U, et al. The effect of graded immersion on heart volume, central venous pressure, pulmonary blood distribution and heart rate in man. *Pflugers Arch.* 1978;374:117.

8. Hurst JW, ed. *The Heart.* 6th ed. New York: McGraw-Hill; 1986:51.

9. McArdle WD, Katch FI, Katch VL. *Exercise Physiology, Energy, Nutrition and Human Performance.* 3rd ed. Philadelphia: Lee & Febiger; 1991:435–436.

10. Haffor AA, Mohler JG, Harrison AC. Effects of water immersion on cardiac output of lean and fat male subjects at rest and during exercise. *Aviat Space Environ Med.* 1991;62:125.

11. Evans BW, Cureton KJ, Purvis JW. Metabolic and circulatory responses to walking and jogging in water. *Res Q Exerc Sport.* 1978;49:442–449.

12. Dressendorfer RH, Morlock JF, Baker DG, Hong SK. Effects of head-out water immersion on cardiorespiratory responses to maximal cycling exercise. *Undersea Biomed Res.* 1976;3:183.

13. McMurray RG, Fieselman CC, Avery KE, Sheps DS. Exercise hemodynamics in water and on land in patients with coronary artery disease. *Cardiopulm Rehabil.* 1988;8:69–75.

14. Balldin UI, Lundgren CEG, Lundvall J. Changes in the elimination of ^{133}xenon from the anterior tibial muscle in man induced by immersion in water and by shifts in body position. *Aerospace Med.* 1971;42:489–493.

15. Epstein M. Cardiovascular and renal effects of head-out water immersion in man. *Circ Res.* 1976;39:620–628.

16. Gleim GW, Nicholas JA. Metabolic costs and heart rate responses to treadmill walking in water at different depths and temperature. *Am J Sports Med.* 1989;17:248–252.

17. Agostoni E, Gurtner G, Torri G, Rahn H. Respiratory mechanics during submersion and negative pressure breathing. *J Appl Physiol.* 1966;21:251–258.

18. Hong SK, Cerretelli P, Cruz JC, Rahn H. Mechanics of respiration during submersion in water. *J Appl Physiol.* 1969;27:535–536.

19. Choukroun ML, Varene P. Adjustments in oxygen transport during head-out immersion in water at various temperatures. *J Appl Physiol.* 1990;68:1475–1480.

20. Connelly TP, Sheldahl LM, Tristani FE, et al. Effect of increased central blood volume with water immersion on plasma catecholamines during exercise. *J Appl Physiol.* 1990;69:651–656.

21. Gwinup G. Weight loss without dietary restriction: efficacy of different forms of aerobic exercise. *Am J Sports Med.* 1987;15:275–279.

22. Kieres J, Plowman S. Effects of swimming and land exercises on body composition of college students. *J Sports Med Phys Fitness.* 1991;31:192–193.

23. *Canadian Olympic Association Report.* Autumn 1982.

24. Cole AJ, Moschetti ML, Eagleston RE. Getting backs in the swim. *Rehabil Manage*. August/September 1992:62–71.

25. Cole AJ, Farrell JP, Stratton SA. Cervical spine athletic injuries: a pain in the neck. In: Press J, ed. *Physical Medicine and Rehabilitation Clinics of North America*. Philadelphia: WB Saunders Company; 1994:37–68.

26. Press JM, Herring SA, Kibler WB. Rehabilitation of musculoskeletal disorders. In: Press JM, Herring SA, Kibler WB, eds. *The Textbook of Military Medicine*. Borden Institute, Office of the Surgeon General. In press.

27. Kibler WB, Chandler TJ, Pace BK. Principles of rehabilitation after chronic tendon injuries. In: Renstrom Per AFH, Leadbetter WB, eds. *Clinics in Sports Medicine*. Philadelphia: WB Saunders Company; 1992:661–672.

28. Herring SA. Rehabilitation of muscle injuries. *Med Sci Sports Exerc*. 1990;22:453–456.

29. Paris S. The spine and swimming. In: Hockschuler S, eds. *Spine: State of the Art Reviews*. Philadelphia: Hanley and Belfus; 1990:351–358.

30. Saal J. Rehabilitation of the injured athlete. In: DeLisa J, ed. *Rehabilitation Medicine: Principles and Practice*. Philadelphia: JB Lippincott Co; 1988:840–864.

31. Saal JA, Saal JS. Later stage management of lumbar spine problems. In: Herring S, ed. *Physical Medicine and Rehabilitation Clinics of North America*. Philadelphia: WB Saunders Company; 1991:205–221.

32. Saal JA. Dynamic muscular stabilization in the nonoperative treatment of lumbar spine pain syndromes. *Orthop Rev*. 1990;19:691–700.

33. Cole AJ, Herring SA. Role of the physiatrist in management of lumbar musculoskeletal pain. In: Tollison DC, ed. *The Handbook of Pain Management*. 2nd ed. Philadelphia: Williams & Wilkins; 1994:85–95.

34. Cole AJ, Moschetti ML, Eagleston RE. Lumbar spine aquatic rehabilitation: a sports medicine approach. In: Tollison DC, ed. *The Handbook of Pain Management*. 2nd ed. Philadelphia: Williams & Wilkins; 1994:386–400.

35. Cole AJ, Eagleston RE, Moschetti ML. Spine injuries in competitive swimmers. In: Watkins R, ed. *The Spine and Sports*. St. Louis: CV Mosby. In press.

36. Cole AJ. *Spine Injuries in the Competitive Swimming Athlete*. Presented at the American College of Sports Medicine Annual Meeting; June 4–5, 1993; Seattle, WA.

37. Cole A, Eagleston R, Moschetti ML, et al. *Lumbar Torque: A New Proprioceptive Approach*. Presented as a poster at the Annual Meeting of the North American Spine Society; August 1–3, 1991; Keystone, CO.

38. Eagleston R. *Aquatic Stabilization Programs*. Presented at the Conference on Aggressive Nonsurgical Rehabilitation of Lumbar Spine and Sports Injuries; March 23, 1989; San Francisco, CA.

39. Cole AJ. *Aquatic Stabilization Strategies*. Presented at the American Academy of Physical Medicine and Rehabilitation Annual Meeting; November 16, 1992; San Francisco, CA.

40. Cole AJ. *The Intrinsic Properties of Water*. Presented at the American Academy of Physical Medicine and Rehabilitation Annual Meeting; November 16, 1992; San Francisco, CA.

41. Cole A, Eagleston R, Moschetti M. Sports specific stabilization training: swimming. In: White A, ed. *Spinal Medicine and Surgery: A Multidisciplinary Approach*. St Louis: CV Mosby. In press.

42. Cole AJ, Moschetti ML, Eagleston RE. Spine pain: aquatic rehabilitation strategies. *J Back Musculoskel Rehabil*. 1994;4:273–286.

43. Brennan DK, Wilder RP. *Aqua Running: An Instructor's Manual*. Houston: Houston International Running Center, 1990.

44. Wilder RP, Brennan DK. Physiological responses to deep water running in athletes. *Sports Med*. 1993;16:374–380.

45. Maglisco E. *Swimming Even Faster*. Sunnyvale, CA.: Mayfield Publishing Co, 1993.

46. American College of Sports Medicine. *Guidelines for Graded Exercise Testing and Prescription*. 4th ed. Philadelphia: Lea & Febiger, 1991:96.

47. Butts NK, Tucker M, Smith R. Maximal responses to treadmill and deep water running in high school female cross country runners. *Res Q Exerc Sport*. 1991;62:236–239.

48. Butts NK, Tucker M, Greening C. Physiologic responses to maximal treadmill and deep water running in men and women. *Am J Sports Med*. 1991;19:612–614.

49. Svedenhag J, Seger J. Running on land and in water: comparative exercise physiology. *Med Sci Sports Exerc*. 1992; 24:1155–1160.

50. Navia AM. *Comparison of Energy Expenditure between Treadmill Running and Water Running*. Birmingham: University of Alabama at Birmingham; 1986. Thesis.

51. Town GP, Bradley SS. Maximal metabolic responses of deep and shallow water running in trained runners. *Med Sci Sports Exerc*. 1991; 23:238–241.

52. Bishop PA, Frazier S, Smith J, Jacobs D. Physiologic responses to treadmill and water running. *Physician Sportsmed*. 1989;17:87–94.

53. Ritchie SE, Hopkins WG. The intensity of exercise in deep water running. *Int J Sports Med*. 1991;12:27–29.

54. Yamaji K, Greenley M, Northey DR, Hughson RL. Oxygen uptake and heart rate responses to treadmill and water running. *Can J Sports Sci*. 1990;15:96–98.

55. Michaud TJ, Brennan DK, Wilder RP, Sherman NW. Aqua running and gains in cardiorespiratory fitness. *J Strength Conditioning Res*. 1995; 9:78–84.

56. Eyestone ED, Fellingham G, George J, Fisher AG. Effect of water running and cycling on maximum oxygen consumption and two-mile run performance. *Am J Sports Med*. 1993;21:41–44.

57. Wilber RL, Moffat RJ, Scott BE, et al. Influence of water run training on the maintenance of physiological determinants of aerobic performance. *Med Sci Sports Exerc*. 1995;20:1056–1062.

58. Bushman BA, Flynn MG, Andres FF, et al. Effect of four weeks of deep water run training on running performance. *Med Sci Sports Exerc*. In press.

59. Borg GV. Psychophysical basis of perceived exertion. *Med Sci Sports Exerc*. 1982;14:377–387.

60. Carlton RL, Rhodes EC. Critical review of the literature on ratings scales for perceived exertion. *Sports Med*. 1985;2:198–222.

61. Wilder RP, Brennan DK, Schotte DE. A standard measure for exercise prescription for aqua running. *Am J Sports Med*. 1993;21:45–48.

CHAPTER 10

Functional Rehabilitation of Cervical Spine Athletic Injuries

Andrew J. Cole, Joseph P. Farrell, and Steven A. Stratton

INTRODUCTION

Interest and participation in recreational and competitive sports have increased over the past several decades. Approximately 25 million Americans run and jog regularly, 110 million swim, 65 million bicycle, 26 million play softball, 25 million ice skate, and 1.3 million participate in interscholastic football programs each season.[1,2] Each year, roughly 17 million Americans seek medical care for sports injuries, the majority of which involve the musculoskeletal system.[2,3] Although injuries to the cervical spine and head are the most frequent catastrophic sports injuries,[4] they do not occur very often.[2] The majority of cervical spine injuries are due to soft tissue and mechanical dysfunction of the spine and its supporting elements.[4] Epidemiologic, clinical, and basic sports medicine research has vastly improved our understanding of the specific risk factors, mechanisms, and pathomechanics of those sports that place athletes at high risk for cervical spine injuries.[5] Thorough training in musculoskeletal medicine and the principles of functional rehabilitation is important to diagnose and treat athletic injuries, including those of the cervical spine.[6] Physical therapists and athletic trainers play a critical role by providing physical therapeutic treatment that can help define and confirm a patient's diagnosis (J.P. Farrell, personal communication, April 1993). Although this chapter reviews sports-related epidemiology, anatomy, and biomechanics of the cervical spine, its focus is the rehabilitation of cervical soft-tissue and mechanical dysfunctions using the vicious cycle of tissue overload injury model as its basis.

EPIDEMIOLOGY OF CERVICAL SPINE SPORTS INJURIES

Epidemiology is the study of the distribution and causes of disease and injury in human populations. Epidemiologic research has helped identify risk factors for sports injuries and has provided information regarding the frequency and pattern of athletic injury.[7] This information has been successfully used to help reduce the number and severity of sports-related injuries.[8]

In the epidemiology of sports injuries, cervical spine and head injuries caused in football have probably received the most study because of the severity of the injuries and the attendant media coverage.[4,9–13] Since the 1950s, approximately 90% of all traumatic football fatalities have involved the head or neck, and the majority of serious cervical spine injuries has been caused by axial loading.[9] After the introduction of the modern football helmet and face mask in the 1950s and 1960s, a significant increase in deaths from head injuries was noted, whereas deaths from cervical injuries remained roughly the same. Helmet use caused players to begin using their heads to "spear" block and tackle their opponents, placing their cervical spines at increased risk of serious injury.[9] Shortly after the introduction of uniform helmet standards and rule changes, an educational program against spear block and tackle techniques was offered. Head injury fatalities decreased to the same level as fatal neck injuries,[2,9] and serious cervical spine injuries declined dramatically.[8] Yet,

Source: Reprinted with permission from A. Cole, Cervical Spine Athletic Injuries: A Pain in the Neck, *Physical Medicine and Rehabilitation Clinics of North America,* Vol. 5, pp. 37–67, Copyright © 1994, W.B. Saunders Company.

The authors wish to thank Marcus G. Calahan and Joyce Heiser for helping to prepare the manuscript and Carolyn A. Cole, MS, for her editorial assistance. The authors would also like to thank the staff of the Scientific Publications Office for their editorial assistance.

after the new standards for helmets and block and tackle techniques took effect, illegal spear block and tackle techniques accounted for the majority of vertebral injuries to the cervical spine resulting in quadriplegia.[4] The rule changes that outlawed the spear block and tackle techniques and brought about a return to shoulder blocking techniques did not result in an increase in brachial plexus injuries,[9] nor was the face mask, type or brand of helmet, or playing surface found to be responsible for cervical neurotrauma.[9]

The mechanism of axial loading has been found to be the most common cause of athletic cervical spine injury in other sports, such as diving,[14] ice hockey,[15] rugby,[16] wrestling,[17,18] and trampolining.[13] The forces that players generate have increased with their greater size, speed, strength, and self-confidence—some of the latter due to better protective equipment. These increased forces could account for the greater numbers of spinal fractures seen in hockey players. The increased number of spinal fractures may also be a warning to other athletes of a clear and present danger.[11,19–22] To create the strength, flexibility, and endurance that provide a player with the controlled spinal motion needed to buffer the forces applied to the cervical spine, renewed emphasis must be placed on appropriate training techniques and conditioning. Mandatory preseason screening evaluations by team physicians identify the injuries and strength or flexibility deficits that would keep an athlete from competition or would require thorough rehabilitation prior to full training or competition.

Sports equipment must be constantly scrutinized for defects. The equipment must also meet established standards for player protection and must not create new types of injuries, exacerbate existing injuries, or increase the frequency of routinely treated problems. These same considerations are important when evaluating any type of athletic injury. Rule changes should always be coupled with adequate education of the players and the coaching, training, and medical staffs. Additional epidemiologic research for all types of sporting activities is necessary to define the frequency of different types of injuries. Outcome studies also are needed to evaluate the efficacy of the factors that control numbers and severity of athletic injuries.

FUNCTIONAL ANATOMY AND BIOMECHANICS

The seven cervical vertebrae connect the head to a relatively immobile thorax. The cervical spine and its supporting elements provide the stability and flexibility needed to control motion and distribute forces applied to the spine. Although cervical vertebrae increase in size with caudal progression to help support increasing loads,[23,24] the cervical vertebral canal is more capacious than the canal at any other part of the spine. Though variable, the transverse diameter decreases with caudal progression. The sagittal diameter decreases slightly down to the third cervical vertebra, then remains relatively constant. When making a diagnosis of instability or cervical spinal stenosis in an athlete, important anatomic information is found on both static and dynamic cervical spine radiographic images. Equally important is the relationship of the sagittal diameter of the central spinal canal to the sagittal diameter of the vertebral bodies.[25,26]

The first and second cervical vertebrae are unique in both appearance and function, whereas the third, fourth, fifth, sixth, and seventh cervical vertebrae are similar.[27–30] The first cervical vertebra, the *atlas*, lacks a vertebral body, having been absorbed into the structure of the axis. The atlas is a ring of bone composed primarily of an anterior arch, lateral masses, posterior arch, and bilateral inward projections of bone called *tubercles* that give rise to the transverse ligament. The atlas can be viewed as a "washer" between the occiput and *axis,* that is, C2.[29] Weight-bearing occurs through the right and left lateral masses.[27–29,31] The superior kidney-shaped concave facet surfaces face upward and inward to support and articulate with the paired convex occipital condyles, which face downward and outward.[27–29,32] Active flexion around the transverse axis of the occipitoatlantal joint has a 15-degree range, whereas active extension has a range of 20 degrees. This occipitoatlantal flexion and extension represent approximately 50% of all flexion and extension occurring in the cervical spine. Impingement of the anterior margin of the foramen magnum on the dens creates a bony limit to further flexion. Smaller amounts of active side bending occur around a sagittal axis and measure approximately 5 degrees. Minor amounts of active rotation may also occur and have been reported to be up to 8 degrees.[29,30,33–38] Stability for this joint is provided by the occipitoatlantal joint configuration, its capsule, and the ligamentum nuchae, as well as the tectorial membrane, the alar, and possibly apical ligaments.[30] The ligaments of the cervical spine, in general, provide stability to joints and significant proprioceptive feedback during physiologic motion; they also help absorb energy during trauma.[39,40]

The second cervical vertebra, the *axis*, has a large body that gives rise to the odontoid process, also called the *dens.* The dens is the phylogenetically displaced body of the atlas. The dens serves as a pivot around which the atlas rotates. The transverse ligament keeps the odontoid process confined to the anterior third of the atlantal ring and permits free rotation of the atlas on the dens and axis as well as ensuring stability during flexion, extension, and lateral bending. The right and left alar ligaments connect the lateral aspect of the apex of the dens to the ipsilateral medial aspect of the occipital condyle and anchor the skull to the axis. They help control excessive lateral and rotational motions, but not flexion or extension. The alar ligaments provide the next line of support against any further anterior translation of the atlas on the axis after rupture of the transverse ligament. If the alar ligaments fail, there remains no other significant barrier to prevent spinal cord compression.[24,27,41,42] Rupture of the transverse ligament should be suspected in an athlete who has a transverse diameter of the atlas 7 mm or greater than the transverse diameter of the axis on anteroposterior (AP) open-mouth projection of C1–C2. This rupture can be encountered in the athlete who sustains a comminuted burst fracture of the atlas.[30,43] A severe cervical flexion injury may cause an atlantoaxial dislocation and rupture of the transverse and alar ligaments. This allows the atlas to translate anteriorly, resulting in impingement of the spinal cord between the posterior aspect of the odontoid process and the posterior rim of the atlas. Rupture of the transverse ligament creates a very unstable spine and can potentially be a fatal injury. Lateral radiographic views of the atlantoaxial articulation show an increase of the atlanto-dens interval and a decrease in the space available for the spinal cord.[43,44] The transverse processes of the atlas (C1), axis (C2), C3, C4, C5, C6, and, usually, C7 have foramen transversarium that house and protect the vertebral arteries. The transverse processes of the atlas and axis also provide attachment sites for the longissimus cervicis, splenius cervicis, and other muscles.[28,29,45]

The superior articular facets of the axis are oriented superiorly and laterally. These facets are convex anteroposteriorly and flat transversely. They articulate with the flat inferior facets of the atlas, which face downward and inward.[31] The plane of the atlantoaxial joint is almost horizontal and is well designed to allow rotary motion. Approximately 40–50 degrees of rotation can occur to each side. This range constitutes half of the total rotation of the cervical spine. Approximately 60% of the axial rotation of the entire cervical spine and occiput occurs in the upper cervical spine, that is, in the occipitoatlantal and atlantoaxial joints.[36,46] Rotation at the atlantoaxial joint is limited primarily by the alar ligaments.[24]

Approximately 10–15 degrees of flexion and rotation occur in the atlantoaxial joint. This range of motion is limited by bony geometry and the securing ligaments. Given the shape of the facet surfaces, rotation produces a telescoping effect and, thus, some joint space widening. This widening is visible on rotational radiographic views and should not be mistaken for instability of the joint. Because the joint capsule is loose, which contributes to the mobility of the atlantoaxial joint, the mobility of this joint is the greatest of any joint in the spine.[27–29] The large amount of rotation that occurs at the atlantoaxial joint can result in traction or kinking of the vertebral artery that passes through the foramen transversarium. After 30 degrees of rotation, kinking of the contralateral vertebral artery may occur, and at 45 degrees of rotation, the ipsilateral vertebral artery may also kink. Reduced circulation to the brain stem and upper spinal cord may result in symptoms and signs of vertibrobasilar insufficiency.[36,47–49] Kinking and consequent reduced circulation may develop iatrogenically because of a traumatic sports injury,[50] inappro-

priate cervical manipulation,[47,49,51] cervical traction,[52] or a therapeutic exercise that creates a rotational subluxation or dislocation of the atlas on the axis.[47,50] Stability of the atlantoaxial joint is provided primarily by the dens and the ring of structures surrounding it; that is, by the osseous portion of the atlas anteriorly and laterally, and the transverse ligament posteriorly.[30]

The third through seventh cervical vertebrae are similar in appearance and function. The vertebral bodies are ovoid and are wider than they are tall. The bilateral raised uncinate processes (or hooks) that are located posterolaterally correspond to similar beveled surfaces, the echancrure (or anvil), located on the inferior aspect of the superior vertebral body. These "uncovertebral joints," also known as *joints of Luschka*, are not present in the embryologic development of the cervical spine but arise as a consequence of the degenerative and adaptive changes of annular tissue to loads and stresses.[27–29]

Intervertebral discs, made up of an outer annulus fibrosis and an inner nucleus pulposus, are located at each motion segment distal to the axis. They are biconvex and conform to the concavity of the vertebral bodies. These discs are thicker anteriorly and, thus, contribute to normal cervical lordosis. The thickest disc is located at C6–C7. Only the outer one-third to one-half of the annular fibers in adults has a vascular supply. The remainder of the annulus and the entire nucleus pulposus are avascular. Nutrition of the inner annular fibers and the nucleus pulposus must, therefore, occur by alternative compression, dehydration, diffusion, and imbibition of fluids.[53,54] The annular fibers that contain the disc are made up of 10–20 circumferential collagenous lamellae. Although the direction of inclination alternates with each lamella, the fibers within each lamella are oriented 35 degrees from the horizontal. Therefore, rotation and translation are more likely to injure the annulus because resistance can be offered by only half of the available lamellae—those with their fibers oriented in the direction of motion.[53] The annulus, particularly the middle third, has been found to be innervated by both nociceptors and mechanoreceptors.[55,56] Painful stimuli, generated by structural disruption of the intervertebral disc itself or possibly created by the chemically mediated inflammatory effect of phospholipase A_2, are mediated by these receptors. Proprioceptive information is thought to be transmitted by the pacinian corpuscles and Golgi tendon organs, which are particularly numerous in the posterolateral region of the outer third of the annulus.[26,53,54,56–59] The intervertebral disc transmits compressive loads throughout a range of motion, but it prevents excessive stress concentrations by slowing the rate at which an applied force is transmitted through the cervical spine. The disc diverts some of the force by temporarily stretching annular fibers, thus protecting each of the underlying vertebrae from receiving the entire force at one time. Stress concentrations are also minimized by a posterior nuclear shift during flexion and an anterior nuclear shift during extension.[24,32,53,54]

The cervical facet joints are synovial joints. Their fibrous capsules are lined with synovium, and their articular surfaces are covered with hyaline cartilage. The facet capsule is richly innervated by both nocioceptors and mechanoreceptors. There are even more mechanoreceptors in the cervical facet capsules than in their lumbar counterparts, thus enhancing cervical proprioception.[53,54,60] The orientation of the cervical facet joints allows them to provide resistance to anterior translation and also to play a weight-bearing role.[24,54,61] From C2–C3, the facet joints' articular planes are oriented at approximately 45 degrees from the horizontal, and with caudal progression, this inclination increases slightly. The articular planes of the facet joints are oriented 70–85 degrees to the sagittal plane. The C2–C3 facet is considered transitional anatomically and biomechanically because of its location between two parts of the cervical spine that move differently. The atlantoaxial joint moves in rotation, and the lower cervical spine both flexes and extends.[24,29,62] Because of the roughly 45 degrees of inclination of the cervical facet joints, lateral bending from C2 to C3 distally is always coupled with rotation in the same direction (Figure 10–1). Pure rotation or side bending is not possible. The relative amount of rotation or side bending that occurs depends on the obliquity of the articular surfaces in the frontal plane. The more horizontal the joint surface, the more the rotation is coupled; and the more vertical, the more side bending is coupled.[27,29,32,62] Cervical facet menisci undergo regressive changes with age. The meniscus narrows and retracts between childhood and the fourth decade.[63] The meniscus is thought to help increase the surface area of contact when articular fac-

ets come together, thus helping to transmit some of the force.[64]

The principal ligaments supporting the middle and lower portions of the cervical spine include the posterior and anterior longitudinal ligaments, the interspinous ligament, the ligamentum nuchae, and the ligamentum flavum. The anterior longitudinal ligament runs from the sacrum to the axis, where it then merges with the anterior atlanto-occipital membrane. The posterior longitudinal ligament also runs the length of the spine and is widest in the cervical spine. The posterior longitudinal ligament widens posterior to the axis and atlas. From this area proximally, the ligament is called the *tectorial membrane*. The tectorial membrane attaches to the clivus and basilar portion of the occipital bone. The anterior and posterior longitudinal ligaments provide significant stability to the intervertebral joints. The posterior longitudinal ligament limits flexion and distraction.[24,28,46] The articulations between the vertebral arches are maintained by the supraspinous ligaments, which evolve into the ligamentum nuchae; the interspinous ligaments, which are poorly developed in the cervical spine; and the segmental ligamentum flavum. The ligamentum nuchae and interspinous ligaments limit flexion and anterior horizontal displacement. Because it has a great deal of elastic tissue, the ligamentum flavum helps limit flexion of the cervical spine.[24,28,46,65,66] The anterior and posterior longitudinal ligament and the interspinous ligaments have a nerve supply that may be similar to their lumbar counterparts.[67–69] The ligamentum flavum does not have a nerve supply.[70]

The cervical spinal cord is somatotopically arranged. This arrangement facilitates the diagnosis of upper motoneuron injury. A regular series of dorsal rootlets, or fila, arises from

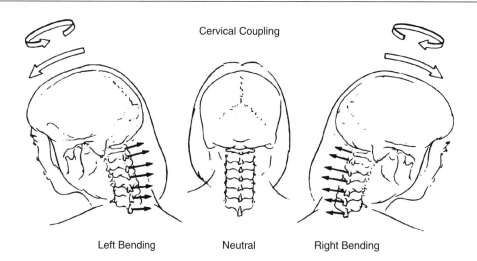

Cervical Coupling

Left Bending   Neutral   Right Bending

Figure 10–1 An important cervical spine coupling pattern. When the head and neck are bent to the left, the spinous processes go to the right. The converse is also shown. *Source:* Reprinted with permission from A.A. White and M.M. Panjabi, Kinematics of the Spine, in White, A.A., Panjabi, M.M., *Clinical Biomechanics of the Spine,* 2nd ed., p. 100, © 1990, J.B. Lippincott.

the dorsolateral sulcus of the spinal cord, and a less regular series of ventral rootlets arises from the ventrolateral aspect of the spinal cord. These rootlets form the dorsal and ventral spinal nerve roots. To help stabilize the spinal cord, the denticulate ligaments anchor lateral expansions of the pia mater surrounding the spinal cord to the internal aspect of the dural sac. The dorsal and ventral roots are also invested with pia mater and are surrounded by an arachnoid sleeve, which is inside the overlying dural sleeve. These two roots are enclosed within a funnel-shaped dural sac that tapers toward the intervertebral foramen. The dorsal and ventral nerve roots become separately enclosed in arachnoid and dural sleeves at the entrance to the foramen. At the level of the dorsal root ganglion, which is located near the outer orifice or just lateral to the foramen, the arachnoid layer ends, allowing spinal fluid within the subarachnoid space to surround the nerve slightly past the interforaminal level.[27,70,71] The mixed spinal nerve has only a dural sheath that then blends imperceptibly into the epineurium. The epineurium gives rise to the perineurium and endoneurium. These tissues invest the spinal nerve and provide it with structural integrity. The dorsal and ventral roots within the dural sheath are supported only by the pia mater that surrounds them. The spinal nerves divide into anterior and posterior rami. The cervical posterior rami supply the intrinsic spinal musculature and the overlying skin. The fifth through eighth cervical anterior primary rami and first thoracic anterior primary rami form the brachial plexus. The epineurium of the fourth, fifth, and sixth cervical anterior primary rami is anchored to the periosteum of the transverse processes at the same level and one level above the fascial prolongation of the posterior longitudinal ligament, the scalene muscle group, and the adventitial coating of the vertebral artery that fixes the spinal nerve against the transverse process.[27,70–73]

The cervical spine is innervated posteriorly by the branches of the dorsal rami of the spinal nerves and anteriorly by the ventral rami. The C1 dorsal ramus supplies the suboccipital muscles. There may be communication with C2. Inconsistently, cutaneous branches are found that may join the greater occipital nerve. The C2 dorsal ramus arises dorsal to the lateral atlantoaxial joint and supplies the splenius capitis and semispinalis capitis. The medial branch, also known as the *greater occipital nerve*, travels cephalad and receives a branch from the third occipital nerve. It pierces the semispinalis capitis deep into the trapezius, then emerges onto the scalp. The C2 lateral branch and communicating branches supply the posterior musculature. The C3 dorsal ramus divides into a lateral, communicating and large medial branch, also known as the *third occipital nerve*. The third occipital nerve curves dorsally and medially around the superior articular process of C3 and crosses the C2–C3 facet joint just below or across the joint margin. It provides innervation to C2–C3 before becoming cutaneous.

The C3–C7 dorsal rami cross the root of the ipsisegmental transverse process and divide into lateral and medial branches. The lateral branch supplies the more superficial posterior neck muscles. The relationship of the medial branch to bone is constant. It is bound to fascia and held against the pillar by the tendons of the semispinalis capitis. The medial branch winds around the middle of the articular pillar at its waist and supplies the facet joint above and below before innervating the multifidus and semispinalis cervices.

The cervical facets from C3–C4 to C7–T1 receive dual innervation from the medial branches of the dorsal rami a level above and below the joint. This is in contrast to the triple innervation of the lumbar facets. The C2–C3 facet is supplied by the third occipital nerve and from a C3-communicating loop at the posterior aspect of the joint. The occipitoatlanto and atlantoaxial joints receive innervation from the C1 and C2 ventral rami. There is no dorsal ramus innervation to these joints.[54]

The cervical sympathetic system consists solely of gray postganglionic unmyelinated fibers derived from preganglionic fibers from the thoracic sympathetic trunk. The cervical postganglionic fibers can travel to three different locations. First, they can travel peripherally with the somatic nerves to the upper extremity and, therefore, may be responsible for sympathetically mediated pain syndromes, such as reflex sympathetic dystrophy or the "coldness" commonly complained of in the upper extremity of a patient with a cervical radicular syndrome. Second, postganglionic sympathetic fibers can travel to the eyes, cranial nerves, carotid plexus, and arteries of the head and neck. This component of the sympathetic system may, therefore, be responsible for a sense of nasal stuffiness, ear clogging, and other pseudo–brain-stem- or midbrain-type symptoms. Third, with the ventral root communicating with the recurrent meningeal nerve, some postganglionic fibers may travel back through the intervertebral foramen. This nerve supplies the anterior aspect of the dura, posterior discs, and posterior longitudinal ligament. Another component of the sympathetic system in the cervical spine involves the vertebral nerve that travels with and provides a nerve supply to the vertebral artery within the foramen transversarium. Irritation of this vasomotor nerve can cause headache, vertigo, tinnitus, nasal disturbance, facial pain and flushing, and pharyngeal paresthesias.[54,70]

"Burners" and "stingers," the most common athletic neurologic injury, are most frequently caused by traction forces that increase the acromion-to-head distance and result in traction to the cervical roots or to the brachial plexus. Although less common, burners and stingers may also be caused by compression created by dynamic narrowing of the neural foramen with cervical extension, lateral bending, or rotation and axial loading.[74,75] Normal cervical anatomy affords two distinct mechanisms that protect nerves from moderate traction injury. With lateral traction, the funnel-shaped dural sac impacts into the inner aspect of the intervertebral foramen, providing resistance to further lateral displacement of the nerve.[27,70–72] Another way the nerve is protected is by the anchoring of the epineurium to the transverse processes, posterior longitudinal ligament, and the scalene muscle groups. This anchoring also provides resistance to lateral traction forces.[27,70–72] Because it lacks a perineurium, the weakest portion of the peripheral nerve is located at the junction of the spinal cord with the dorsal and ventral rootlets. If traction forces are excessive, nerve rootlet avulsion, a preganglionic lesion, can occur. Unlike postganglionic lesions, which are amenable to surgical repair, preganglionic lesions have no significant possibility of successful surgical repair.[76]

The muscles that create cervical spine movement can be divided into two functional groups: the capital movers, which flex and extend the head; and the cervical movers, which flex and extend the cervical spine. Other muscle groups contribute to cervical rotation and lateral flexion.[20,70,77] A list of these muscles is presented in Exhibit 10–1.

The *capital flexors* flex the head on the neck and include the longus capitis, rectus capitis anterior and lateral, and hyoid and suprahyoid muscles. The *capital extensors* include the rectus capitis posterior minor, rectus capitis posterior major, obliquus capitis superior, obliquus capitis inferior,

longissimus capitis, semispinalis capitis, and splenius capitis. They attach to the skull and move the head on the neck.[28,70,78]

The *cervical flexors,* that is, the sternocleidomastoid and the anterior scalene and middle scalene, flex the cervical spine. The *cervical extensors* originate on the cervical spine and attach to the cervical spine and upper thoracic vertebrae and ribs. They can extend the cervical spine and alter its curvature. The extensors include the splenius cervicis, longissimus cervicis, and the semispinalis cervicis.[28,70,78]

Because the main mass of the extensor groups overlies the atlantoaxial area as well as the C6–T1 levels, and because the bulk of flexor muscle groups are at the C4–C5 level, these muscle groups are thought to be sites of major stress.[8] The muscle groups that rotate and laterally flex the cervical spine include the sternocleidomastoid, scalene group (anterior, middle, posterior), splenius capitis, splenius cervicis, longissimus capitis, levator scapulae, longus colli, iliocostalis cervicis, multifidi, intertransversarii, obliquus capitis inferior, obliquus capitis superior, and rectus capitis lateralis.[28,78]

Motion of the lower cervical spine occurs in conjunction with that of the upper thoracic spine. Cervical spine motion mediated by the splenius, longissimus, semispinalis cervicis, and semispinalis capitis muscles creates stress and motion of

---

Exhibit 10–1 The Muscles Controlling Cervical Motion

Capital Extensors
- Rectus capitis posterior minor
- Rectus capitis posterior major
- Obliquus capitis superior
- Obliquus capitis inferior
- Longissimus capitis
- Semispinalis capitis
- Splenius capitis

Cervical Extensors
- Splenius cervicis
- Longissimus cervicis
- Semispinalis cervicis

Capital Flexors
- Longus capitis
- Rectus capitis anterior and lateralis
- Lateral
- Hyoid
- Suprahyoid

Cervical Flexors
- Sternocleidomastoid
- Scalene medius and anterior

Rotation and Lateral Flexion
- Sternocleidomastoid
- Scalene group
- Splenius capitis
- Splenius cervicis
- Longissimus capitis
- Levator scapulae
- Longus colli
- Iliocostalis cervicis
- Multifidi
- Intertransversarii
- Obliquus capitis inferior
- Obliquus capitis superior
- Rectus capitis lateralis

Source: Data from Parke W.W., Sherk H.H. Normal adult anatomy. In: Sherk H.H., et al. eds. *The Cervical Spine,* 2nd ed. Philadelphia: J.B. Lippincott Co., 1989; 16; and Calliet R. Functional anatomy. In: Calliet R. *Neck and Arm Pain,* 2nd ed. Philadelphia: F.A. Davis, 1981; 22.

the upper thoracic spine from T1 to T6 because of their distal attachment to these vertebrae.[29,78] Based on our experience, this is one reason that cervical spine dysfunction, particularly postural abnormalities, can create thoracic spine dysfunction and pain, and vice versa.

Athletic trauma and the normal degenerative process can compromise a cervical motion segment's biomechanical properties that handle applied forces. Cervical spondylosis is found most often at the C5–C6 level, less at the C6–C7 level, and even less at the C4–C5 level. Because of the spondylosis at those levels, central and foraminal stenosis may occur. These degenerative changes may also result in progressive thinning of the facet joint articular cartilage. In addition, sclerosis and reactive bone formation of the facet joints may also occur. The annulus may become stiff and break down with the desiccation of the nucleus pulposus and with changes in the annular collagen type. Annular fissures and a herniated nucleus pulposus may then occur. Herniated discs are most often found posterolaterally, where the rate of curvature of the annulus is greatest and the strong posterior longitudinal ligament is most vulnerable. Excessive stress concentrations occur at these sites and can increase annular damage, causing a herniated nucleus pulposus.[70,79,80] The development of anterior vertebral body traction spurs, posterior vertebral body osteophytes and bony bar formation, osteophytosis of the uncovertebral joints, thickening of the ligamentum flavum, and calcification of the posterior longitudinal ligament are other degenerative changes that can compromise normal cervical biomechanics.[81–87] How much exercise accelerates or slows this degenerative process is not known. However, exercise may promote improved discal nutrition and collagen alignment, strength, and flexibility. Exercise may also improve muscular strength and flexibility. All of these factors can protect the motion segment from applied forces.[88,89]

THE SPECTRUM OF CERVICAL MUSCULOSKELETAL ATHLETIC INJURIES

The spectrum of cervical musculoskeletal injuries ranges from simple muscle strains or ligamentous sprains to bone and neurovascular injuries that can compromise central or peripheral nervous system function. A *muscular strain,* or *ligamentous sprain,* one of the most common noncatastrophic injuries, can be associated with a restriction of vertebral motion. A cervical strain is produced by an overload injury to the musculotendinous unit due to excessive forces on the cervical spine. Muscular strains are seen most frequently because many cervical muscles, which do not terminate in tendons, attach to bone by myofascial tissue that blends into the periosteum.[90] The precise etiology of vertebral motion restrictions is not known. These restrictions may be the primary source of secondary muscular inflexibility

and pain or may be created by a primary muscular strain. Careful history and physical examinations can help the skilled practitioner determine whether one or both of these components are part of a patient's injury complex.

Muscular strain injuries can be categorized based on the structural and biomechanical integrity of the cervical spine and on the forces that contribute to muscular injury (S.A. Stratton, personal communication, April 1993). Normal forces acting on a normal spine may result in the typical postural dysfunction seen in nonathletes—that is, the forward head posture. Poor postural habits are usually acquired at a young age, when the patient learns that slumping the thoracic spine requires no energy expenditure. Regular athletic training can exacerbate this postural defect. Pain also can contribute to developing a slumping posture when a patient with chronic cervical pain compensates by thrusting the head forward. This dysfunction includes increased kyphosis of the thoracic spine, with secondary increased lordosis of the cervical spine initially, as well as increased capital extension. Later, a decrease in midcervical lordosis results, along with adaptive soft tissue changes as capital extension is maintained. Over time, the body attempts to keep the eyes horizontal, using greater capital extension.[29,91–93] This forward head posture results in muscle length adaptations that alter normal spinal biomechanics—for example, relying on short segmental muscle groups to function as primary movers, rather than as stabilizers. Normal motion undertaken in this poor postural environment produces abnormal muscular strain, particularly of the levator scapulae, upper trapezius, sternocleidomastoid, scalene, and suboccipital muscles. Other adaptations associated with this posture include a retruded mandible, rounded shoulders, and protracted scapulae with tight anterior muscles and stretched posterior muscles.[29,51,94,95] Patients with these postural abnormalities may develop secondary *myofascial pain* that can cause referral zone pain.[96] Myofascial pain syndrome involves pain and autonomic responses referred from active myofascial trigger points[97] with associated soft tissue dysfunction. Myofascial trigger points are hyperirritable areas, usually within a taut band of skeletal muscle or the muscle's fascia, that are painful on compression and can give rise to characteristic referred pain, tenderness, and autonomic phenomena. Normal muscle tissue does not exhibit these characteristics. Direct pressure over a trigger point will create local pain and will also reproduce the referred pain patterns. A tense band of muscle fibers within a shortened and weak muscle can also be identified on physical examination. Pressure over a trigger point may produce a twitch response, which is considered pathognomonic of a trigger point. Myofascial trigger points are thought to begin with muscular strain and later become sites of sensitized nerves with altered metabolism. Active trigger points cause pain, whereas latent trigger points restrict range of motion and produce weakness in the affected muscle. Latent trigger points may persist for years after a patient recovers from an injury, but the latent trigger point may become active and create acute pain in response to minor overstretching, overuse, or chilling of the muscle.[29,98]

Abnormal forces acting on a normal spine can cause a variety of muscle strain and associated injuries—their severity depends on the magnitude of forces involved. For example, a "shoulder pointer," which involves the acromioclavicular joint, or contusion of the trapezius or the deltoid muscle around the shoulder, also may occur if a football player is tackled and his acromion hits the ground. The trapezius fibers may be strained or avulsed where the muscle inserts into the posterior edge of the clavicle near but not at the acromioclavicular joint.[99] With greater forces, a *somatic dysfunction*—that is, a *vertebral motion restriction*, may occur at specific cervical levels. The levels of restriction can be isolated with great accuracy by a skilled manual physical therapist or physician.[72,100] The pathomechanics of these restrictions are not known. Possible explanations include entrapment of synovial material[101] or a meniscoid[102] to hypertonic contracted or contractured musculature[45] to changes in nervous reflex activity, such as a sympathicotonia[103] or gamma bias[104] to abnormal stresses on an unguarded spine.[9] With even greater forces, a burner or stinger may occur. With extreme forces, which overcome the cervical root protective mechanisms already discussed, nerve root avulsion may occur.

Normal forces acting on an abnormal spine can produce a muscular strain injury. For example, a poorly conditioned, middle-aged weekend tennis player who has C5–C6 degenerative disc disease can have the onset of posterolateral neck pain after playing for prolonged periods of time. The repetitive microtrauma of cervical rotation during ground strokes and the combined extension and rotation during serves place relatively normal forces on the cervical muscle groups that have undergone adaptive changes. These adaptations have occurred because of the pain and abnormal mechanics of the underlying C5–C6 degenerative disc disease. The affected muscle groups, including the cervical rotators, extensors, and lateral flexors, become shortened, less flexible, and weak. Tissue overload creates a vicious cycle of further pain and dysfunction. The disc and facet joints of the C5–C6 motion segment may also contribute to part of the patient's overall pain picture.

Abnormal forces acting on an abnormal cervical spine can produce painful spasm of the levator scapulae, upper trapezius, and capital extensor muscle groups. For example, a high-school soccer player with a forward head posture may incur an acute flexion injury of the cervical spine when tackled. The sudden flexion on being tackled results in tissue overload and failure of those muscle groups that were chronically weakened, shortened, and made less flexible by the underlying postural dysfunction.

Repetitive microtrauma or an excessive single load occurrence may cause an *annular fissure* or *herniated nucleus pulposus*.[105] Depending on the size and location of the lesion and the significance of any inflammation[59,106] or compression of local nervous or vascular tissue,[107] the patient may develop axial pain, referral zone pain,[108] radicular pain, *radiculopathy*, or even *myelopathy*, if the spinal cord is compressed. Patients with a herniated nucleus pulposus without radiculopathy will complain of increased pain with cervical flexion or extension and will usually experience relief with traction.[29,109–111] Radiculopathy will include radicular pain and weakness in the appropriate myotome, as well as associated changes of the reflexes. Cervical pain becomes worse with positional foraminal compression maneuvers and with cervical extension and rotation. The pain may be relieved with cervical traction maneuvers. Traction may help provide relief from the pain associated with a radiculopathy if it is performed in approximately 20 degrees of cervical flexion as this posture can increase the diameter of the intervertebral foramen up to 33%. Manual traction seems to be better tolerated than is mechanical traction.[29,109–111] Cervical radiculopathy must be differentiated from peripheral nerve entrapments—for example, from carpal tunnel syndrome. C6 radiculopathy must be differentiated from high median neuropathy; C8 radiculopathy from ulnar neuropathy; C5 radiculopathy from shoulder and hand tendinitis; and C6 or C7 radiculopathy from de Quervain's disease and extensor tendinitis of the wrist.[96]

Patients with cervical myelopathy frequently have difficulties with balance and a stooped, wide-based gait. Patients may experience loss of dexterity, nonspecific weakness, numbness and paresthesia of the upper extremities, and incontinence of the bladder. Lhermitte's sign may be present. Lower motoneuron deficits at the level of the cervical lesion and upper motoneuron signs below the lesion may be found on physical examination. The exact distribution of signs and symptoms will be dictated by the location of the spinal cord lesion.[74,112] *Cervical spinal cord neuropraxia* may occur, particularly given certain predisposing factors that may cause the anteroposterior diameter of the spinal canal to narrow. These factors include developmental spinal stenosis, instability, herniated nucleus pulposus, and spondylosis. Forced hyperflexion or hyperextension injuries of the cervical spine may further decrease the size of an already stenotic central canal. The cervical central canal diameter can be reduced by 2–3 mm during forced extension, due to laxity and secondary thickening of the posterior longitudinal ligament and the ligamentum flavum. These forced injuries may result in brief but abrupt mechanical compression of the spinal cord, causing transient interruption distal to the lesion of motor function, sensory function, or both. Both arms, both legs, or all four extremities may be involved. These bilateral findings help differentiate spinal cord neuropraxia from radiculopathy or from brachial plexus injury, both of which are almost always unilateral. By definition, the neurologic deficit associated with cervical spinal cord neuropraxia is transient and completely reversible.[8,25,74]

Shoulder complex pain syndromes may easily be confused with pain emanating from the cervical spine. Acromioclavicular joint synovitis may recreate C5 pain. Subacromial bursitis may mimic C5 or C6 pain patterns. A rotator cuff tear may mimic neurologic loss associated with C5 or C6 root lesions. Glenohumeral joint synovitis associated with osteoarthritis or adhesive capsulitis may be felt in any radicular pattern. Adverse neural tissue tension also may be a source of pain and can mimic almost any cervical pain pattern, particularly a radiculopathy.[113] These lesions can usually be differentiated from cervical sources of pain, given a careful history, physical examination, physical therapy, and possibly differential contrast-enhanced fluoroscopically guided injections, using an appropriate combination of anesthetic and steroid. The subacromial bursa, acromioclavicular joint, glenohumeral joint, cervical facet, cervical nerve root, or cervical epidural space may be targeted in varying combinations, depending on a physician's working diagnosis.[96,114,115]

Cervical facet pain may mimic cervical disc disease or shoulder pain.[116] Depending on the facet joints involved, different pain patterns will result.[116] The pain will usually be unilateral and may be felt in particular areas of the cervical or scapular region.[116] Dull, aching neck pain is a common complaint from patients with facet pain. Limited range of cervical motion due to soft-tissue dysfunction and restriction, either diffusely or segmentally, will be noticed by the patient and can be easily confirmed on physical examination. The spondylogenic reflex[117,118] may be responsible for the appearance of secondary muscular zones of irritation with tender points or trigger points. The affected tissues may be related to the dysfunctional facet, segmentally and sclerotomally.[117,118] This "facilitated segment" concept was originally described by Korr.[83] If the patient has occipitoatlantal, atlantoaxial, C2–C3, C3–C4, C5–C6 facet involvement or a T4 syndrome,[113,119] he or she may experience headaches.[117,120] Upper cervical headaches may be accompanied by nausea, blurred vision, and dizziness.[117,121] The atlantoaxial joint involvement may also cause ear pain.[117,122] The patient's history, mechanism of injury, pattern of painful and pain-free motion, and response to treatment are helpful in sorting out the source of pain—that is, whether the source of pain is the facet or the disc. The trained clinician, using a manual examination of the cervical spine, will be able to isolate the affected joints with great accuracy. Manual physical therapists are particularly well suited in this regard.[100,113] In some cases, contrast-enhanced fluoroscopically guided facet injections may be required to help advance the patient's rehabilitation program.[117,123]

Vascular injuries in the cervical spine may result, iatrogenically,[37,40,47–50,73,124] from cervical athletic trauma[50,125] or from cervical spondylosis.[84] An acute hyperextension injury, occurring in football,[125] soccer, rugby, and equestrian sports, for example, may produce vertebral artery ischemia or thrombosis. Momentary feelings of paralysis or tingling of the limbs may occur. Compression and spasm of the spinal arteries may produce acute paralysis, numbness, and tingling in the lower limbs and then in the upper limbs. The athlete may recover even before being transported from the field.[125] The vertebral arteries are most vulnerable to compression at the occipitoatlantal area by hyperextension and compression injuries.[4,126,127] Brief neurologic brain stem signs and symptoms secondary to vasospasm, as well as cervicomedullary infarction and death due to thrombosis, have also been reported.[4,127] An internal carotid-middle cerebral transient ischemic attack or stroke may develop if these arterial systems are injured by extreme cervical lateral flexion, extension, or a direct blow to the anterolateral neck.[4]

Thoracic outlet syndrome (TOS) is a constellation of disorders due to compression of the neurovascular bundle that travels through this region. The neurovascular bundle includes the brachial plexus nerve fibers and the subclavian vein and artery.[90] Compression may occur anywhere along the three zones of the cervicoaxillary canal: (1) the interscalene triangle; (2) the costoclavicular triangle; and (3) the subcoracoid space. The lateral border of the thoracic outlet is formed by the first rib, the medial border by the vertebral column, and the anterior border by the claviculomanubrial complex.[54] Thoracic outlet syndrome has been classified as either vascular or neurologic and as combined vascular and neurologic. Each of the categories is further subdivided.[128] Differentiation between thoracic outlet symptoms that most commonly affect the C8 and T1 nerve roots and cervical radicular syndromes that usually affect C5, C6, and C7 can usually be made by taking a careful history and performing a thorough physical examination. Factors contributing to TOS include a true or rudimentary cervical rib, fibrous bands, postural dysfunction, and droopy shoulder syndrome. Thoracic outlet syndrome must also be differentiated from spondylosis, shoulder disorders, and nerve entrapment syndromes.[54,90]

Although burners and stingers have already been discussed, one further point deserves mention. If avulsion of the first thoracic nerve rootlets from the spinal cord occurs, interruption of the preganglionic *sympathetic fibers* that supply the eye can occur. The ocular portion of Horner's syndrome may result.[27] Other problems that can mimic cervical pain or refer pain to the cervical region include *thoracic facet* or *costovertebral joint synovitis*, *spinal cord tumors*, *lung pathology*, and *upper extremity peripheral nerve entrapments*.[96,115,128,129]

A CASE PRESENTATION ILLUSTRATING THE TISSUE INJURY CYCLE AND A COMPREHENSIVE REHABILITATION PLAN

History

The patient is a 20-year-old Division I college swimmer. His events are the 200- and 500-yard freestyle. He has a history of chronic right shoulder rotator cuff tendinitis. This injury has recently had an acute flare. His regular physician prescribed two weeks of rest and oral nonsteroidal antiinflammatory agents. Shortly after the patient resumed regular training, right shoulder pain recurred in conjunction with an acute onset of right-sided upper and lower cervical pain. There was also associated pain in the right upper trapezius and behind his right ear. His pain was exacerbated with right-sided breathing, making breathing and concentration difficult. His racing times increased, which soon prompted him to see a sports medicine physician.

Physical Examination

The physician's physical examination was thorough and focused, and was guided by an understanding of swimming biomechanics. The evaluation also took into account the way in which repetitive microtrauma can damage particular structures in the spine and shoulder complex. The patient had a typical swimmer's posture—the exaggeration of the forward head posture previously described. Notable, however, was the severity of the swimmer's rounded shoulder posture and the degree of lumbar lordosis. Cervical active range of motion was restricted in right rotation, lateral flexion, extension, and extension/rotation, with reproduction of pain in all these planes of motion, but particularly with extension/rotation. Other cervical active range of motion was normal. The patient's cervical pain was decreased with manual traction (with the cervical spine in 20 degrees of flexion) and increased with compression. Manual examination of his cervical spine revealed tenderness to palpation and motion restrictions at the right occipitoatlantal, atlantoaxial, and C5–C6 facet joints, with reproduction of pain on motion and associated overlying soft tissue changes. Decreased soft tissue flexibility[95] was noted in the capital extensors, cervical extensors, scalenes, levator scapulae, upper trapezius, and the humeral internal rotators—especially subscapularis, latissimus dorsi, and pectoralis minor and major. Trigger points and tight bands were palpated in the upper trapezius, cervical extensors, scalenes, levator scapulae, latissimus dorsi, and pectoralis minor and major. There was muscular strength imbalance between the cervical flexors, which were weaker than cervical extensors; however, there was also a muscular strength imbalance between the stronger capital extensors and the weaker cervical extensors.[95]

Evaluation of the patient's right shoulder complex revealed normal right shoulder active range of motion, with pain in the anterolateral acromial region at roughly 90 degrees of abduction, as well as pain at the end ranges of forward flexion and abduction. Passive range of motion was already tested and noted above. Anterior glenohumeral instability was present. Scapulothoracic mechanical dysfunction was noted, and the patient had an abnormal slide test.[130] Significant muscular strength imbalances were identified with particularly weak scapular depressors—for example, the lower trapezius; weak scapular retractors—for example, the rhomboid minor and major as well as middle trapezius; and humeral external rotators—for example, the teres minor and infraspinatus. With the exception of the strength imbalances noted, the patient's neurologic examination was completely normal in both his upper and lower extremities.

Radiographic evaluation was deferred, as the patient had a recent set of shoulder films from his last episode of shoulder pain. There was no significant indication for cervical films, based on the physician's initial cervical evaluation.

The Tissue Injury Cycle

The tissue injury cycle assisted the physician in defining all aspects of this patient's total injury complex. The patient's response to rehabilitation will further clarify and define the total extent of the injury. The patient had an acute cervical facet injury superimposed on a chronic postural dysfunction. The cervical facet injury was also superimposed on an acute exacerbation of a chronic rotator cuff tendinitis that was due to extrinsic impingement secondary to glenohumeral instability. His cervical and postural *tissue overload complex* consisted of eccentric overload of the capital and cervical flexors, scalene muscles, thoracic spinal extensors, humeral external rotators, and scapular depressors and retractors. Concentric overload of the capital and cervical extensors, humeral internal rotators, scapular protractors, upper trapezius, and levator scapulae also characterized this patient's injury. Included in this complex were the posterior occipitoatlantal fascia and intermuscular fascia surrounding the named muscle groups. The joint capsules of the right occipitoatlantal, atlantoaxial, and C5–C6 facet joints were also involved.

The postural and cervical tissue injury complex included a synovitis and capsulitis of the right occipitoatlantal, atlantoaxial, and C5–C6 facet joints. Additional components of the tissue injury complex included myofascial changes in the upper trapezius, cervical extensors, scalenes, levator scapulae, latissimus dorsi, and pectoralis minor and major muscle groups.

The *clinical sign and symptom complex* included myofascial pain, trigger points, and tight bands in those muscles subserving the postural abnormality. These myofascial changes especially affected the upper trapezius, cervical extensors, scalenes, levator scapulae, latissimus dorsi, and pectoralis minor and major muscle groups. Other components of this complex were pain, tenderness, and segmental motion restrictions localized to the right occipitoatlantal, atlantoaxial, and C5–C6 facet joints. The right occipitoatlantal, atlantoaxial, and C5–C6 facet joints referred pain to the right cervical spine posterior to the ear, the right upper cervical spine, and the right upper shoulder from C3 to T1 above the level of the scapular spine.

The *functional biomechanical deficits* included decreased cervical active range of motion with extension and the coupled complex motions of right lateral bending, right rotation, and right extension/rotation. Tight humeral internal rotators and capital and cervical extensors also were part of the functional biomechanical deficit complex. The tight humeral internal rotators and forward position of the scapula due to the shortened pectoralis minor created a functional narrowing of the supraspinous outlet exacerbating the dynamic subacromial impingement. Strength imbalances with weak cervical flexors compared with cervical and usually stronger capital extensors; weak scapular depressors—for example, lower trapezius compared with scapular elevators; weak scapular retractors—for example, rhomboid minor and major as well as middle trapezius compared with scapular protractors; and weak humeral external rotators—for example, teres minor and infraspinatus compared with very powerful humeral internal rotators, for example; subscapularis, pectoralis major, and latissimus dorsi also affected the swimmer's performance.

The *subclinical adaptation complex* included an increased body roll to enhance access of the mouth to air, a decreased but maximum cervical suboccipital spinal extension and cervical rotation, and an increased mid- and lower cervical and upper thoracic extension to ensure that the patient's head rode higher out of the water. All these subclinical adaptations ensured the patient's adequate access to air. These changes in stroke biomechanics resulted in increased head drag[131] and ultimately slowed the patient's swimming speed, thus increasing his performance times.

The patient's shoulder injury complex was also noted by the physician. The *tissue overload complex* consisted of tensile loading of the posterior shoulder capsule and muscles, as well as the scapular stabilizers. The *tissue injury complex* included rotator cuff tendon dynamic impingement, anterior glenoid labrum attrition, and anterior capsule stretch and inflammation. The *clinical sign and symptom complex* included dynamic subacromial impingement pain and anterior-superior glenohumeral instability. The *functional biomechanical deficits* were tight internal rotators, rounded shoulders, and strength deficits in the right shoulder scapular stabilizers. Decreased strength in the external rotators was found when the external and internal rotators were compared, indicating a strength differential that created a muscle strength imbalance. The *subclinical adaptation complex* included a recovery phase using a shortened and lowered right arm and a shortened and less powerful pull phase, with decreased internal rotation of the shoulder. Entry, pull, and recovery phases made with right arm lateral drift from the midline and continued humeral external rotation of the right arm also were part of this complex.[115]

The tissue injury cycle helped the physician to understand the relationship between the three components of the patient's examination. The patient's chronic postural dysfunction produced tight humeral internal rotators. The tight, shortened pectoralis minor, in particular, caused the patient's scapula to assume a forward, protracted position, which created a functional narrowing of his supraspinous outlet. When he began regular swim training, the patient developed laxity in his anterior glenohumeral capsule. The glenohumeral laxity superimposed on the functional narrowing of his supraspinous outlet yielded extrinsic impingement secondary to glenohumeral instability, which was the source of the patient's recurring shoulder pain.[71] The altered shoulder mechanics superimposed on the patient's postural dysfunction resulted in his newest problem, the facet injury complex, which caused his cervical pain.

This patient's freestyle stroke underwent many adaptations to avoid further pain as a result of impingement. A description of the freestyle stroke phases can be found in Exhibit 10–2. The patient lowered his arm above water during the recovery phase and externally rotated his humerus, thus allowing his hand to enter the water palm down rather than thumb down. The patient also allowed his hand to enter the water farther away from the midline. By lowering his arm during the recovery phase, the patient increased upper body roll in order to breathe. In an effort to moderate the amount of segmental roll through his spine to gain access to suffi-

---

Exhibit 10–2 Swimming Stroke Phases (Freestyle)

  I. Entry Phase
   II. Hand entry
  III. Hand submersion ("ride")
 IV. Pull Phase
   V. Insweep
  VI. Outsweep
 VII. Finish
VIII. Recovery Phase
  IX. Exit
   X. Arm swing

Source: Courtesy of Aquatechnics Consulting Group, Inc., Aptos, California.

cient air to right-side breathe, he began to right "crane" breathe; that is, the patient increased his capital and cervical spine extension and rotation. An example of crane breathing can be found in Figure 10–2. The patient was attempting to moderate the amount of segmental roll developed in his spine by using crane breathing. Segmental roll increases head-drag forces and reduces swimming speed.[6,114,131–134] Owing to his underlying postural dysfunction, the patient was already functioning at near-end-range capital and cervical extension. The additional stress placed on his tight and weak capital and cervical extensors and rotators due to crane breathing allowed the patient to function at end-range active motion for a short period of time. Soon, he began to strain the noncontractile tissue supporting those joints that allow crane breathing to occur—the facet capsules of the right occipito-atlantal, atlantoaxial, and C5–C6 facet joints. Roughly half of the cervical spine extension and rotation occurs at the occipitoatlantal and atlantoaxial joints.[29,30,33–35,37,135] The patient recruited his C5–C6 joint to increase his cervical extension and rotation more than was already being provided by the occipitoatlantal extension and atlantoaxial rotation. The tissue overload of the occipitoatlantal, atlanto-occipital, and C5–C6 facet joints created a capsulitis and synovitis in them. These inflamed facet tissues referred pain as previously noted. These distributions correspond to the referral zones reported in the literature.[116] The result of increased body roll, however, had additional biomechanical consequences. The patient found it impossible to move the lumbar, thoracic, and cervical parts of his spine as a unit, that is, using log roll or nonsegmental motion. This biomechanical adaptation re-

sulted in an increase in segmental rotation through his lumbar spine. Because the patient externally rotated his humerus to minimize further loss of supraspinous outlet space and to minimize his subacromial impingement, his hand entered the water palm down, resulting in an increased amount of segmental motion, that is, twist, through his lumbar spine. Widening the entry phase position caused the patient's trunk to rotate away from the entry phase side, thus increasing lateral flexion and segmental motion through the lumbar spine. The patient also adopted a crossover kick to offset the segmental rotation produced through his lumbar spine. Unfortunately, the crossover kick served only to further increase the amount of lateral flexion and segmental motion through the patient's lumbar spine.[6,114,132–134,136]

In summary, this swimmer's postural dysfunction created a number of soft-tissue and biomechanical deficits that placed his shoulder complex at increased risk for developing impingement and rotator cuff tendinitis. This same postural dysfunction, with the contribution of the glenohumeral impingement and rotator cuff tendinitis, then created the opportunity for the cervical facet dysfunction to occur.

Most swimmers and other athletes will experience a myriad of functional adaptations at sites distant from the initial musculoskeletal injury. The motion cascade (Figure 10–3), originally described by Cole et al.,[6,114,132,133] describes the relationship between the spine and peripheral joints. The cascade helps the clinician understand how injuries in one part of the kinetic chain can create both primary and secondary sites of pain and dysfunction. For example, a shoulder injury such as rotator cuff tendinitis results in guarding and decreased shoulder range of motion.[39,61,70,113,137] The swimmer's arm cannot abduct and extend as it normally would[77] during recovery, resulting in decreased body roll, increased lumbar segmental motion, and an abnormally low head position from which to breathe.[47] Compensatory adaptive changes then occur. These adaptive changes include crane breathing (increased cervical suboccipital extension [OA] and rotation [AA], cervical extension [C2–C7]) and cervical rotation [C2–C7] (see Figure 10–3), as well as even more extension and rotation from C3 to C5.[47] The C5–T1 segments ultimately become hypomobile to compensate, and mid- and low cervical pain results. Compensatory hypermobility from T2 to T5 and hypomobility from T5 to T7 and T10 to L1 begin. Primary cervical, thoracic, and lumbar injuries and pain influence the spinal axis in a similar fashion. Hip,[4] pelvis, and lumbar spine pain result in hypomobility at L4–S1 and, ultimately, at the T10–L1 transition zone. Adaptive changes then proceed up the axis and may even set the stage for a compensatory change in shoulder mechanics and, ultimately, cause a shoulder injury. Identification of the initial injury is important so that treatment can eliminate that problem, as well as the secondary compensatory sites of dysfunction.[39,61,138] Therefore, an initial tis-

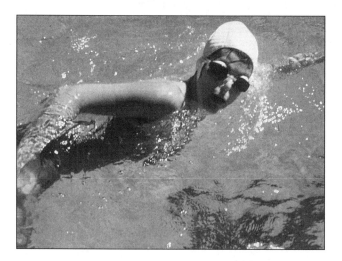

Figure 10–2 Crane breathing. A biomechanical adaptation that improves access to air by increasing capital and cervical spine extension and rotation. It can occur due to a variety of reasons, most commonly poor body roll. *Source:* Courtesy of Aquatechnics Consulting Group, Inc., Aptos, California.

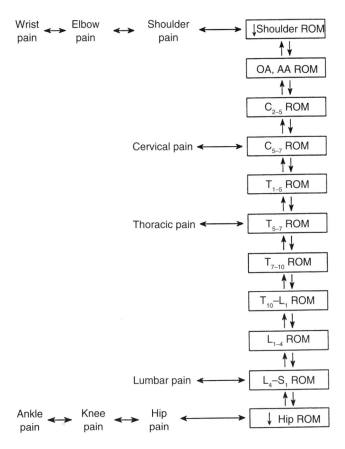

Figure 10–3 The motion cascade. $\downarrow$, decreased; *C*, cervical; *L*, lumbar; $\uparrow$, increased; *T*, thoracic; *S*, sacral; *ROM*, range of motion; *AA*, atlantoaxial; *OA*, occipitoatlantal. *Source:* Aquatechnics Consulting Group, Inc., Aptos, California.

sue injury should not be viewed and treated in isolation but should be seen as having the potential to create a cascading effect that can produce or exacerbate other painful musculoskeletal injuries or dysfunctions.

The Rehabilitation Program

According to Kibler et al.,[130] the rehabilitation of soft-tissue injuries and their associated deficits can be divided into three parts: (1) an acute phase, (2) a recovery phase, and (3) a maintenance phase. Each phase is designed to sequentially address specific aspects of the tissue injury cycle. The next section describes the rehabilitation process for this patient's constellation of injuries. However, the details of the rehabilitation process of rotator cuff tendinitis in a competitive swimmer have been previously described and, therefore, will not be repeated. It is most important to realize that the rotator cuff tendinitis program, as well as the posture and cervical spine program, must occur in a coordinated and simulta-

neous manner to address all components of the patient's injury and to minimize the chance for a recurrence.[6,132]

Acute Phase of Rehabilitation

During the acute phase of rehabilitation, the tissue injury and clinical signs and symptoms complexes are treated. A description of the acute phase of rehabilitation is presented in Exhibit 10–3. The goals of this phase are to reduce pain and inflammation, reestablish nonpainful range of motion, improve neuromuscular cervical spine postural control, and retard the development of any muscular atrophy of the cervical spine muscle groups, postural muscles, and muscle groups subserving the upper extremity and scapulothoracic articulation.

Pain and inflammation can be reduced by the judicious use of nonsteroidal antiinflammatory drugs (NSAIDs) that are prescribed by the physician. The antiprostaglandin effect of NSAIDs may control an injury's inflammatory response and provide pain relief. The duration of an NSAID's analgesic effect may be different than its antiinflammatory effect.[139] Some investigators have expressed concern that NSAIDs may actually interfere with the later stages of tissue repair and remodeling, when prostaglandins still help mediate debris cleanup.[140] The dosage, timing, and potential side effects of NSAIDs should be evaluated. Patient responses to a particular NSAID cannot be predicted based on its chemical class or pharmacokinetics.[141]

The physical therapist has a variety of techniques available to control further inflammation and pain. Acute injury is best treated by therapeutic cold, which decreases pain and muscle spasm and causes arteriolar and capillary blood flow to diminish, thus helping to control edema. The time required to cool an injured structure is directly dependent on the depth of intervening fat and may vary from 10 to 30 minutes.[142–144] Cryotherapy is easily applied to the cervical spine at home or in the clinic and may be used in conjunction with other treatment techniques. In addition to providing pain relief and controlling inflammation, physical modalities have other benefits. Ultrasound can stimulate tissue regeneration, promote soft-tissue repair, increase blood flow to damaged tissue to provide needed nutrients to the healing tissue, and aid in the removal of inflammatory byproducts, increase soft-tissue distensibility, and decrease muscle spasm and pain.[52,145–147]

Electrical stimulation is another extremely useful modality that is particularly helpful in modulating acute pain. It also can help decrease muscle spasm by inducing posttetanic relaxation, as well as increasing circulation, which helps remove inflammatory waste products.[148] Electrical stimulation techniques, including transcutaneous electrical nerve stimulation (TENS), high-voltage pulsed galvanic stimulation (HVPGS), interferential electrical stimulation, and minimal

Exhibit 10–3 Acute Phase of Rehabilitation

Complexes Involved
- Tissue injury
- Clinical sign and symptom

Therapeutic Activities
- Active rest
- Conditioning of other areas
- NSAIDs
- Physical therapy modalities
- Manual therapy approaches
- Protected range of motion/stabilization
- Isometric muscle strengthening

Criteria for Advancement
- Increased cervical range of motion
- Decreased cervical pain
- Decreased muscle spasm
- Decreased adaptive muscle and other soft tissue changes

Source: Courtesy of Aquatechnics Consulting Group, Inc., Aptos, California.

electrical noninvasive stimulation (MENS), have been reported to promote analgesia, muscle relaxation, resolution of edema, and wound healing, as well as to retard inflammation and muscle atrophy.[128]

The recent application of electro-acuscope and low-energy lasers, which are newer and less traditional modalities for the management of pain associated with sports injuries, awaits well-controlled prospective studies to determine their mechanism of action and their efficacy.[149]

Joint protection techniques offer another way to help reduce pain by minimizing repetitive cervical motion into painful ranges of motion. This can be accomplished passively by providing a soft cervical collar that can be worn for as long as 10–12 days, then weaning the patient as rapidly as possible to help avoid psychologic dependence and to help prevent further muscular weakness and decreased soft-tissue flexibility. Weaning should allow increasing daytime removal, with continued use at night to prevent injury during sleep.[90,150] Once the patient has been weaned from daytime collar use, nighttime use also may be discontinued. Active joint protection techniques are part of the initial phase of a cervicothoracic stabilization program. Cervicothoracic stabilization training is a specific type of therapeutic exercise that can help the patient to (1) gain dynamic control of cervicothoracic spine forces, (2) eliminate repetitive injury to the motion segments, that is, discs, facets, and related structures, (3) encourage healing of an injured segment, and

(4) possibly alter the degenerative process. The underlying premise is that the motion segment and its supporting soft tissues react to minimize applied stress, thereby reducing the risk of injury. During the initial phase of stabilization training, the patient is taught how to find the neutral position or position of optimal function, which is the least painful cervicothoracic spine position that minimizes segmental biomechanical stress. As the patient's condition improves, a series of flexibility and strengthening exercises is initiated to help correct postural dysfunction, inflexibilities, and muscle strength deficits and imbalances.[151]

Manual therapy techniques also can help decrease pain and improve mobility and function to the point that the patient may begin to exercise in a painless manner. The techniques may also be used to help determine the source and relative contribution of various aspects of a patient's pain and dysfunction. These techniques include massage of the soft tissues, manually sustained or rhythmically applied muscle stretching, traction applied in the longitudinal axis of the spine, passive joint mobilization, and, as the patient's pain begins to subside, specific or general high-velocity manipulation.[152–154] High-velocity manipulation can be particularly helpful to treat painful dysfunctions that are aggravated by repetitive oscillatory movements (J.P. Farrell, personal communication, April 1993). Manual therapy techniques would be targeted to this patient's occipitoatlantal, atlantoaxial, and C5–C6 facets, as well as all their supporting structures in the cervical and thoracic spine and associated joints, including the glenohumeral joint and scapulothoracic articulation. The neurologic effects of manual therapy that can help attenuate pain include restoration of axonal transport due to mechanically induced deformation of spinal nerves,[152,155] stimulation of large-fiber joint afferents conveyed by joint receptors that depend on the gate control theory,[152,156] and stimulation of clinically effective levels of endorphins.[152,157] Increased intraosseous pressure can cause pain, and this pressure may be influenced by both joint position and intra-articular pressure. End-range passive mobilization techniques may help decrease intra-articular pressure, thereby reducing pain.[137,152,158–162]

There are other benefits of manual therapy. Repetitive passive joint oscillations carried out at the limit of the joint's available range can have a mechanical effect on joint mobility, thus improving a vertebral motion restriction.[152,162–165] Mechanically controlled passive or active movements of joints can improve the remodeling of local connective tissue, the rate of tendon repair, and gliding function within tendon sheaths during the repair process.[84,138,152,166,167] Passive joint motion has been shown to stretch joint capsules and lubricate tissues, and to induce metabolic changes in soft tissue, cartilage, and bone.[106,152] Manipulation, if needed, would most likely involve the occipitoatlantal, atlantoaxial, and C5–C6 facets.

If the patient's pain is not significantly relieved during the acute phase of the rehabilitation program, trigger point injections may help lessen trigger zone and referred pain, and may help improve muscular flexibility.[11,168] Oral steroids may also be used; contrast-enhanced, fluoroscopically guided facet injections using a combination of steroid and local anesthetic at the site of pain may help to significantly decrease the patient's pain. These injections may allow rehabilitation to progress more rapidly.[54,84,90,123,169]

The second goal of this patient's acute phase of rehabilitation is to reestablish nonpainful active and passive ranges of motion of the cervical spine, thoracic spine, and associated joints, including the glenohumeral joint and scapulothoracic articulation. Passive joint mobilization techniques are usually the most successful during the early portion of the acute phase of rehabilitation. Then, as the patient's condition improves, a gradual shift to an active program is made to ensure rapid recovery and patient independence. Passive mobilization of the occipitoatlantal, atlantoaxial, C2–C3, and C5–C6 vertebral motion segments mobilizes their respective facet joints and stretches their facet capsules, and is initiated for reasons previously cited.[152] Soft-tissue techniques, including lateral stretching, linear stretching, deep pressure, traction, and separation of muscle origin and insertion,[170,171] can help to decrease pain, muscle spasm, and soft-tissue inflexibility, as well as to improve circulation and remove inflammatory byproducts.[171,172] Myofascial techniques can be used to help stretch the noncontractile portion of the soft tissue.[173] Inhibition techniques, such as positional release, can help to modify increased muscle tone, thus helping to restore balanced muscular flexibility and strength.[174–176] Varying combinations of these techniques would be directed primarily at those muscles that have become tight and painful secondary to the acute underlying facet pain. Treatment would also be directed to the muscles and other soft tissues chronically affected by poor posture to help restore them to normal length and flexibility. These muscles include those that are shortened, less flexible, and weak—the capital and cervical extensors, sternocleidomastoid, upper trapezius, and levator scapulae. These techniques could also be used to help restore normal flexibility, strength, and length to the muscles that have been eccentrically lengthened and are weak—the scalenes, cervical and capital flexors, middle and lower traezius, and the rhomboid minor and major. The muscles, fascia, and other soft-tissue components responsible for creating a functionally narrowed supraspinous outlet and the rounded shoulder posture should be treated: pectoralis minor and major, subscapularis, serratus anterior, latissimus dorsi, anterior deltoid, and thoracic musculature. Particular care should be taken while stretching these muscles to avoid inadvertently stretching the anterior glenohumeral joint capsule and ligaments so that the patient's anterior glenohumeral instability is not worsened. Finally, an active stretching program for those muscles that stabilize and support the lumbar spine will be implemented at this stage of rehabilitation.[88,177]

The last two goals of this patient's acute phase of rehabilitation must also be addressed—improving neuromuscular control of the cervical spine and retarding weakness and increasing the strength of the cervical spine muscle groups and those that support the glenohumeral joint and scapulothoracic articulation. Improved neuromuscular control is developed for static positions first and then progressed to include control during dynamic and functional activities. This type of training is included in the cervicothoracic dynamic stabilization program.[151] Various proprioceptive neuromuscular facilitation techniques can be performed within the pain-free portion of the weakened or limited cervical and shoulder complex range of motion. As the patient improves, the extent of the movement pattern is increased, both for range of motion and the amount of resistance that is manually applied.[151,178]

Cervical spine strengthening should begin with isometric exercises in the neutral position, determined during previous stabilization training. Single-plane isometric strengthening with resistive forces applied perpendicularly to the head to strengthen the cervical flexors, extensors, rotators, and lateral flexors is initiated with the patient supine, then progressed to the seated then standing positions. By varying the patient's positioning and direction relative to gravity, direct stabilization of the cervical spine results.[90,151] As the patient's pain permits, an increasing range of isometric strengthening occurs.

When progressed to isotonic strengthening, care should be taken during the initiation of combined cervical movements, such as lateral bending and rotation, to avoid an increase in symptoms that are due to the increased facet joint and muscular requirements needed to perform these movements. When symptoms permit, concentric isotonic strengthening of all the cervical spine muscles should begin and should emphasize those muscle groups that have been stretched and weakened because of poor posture—the cervical and capital flexors and scalenes—thus providing improved muscular balance and flexibility with the cervical and capital extensors.

Strengthening programs must also include the thoracic muscle groups, middle and lower trapezius, and rhomboid minor and major to provide strength to the thoracic spine and scapulothoracic articulation helping to lessen postural thoracic kyphosis and scapular protraction and elevation. Balanced flexibility and strength will allow the patient to assume a more mechanically correct posture from which he can develop further segmental mobility and dynamic functional strength. Finally, special emphasis should be placed on strengthening the humeral external rotators, including teres minor, infraspinatus, and latissimus dorsi. This strengthening will improve strength balance with the disproportionately strong internal rotators of swimmers that also contribute to poor posture and functional narrowing of the supraspinous outlet (also, R. Eagleston, personal communication, September 30, 1989).[24,132]

A low-level program of aerobic conditioning may be instituted, depending on the patient's level of pain and function. This low-level program can help the patient avoid significant cardiovascular deconditioning. Stationary bike, treadmill, or StairMaster™ (Tri-Tech, Inc, Tulsa, Oklahoma) training provides excellent cardiovascular training without requiring upper-extremity involvement. Aqua running using only the legs is particularly appropriate because it involves only the lower extremities. These low-level programs will allow this athlete to continue training in his competitive environment without potentially compromising his shoulder function.

The patient should be advanced to the recovery phase when his cervical pain has almost completely resolved, when his passive and active cervical range of motion and neuromuscular control have significantly improved, and when the muscles and other tissue maintaining his postural adaptive changes have improved.

Recovery Phase of Rehabilitation

The recovery phase of rehabilitation addresses the tissue overload and functional biomechanical deficit complexes. A description of the recovery phase of rehabilitation is presented in Exhibit 10–4. The goals of this phase are to completely eliminate the patient's pain; improve and normalize his cervical, thoracic, glenohumeral, and scapulothoracic passive and active ranges of motion; improve and normalize his cervical, thoracic, glenohumeral, and scapulothoracic strength and neuromuscular control; continue to improve his posture; and initiate swim training progressions. Complete resolution of the tissue injury and clinical symptom complexes is necessary in the early recovery phase. NSAIDs are probably unnecessary in this phase. Manual therapy, including manipulative and soft-tissue techniques, may still be needed to help eliminate vertebral motion restrictions and to improve the flexibility, length, and motion of the soft tissues so that cervical, thoracic, glenohumeral, and scapulothoracic active and passive ranges of motion are normalized. The improved active and passive ranges of motion permit further normalization of the patient's posture as muscular strength and balance are enhanced to help maintain the improved posture during daily activities, as well as during athletic training and competition. Strength training using independent single-plane and complex multiple-plane coordinated motions are performed using varying combinations of concentric and eccentric isotonic, isokinetic, tube, pulley, and isolation exercises. Theraband (Hygenic Co., Akron, Ohio) or Sportscord (Sport Cord, Inc., Irvine, California) can be used to allow training at home. The specific type of strengthening depends

Exhibit 10-4 Recovery Phase of Rehabilitation

Complexes Involved
- Tissue overload
- Functional biochemical deficit

Therapeutic Activities
- Appropriate loading
- Protected range of motion
- Resistive exercise
  - Local
  - Balance
  - Kinetic chain
- Functional exercises

Criteria for Advancement
- Full nonpainful range of motion
  - Cervical
  - Thoracic
  - Lumbar
  - Scapulothoracic
  - Glenohumeral
- Improved spine posture
  - Cervical
  - Thoracic spine
- Improved cervical, thoracic, scapulothoracic
  - Neuromuscular control
  - Strength
- Improved strength and flexibility of the supporting
  - Muscles
  - Joints
- Improved stroke mechanics

Source: Courtesy of Aquatechnics Consulting Group, Inc., Aptos, California.

on the joint and particular muscles targeted. Emphasis is placed first on improving the strength, balance, and neuromuscular control of the force couples that govern proper cervical, thoracic, glenohumeral, and scapulothoracic mechanics. For example, cervical and capital flexor and extensor strength balance is improved, then those force couples that control the scapulothoracic articulation improve, including the scapular protractors and retractors, elevators, and depressors. Upward rotators and downward rotators are trained before the force couples that govern glenohumeral mechanics, including humeral internal and external rotators, abductors and adductors, elevators, and depressors. These training techniques are extended to the entire kinetic chain.[115,179,180] Appropriate strength should be developed throughout a particular range of motion to help minimize the potential for future injury.[179] Multiple-plane and combined motions that create cervicothoracic, scapulothoracic, and glenohumeral rhythms are emphasized to help improve general and sports-specific coordination and strength.[29] Muscular reeducation may be necessary to help the patient isolate individual muscles and coordinate the firing of muscles involved in complex rhythmic sequences.[178] Muscular reeducation should be done early in strength training to ensure that proper muscle firing patterns and neuromuscular control are maintained during higher-level function. This reeducation can be facilitated with a variety of electronic biofeedback devices that use surface electrodes to monitor muscular activity. Strengthening techniques that simulate the freestyle stroke are initiated later in this phase of treatment.

Toward the end of this phase of rehabilitation, while continuing the aerobic cross-training begun during the acute phase of rehabilitation, the patient begins freestyle specific retraining progressions. First, while lying on a bench, the patient simulates the freestyle stroke with his coach, physical therapist, trainer, and physician present. Retraining of his stroke mechanics is initiated, with special emphasis on head position during breathing to ensure that crane breathing is eliminated and cervical rotation and nonsegmental body roll are incorporated. This retraining will help prevent reinjury of the patient's cervical facets. The normal engram for proper arm mechanics is established to help avoid an exacerbation of the patient's rotator cuff tendinitis. After his land-based swim stroke mechanics are normalized, the patient begins aquatic retraining. At first, a mask and snorkel are used to avoid a struggle for air, so that arm and body mechanics can be trained. Then the mask and snorkel are removed, and hypoxic training is begun. Hypoxic training limits the number of breaths per length so that the mechanics of each breathing cycle can be analyzed and perfected. Finally, the patient is trained to breathe on alternate sides to minimize the repetitive microtrauma from single-side breathing. Because the patient uses all four competitive strokes—freestyle, backstroke, breaststroke, and butterfly—during training, review of the mechanics of these strokes also is imperative to ensure that reinjury does not occur as a result of the biomechanical consequences of a different stroke's mechanics. Criteria for advancement to the maintenance phase of rehabilitation include full, nonpainful, active and passive cervical, thoracic, glenohumeral, and scapulothoracic ranges of motion, significantly improved posture, normal neuromuscular control, significantly improved strength and strength balance, and improved stroke mechanics.

Maintenance Phase of Rehabilitation

Maintenance is the final phase of rehabilitation. A description of the maintenance phase of rehabilitation is presented in Exhibit 10–5. The goals of this phase are to increase and improve balance, power, and endurance of the cervical, thoracic, scapulothoracic, and glenohumeral

Exhibit 10–5 Maintenance Phase of Rehabilitation

Complexes Involved
- Functional biochemical deficit
- Subclinical adaptation

Therapeutic Activities
- Strength and flexibility balance
- Endurance
- Functional aquatic progressions

Criteria for Return to Play
- Normal cervical coupled multiplane active range of motion
- Normal cervical muscular strength and muscle balance
- Normal cervical, thoracic, glenohumeral, and scapulothoracic
- Muscular passive range of motion
- Active range of motion
- Negative clinical examination, including negative provocative tests
  –Quadrant testing
  –Overpressure testing
- Normal and balanced strength and neuromuscular control
  –Shoulder complex
  –Upper extremities
  –Thoracic spine and associated structures

Source: Courtesy of Aquatechnics Consulting Group, Inc., Aptos, California.

muscle groups, as well as other muscles in the kinetic chain; to normalize posture; to normalize multiplane-coupled neuromuscular control and eliminate subclinical adaptations; and to enable the patient to return to unrestricted, sport-specific aquatic activities.

Soft-tissue flexibility and proper balance of flexibility and strength are emphasized to allow the patient to assume and maintain a biomechanically correct posture. Power and endurance training are initiated and focus on maintaining normal multiplane-coupled cervical motion and normal scapulothoracic and glenohumeral joint mechanics and control. Patterned motion training using tubing is particularly helpful because it permits enough freedom of movement to mimic swimming patterns. These activities can be performed in front of a wall mirror to further enhance proprioceptive feedback. The Biokinetic Fit Lab (Biokinetic Fitness Laboratories, Berkeley, California), a particular type of land-based swim training equipment, can be used to develop strength, endurance, and specific stroke mechanics. Continued used of tubing and Theraband or Sportscord is recommended for home use. Freestyle, backstroke, breaststroke, and butterfly stroke retraining continues with increased workout times and difficulty. Bilateral breathing is maintained for the freestyle. Starts and turns are reviewed to ensure that proper mechanics are used to avoid reinjury.

Criteria for this patient's return to unrestricted competition include no pain, normal physical examination that ensures that provocative testing, such as the cervical quadrant and overpressure tests,[29] do not produce the patient's symptoms, normalized posture, and normal stroke mechanics.

CONCLUSION

Prevention, evaluation, and treatment of athletic cervical spine injuries require thorough understanding of athletic epidemiology and anatomy and biomechanics not only of the cervical spine but also of the shoulder, thoracic spine, and all other structures in their kinetic chains. Understanding the sport-specific biomechanics of the involved and contiguous structures is equally as important, so that all aspects of the injury mechanism and tissue overload complex are discerned. The clinician can then use the tissue injury cycle model to ensure that all aspects of a patient's tissue injury complex, sign and symptom complex, functional biomechanical deficit, and subclinical adaptation complex are identified and that an appropriate rehabilitation program is prescribed. The rehabilitation program is then implemented by the physical therapist and customized, depending on the patient's response to various aspects of the treatment program. Customizing a program allows the physical therapist not only to treat the patient's entire injury complex but also to provide the physician with important clinical information that will aid in determining what additional, if any, diagnostic and therapeutic procedures may be required to most rapidly rehabilitate the injured athlete.

REFERENCES

1. Nicholas J. What sportsmedicine is about. *Community Med.* 1978; 42:4.

2. Torg J. Anecdotal observations. In: Torg JS, ed. *Athletic Injuries to the Head, Neck, and Face.* 2nd ed. St Louis: Mosby–Year Book; 1991: 3–14.

3. Nicholas J. *Hippocrates, the Father of Sports Medicine.* Lenox Hill Hospital, Institute of Sports Medicine and Athletic Training, 1975.

4. Cantu R. Head and neck injuries. In: Mueller FO, Ryan AJ, eds. *Prevention of Athletic Injuries: The Role of the Sports Medicine Team.* Philadelphia: FA Davis; 1991:201–213.

5. Mueller FO, Ryan AJ. Epidemiologic research for injury prevention programs in sports. In: Mueller FO, Ryan AJ, eds. *Prevention of Athletic Injuries: The Role of the Sports Medicine Team.* Philadelphia: FA Davis; 1991:11–25.

6. Cole AJ, Herring SA. Role of the physiatrist in management of lumbar musculoskeletal pain. In: Tollison DC, ed. *The Handbook of Pain Management.* 2nd ed. Baltimore: Williams & Wilkins; 1994:85–95.

7. Morton RF, Hebel JR, McCarter RJ. Investigation of an epidemic. In: *A Study Guide to Epidemiology and Biostatistics.* Gaithersburg, MD: Aspen Publishers; 1989:1–19.

8. Torg J, Vegso M, O'Neill M, et al. The epidemiologic, pathologic, biomechanical, and cinematographic analysis of football-induced cervical spine trauma. *Am J Sports Med.* 1990;18:50–57.

9. Clarke K. An epidemiologic view. In: Torg JS, ed. *Athletic Injuries to the Head, Neck, and Face.* 2nd ed. St. Louis: Mosby–Year Book; 1991:15–27.

10. Kraus J, Conroy C. Mortality and morbidity from injuries in sports and recreation. *Ann Rev Public Health.* 1984;5:163.

11. Reynolds M. Myofascial trigger point syndromes in the practice of rheumatology. *Arch Phys Med Rehabil.* 1981;6:111–113.

12. Torg J. The epidemiologic, biomechanical, and cinematographic analysis of football-induced cervical spine trauma and its prevention. In: Torg JS, ed. *Athletic Injuries to the Head, Neck, and Face.* 2nd ed. St Louis: Mosby–Year Book; 1991:97–111.

13. Torg J. Trampoline-induced cervical quadriplegia. In: Torg JS, ed. *Athletic Injuries to the Head, Neck, and Face.* 2nd ed. St Louis: Mosby–Year Book; 1991:85–96.

14. Torg J. Injuries to the cervical spine and spinal cord resulting from water sports. In: Torg JS, ed. *Athletic Injuries to the Head, Neck, and Face.* 2nd ed. St Louis: Mosby–Year Book; 1991:157–173.

15. Tator C. Injuries to the cervical spine and spinal cord resulting from ice hockey. In: Torg JS, ed. *Athletic Injuries to the Head, Neck, and Face.* 2nd ed. St Louis: Mosby–Year Book; 1991:124–132.

16. Taylor KF, Coolican MR. Spinal cord injuries in football-rugby union, rugby league and Australian rules. In: Torg JS, ed. *Athletic Injuries to the Head, Neck, and Face.* 2nd ed. St Louis: Mosby–Year Book; 1991:174–197.

17. Cloward R. Acute cervical spine injuries. *Clin Symp.* 1980;32:2–32.

18. Wu W, Lewis R. Injuries of the cervical spine in high school wrestling. *Surg Neurol.* 1985;23:143–147.

19. Allan D, Reid D, Saboe L. Off-road recreational motor vehicle accidents: hospitalization and deaths. *Can J Surg.* 1988;31:233–236.

20. Perry J, Nickel V. Total cervical-spine fusion for neck paralysis. *J Bone Joint Surg Am.* 1959;41:37–60.

21. Tator C, Edmonds V. National survey of spinal injuries in hockey players. *Can Med Assoc J.* 1984;30:875–880.

22. Tator C, Edmonds V. Sports and recreation are a rising cause of spinal cord injury. *Phys Sports Med.* 1986;14:157–167.

23. Panjabi M, Duranceau J, Goel V, et al. Cervical human vertebrae quantitative three-dimensional anatomy of the middle and lower regions. *Spine.* 1991;16:861–869.

24. Panjabi M, Vasavada A, White A. Cervical spine biomechanics. *Semin Spine Surg.* 1993;5:10–16.

25. Herzog RJ, Wiens JJ, Dillingham MF, et al. Normal cervical spine morphometry and cervical spinal stenosis in asymptomatic professional football players plain film radiography, multiplanar computed tomography, and magnetic resonance imaging. *Spine.* 1991;16(suppl 6):S178–S188.

26. Hickey D, Hukins S. X-ray diffraction studies of the arrangement of collagen fibres in human fetal intervertebral disc. *J Anat.* 1980; 131:81–90.

27. Johnson R. Anatomy of the cervical spine and its related structures. In: Torg JS, ed. *Athletic Injuries to the Head, Neck, and Face.* 2nd ed. St Louis: Mosby–Year Book; 1991:371–383.

28. Parke WW, Sherk HH. Normal adult anatomy. In: Sherk HH, Dunn EJ, Eismon FJ, et al, eds. *The Cervical Spine.* 2nd ed. Philadelphia: JB Lippincott Co; 1989:11–32.

29. Stratton SA, Bryan JM. Dysfunction, evaluation, and treatment of the cervical spine and thoracic inlet. In: *Orthopaedic Physical Therapy.* 2nd ed. New York: Churchill Livingstone; 1993:77–122.

30. White AA, Panjabi MM. *Clinical Biomechanics of the Spine.* 2nd ed. Philadelphia: JB Lippincott Co; 1990.

31. Dvorak J, Dvorak V. *Manual Medicine Diagnostics.* New York: Thieme-Stratton, 1984.

32. Kapandji I. *The Physiology of the Joints: The Trunk and Vertebral Column.* 2nd ed. Edinburgh: Churchill Livingstone; 1974:170–251.

33. Clark C, Goel V, Galles K, et al. Kinematics of the occipito-atlanto-axial complex. *Trans Cervical Spine Res Soc.* 1986.

34. Depreux R, Mestdagh H. Anatomic functionelle de l'articulation sousoccipitale. *Lille Med.* 1974;19:122.

35. Dvorak J, Panjabi M, Gerber D, et al. Functional diagnostics of the rotary instability of the upper cervical spine; an experimental study in cadavers. *Spine.* 1987;12:197.

36. Field J, Hawkins R, Hensinger R, et al. Deformities. *Orthop Clin North Am.* 1978;9:955.

37. Fielding J. Cineroentgenography of the normal cervical spine. *J Bone Joint Surg Am.* 1957;39:1280.

38. White A, Panjabi M. The basic kinematics of the human spine. *Spine.* 1978;3:13.

39. Brand RA. Knee ligaments: a new view. *J Biomech Eng.* 1986;108:106–110.

40. Panjabi M, Oxland T, Parks E. Quantitative anatomy of cervical spine ligaments. I. Upper cervical spine. *J Spinal Disord.* 1991;4:270–276.

41. Dvorak J, Froelich D, Penning L, et al. Functional radiographic diagnosis of the cervical spine: flexion/extension. *Spine.* 1988;13:748–755.

42. Dvorak J, Panjabi M, Novotny J, et al. In vivo flexion/extension of the normal cervical spine. *J Orthop Res.* 1991;9:828–834.

43. Glasgow S. Upper cervical spine injuries (C1 and C2). In: Torg JS, ed. *Athletic Injuries to the Head, Neck, and Face.* 2nd ed. St Louis: Mosby–Year Book; 1991:457–468.

44. Steel H. Anatomical and mechanical considerations of the atlanto-axial articulations. *J Bone Joint Surg Am.* 1968;50:1481–1482.

45. Janda V. Muscles, central nervous regulation and back problems. In: Korr IM, ed. *Neurobiologic Mechanisms in Manipulative Therapy.* New York: Plenum Publishing; 1978.

46. White AA, Panjabi MM: The problem of clinical instability in the human spine: a systematic approach. In: White AA, Panjabi MM, eds. *Clinical Biomechanics of the Spine.* 2nd ed. Philadelphia: JB Lippincott Co; 1990:277–378.

47. Barton J, Margolis M. Rotational obstruction of the vertebral artery at the atlantoaxial joint. *Neuroradiology.* 1975;9:117.

48. Selecki B. The effects of rotation of the atlas on the axis: experimental work. *Med J Aust.* 1969;1:1012.

49. Miller R, Burton R. Stroke following chiropractic manipulation of the spine. *JAMA.* 1974;229:189.

50. Weinstein S, Cantu R. Cerebral stroke in a semi-pro football player: a case report. *Med Sci Sports Exerc.* 1991;23:1119–1121.

51. Schellas K, Latchaw R, Wendling L, et al. Vertebrobasilar injuries following cervical manipulation. *JAMA.* 1980;244:1450.

52. Gann N. Ultrasound: current concepts. *Clin Manage.* 1991;11:64–69.

53. Bogduk N, Twomey LT. *Clinical Anatomy of the Lumbar Spine.* 2nd ed. New York: Churchill Livingstone; 1991.

54. Dreyfus P. The cervical spine: non-surgical care. Presented at the Tom Landry Sports Medicine and Research Center; April 8, 1993; Dallas, TX.

55. Bogduk N, Windsor H, Inglis A. The innervation of the cervical intervertebral discs. *Spine.* 1988;13:2–8.

56. Mendel T, Wink CS, Zimny M. Neural elements in human cervical intervertebral discs. *Spine.* 1992;17:132–135.

57. Franson R, Saal J, Saal J. Human disc phospholipase A2 in inflammatory. *Spine.* 1992;17(suppl 6):S129–S132.

58. Hickey D, Hukins D. Relation between the structure of the annulus fibrosus and the function and failure of the intervertebral disc. *Spine.* 1980;5:100–116.

59. Saal J, Franson R, Dobrow R, et al. High levels of inflammatory phospholipase A2 activity in lumbar disc herniations. *Spine.* 1990;15:674–678.

60. Benzon HT. Epidural steroids for lumbosacral radiculopathy. *Adv Pain Res Ther.* 1990;13:231.

61. Bland JH. *Disorders of the Cervical Spine.* Philadelphia: WB Saunders Company; 1987.

62. Lysell E. Motion in the cervical spine. *Acta Orthop Scand.* 1969;123(suppl):54.

63. Yu S, Sether L, Haughton V. Facet joint menisci of the cervical spine: correlative MR imaging and cryomicrotomy study. *Radiology.* 1987;164:79–82.

64. Lewin T, Moffet B, Viidik A. The morphology of the lumbar synovial intervertebral joints. *Acta Morphol Neerl Scand.* 1962;4:299–319.

65. Dvorak J, Panjabi M. Functional anatomy of the alar ligaments. *Spine.* 1987;12:183–189.

66. Jia L, Shen Q, Chen D, et al. Dynamic changes of the cervical ligamental flavum in hyperextension-hyperflexion movement and their measurement. *Chin Med J.* 1990;103:66–70.

67. Jackson H, Winklemann R, Bickel W. Nerve endings in the human lumbar spine and related structures. *J Bone Joint Surg Am.* 1966;48:1272–1281.

68. Roofe P. Innervation of annulus fibrosus and posterior longitudinal ligaments. *Arch Neurol Psychiatry.* 1940;44:100.

69. Wyke B, Polacek P. Articular neurology: the present position. *J Bone Joint Surg Br.* 1975;57:401.

70. Calliet R. Functional anatomy. In: Calliet R, ed. *Neck and Arm Pain.* 2nd ed. Philadelphia: FA Davis; 1981:1–41.

71. Frykholm R. Cervical nerve root compression resulting from disc degeneration and root-sleeve fibrosis: a clinical investigation. *Acta Chir Scand.* 1951(suppl):160.

72. Sunderland S. Meningeal-neural relations in the intervertebral foramen. *J Neurosurg.* 1974;40:756.

73. Herring SA, Weinstein SM. Electrodiagnosis in sports medicine. *Phys Med Rehabil.* 1989;3:809–822.

74. Gamburd RC. Sports related cervical injuries of the cervical and lumbar spine. Presented at the State of the Art '91; March 24, 1991; San Francisco: The San Francisco Spine Institute.

75. Marks MR, Bell GR, Boumphrey FR. Cervical spine injuries and their neurologic implications. *Clin Sports Med.* 1990;9:263–278.

76. Saal JS. *Brachial Plexus Injuries at the Cervical Spine and Upper Extremity in Sports and Industry.* San Francisco: The San Francisco Spine Institute, April 2, 1990.

77. Calliet R. *Neck and Arm Pain.* Philadelphia: FA Davis; 1981.

78. Warwick R, Williams PL, eds. *Gray's Anatomy.* 35th ed. (British). Philadelphia: WB Saunders Company; 1973.

79. Krag, M. Biomechanics of the cervical spine: including bracing, surgical constructs, and orthoses. In: Frymoyer JW, ed. *The Adult Spine: Principles and Practice.* New York: Raven Press; 1991:929–965.

80. Wilder D, Pope M, Frymoyer J. The biomechanics of lumbar disc herniation and the effect of overload and instability. *J Spinal Disord.* 1988;1:16–32.

81. Friedenberg Z, Miller W. Degenerative disc disease of the cervical spine. *J Bone Joint Surg Am.* 1963;45:1171.

82. Kelsey J, Githens P, Walter S, et al. An epidemiological study of acute prolapsed cervical intervertebral disc. *J Bone Joint Surg Am.* 1984; 66:907.

83. Kondo K, Molgaard C, Kurland L, et al. Protruded intervertebral cervical disc. *Minn Med.* 1981;64:751.

84. Lester JP, Windsor RE, Dreyer SJ. *Medical Management of the Cervical Spine.* New York: Churchill Livingstone. In press.

85. Lestini W, Wiesel S. The pathogenesis of cervical spondylosis. *Clin Orthop.* 1989;239:69.

86. Parke W. Correlative anatomy of cervical spondylotic myelopathy. *Spine.* 1988;13:831.

87. Saal JS. *Pathophysiology of the Degenerative Cascade at the Cervical Spine and Upper Extremity in Sports and Industry.* San Francisco: The San Francisco Spine Institute, April 1, 1990.

88. Saal J. Flexibility training. In: Saal JA, ed. *Physical Medicine and Rehabilitation: Rehabilitation of Sports Injuries.* Philadelphia: Hanley & Belfus; 1987:537–554.

89. Smith W. Exercise and the intervertebral disc. In: Hochschuler SH, ed. *The Spine in Sports.* Philadelphia: Hanley & Belfus; 1990:3–10.

90. Press JM, Herring SA, Kibler WB. Rehabilitation of musculoskeletal disorders. In: Press JM, Herring SA, Kibler WB, eds. *The Textbook of Military Medicine.* Borden Institute, Office of the Surgeon General. In press.

91. Grieve G. *Common Vertebral Joint Problems.* Edinburgh: Churchill Livingstone; 1979.

92. Kendall FP, Kendall-McCreary E. *Muscles: Testing and Function.* 3rd ed. Baltimore: Williams & Wilkins; 1983.

93. Rocabado M. *Diagnosis and Treatment of Abnormal Craniocervical and Craniomandibular Mechanics.* Knoxville, TN: Rocabado Institute; 1981.

94. Grieve G. Common patterns of clinical presentation. In: *Common Vertebral Joint Problems.* 2nd ed. London: Churchill Livingstone; 1988.

95. Janda V. *Muscle Function Testing.* London: Butterworths, 1983.

96. Saal JA. Diagnostic decision making—where do all the pieces fit? Presented at the Cervical and Lumbar Spine: State of the Art '91; March 24, 1991; San Francisco: The San Francisco Spine Institute.

97. Hubbard DR, Berkhoff GM. Myofascial trigger points show spontaneous needle EMG activity. *Spine.* 1993;18:1803–1807.

98. Travell JH, Simons DG. *Myofascial Pain and Dysfunction: Trigger Point Manual.* Baltimore: Williams & Wilkins, 1983.

99. Kulund D. The shoulder. In: Kulund D, ed. *The Injured Athlete.* 2nd ed. Philadelphia: JB Lippincott Co; 1988:301–355.

100. Jull G, Bogduk N, Marsland A. The accuracy of manual diagnosis for cervical zygapophyseal joint pain syndromes. *Med J Aust.* 1988; 148:233–236.

101. Bogduk N, Engel R. The menisci of the lumbar zygapophyseal joints: a review of their anatomy and clinical significance. *Spine.* 1984; 9:454–460.

102. Kos J, Wolf J. Die "Menisci" der Zwischenwirbelgelenke und ihre mogliche Role bei Wirbelblockierung. *Manuelle Med.* 1972;10:105.

103. Korr I. Sustained sympathicotonia as a factor in disease. In: Korr IM, ed. *Neurobiologic Mechanisms in Manipulative Therapy.* New York: Plenum Publishing; 1978.

104. Korr I. Proprioceptors and somatic dysfunction. *J Am Osteopath Assoc.* 1975;74:638.

105. Saal J, Saal J, Herzog R. The natural history of lumbar intervertebral disk extrusions treated nonoperatively. *Spine.* 1990;15:683–686.

106. Frank C, Akeson W, Woo S, et al. Physiology and therapeutic value of passive joint motion. *Clin Orthop Rel Res.* 1984;185:113–125.

107. Rydevik B, Brown M, Lundborg G. Pathoanatomy and pathophysiology of nerve root compression. *Spine.* 1984;9:7–15.

108. Cyriax JH, Cyriax PJ. *Illustrated Manual of Orthopaedic Medicine.* Boston: Butterworth; 1983.

109. Colachis S, Strohm B. A study of tractive forces and angle of pull on vertebral interspaces in the cervical spine. *Arch Phys Med Rehabil.* 1965;46:820.

110. Colachis S, Strohm B. Cervical traction: relationship of traction time to varied tractive force with constant angle of pull. *Arch Phys Med Rehabil.* 1965;46:815.

111. Valtonen E, Kiurn E. Cervical traction as a therapeutic tool: a clinical analysis based on 212 patients. *Scand J Rehabil Med.* 1970;2:29.

112. Bernhardt M, Hynes R, Blume H, et al. Cervical spondylotic myelopathy. *J Bone Joint Surg Am.* 1993;75:119–128.

113. Butler D. Adverse neural tension disorders based on the spinal canal. In: *Mobilization of the Nervous System.* Melbourne: Churchill Livingstone; 1991:231–246.

114. Cole AJ, Moschetti ML, Eagleston RE. Lumbar spine aquatic rehabilitation: a sports medicine approach. In: Tollison DC, ed. *The Handbook of Pain Management.* 2nd ed. Baltimore: Williams & Wilkins; 1994:386–400.

115. Cole A, Reid M. Clinical assessment of the shoulder. *J Back Musculoskel Rehabil.* 1992;2(2):7–15.

116. Dwyer A, Aprill C, Bogduk N. Cervical zygapophyseal joint pain patterns. I: A study in normal volunteers. *Spine.* 1990;15:453.

117. Dreyfus P, Calodnex A. Cervical facet pain. *Pain Digest.* 1993;3:197–201.

118. Dvorak J, Dvorak V. Differential diagnosis and definition of the radicular and spondylogenic (nonradicular) pain syndromes. In: *Manual Medicine—Diagnostics.* 2nd ed. New York: Thieme; 1990: 63–64.

119. McGuckin J. The T4 syndrome. In: Grieve GP, ed. *Modern Manual Therapy of the Vertebral Column.* Edinburgh: Churchill Livingstone; 1986.

120. Bogduk N. Back pain: zygapophysial joint blocks and epidural steroids. In: Cousins MJ, Bridenbaugh PO, eds. *Neural Blockade in Clinical Anesthesia and Pain Management.* 2nd ed. Philadelphia: JB Lippincott Co; 1990:935–954.

121. Rossi U, Pernak J. Low back pain: the facet syndrome. *Adv Pain Res Ther.* 1990;13:231–244.

122. Haldeman S. Spinal manipulative therapy in sports medicine. *Clin Sports Med.* 1986;5:277–293.

123. Derby R. Cervical injection procedures at the cervical and lumbar spine. Presented at the State of the Art '91; March 24, 1991. San Francisco, The San Francisco Spine Institute.

124. Geiringer SR, Kincaid CB, Rechtein JJ. Traction, manipulation and massage. In: Delisa JA, ed. *Rehabilitation Medicine: Principles and Practice.* Philadelphia: JB Lippincott Co; 1988:276–294.

125. Kulund D. Athletic injuries to the head, face, and neck. In: Kulund D, ed. *The Injured Athlete*. 2nd ed. Philadelphia: JB Lippincott Co; 1988:267–299.

126. Schneider R, et al. Serious and fatal football injuries involving the head and spinal cord. *JAMA*. 1961;177:362.

127. Schneider R, Gosch H, Norrell H. Vascular insufficiency and differential distortion of brain and cord caused by cervicomedullary football injuries. *J Neurosurg*. 1970;33:363.

128. Wilbourn AJ, Porter JM: Thoracic outlet syndromes. *Spine*. 1988;2:597–625.

129. Karas S. Thoracic outlet syndrome. *Clin Sports Med*. 1990:297–310.

130. Kibler WB, Chandler TJ, Pace BK. Principles of rehabilitation after chronic tendon injuries. In: Renstrom Per AFH, Leadbetter WB, eds. *Clinics in Sports Medicine Tendonitis II: Clinical Considerations*. Philadelphia: WB Saunders Company; 1992:661–672.

131. Martin R. Swimming: forces on aquatic animals and humans. In: Vaughan CL, ed. *Biomechanics of Sport*. Boca Raton, FL: CRC Press; 1989:35–51.

132. Cole A, Eagleston R, Moschetti M. Sports specific stabilization training: swimming. In: White A, ed. *Spinal Medicine and Surgery: A Multidisciplinary Approach*. St Louis: Mosby–Year Book. In press.

133. Cole A, Moschetti M, Eagleston R. Getting backs in the swim. *Rehabil Manage*. August/September 1992:62–71.

134. Cole AJ, Moschetti ML, Eagleston RE. Aquatic rehabilitation applications for spine pain. *J Back Musculoskel Rehabil*. Accepted for publication, October 1994.

135. Lehmkuhl LD, Smith LK. Head, neck, and trunk. In: Lehmkuhl LD, Smith LK, eds. *Brunnstrom's Clinical Kinesiology*. 2nd ed. Philadelphia: FA Davis; 1983:337–359.

136. Sander R, Stewart A. Principles relating to reducing resistive forces. *Swim Tech*. 1991;29:21–23.

137. Bustrode C. Why are osteoarthritic joints painful? *J R Nav Med Serv*. 1976;62:5–16.

138. Cantu R, Grodin A. *Myofascial Manipulation: Theory and Clinical Application*. Gaithersburg, MD: Aspen Publishers, 1992.

139. Huskisson E. Non-narcotic analgesics. In: Wall PD, Melzach R, eds. *Text Book of Pain*. New York: Churchill Livingstone; 1984:505–513.

140. Kellett J. Acute soft tissue injuries—a review of the literature. *Med Sci Sports Exerc*. 1986;18:489.

141. Dahl S. Nonsteroidal anti-inflammatory agents: clinical pharmacology/adverse effects/usage guidelines. In: Williams RF, Dahl SL, eds. *Therapeutic Controversies in the Rheumatic Diseases*. Orlando, FL: Grune & Stratton; 1987:27–68.

142. Eldred E, Lindsky D, Buchwald J. The effect of cooling on mammalian muscle spindles. *Exp Neurol*. 1960;2:144–157.

143. Lehmann J. Therapeutic heat and cold. *Clin Orthop*. 1974;99:207.

144. Lehmann J, deLateur BJ. Diathermy and superficial heat and cold therapy. In: Kottke EJ, Stillwell GK, Lehmann JF, eds. *Krusen's Handbook of Physical Medicine and Rehabilitation*. Philadelphia: WB Saunders Company; 1982:275–350.

145. Cole A, Eagleston RE. The benefits of deep heat: ultrasound and electromagnetic diathery. *Phys Sports Med*. February 1994;22(2):77–88.

146. Dyson M. Therapeutic applications of ultrasound. In: Nyberg WL, Ziskin MC, eds. *Biological Effects of Ultrasound: Clinics in Diagnostic Ultrasound*. New York: Churchill Livingstone, 1985:121–133.

147. Ziskin MC, McDiarmid T, Michlovitz SL. Therapeutic ultrasound. In: Michlovitz SL, ed. *Thermal Agents in Rehabilitation*. Philadelphia: FA Davis; 1990:134–169.

148. Windsor RE, Lester JP, Herring SA. Electrical stimulation in clinical practice. *Phys Sports Med*. 1993;21:85–93.

149. Dreyfus P, Stratton S. The use of the low energy laser, electroacuscope, and neuroprobe in sports medicine: a current review. *Phys Sports Med*. 1993;21:47–56.

150. Shelokov A. Evaluation, diagnosis and initial treatment of general disc disease. *Spine*. 1991;5:167–176.

151. Sweeney T, Prentice C, Saal J, et al. Cervicothoracic muscular stabilization techniques. *Phys Med Rehabil. State of the Art Rev*. 1990; 14:335–359.

152. Farrell JP. Cervical passive mobilization techniques: the Australian approach. *Phys Med Rehabil*. 1990;4:309–334.

153. Farrell JP, Soto J, Tichenor CJ. The role of manual therapy in spinal rehabilitation. In: White A, ed. *Spinal Medicine and Surgery: A Multidisciplinary Approach*. St Louis: Mosby–Year Book. In press.

154. Nyberg R, Basmajian JV. Rationale for the use of spinal manipulation. In: Basmajian JV, Nyberg R, eds. *Rational Manual Therapies*. Baltimore: Williams & Wilkins; 1993:451–467.

155. Korr I. Neurochemical and neurotrophic consequences of nerve deformation. In: Glasgow EF, Twomey LT, Skull ER, et al., eds. *Aspects of Manipulative Therapy*. Melbourne: Churchill Livingstone; 1985: 64–71.

156. Wyke B. The neurological basis of thoracic spinal pain. *Rheum Phys Med*. 1970;10:356–367.

157. Ward R. Headache: an osteopathic perspective. *J Am Osteopath Assoc*. 1982;81:458–466.

158. Arnoldi C, Reimann I, Christensen S, et al. The effect of joint position in juxtaarticular bone marrow pressure. *Acta Orthop Scand*. 1980;51:893–897.

159. Ferrel W, Nade S, Newbold P. Inter-relation of neural discharge; intraarticular pressure, and joint angle in the knee of the dog. *J Physiol*. 1986;373:353–365.

160. Giovanelli-Blacker B, Elvey R, Thompson E. *The Clinical Significance of Measured Lumbar Zygoapophyseal Intra-Capsular Pressure Variation*. Proceedings of Manipulative Therapists Association of Australia. Brisbane, Australia: 1985.

161. Levick J. An investigation into the validity of subatmospheric pressure recordings from synovial fluid and their dependence on joint angle. *J Physiol*. 1979;289:55–67.

162. Paris S. Mobilization of the spine. *Phys Ther*. 1979;59:988–995.

163. Maitland G: *Vertebral Manipulation*. 2nd ed. London, Butterworth; 1986.

164. Mennel J. *Back Pain*. Boston: Little, Brown and Company; 1960.

165. Wright V, Dawson N. Biomechanics of joint function. In: Holt PLJ, ed. *Current Topics in Connective Tissue Disease*. Edinburgh: Churchill Livingstone; 1975:115.

166. Kvist M, Jarvenen M. Clinical, histochemical and biochemical features in repair of muscle and tendon injuries. *Int J Sports Med*. 1982;3:12–14.

167. Woo S, Gomez M, Amiel D, et al. The effects of exercise on the biomechanical and biochemical properties of swine digital flexor tendon. *J Biomech Eng*. 1981;103:51–56.

168. Simons D. Myofascial trigger points: a need for understanding. *Arch Phys Med Rehabil*. 1981;62:97–99.

169. Cousins MJ, Bromage PR. Epidural neural blockage. In: Cousins MJ, Bridenbaugh PO, eds. *Neural Blockage in Clinical Anesthesia and Management of Pain*. New York: JB Lippincott Co; 1988.

170. Ward RC, Sprafka S. Glossary of osteopathic terminology. *J Am Osteopath Assoc*. 1981;80:552–567.

171. Greenman P. Principles of soft tissue and articulatory (mobilization without impulse) technique. In: *Principles of Manual Medicine*. Baltimore: Williams & Wilkins; 1989:71–87.

172. Cantu R, Grodin A. Soft tissue mobilization. In: Basmajian JV, Nyberg R, eds. *Rational Manual Therapies*. Baltimore: Williams & Wilkins; 1993:199–221.

173. Ward R. Myofascial release concepts. In: Basmajian JV, Nyberg R, eds. *Rational Manual Therapies*. Baltimore: Williams & Wilkins; 1993:451–467.

174. Jones L. Spontaneous release by positioning. *DO*. 1964;4:109–116.

175. Jones L. *Strain and Counterstrain*. Newark, OH: American Academy of Osteopathy; 1981.

176. Kusunose R. Strain and counterstrain. In: Basmajian JV, Nyberg R, eds. *Rational Manual Therapies*. Baltimore: Williams & Wilkins; 1993:323–333.

177. McClure M. Flexibility training. In: Basmajian JV, Nyberg R, eds. *Rational Manual Therapies*. Baltimore: Williams & Wilkins; 1993:359–386.

178. Saliba VL, Johnson GS, Wardlaw CF. Proprioceptive neuromuscular facilitation. In: Basmajian JV, Nyberg R, eds. *Rational Manual Therapies*. Baltimore: Williams & Wilkins; 1993:243–284.

179. Cole A, Kadaba M, McCann P, et al. Electromyographic study of the subscapularis. *Arch Phys Med Rehabil*. 1990;71:790.

180. Inman V, Sanders J, Abbott L. Observations of the function of the shoulder joint. *J Bone Joint Surg Am*. 1944;26:1–30.

CHAPTER 11

Rehabilitation of the Shoulder

W. Ben Kibler

INTRODUCTION

Knowledge of normal shoulder function is essential for implementing efficacious shoulder rehabilitation. Protocols that emphasize restoration of normal motions, force couples, and biomechanics will allow soonest return to activity. This chapter reviews the current knowledge of the biomechanics and physiology of the shoulder, then describes evaluation frameworks and specific rehabilitation protocols.

MOBILITY VERSUS STABILITY

The shoulder functions most effectively in a relatively limited set of anatomic conditions that create a balance between the mobility necessary to achieve the wide ranges of joint motion and disparate joint and bone positions necessary for athletic activity (Table 11–1), and the stability necessary to allow a normal path of the instant center of joint motion in the face of large forces and translatory and distraction loads that occur in normal throwing or serving (Table 11–2).

Mobility is possible because of the "large ball/small socket" bony arrangement and the voluminous glenohumeral joint capsule that does not restrict motion except at the extremes of motion. The scapula is also highly mobile, due to the limited bony constraint of the clavicle. The scapula can, therefore, retract and protract on the thoracic wall to follow the moving humerus and rotate and elevate to avoid humeral impingement.

Stability is conferred by the interaction of bony, ligamentous, and muscular constraint systems that control the movement of the instant center of motion of the glenohumeral joint. Studies on the movement show that in the midranges of motion, very little translation of the humerus occurs on the glenoid, but at the extremes of motion in flexion, abduction, or rotation, translation occurs within certain limits. This means that, despite the anatomic "small socket/large ball" discrepancy, the glenohumeral joint does function as a ball-and-socket joint in most positions during throwing or serving, being stabilized by the ligaments mainly at the extremes of motion.

CONSTRAINT SYSTEMS AROUND THE SHOULDER

The bony constraints do contribute to stability. The geometry of the joint surfaces allows smooth conformity of the two bones. The glenoid is enlarged and deepened by the labrum, which will increase the conformity. This increases the "concavity-compression" effect to control translation. The conformity is maximized by a proper positioning of the scapula with the glenoid, in relation to the moving arm. This positioning will depend on proper scapular muscle activity. The glenohumeral joint has been statically compared to a "golf ball on a tee" in terms of its size relationships. A more appropriate description of the dynamic situation would be Rowe's comparison to a "ball on the seal's nose." As the ball (humerus) moves, the seal (scapula and glenoid) moves to maintain the balanced relationship.

The ligamentous constraints are the primary stabilizers at extremes of motion in rotation, abduction, or flexion. They control both anterior/posterior and superior/inferior translation, and control "coupled translation," or translation that occurs at the limit of normal rotation. Different parts of the ligamentous structures are the main restraints at different glenohumeral positions. The ligaments work in a static fashion to limit translation and rotation, but their stiffness and torsional rigidity are increased with concomitant muscle activity. Both rotator cuff activity and biceps activity have been shown to stiffen the capsule and to decrease glenohumeral translation.

Table 11–1   Normal Joint Motions and Bony Positions around the Shoulder Joint

Scapula

- Rotation through arc of 65 degrees with shoulder abduction
- Translation on thorax up to 15 cm

Glenohumeral

• Abduction	140 degrees
• Internal/External Rotation	90 degrees/90 degrees
• Translation:	
–Ant/Post	5 mm–10 mm
–Inf/Sup	4 mm–5 mm
• Total Rotations:	
–Baseball	185 degrees
–Tennis	165 degrees

The muscular constraints work in several ways to allow stability. First, as has already been mentioned, they contribute to the other constraint systems by dynamic positioning of the scapula and by increasing capsuloligamentous stiffness. Second, they can act as dynamic ligaments when their passive elements are used to limit joint excursion as the muscles are put on stretch. Third, and most importantly, they act as parts of force couples around the joint by controlling the joint motion, controlling the position of the bones and joint, or controlling and directing the force through the joint. Two types of force couples work around the shoulder joint (Exhibit 11–1). The first is coactivation, or coordinated simultaneous activation of agonist and antagonist muscles about a

Table 11–2   Forces and Loads on the Shoulder in Normal Athletic Activity

• Rotational Velocities:	
–Baseball	7,000 deg/sec
–Tennis Serve	1,500 deg/sec
–Tennis Forehand	245 deg/sec
–Tennis Backhand	870 deg/sec
• Angular Velocities:	
–Baseball	1,150 deg/sec
• Acceleration Forces:	
–Internal Rotation	60 nm
–Horizontal Adduction	70 nm
–Anterior Shear	400 nm
• Deceleration Forces:	
–Horizontal Abduction	80 nm
–Posterior Shear	500 n
–Compression	70 nm

Exhibit 11–1   Force Couples around the Shoulder

COORDINATED COACTIVATION
- Low net torque
- Increased joint control
- Small number of muscles, close to joint
- Dependent upon length changes in muscles

EXAMPLES
- Upper trapezius/levator scapulae: lower trapezius/serratus anterior to control scapular rotation
- Deltoid: subscapularis/infraspinatus/teres minor to control glenohumeral rotation
- Subscapularis: infraspinatus/teres minor to control glenohumeral movement

AGONIST/ANTAGONIST
- Increase joint torque and motion
- Larger number of muscles, distant and local to joint
- Coordinated sequencing
- Dependent on force changes of the activity

EXAMPLES
- Trapezius/rhomboids: serratus to control scapular retraction and protraction
- Pectoralis/latissimus dorsi: posterior deltoid/infraspinatus/teres minor to control upper arm internal rotation

---

joint. This creates low net torque around the joint but creates increased control of motion. These activations are confined to muscles near the joint. They involve a small number of muscles and are controlled by and respond to length changes in the muscles. Their major function is to control pertubations of the joint. Examples of this type would be upper trapezius/levator scapulae working with lower trapezius/serratus anterior to control scapular rotation, deltoid working with subscapularis/infraspinatus/teres minor to control glenohumeral rotation, and subscapularis working with infraspinatus/teres minor to control glenohumeral movement in the transverse plane.

The second force couple is an agonist/antagonist activity, with coordinated activation of the agonist and inhibition of the antagonist muscles. This will increase joint torque and motion, will increase forces through the joint, and will allow transfer of forces through the joint. These activations are usually part of a sequence of activations involving many often distant muscles and are controlled by and respond to force demands of the activity. Examples would include trapezius/rhomboids working with serratus anterior to control scapular retraction and protraction and pectoralis/latissimus dorsi working with posterior deltoid/infraspinatus/teres minor to control upper-arm internal rotation.

Sequential coordinated muscle activation is necessary to produce the torques and accelerations around the shoulder necessary to throw or serve. The intrinsic shoulder musculature does not have the capability to generate the recorded velocities. Studies have shown that the cross-sectional area of the muscles is not large enough to generate the torques, that optimum arm velocity is not related to shoulder muscle strength, that peak torques and maximal velocities of the shoulder or of thrown objects decrease by about 50% as body parts are eliminated from the normal sequencing, and that peak velocity in female tennis players is more highly correlated with leg strength than with arm strength. Mathematical analysis based on measured velocities throughout the tennis serve in elite players shows that the shoulder link contributes about 13% of the total kinetic energy of the service motion and is contributing 10% of the total forward arm velocity at the moment of ball impact.

The sequential activation that occurs to assist the shoulder in most throwing or serving activities is a proximal-to-distal activation of the links in a kinematic chain. The simplest representation of this chain is a kinetic chain, where each link is isolated and stops its function before the next link works. In actuality, the activation is more complex, with link activity overlapping. However, from a standpoint of performance and rehabilitation, it is correct to say that this proximal-to-distal sequencing allows generation, summation, and transfer of velocities, energy, and accelerations from the proximal segments of the legs and back through the shoulder to be added to the contributions of the distal segments of the arm. The primary pattern of muscle activation for this link sequencing is a force-dependent, agonist/antagonist pattern, with each link being activated in the specific sequence for the shoulder activity. The shoulder functions not only as a small energy generator in this sequence, but also as a funnel for the transfer and concentration of the forces generated from the proximal links. The efficiency with which this is accomplished depends on the stability of the joint.

It appears that the primary force couple activation pattern of local muscles around the shoulder joint to allow this stability is the length-dependent, coordinated coactivation, stabilization pattern. This pattern would regulate the transferred forces, allow humeral head compression, allow ball-and-socket motion in the midranges of motion, and help stiffen the capsule at the extremes of motion.

As can be seen, the muscles around the shoulder, both locally and regionally, have major input into normal shoulder function, both as part of the muscular constraint system and in complementing the other constraint systems. This has important implications for shoulder rehabilitation because muscles can be rehabilitated and conditioned in many effective ways.

IMPLICATIONS FOR REHABILITATION— GENERAL PRINCIPLES

From a rehabilitation perspective, the shoulder is a highly muscular-dependent joint and is dependent on both local and distant input for normal function. Once the clinical pathology has been treated, rehabilitation should be designed from these two perspectives to allow the normal functions.

Pain must be kept to a minimum because of the marked inhibitory effect on muscle peak torque and muscle coactivation. Modalities, medications, and judicious injections may be used.

Deficits in range of motion restrict normal shoulder function in several ways. Restricted glenohumeral internal rotation alters coupled translation, allowing anterior translation in the midranges of motion; changes the activation of the length-dependent force couple patterns; and interferes with upper-arm internal rotation—the most significant contributor to forward arm velocity in both the serve and the forehand. These deficits must be identified and objectively measured by goniometric evaluation to get a true measure of glenohumeral range of motion.

The only way that muscles can be organized to repetitively function well with precision through such rapid speeds and high loads is through learned motor patterns. These patterns position the body links in certain predetermined ways and activate muscles in precise agonist/antagonist force-dependent patterns and coordinated coactivation length-dependent patterns, depending on the demands of the activity. These motor patterns are more efficient—in terms of shoulder duration, higher amplitude, and smoother coordination—in more skilled athletes, but are also more "fragile" and can be altered with relatively minor injuries. Therefore, rehabilitation will be more effective if it recognizes the alterations and focuses on reestablishing these patterns early in the rehabilitation protocol. Cocontraction muscle activation patterns for the scapula and shoulder should be employed as these are directly related to the normal physiologic function of the shoulder. Finally, functional progressions of throwing or serving, employing the same motions as are present in the sport, complete the rehabilitation for normal shoulder function.

In addition to local treatment, evaluation and possible rehabilitation of the distant contributors to shoulder function should be done. Deficits in strength, strength balance, and flexibility in the legs, hips, and trunk should be sought. Restrictions of hip and neck motion are common in throwing athletes and should be included in the rehabilitation protocols. Maintenance of fitness of all of the other links of the kinematic chain can be done while early shoulder healing is progressing; they can then be integrated into the shoulder rehabilitation program to allow normal force generation and transfer.

PATHOLOGY IN THE SHOULDER

In either the macrotrauma or microtrauma situation, the pathologic process alters the normal bony, ligamentous, or muscular systems so that the normal path of the instant center of rotation is not constrained (Exhibit 11–2). Pathology may involve only one of the constraint systems but, due to the interaction of the constraint systems in allowing mobility while conferring stability, there is usually some involvement of several constraints. The constraint systems may fail individually (one system only), concurrently (two or three at the same time), or consecutively (failure of one followed by failure of others) (Exhibit 11–3). The initiating factor in the pathology is commonly local, but alterations in other parts of the kinematic chain may produce loads or stresses that have clinical expression at the shoulder, due to the shoulder's role as a funnel for developed forces.

From a rehabilitation standpoint, alterations in the muscular constraint system are the most important, as they can be modified and improved by appropriate protocols and because of the muscular system's important role in complementing and increasing the efficiency of the other constraint systems. Alterations in muscle may be either anatomic or neurologic.

Anatomic alterations may be due to direct-blow trauma and muscle damage, but these injuries are rare, and their effect on shoulder function is small. Disuse or altered use is the most common factor in anatomic alterations. The muscle requires a certain level of activation and feedback to maintain normal size and physiologic function. Immobilization and disuse cause severe loss of muscle size over short periods of time. Because muscle strength is proportional to muscle mass, ability to generate torque or to absorb a load is similarly diminished.

If a muscle is immobilized in a shortened position, is not used in ways that allow full repetitive motion, or is shortened due to inflexibility, the normal length/tension relationship is shifted, resulting in decreased maximum tension and strength-generating capacity.

Neurologic alterations affect the muscular constraint system by altering local strength development and by altering the organization of the motor firing patterns necessary for force-dependent kinematic chain activity. Most of the muscle weakness seen in the postoperative or postinjury period is due to decreased "neural drive" or the activation and coordination of muscle firing patterns. Many factors, including joint effusions, pain from any source, disuse, and different abnormalities such as altered proprioception decrease the neural drive stimulus. It appears that maximum strength output is highly related to available neural drive for months after the injury.

The force-dependent motor patterns that are responsible for smooth generation and transfer of force through a coordinated succession of joint positions and movements are highly dependent on the neurologic integrity of each of the joints. If the length-dependent patterns that operate around individual joints are not working right due to weakness, inhibition, or other problems with neural drive, the force-dependent patterns break down and are altered, thereby decreasing

Exhibit 11–2 Acute Macrotrauma and Chronic Microtrauma

ACUTE MACROTRAUMA
- One-time event
- Normal tissues → abnormal tissues with clinical symptoms
  –Fracture of clavicle
  –Acute traumatic shoulder dislocation
  –AC joint sprain

CHRONIC MICROTRAUMA
- Process
- Normal tissue → abnormal but asymptomatic tissues → abnormal clinically symptomatic tissues
  –Rotator cuff tendinitis
  –Nontraumatic capsuloligamentous instability
  –Attritional labral tears

AC, acromioclavicular.

Exhibit 11–3 Methods of Constraint System Failure

CONSTRAINT SYSTEM FAILURE

Individual

- Fractures clavicle (bony)
- Acute Bankhart lesion (ligamentous)

Concurrent

- Rotator cuff tear (muscular) with anterior dislocation (ligamentous)
- Bony Bankhart lesion (bony) and capsular stretch (ligamentous)

Consecutive

- Rotator cuff weakness (muscular) → decreased capsular stiffness and laxity (ligamentous)
- Posterior cuff weakness and inflexibility (muscular) → anterior humeral translation and labral tear (ligamentous)

the efficiency and maximal force production from that pattern.

Both anatomic and neurologic alterations in muscle are present at the same time during the pathologic process. Their clinical effect is to decrease the amount and effectiveness of muscle strength production. They are widespread in a muscle-dependent joint like the shoulder and should be checked for closely.

Scapular muscle failure is commonly seen in shoulder pathology. This appears to be a nonspecific response to glenohumeral pain, injury, or pathology and appears in 68–100% of cases. Disruption of the force couples has deleterious effects on the four purposes of the scapula in overhead activities. Lack of acromial elevation due to upper trapezius weakness increases impingement with abduction. Trapezius, rhomboid, and serratus anterior weakness impairs the scapula's ability to position itself as a congruent socket for the moving humerus; to stabilize itself as an anchor for origins of the rotator cuff, deltoid, biceps, and triceps; and to move smoothly from retraction to protraction during the throwing motion. Finally, this weakness will serve as a break in the kinematic chain that disrupts funneling of velocity and force, and does not allow a stable base for the arm to work.

Rotator cuff injury, due to either impingement or partial- or full-thickness tears, results in failure of energy and force production, but its most deleterious effects are upon the force couples that position and stabilize the glenohumeral joint. Supraspinatus weakness decreases capsular stiffness and concavity/compression. Infraspinatus/teres minor weakness alters the deltoid force couple for abduction, leading to excessive superior translation. Subscapularis weakness can lead to overstretching of the anterior capsular structures and cause excessive anterior translation. Internal/external rotation force couple imbalance, with relatively strong internal rotators and relatively weak external rotators, is another common problem. This imbalance decreases concavity/compression and, in concert with restricted glenohumeral internal rotation, increases anterior translation.

Pathology in other links of the kinematic chain may affect the muscular constraints. Biomechanical flaws or anatomic injuries such as ankle sprains, knee pathology, or back inflexibility or weakness create a "catch-up" situation if the distal kinematic links have to increase their energy or force production to maintain normal force production at the hand. The arm muscles, with their smaller cross-sectional area, cannot initiate or maintain this higher level of activity well, thereby putting them at risk of fatigue and injury. Our studies have shown that in a mathematical model, a decrease of 10% of trunk/leg kinetic energy requires an 18.5% increase in shoulder velocity or a 40% increase in shoulder mass to achieve the same resultant energy at the hand.

CLOSED-CHAIN REHABILITATION

There are differences in muscle recruitment and joint motion when the distal arm or leg meets considerable resistance, compared to when it is free to move. A "closed-chain" type of movement occurs when the distal end of a linked system meets considerable resistance. The operational definition of the movement pattern that occurs in this event is that a closed chain exists when there is a sequential combination of joints and that the translation of the instant centers of motion of the specific joints occurs in a predictable manner that results from the generation and distribution of forces from a base of support through the links.

Although most overhead throwing functions seem to involve open-chain patterns, there are several reasons that exercises based on closed-chain principles should be used in shoulder rehabilitation. First, the shoulder's function as a funnel—transferring forces from the stable base of the trunk and scapula in a predictable sequence—fits the definition of a closed-chain activity. Second, these exercises, by promoting coactivation force couples around the scapula and glenohumeral joint, enhance the muscle's primary role as shoulder stabilizers. Third, by fixing the hand, these exercises allow more muscle activity at the scapula. Fourth, strengthening of the muscles in a closed-chain, coactivation sequence at 90 degrees of abduction decreases tensile stresses on the capsular ligaments and rotator cuff tendon and decreases the effect of the deltoid component of the abduction force couple. Fifth, proprioceptive activity is enhanced by emphasis on stability and coactivation. Finally, closed-chain exercises result in muscle loads and activation levels that are safe enough to be used early in rehabilitation. The muscle firing activity is between 10% and 40% of maximum.

Closed-chain exercises, therefore, should be used as part of a shoulder rehabilitation program. They simulate and enhance most of the important functions of the shoulder joint, recreate the motor patterns necessary for scapular and glenohumeral stability, and are safe to use. They are particularly suited for the earlier stages of rehabilitation, when neurologic retraining is important, when a scapular base should be established, and when minimal tension and shear should be placed across the injured or repaired tissues.

SPECIFIC PROTOCOLS

Implementation of specific rehabilitation protocols for the shoulder must be based on basic science knowledge and must be used in a logical diagnosis or activity-specific progression to achieve maximum efficiency. The goal of the rehabilitation program—functional restoration—is the same for each condition, but the starting point is widely variable, depending on the pathologic process (macrotrauma, microtrauma), type of treatment (rest, immobilization, surgery), and associated alterations (other injuries, inflexibility, strength deficit). This point reinforces the need for a complete and accurate diagnosis as a starting point for rehabilitation.

EVALUATION BEFORE REHABILITATION

Evaluation of the shoulder should include evaluation of the kinematic chain, as well. The hips and knees should be assessed for any incompletely resolved injury. Special attention should be focused on hip rotation and flexion, especially on the nondominant side, as these areas have been shown to be tight. Lumbar flexibility, both in flexion and lateral bending, should be measured, lumbar lordosis should be checked, and trunk musculature strength should be evaluated. Finally, the thoracic spine should be evaluated for scoliosis or kyphosis. Both of these conditions can alter spine motion in throwing but may also disrupt normal scapulothoracic motion.

Evaluation of the scapula should be done from the back. Abnormalities of the scapular position, such as winging or excessive prominence, should be noted (Figure 11–1). Scapular motion should be observed in both arm flexion and arm abduction (Figure 11–2). Smooth symmetrical motion in both the ascending phase and the descending phase should be observed. Asymmetry, which is usually noted in the descending phase, suggests weakness in the scapula force couple. Scapular stabilizer strength may be assessed by wall push-ups or by the "lateral slide" measurement (Figure 11–3). Both of these tests measure the ability of the scapular muscles to stabilize the scapula on the thoracic wall in response to an imposed load.

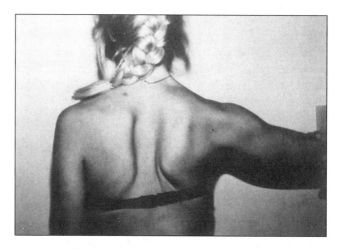

Figure 11–2 Scapular winging with resisted abduction.

The acromioclavicular joint is important as a stabilizing strut and as a load-bearing joint when the arm is in the overhead position. Palpation for tenderness, swelling, or crepitus should be done, and motion of the joint in both anterior/posterior and superior/inferior directions may be evaluated by stabilizing the scapula and moving the clavicle by direct pressure.

Evaluation of the glenohumeral joint should include range of motion, strength, and provocative testing. Glenohumeral motion is a sensitive measure of shoulder pathology and should be measured accurately by a goniometer, rather than by estimating spinous process levels. The shoulder should be placed in the scapular plane, with the goniometer centered along the axis of rotation (Figure 11–4). Abduction and horizontal abduction/adduction may be measured in the same fashion.

Glenohumeral strength can be estimated by manual muscle testing or can be objectively described by isokinetic testing. Manual muscle testing is much better for evaluation of the individual components of the rotator cuff, which cannot be accurately evaluated by isokinetics.

Provocative tests for glenohumeral stability should be done to assess the competence of the ligamentous constraints after either treatment or surgery, so that full range of motion exercises and muscular loading can be done safely.

PHASES OF REHABILITATION

Our functional rehabilitation program is divided into three phases, each based on the resolution of certain aspects of the tissue injuries or alterations that exist in the shoulder problem (Exhibit 11–4, Figure 11–5). These are specific goals, activity progressions, and criteria for movement to the next

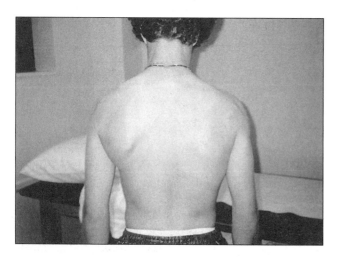

Figure 11–1 Scapular prominence with arm at rest.

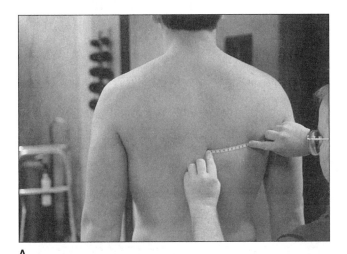

A

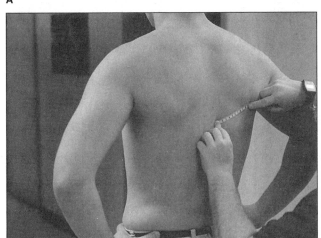

B

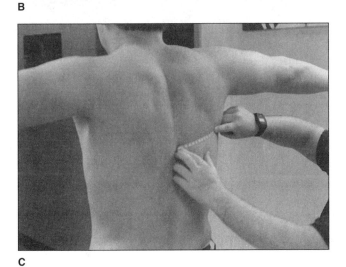

C

Figure 11–3 Lateral slide measurement. Measurements are taken from the inferior medial tip of the scapula to the nearest spinous process. (*A*) Position 1, with arms at rest at the side. (*B*) Position 2, with hands on hips. (*C*) Position 3, with arms abducted to 80 to 90 degrees, and maximum glenohumeral internal rotation. This position places maximal load on the scapular stabilizers.

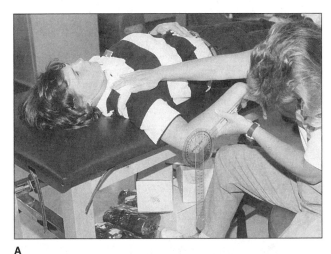

A

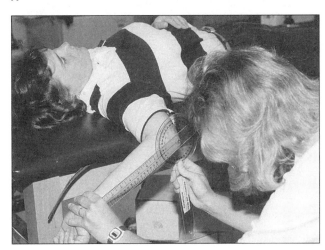

B

Figure 11–4 Goniometric measurement of glenohumeral rotation. (*A*) Internal rotation. (*B*) External rotation.

phase. Because this is a function-based program, all of the protocols tend to progress to some common end points in the later phases, regardless of the starting point.

Acute Phase

The acute phase begins with the onset of clinical symptoms of injury or when the patient is seen for rehabilitation. Patient injuries will vary widely, from acute fracture or dislocation to a postoperative rotator cuff repair, to an overload tendinitis. In each instance, attention will focus on resolving the clinical symptoms and the tissue injuries. This phase will be the most diverse because of the wide spectrum of clinical symptoms and tissue injuries, and the variety of treatments that are necessary. The objective of this phase is to create stable, healing tissues and to improve joint health, allowing more advanced rehabilitation.

Exhibit 11–4 Phases of Rehabilitation and Complexes Addressed in Each Phase

Acute Phase

• Clinical symptom complex
• Tissue injury complex

Recovery Phase

• Tissue injury complex
• Tissue overload complex
• Functional biomechanical deficit complex

Functional Phase

• Functional biomechanical deficit complex
• Subclinical adaptation complex

Recovery Phase

The recovery phase will continue rehabilitation of the tissue injury complex but will address the tissue overloads and functional biomechanical deficits. Entry into this phase assumes that the injured tissues may be loaded in tension and compression so that normal strength and flexibility may be reached. This phase is frequently the longest and most complex because of the large amount of work required to restore all of the alterations, both locally and distantly. Force couple restoration, full range of motion, scapular stability, and kinematic chain restoration are addressed in this phase. By the end of this phase, most of the protocols will be merging toward the common goals of gaining full motion and muscular balance.

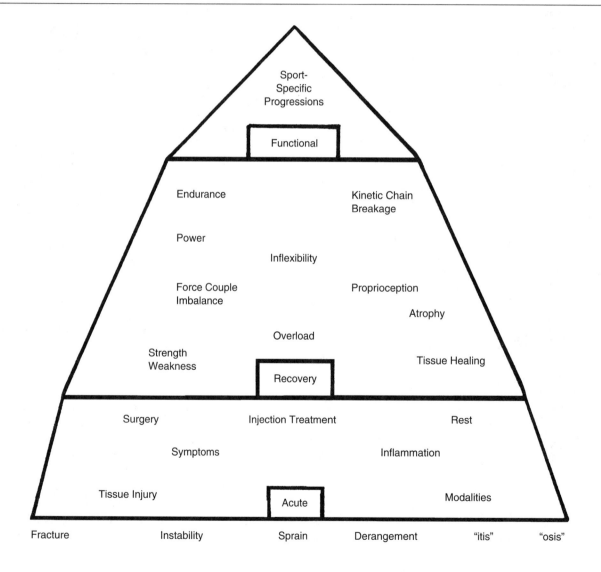

Figure 11–5 Rehabilitation phases.

Functional Phase

The functional phase will address any of the remaining functional biomechanical deficits, correct any subclinical adaptations that may have developed, and use functional progressions to return to play. This is the final common pathway of all of the protocols. The athlete may start some modified athletic activity, such as hitting ground strokes only or throwing a limited number of pitches, but functional progressions of throwing, hitting, or serving should be completed before full competition is allowed. These progressions test all of the mechanical parts of the normal overhead throwing or serving motion. Very few deviations from normal mechanics should be allowed as these deviations will create extra stress when the athlete has to meet the normal demands inherent in the sport.

The functional phase should also be used to instruct the athlete in preventive activities, or "prehabilitation." The athlete who is injured as a result of participating in a sport will usually return to that sport and its demands after the injury is rehabilitated. A maintenance program of stretching, muscle balance exercises, power exercises, and kinematic chain exercises—all designed to improve the athlete's ability to withstand sports demands—is the best method of conditioning to prevent the overload injuries that are common around the shoulder.

REHABILITATION PROTOCOLS

Postoperative Rehabilitation Protocol

This general protocol illustrates principles for rehabilitation of any postoperative problem. The specific protocols are outlined at the end of the chapter. This protocol assumes stable repair of the labrum, capsule, or rotator cuff, and ability to achieve 90 degrees of abduction without impingement or excessive capsular stretch at the time of the operation. We try to get our postoperative labral repairs, shoulder reconstructions, and acromioplasties to 90 degrees of passive or active assisted abduction by three weeks and our rotator cuff repairs to 90 degrees of passive or active assisted abduction by four to six weeks.

Acute Phase

I. GOALS:
1. Tissue healing
2. Reduce pain and inflammation
3. Reestablish nonpainful range of motion below 90 degrees of abduction
4. Retard muscle atrophy
5. Scapular control
6. Maintain fitness of other components of kinematic chain

II. TISSUE HEALING:
Combination of
1. Rest
2. Short-term immobilization
3. Modalities
4. Surgery

III. PAIN AND INFLAMMATION:
Aggressive treatment to control pain to decrease inhibition-based muscle atrophy and scapular instability due to serratus and/or trapezius inhibition.
1. Medications, nonsteroidal or judicious use of steroids orally or by injection
2. Modalities, usually ultrasound, 2/wk × 2 wk
3. Cold compression devices
4. Joint protection, usually by sling or swathe, with gradual progression out of sling

IV. RANGE OF MOTION:
Should be started in pain-free arcs, kept below 90 degrees of abduction, and may be passive or active assisted. The degree of movement will be guided by the stability of the operative repair.
1. Codman's or other pendulum exercises
2. Manual capsular stretching and cross-fiber massage
3. T-bar or ropes and pulleys (Figure 11–6)

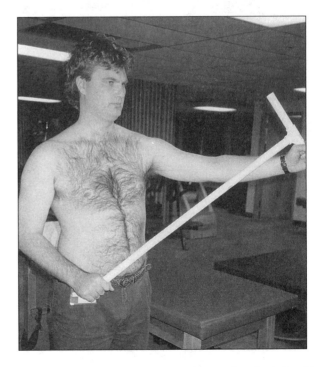

Figure 11–6 Acute phase active assisted range of motion below 90 degrees.

V. MUSCLE ATROPHY:

1. Isometric exercises, with arm below 90 degrees of abduction and 90 degrees of flexion. These should be done in labral or capsular repair patients, but not in rotator cuff patients.

VI. SCAPULAR CONTROL:

1. Isometric scapular pinches and scapular elevation
2. Closed-chain weight shifts, with hands on table, shoulder flexed <60 degrees, abducted <45 degrees (Figure 11–7)
3. Tilt board or circular board weight shifts with same limitations

VII. FITNESS OF REST OF KINEMATIC CHAIN:

1. Aerobic exercises such as running, bicycling, or stepping
2. Anaerobic agility drills
3. Lower extremity strengthening by machines, squat exercises, or open-chain leg lifts
4. Elbow and wrist strengthening by isometrics or rubber tubing
5. Flexibility exercises, especially areas that are shown to be tight on the evaluation

6. Integration of the kinematic chain by leg and trunk stabilization on a ball, employing rotational and oblique patterns of contraction (Figure 11–8)

VIII. CRITERIA FOR MOVEMENT OUT OF ACUTE PHASE:

1. Progression of tissue healing (healed or sufficiently stabilized for active motion and tissue loading)
2. Passive range of motion 66–75% of opposite side
3. Minimal pain
4. Manual muscle strength in nonpathologic areas 4+/5
5. Scapular control, with dominant side/nondominant side scapular asymmetry <1.5 cm
6. Kinematic chain function and integration

Recovery Phase

I. GOALS:

1. Normal active and passive shoulder and glenohumeral motion
2. Improved scapular control
3. Normal upper-extremity strength and strength balance
4. Normal shoulder arthrokinematics in single, then multiple planes of motion
5. Normal kinematic chain and force generation patterns

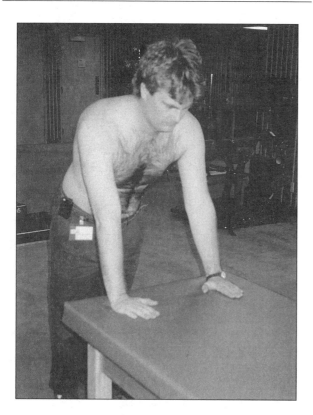

Figure 11–7 Acute phase closed-chain weight shifts. Arms are kept below 60 degrees of abduction.

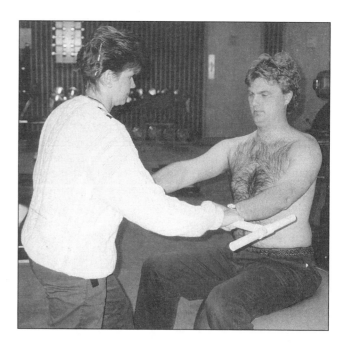

Figure 11–8 Acute phase ball exercises. They start integration of the trunk into shoulder rehabilitation.

II. RANGE OF MOTION:

1. Active assisted motion above 90 degrees of abduction with wand (Figure 11–9)
2. Active assisted, then active motion in internal and external with scapula stabilized (Figure 11–10). In this manner, glenohumeral rotation is normalized without substitution movements from the scapula

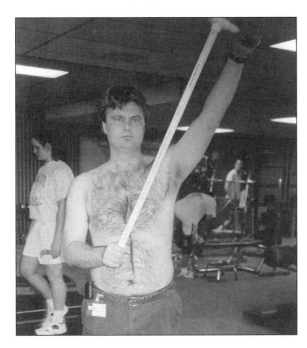

Figure 11–9 Recovery phase active assisted range of motion in rotation.

III. SCAPULAR CONTROL:

1. Scapular proprioceptive neuromuscular facilitation (PNF) patterns, in diagonals
2. Closed-chain exercises at 90 degrees of flexion/ 90 degrees of abduction—scapular retraction/protraction and scapular elevation/depression (Figure 11–11)
3. Modified push-ups
4. Regular push-ups
5. Medicine ball catch and push
6. Dips

IV. UPPER-EXTREMITY STRENGTH AND STRENGTH BALANCE:

1. Glenohumeral PNF patterns (Figure 11–12)
2. Closed-chain exercises at 90 degrees of flexion, then 90 degrees of abduction—glenohumeral depressors and glenohumeral internal/external rotators
3. Forearm curls
4. Isolated rotator cuff exercises
5. Machines or weights for light bench press, military press, and pull downs. The resistance should initially be light, then progress as strength improves. Emphasis is placed on proper mechanics, proper technique, and joint stabilization.

V. NORMAL SHOULDER ARTHROKINEMATICS:

1. Range of motion with arm at 90 degrees of abduction. This is the position where most throwing and serving activities occur. The periarticular soft tissues must be completely loose and balanced at this position.

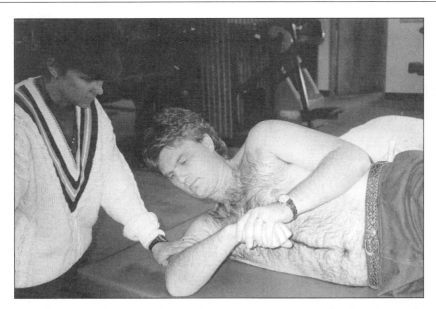

Figure 11–10 Recovery phase glenohumeral rotation with scapula stabilized to stretch posterior shoulder capsule.

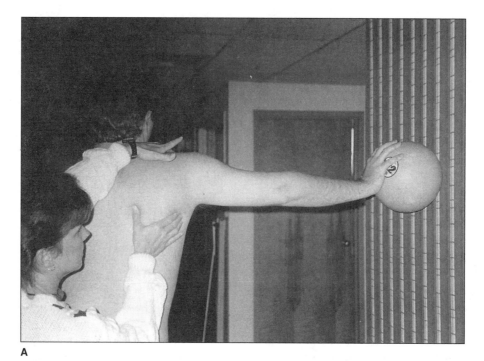

A

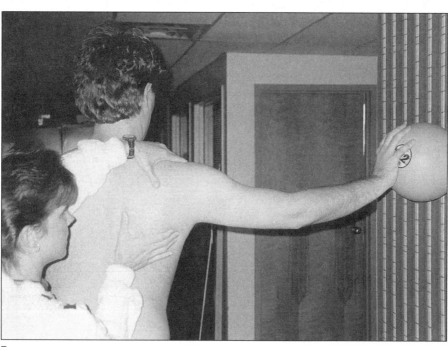

B

Figure 11–11 Recovery phase closed-chain exercises for scapular control. (*A*) Scapular elevation. (*B*) Scapular depression.

2. Muscle activity at 90 degrees of abduction. Normal muscle firing patterns must be reestablished at this position, both in organization of force generation and force regulation patterns, and in proprioceptive sensory feedback. Closed-chain patterns are an excellent method to reestablish the normal neurologic patterns for joint stabilization.

3. Open-chain exercises, including mild pyelometric exercises, may be built on the base of the closed-chain stabilization to allow normal control of joint mobility.

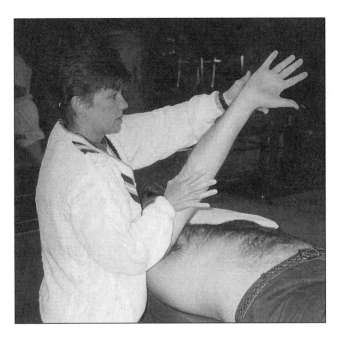

Figure 11–12 Recovery phase glenohumeral PNF patterns.

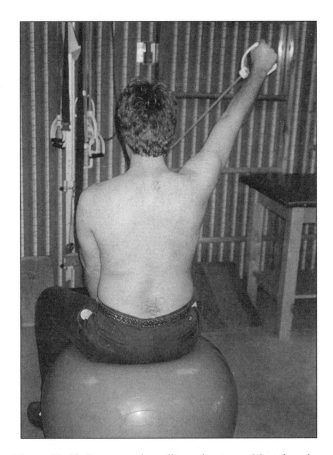

Figure 11–13 Recovery phase diagonal patterns. Most throwing activities involve diagonal force generation and force regulation, starting from the legs, through the trunk, to the arm.

VI. NORMAL KINEMATIC CHAIN AND FORCE GENERATION:

1. Normalization of all inflexibilities throughout chain
2. Normal agonist-antagonist force couples in legs by squats, pyelometric depth jumps, lunges, and hip extensions
3. Trunk rotation exercises with medicine ball or tubing
4. Integrated exercises with leg and trunk stabilization—rotations, diagonal patterns from hip to shoulder (Figure 11–13), and medicine ball throws (Figure 11–14)
5. Rotator cuff strength 4+/5 or higher
6. Normal kinematic chain function

Functional Phase

I. GOALS:

1. Increase power and endurance in the upper extremity
2. Increase normal multiple-plane neuromuscular control; locally, regionally, and in entire kinematic chain
3. Instruction in prehabilitation activities
4. Sports specific activity

II. POWER AND ENDURANCE IN UPPER EXTREMITY:

Power is the rate of doing work. Work may be done to move the joint and the extremity, or it may be done to absorb a load and stabilize the joint or extremity. Power has a time component, and for shoulder activity, quick movements and quick reactions are the dominant ways of doing work. These exercises should, therefore, be done with relatively rapid movements in planes that approximate normal shoulder function (i.e., 90 degrees of abduction in shoulder, trunk rotation and diagonal arm motions, and rapid external/internal rotation).

1. Diagonal and multiplanar motions with tubing, light weight, small medicine balls, and isokinetic machines
2. Pyelometrics—wall push-ups, corner push-ups, weighted ball throws, and tubing. Tubing exercises may be used to mimic any of the needed motions in throwing or serving. Medicine balls are very effective pyelometric devices (Figure 11–14). The weight of the ball creates a prestretch and an eccentric load when it is caught, creates a resistance, and demands a powerful agonist contraction to propel it forward again.

III. INCREASE MULTIPLE-PLANE NEUROMUSCULAR CONTROL:

The force-dependent motor firing patterns should be reestablished. No subclinical adaptations, such as "opening up" (trunk rotation too far in front of shoulder rotation), 3/4 arm positioning on throwing, or excessive wrist snap, should be

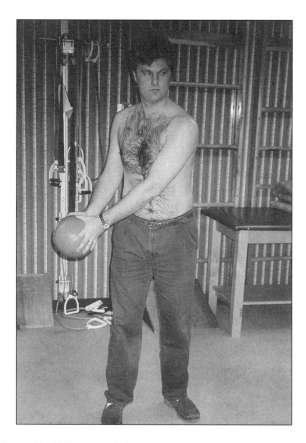

Figure 11–14 Functional phase medicine ball pyelometrics. Power should be emphasized, catching the ball, then throwing it back with a powerful thrust. Using the ball allows integration of the kinetic chain.

allowed. Help in this area can be obtained by watching preinjury videos or by using a knowledgeable coach in the particular sport. Special care must be taken to integrate completely all of the components of the kinematic chain to generate and funnel the proper forces to and through the shoulder.

IV. PREHABILITATION:

The athlete who is injured while playing a sport will most likely be going back to the same sport and will be facing the same sports demands. The body should not only be healed from the symptomatic standpoint, but should be prepared for resuming the stresses inherent in playing the sport. A maintenance program is the best way to condition and to prevent overload injuries and further problems in sport.

1. Flexibility—general body flexibility, with emphasis on sport-specific problems (shoulder internal rotation and elbow extension in the arm, low back, hip rotation, and hamstrings in the legs)
2. Strengthening—appropriate amount and locations of strength for sport-specific activities (quadriceps/ham-

string strength for force generation, trunk rotation strength, strength balance for the shoulder)
3. Power—rapid movements in appropriate planes with light weights
4. Endurance—mainly anaerobic exercises due to short duration and explosive and ballistic activities seen in throwing and serving. These exercises should be based on the periodization principle of conditioning.

V. SPORT-SPECIFIC ACTIVITY:

Functional progressions of throwing or serving must be completed before full completion is allowed. These progressions will gradually test all of the mechanical parts of the throwing or serving motion. Very few deviations from normal parameters of arm motion, arm position, force generation, smoothness of all of the kinematic chain, and from preinjury form should be allowed as most of these adaptations will be biomechanically inefficient. The athlete may move through the progressions as rapidly as possible.

VI. CRITERIA FOR RETURN TO PLAY:

1. Normal clinical examination
2. Normal shoulder arthrokinematics
3. Normal kinematic chain integration
4. Completed progressions

Arthroscopic Glenoid Labral Repair

- *Method of Presentation*—Mainly chronic microtrauma from overhead throwing; also may be acute presentation after a fall on the arm or acute exacerbation of chronic pain with a "pop" on overhead throwing.
- *Clinical Symptom Complex*—Pain, often localized precisely over the anterior superior glenohumeral joint area; clicking or popping on throwing, usually in midranges of motion; impingement or other rotator cuff symptoms; positive anterior slide test or O'Brien maneuver.
- *Tissue Injury Complex*—Superior glenoid labrum, +/– the biceps root; sometimes the undersurface of the rotator cuff; occasionally the anterior inferior labrum.
- *Tissue Overload Complex*—Rotator cuff (manifested by weakness); posterior capsule (manifested by internal rotation inflexibility), scapular muscles (manifested by scapular dyskinesis).
- *Functional Biomechanical Deficit Complex*—Internal rotation inflexibility; stiffness from postoperative immobilization; force couple weakness.
- *Subclinical Adaptation Complex*—Trapezial elevation to avoid impingement; 3/4 arm position.

After surgery, the shoulder should be protected from active movement, especially elbow extension, which creates tension on the labrum, and shoulder abduction, which produces anterior shear, for 3–4 weeks. Passive range of motion may be started at 7–10 days below 60 degrees of abduction. After 3–4 weeks, when the repair is healed enough to allow loading, the athlete may participate in the postoperative protocol (Exhibit 11–5).

Shoulder Instability Repair

* *Method of Presentation*—Acute macrotrauma with fall on the arm or sudden external rotation movement; or chronic microtrauma overload from throwing or serving.
* *Clinical Symptom Complex*—Overt instability with one-time or recurrent dislocation; mild instability with one dislocation and other subluxations; or covert instability with no dislocation, mild subluxability but predominant pain with throwing, either in cocking or at ball impact or ball release.
* *Tissue Injury Complex*—Anterior, anterior/inferior, or posterior/inferior capsuloligamentous complex; inferior glenohumeral ligament; occasionally rotator cuff.
* *Tissue Overload Complex*—Inferior glenohumeral ligament (manifested by increased humeral translation); rotator cuff (manifested by strength weakness or partial tear); scapular stabilizers (manifested by scapular dyskinesis).
* *Functional Biomechanical Deficit Complex*—Lack of anterior shoulder muscular stabilization; joint stiffness due to postoperative immobilization; scapular dyskinesis; generalized shoulder girdle muscle weakness.
* *Subclinical Adaptation Complex*—Decreased glenohumeral external rotation; abnormal position of scapula to avoid subluxation.

At the time of surgery, the damaged capsule, ligaments, and bone should be repaired so that the joint is stable at 90 degrees of abduction/60 degrees of external rotation and so that the shoulder can reach these positions without excessive tension on the repair (Exhibit 11–6). In this manner, early passive and active assisted range of motion may be instituted at 3–7 days in positions of 60 degrees' abduction and may progress to 90 degrees of abduction by 3 weeks. The patient may then enter the postoperative protocol.

If nonoperative treatment is selected for a first-time acute dislocation, the arm should be protected in a sling for 7–10 days. Pain control measures should be used; then the athlete should be placed in the rotator cuff tendinitis protocol. Many mild instabilities due to chronic microtrauma can also be treated nonoperatively by emphasizing the scapular stabilization protocol, followed by the rotator cuff tendinitis protocol.

Rotator Cuff Repair

* *Method of Presentation*—Usually acute trauma, with fall on an outstretched arm; may also result from chronic microtrauma.
* *Clinical Symptom Complex*—Pain, localized to the anterior or lateral acromion; positive impingement sign; lack of active abduction and/or external rotation; muscle atrophy in chronic cases; pain at night.
* *Tissue Injury Complex*—Rotator cuff, supraspinatus and infraspinatus detachment from greater tuberosity; acromioclavicular (AC) joint; subacromial space.
* *Tissue Overload Complex*—Trapezius (manifested by abnormal scapular motion).
* *Functional Biomechanical Deficit Complex*—Loss of deltoid/rotator cuff force couple, with superior humeral migration and abnormal instant center of rotation.
* *Subclinical Adaptation Complex*—Abnormal scapular elevation with abduction.

The object of the rotator cuff repair is to restore the deltoid/rotator cuff force couple and eliminate subacromial impingement. As soon as the repair will allow, range of motion in safe arcs should be allowed. Closed-chain rehabilitation is especially effective in allowing return of rotator cuff strength without creating excessive shear early in rehabilitation. After 4–6 weeks, when the repair is secure enough to allow maximum tensile loading, the patient may enter the postoperative protocol.

AC Joint Arthrosis or Separation

* *Method of Presentation*—Acute macrotrauma, from fall on point of the shoulder; chronic microtrauma, usually associated with mild separation or weight lifting.
* *Clinical Symptom Complex*—Point-tender pain over AC joint; deformity, due either to separation or to bone spurs; pain on shoulder horizontal adduction; crepitus; decreased strength.
* *Tissue Injury Complex*—AC joint; articular disc; distal clavicle; coracoclavicular ligaments; AC ligaments.
* *Tissue Overload Complex*—Scapular stabilizers (manifested as pain in muscles and scapular dyskinesis).
* *Functional Biomechanical Deficit Complex*—Scapular instability, with dyskinesis and lack of strut; decreased strength due to lack of a stable origin for muscle work; decreased scapular retraction.
* *Subclinical Adaptation Complex*—Short-arming a throw or serve.

Treatment is necessary if AC joint dysfunction, either arthrosis or separation, impairs the clavicle's role as a strut and

Exhibit 11–5 Postoperative Labral Repair Rehabilitation Protocol

I. ACUTE PHASE
  A. Goals
    1. Reestablish nonpainful range of motion
    2. Retard muscle atrophy of entire upper extremity
    3. Neuromuscular control of scapula in neutral glenohumeral position
    4. Reduce pain and inflammation
    5. Maintain other components of kinetic chain
  B. Range of motion
    1. Dependent
      a. Mobilization of glenohumeral, clavicle, and scapulothoracic joints
      b. Manual capsular stretching and cross-friction massage
    2. Independent
      a. Codman's and /or pendulum exercises
      b. Ropes and pulleys
      c. T-bar
    3. Back
      a. Flexion/extension
      b. Rotation
  C. Muscle atrophy/neuromuscular control
    1. Local
      a. Isometrics
      b. Scapular control
      c. Closed-chain activities
    2. Distant
      a. Open chain—nonpathologic areas (elbow, back)
        i. Concentrics
        ii. Eccentrics
    3. Aerobic/anaerobic activities for rest of kinetic chain
  D. Pain and inflammation
    1. NSAIDs 48–96 hrs
    2. Modalities 2–3 wks
    3. Joint mobilization
    4. Joint protection—sling, gradual progression out of sling
  E. Criteria for advancement
    1. No swelling
    2. Level II pain
    3. Manual muscle testing strength 75% of strength in other muscles
    4. Scapular control in neutral position
    5. Back flexibility 75%
    6. Kinetic chain function

II. RECOVERY PHASE
  A. Goals
    1. Regain and improve upper-extremity muscle strength
    2. Improve upper-extremity neuromuscular control
    3. Normalize shoulder arthrokinematics in single planes of motion
    4. Improve active/passive range of motion flexibility

    5. Normal back and hip flexibility, normal kinetic chain
  B. Strengthening
    1. Dependent
      a. Scapular proprioceptive neuromuscular facilitation
      b. Glenohumeral proprioceptive neuromuscular facilitation
    2. Independent single-plane motions
      a. Concentric and eccentric isotonics
      b. Isokinetics
      c. Tubing
      d. Rotator cuff isolation exercises (Jobe)
      e. Hip rotation
      f. Back flexion/extension
  C. Neuromuscular control
    1. Proprioceptive neuromuscular facilitation
    2. Closed chain—emphasis on force couples
      a. Scapular retractors/protractors
      b. Glenohumeral elevators/depressors
      c. Glenohumeral internal/external rotators
      d. Back/trunk rotation—"Swiss ball"
  D. Arthrokinematics
    1. Joint mobilization
    2. Kinetic chain movement patterns—rotation, stretch-shortening
  E. Criteria for advancement
    1. Full nonpainful scapulothoracic motion
    2. Almost full nonpainful glenohumeral motion
    3. Normal scapular stabilizer strength (lateral slide asymmetry <0.5 cm)
    4. Normal back motion
    5. Rotator cuff strength 75% of normal
    6. Normal throwing motion in rest of kinetic chain

III. FUNCTIONAL PHASE
  A. Goals
    1. Increase power and endurance in upper extremity
    2. Increase normal multiple-plane neuromuscular control (eliminate subclinical adaptations)
    3. Sports-specific activity
  B. Power and endurance
    1. Multiple-plane motions—tubing, light weights
    2. Pyelometrics
      a. Wall push-ups
      b. Ball throws
      c. Tubing or other elastic resistance
      d. Medicine ball
    3. Advanced closed chain
    4. Advanced open chain
    5. Conditioning based on principles of periodization
  C. Sports-specific functional progression
    1. Long toss—short toss
    2. Serving
    3. Other

continues

Exhibit 11–5 continued

IV. **CRITERIA FOR RETURN TO PLAY**
  A. **Normal arthrokinematics in multiple planes**
  B. **Isokinetic strength 90% of normal**

C. **Completed progressions**
D. **Negative clinical examination**

Courtesy of Lexington Clinic, Lexington, KY.

Exhibit 11–6 Postoperative Shoulder Instability Rehabilitation Protocol

I. **ACUTE PHASE**
  A. **Goals**
    1. Reestablish nonpainful range of motion
    2. Retard muscle atrophy of entire upper extremity
    3. Neuromuscular control of scapula in neutral glenohumeral position
    4. Reduce pain and inflammation
    5. Maintain other components of kinetic chain
  B. **Range of motion**
    1. Dependent
      a. Scapular, neck, and clavicle mobilization
      b. Elbow mobilization
    2. Independent
      a. Codman's and pendulum exercises
  C. **Muscle atrophy/neuromuscular control**
    1. Local
      a. Isometrics
      b. Scapular pinches and shrugs
      c. Closed chain, abduction ≤ 45 degrees
    2. Distant
      a. Open chain for kinetic chain
      b. Aerobics for legs
      c. Anaerobics as tolerated
  D. **Pain and inflammation**
    1. Cryocuff postoperatively and after therapy
    2. Modalities 2–3 weeks
    3. Joint protection—sling, or arm at less than 60 degrees of abduction/40 degrees of external rotation
  E. **Criteria for advancement**
    1. Tissue healing
    2. No swelling
    3. Level II pain
    4. Scapular control to neutral position
    5. Back and leg flexibility
    6. Kinetic chain function

II. **RECOVERY PHASE**
  A. **Goals**
    1. Regain and improve upper-extremity muscle strength
    2. Improve upper-extremity neuromuscular control

Courtesy of Lexington Clinic, Lexington, KY.

    3. Normalize shoulder arthrokinematics in single planes of motion
    4. Improve active/passive range of motion flexibility
    5. Normal back and hip flexibility, normal kinetic chain
  B. **Range of motion**
    1. Wand-assistive abduction, external/internal rotation
    2. Active ROM flexion/extension, progressing to abduction/external rotation
  C. **Strengthening**
    1. PNF
      a. Scapulothoracic
      b. Glenohumeral
    2. Independent single-plane motions
      a. 45 degrees' abduction
      b. 60 degrees' abduction
      c. 90 degrees' abduction
      d. Isotonics
      e. Tubing
  D. **Neuromuscular control**
    1. Closed chain—force couples
      a. Scapular retractors/protractors
      b. Glenohumeral elevators/depressors
      c. Glenohumeral internal/external rotators
    2. Back flexion/extension
  E. **Arthrokinematics**
    1. Joint mobilization and cross-fiber friction massage
    2. Capsular stretching
    3. Kinetic chain movement patterns
      a. Back and leg
      b. Scapula
      c. Shoulder and elbow
  F. **Criteria for advancement**
    1. Full scapulothoracic motion and stability
    2. Glenohumeral ROM 90 degrees' abduction, 60–80 degrees' external rotation
    3. Scapular side, 0.5 cm

III. **FUNCTIONAL PHASE**
  A. **Same as for labral repair, rotator cuff tendinitis, or scapular instability**

a guide for the scapula. Operative treatment may be necessary for joint debridement, repair, or reconstruction. The patient may then be started on the postoperative protocol.

NONOPERATIVE SHOULDER PROTOCOLS

Protocols for nonoperative problems such as impingement, scapular dyskinesis, or rotator cuff tendinitis/tendinosis vary from the postoperative protocol mainly in the methods used in the acute phase. More emphasis is placed on resolving the symptoms of pain, swelling, or mechanical derangement. Medications, injections, ultrasound or other modalities, and relative rest are commonly used in the acute phase. We direct most of our attention to resolving pain because of its major effect on all shoulder function. We try to implement the other aspects of the acute care protocol as soon as symptoms and tissue integrity will allow. After the acute symptoms have been resolved, entry into the recovery phase will be implemented. The protocols are basically the same from this point, differing only by whatever tissue overloads or biomechanical deficits are discovered on the prerehabilitation evaluation.

Rotator Cuff Tendinitis/Tendinosis

* *Method of Presentation*—Chronic repetitive microtrauma, usually with gradual onset of symptoms.
* *Clinical Symptom Complex*—Pain over anterior and lateral acromion; pain with elevation, abduction, or rotation; pain upon internal rotation; "painful arc" of motion 60–120 degrees of abduction; positive impingement sign; decreased strength with abduction and/or external rotation; pain at night.
* *Tissue Injury Complex*—Rotator cuff, usually supraspinatus; occasionally superior labrum; occasionally anterior capsuloligamentous structures.
* *Tissue Overload Complex*—Rotator cuff; posterior capsule (manifested by internal rotation inflexibility); scapular stabilizer muscles (manifested by scapular dyskinesis); occasionally hip and trunk muscles (manifested by back or hip inflexibility).
* *Functional Biomechanical Deficit Complex*—Force couple imbalance, deltoid/rotator cuff; internal rotation deficit; external rotator muscle weakness; "scapular slide" and scapular dyskinesis; occasionally kinetic chain breakage due to hip or trunk inflexibility.
* *Subclinical Adaptation Complex*—Three-quarter position of arm on throwing or serving; excessive wrist snap on ball release; "opening up" of trunk (see Exhibit 11–7).

Impingement Syndrome

* *Method of Presentation*—Gradual onset associated with chronic microtrauma.
* *Clinical Symptom Complex*—Positive impingement sign with pain upon abduction, rotation, or horizontal adduction; positive impingement test with decrease in symptoms after Xylocaine injection into the subacromial space; other symptoms due to associated pathology (rotator cuff injury, labral tear, AC joint arthrosis).
* *Tissue Injury Complex*—Rotator cuff, either superior or inferior surface; AC joint; superior glenoid labrum; subacromial bursa.
* *Tissue Overload Complex*—Rotator cuff (manifested as weakness); scapular stabilizers (manifested by dyskinesis); anterior or superior labrum inflexibility (manifested by mild instability); posterior capsule (manifested by internal rotation).
* *Functional Biomechanical Deficit Complex*—Decreased abduction; internal rotation inflexibility; force couple imbalance.
* *Subclinical Adaptation Complex*—Decreased abduction; more elbow and wrist motion.

Impingement, especially in athletes under 35–40 years old, is most frequently a clinical sign or symptom rather than a diagnosis. Impingement is occurring secondary to some other pathology, such as anterior instability, labral tears, or muscle weakness and imbalance. Primary impingement is due to true subacromial pathology, such as AC joint arthrosis, subacromial spurs, or subacromial bursitis. Treatment should address the underlying causes of the impingement. If treatment is surgical, the patient may then start the postoperative protocol. If nonoperative treatment is recommended, the athlete should be placed in the rotator cuff tendinitis/tendinosis protocol.

Scapular Instability and Dyskinesis

* *Method of Presentation*—Acute after nerve or muscle injury; chronic if secondary to other glenohumeral pathology.
* *Clinical Symptom Complex*—Winging; painful snapping or crepitus; abnormal motion and prominence with shoulder flexion or abduction; impingement.
* *Tissue Injury Complex*—Long thoracic nerve; spinal accessory nerve; glenohumeral pathology (rotator cuff, labrum, instability).
* *Tissue Overload Complex*—Serratus anterior, upper and lower trapezius (manifested by scapular prominence and dyskinesis).
* *Functional Biomechanical Deficit Complex*—Decreased acromial elevation with impingement; lack of scapular

Exhibit 11–7 Rotator Cuff Tendinitis Rehabilitation Protocol

I. ACUTE PHASE
A. Goals
1. Reestablish nonpainful range of motion
2. Retard muscle atrophy of entire upper extremity
3. Neuromuscular control of scapula in neutral glenohumeral position
4. Reduce pain and inflammation

B. Range of motion
1. Dependent
   a. Mobilization of glenohumeral, clavicle, and scapulothoracic joints
   b. Manual capsular stretching and cross-friction massage
2. Independent
   a. Codman's and/or pendulum exercises
   b. Ropes and pulleys
   c. T-bar

C. Muscle atrophy/neuromuscular control
1. Local
   a. Isometrics
   b. Scapular control
   c. Closed chain activities
2. Distant
   a. Open chain—nonpathologic areas (elbows, back)
      1) Concentrics
      2) Eccentrics
3. Aerobic/anaerobic activities

D. Pain and inflammation
1. NSAIDs 48–92 hrs
2. Modalities 2–3 weeks
3. Joint mobilization
4. Joint protection

E. Range of motion
1. Passive flexibility
2. Active flexibility

F. Criteria for advancement
1. No swelling
2. Level II pain
3. Manual muscle testing strength 75% of strength in other muscles
4. Scapular control in neutral position

II. RECOVERY PHASE
A. Goals
1. Regain and improve upper extremity muscle strength
2. Improve upper extremity neuromuscular control
3. Normalize shoulder arthrokinematics in single planes of motion
4. Improve active/passive range of motion flexibility

B. Strengthening
1. Dependent
   a. Scapular proprioceptive neuromuscular facilitation
   b. Glenohumeral proprioceptive neuromuscular facilitation
2. Independent single-plane motions
   a. Concentric and eccentric isotonics
   b. Isokinetics
   c. Tubing
   d. Rotator cuff isolation exercises (Jobe)

C. Neuromuscular control
1. Proprioceptive neuromuscular facilitation
2. Emphasis on force couples
   a. Scapular retractors/protractors
   b. Glenohumeral elevators/depressors
   c. Glenohumeral internal/external rotators

D. Arthrokinematics
1. Joint mobilization
2. Kinetic chain movement patterns

E. Criteria for advancement
1. Full nonpainful scapulothoracic motion
2. Almost full nonpainful glenohumeral motion
3. Normal scapular stabilizer strength (later slide asymmetry ≤0.5 cm)
4. Rotator cuff strength 75% of normal
5. Normal throwing motion

III. FUNCTIONAL PHASE
A. Goals
1. Increase power and endurance in upper extremity
2. Increase normal multiple-plane neuromuscular control (eliminate subclinical adaptations)
3. Sport-specific activity

B. Power and endurance
1. Multiple-plane motions
2. Pyelometrics
   a. Wall push-ups
   b. Ball throws
   c. Tubing or other elastic resistance
   d. Medicine ball
3. Conditioning based on principles of periodization

C. Sport-specific functional progression
1. Long toss—short toss
2. Throwing
3. Pitching

IV. CRITERIA FOR RETURN TO PLAY
A. Normal arthrokinematics in multiple planes
B. Isokinetic strength 90% of normal
C. Negative clinical examination

Courtesy of Lexington Clinic, Lexington, KY.

retraction/protraction; lack of stable anchor for muscle origins; kinetic chain breakage due to lack of stable base for the arm.
- *Subclinical Adaptation Complex*—Excessive hip and trunk rotation; 3/4 arm positioning.

Scapular dyskinesis is very common in shoulder injuries. Very rarely is there direct nerve involvement. The most common etiology for scapular dyskinesis is muscle inhibition secondary to some other pain generator. Treatment of the underlying problem relieves the inhibition and allows the patient to enter the scapular stability protocol. This may be done in coordination with the treatment protocols for the underlying pathology. Scapular stability may be difficult to restore and often takes two to three months (Exhibit 11–8).

CONCLUSIONS

The negative feedback vicious cycle can be used to identify all of the alterations that may exist to create the abnormal function that characterizes shoulder pathology. Just as normal function is the result of many anatomic, physiologic, and biomechanical factors working in a coordinated fashion, pathology may result in abnormalities at many levels of the local and distant kinetic chains. The complete and accurate diagnosis must be made to allow effective rehabilitation. Most rehabilitation protocols are variations of a postoperative or a nonoperative protocol, once the acute symptoms and tissue injuries have been stabilized. Scapular dyskinesis and instability is very common and must be evaluated and rehabilitated along with glenohumeral alterations.

SUGGESTED READING

Chandler TJ, Kibler WB. Muscle training in injury prevention. In: Renstrom PFH, ed. *Sports Injuries—Basic Principles of Prevention and Care.* Oxford: Blackwell; 1993:252–261.

Kibler WB. The role of the scapula in the overhead throwing motion. *Contemp Orthop.* 1991;22:525–532.

Kibler WB. Evaluation of sports demands as a diagnostic tool in shoulder disorder. In: Matson FA, Fu FH, Hawkins RJ, eds. *The Shoulder: A Balance of Mobility and Stability.* Rosemont, IL: AAOS; 1994: 379–399.

Kibler WB, Chandler TJ, Pace BK. Principles of rehabilitation after chronic tendon injuries. *Clin Sports Med.* 1992;11:661–673.

Kibler WB, Livingston BK, Bruce R. Current concepts in shoulder rehabilitation. *Adv Operative Orthop.* 1996;3:249–300.

Pink M, Screnar PM, Tollefson KD. Injury prevention and rehabilitation in the upper extremity. In: Jobe FW, ed. *Operative Techniques in Upper Extremity Sports Injuries.* St Louis: Mosby; 1996:3–14.

Sobel J. Shoulder rehabilitation. In: Pettrone FA, ed. *Athletic Injuries of the Shoulder.* New York: McGraw-Hill; 1994:245–270.

Wilk KE. *Preventative and Rehabilitative Exercises for the Shoulder and Elbow.* Birmingham: ASMI; 1991.

Wilk KE, Arrigo C, Andrews JR. Current concepts in the rehabilitation of the athlete's shoulder. *J South Orthop Assoc.* 1994;3:216–231.

Exhibit 11–8 Shoulder and Functional Scapular Stability Rehabilitation Protocol

The purpose of this protocol is to describe the basis for rehabilitation of scapular and shoulder dysfunction occurring in upper-extremity athletic injuries. This program is based on scientific principles of anatomy, physiology, biomechanics, and kinesiology.

I. PHASE OF REHABILITATION

A. Acute
1. Goals
   a. Reestablish nonpainful ROM
   b. Retard muscle atrophy of the entire upper extremity complex
   c. Neuromuscular control of the scapula in neutral glenohumeral positions
   d. Decrease pain and inflammation
2. Progressions in phase I
   a. ROM
      1. Dependent
         a) Grade I and II mobilization of the glenohumeral, sternoclavicular, acromioclavicular, and scapulothoracic joints
         b) Manual capsular stretching and cross-friction massage
      2. Independent
         a) Codman's and/or pendulum exercises
         b) Ropes and pulleys
         c) T-bar exercises
         d) Active and passive flexibility exercises
   b. Muscle atrophy/neuromuscular control
      1. Types
         a) Isometrics
         b) Scapular PNF
         c) Closed-chain activities (weight shift)
         d) Open chain and isotonics (non-pathologic area)
            1) Concentrics
            2) Eccentrics
   c. Pain and inflammation
      1. Modalities
      2. Joint mobilization
3. Criteria for progression from acute to recovery
   a. Full passive ROM
   b. Minimal pain and tenderness
   c. MMT strength in the nonpathologic area 4/5, and scapular control (no scapular slide) in the neutral glenohumeral posture

B. Recovery
1. Goals
   a. Regain and improve upper-extremity muscular strength
   b. Improve neuromuscular control of the entire upper-extremity complex
   c. Normalize arthrokinematics of the shoulder in single planes of motion

2. Progressions in phase II
   a. Strengthening
      1. Dependent
         a) PNF of the scapula and the glenohumeral areas
      2. Independent
         a) Single planes of motion exercise
            1) Isotonics—concentric, eccentric
            2) Isokinetics
            3) Tubing exercises
            4) Jobe exercises
         b) Neuromuscular control
            1) PNF
         c) Arthrokinematics
            1) Joint mobilization
            2) Recognize the importance of movement patterns of the other joints that make up the shoulder complex
   3. Criteria for progression from recovery to functional
      a) Full nonpainful active and passive ROM
      b) No pain or tenderness
      c) Strength 75% of the other side
      d) Negative lateral or anterior side

C. Functional
1. Goals
   a. Increase power and endurance of the upper-extremity complex
   b. Increase neuromuscular control in multiple planes of motion
   c. Prepare for return to the sport-specific activity
2. Progression in functional phase
   a. Power and endurance
      1. Multiple planes of motion exercise with concentration on power and endurance
      2. Begin pyelometrics
         a) Wall push-ups to ball push-ups
         b) Tubing exercises
         c) Medicine ball
      3. Periodization training program return
   b. Neuromuscular control
   c. Sport-specific activity
3. Criteria for progression from functional phase to return to play
   a. Normal arthrokinematics in multiple-plane activities
   b. Isokinetic test 90% of the other side
   c. Satisfactory clinical exam by physician

D. Return to play
1. Goals
   a. Sport-specific training to full return of athletic activity
2. Progression in return to play
   a. Functional progression sport-specific

continues

Exhibit 11–8 continued

II. SCAPULAR DEPRESSION
A. Side lying
1. PNF patterns. Perform in glenohumeral neutral position. Progress by varying the degree of flexion and abduction at the glenohumeral joint.
2. Arm over the ball. Progress by moving anywhere from 0–90 degrees of shoulder flexion.

B. Sitting/standing
1. Isometrics. Push elbow down into a chair.
2. Isotonics
   a. Weights in hand.
   b. Wall slides. Scapula against wall with arms in a 90/90 position.
   c. Arms forward flexed and depression of the scapula so arm is lifted away from the wall.
   d. Utilize tubing with pull-back with elbow at 90 degrees of flexion. Progress to performing the exercise with elbows straight.

C. Prone
1. Begin in a glenohumeral neutral position and progress to arms in a 90/90 position. Further increase the difficulty by adding weights to the hand.
2. Arms forward flexed so that they are beside head and lift arms. The difficulty of this can be increased by trying various degrees of glenohumeral rotation.
3. With hand in small of back, elbows are lifted away from the body. The difficulty of this can be increased by adding a weight on the elbow or by performing this in varying degrees of rotation.

III. SCAPULAR RETRACTION
A. Side lying
1. PNF patterns to begin in glenohumeral neutral position, progressing to varying degrees of shoulder flexion and abduction.
2. Arm over the ball and moving through various degrees of shoulder flexion from 0–90.

B. Sitting/standing
1. Isometrics. The difficulty can be varied from glenohumeral neutral to 90 degrees of abduction/external rotation.
2. Isotonics
   a. Free weights can be utilized in a glenohumeral neutral position to 90 degrees of abduction.

   b. Tubing utilized with the same variations for degree of difficulty.

C. Prone
1. Glenohumeral neutral retraction, progressing to a 90/90 position, weights in hand.
2. Retraction with a longer lever arm (meaning elbow is straight) and increasing difficulty by adding weight in hands.
3. Scapular retraction with 90 degrees of elbow flexion, weight in hands to increase difficulty.

IV. SCAPULAR PROTRACTION
A. Side lying
1. PNF patterns in a glenohumeral neutral position, progressing to various degrees of shoulder flexion and abduction.
2. Arm over ball, progressing the difficulty from 0–90 degrees of shoulder flexion.

B. Sitting/standing
1. Isometric wall push-ups.
2. Isotonics with tubing or with weights. Varying the degrees of glenohumeral abduction to flexion from 0–90 degrees will increase the difficulty of these exercises.

C. Supine
1. Bench protraction with progressive resistance.

V. SCAPULAR ELEVATION
A. Side lying
1. PNF patterns in a glenohumeral neutral position to progress to various degrees of flexion/abduction.
2. Arm over the ball, moving it to progress from 0–90 degrees of shoulder flexion.

B. Sitting/standing
1. Isometrics.
2. Isotonics with weights or tubing to perform an upright row or shrugs.

C. Supine
1. Elevate utilizing weights/tubing in a glenohumeral neutral position.

D. Prone
1. Glenohumeral neutral
2. Various degrees of abduction and flexion
3. Various degrees of external rotation utilizing tubing and/or weights

Courtesy of Lexington Clinic, Lexington, KY.

CHAPTER 12

Rehabilitation of the Elbow

W. Ben Kibler and Joel M. Press

GENERAL PRINCIPLES

Biomechanically, the elbow is a hinged joint and, as long as the hinge function in flexion and extension is maintained, very few sports medicine problems exist. However, because of the forces placed on the elbow and the positions used in throwing a baseball or javelin, in hitting a tennis ball, or when the elbow is being used as a weight-bearing surface, such as in gymnastics, shear loads and valgus-varus loads are also placed on the elbow. In these situations, injury can occur.

BIOMECHANICS

The elbow joint does not act in isolation but is an integral component of the upper extremity kinetic chain. Events and forces occurring at either the shoulder or the hand will ultimately involve the elbow as well.[1] The ability of the elbow to precisely and painlessly shorten or lengthen the upper limb is contingent on the integrity of the elbow joint proper, as well as the spine and the sternoclavicular, acromioclavicular, scapulothoracic, and glenohumeral joints. The inability to comfortably lean or bend forward due to lumbar spine-based restrictions necessitates greater elbow extension when reaching downward or forward. Loss of cervicothoracic flexion and rotation requires greater elbow flexion to keep finer manual work in the center of the field of vision. Acromioclavicular or sternoclavicular joint pain limits the weight-bearing tolerance of the "strut" from which the upper limb is suspended, thereby reducing loads that can be dynamically or isometrically supported at varying degrees of elbow flexion. Scapulothoracic dyskinesis and cervicothoracic kyphosis may lead to rotator cuff impingement and glenohumeral joint–based pain, which will also reduce upper limb weight-bearing. Finally, capsular restrictions and loss of internal/external rotation at the shoulder may induce compensatory increases in the amount of forearm pronation/supination employed during repetitive tasks. The same process applies to regions distal to the elbow—loss of wrist extension necessitates greater elbow extension to elevate an object that is held in the hand to the same height. Thus, when analyzing the injured athlete's source of elbow pain, looking beyond the elbow itself is critical. Furthermore, any elbow rehabilitation program must address deficits in the scapular stabilizer muscles, cervicothoracic extensor muscles, and muscles around the glenohumeral joint to be successful. Finally, reestablishment of proper posture with the head centered over the shoulders decreases the activity of the shoulder- and neck-stabilizing muscles and prevents the fatiguing of these muscles, which would lead to new substitution patterns and more musculotendinous overload.

Proper functioning of the elbow allows the hand to be positioned in space and provides a stabilizing role for power production and performance of work and sports activities.[2] Although most activities of daily living require between 30 and 140 degrees of flexion and between 50 degrees of pronation and 50 degrees of supination, the articular orientation of the joint allows for approximately 150 degrees of flexion, 75 degrees of pronation, and 85 degrees of supination for an arc of forearm rotation averaging 160–170 degrees.[3,4] These motions, which are integral to proper elbow rehabilitation, occur at the ulnohumeral, radiohumeral, and proximal and distal radioulnar joints. Restriction in motion or laxity at any of these joints due to ligamentous, capsular, or musculotendinous factors requires proper assessment in the rehabilitation process.[5] Restrictions in motions elsewhere along the kinetic chain can change activities from those performed in the usual range of joint motion to others performed at extremes or limits of permissible joint motion, with accompanying increases in musculotendinous stress.

Locally, elbow motion consists of large flexion and extension rotations and minimal varus and valgus rotations. Included in these local joint biomechanics are forearm pronation and supination, as they affect the radiohumeral joint. Bony stability for the hinge is provided by the tightly conforming ulnohumeral and radiohumeral articulations and the olecranon fossa. Ligamentous stability is conferred by the thick ulnar collateral ligament, especially the anterior band, and the smaller radial collateral ligament. Ligamentous integrity is important to allow bony conformity, especially in extremes of range of motion and in the face of varus or valgus loads.

The elbow is also a link in the kinematic chain of link sequencing, receiving input from the more proximal links and transferring the generated force and velocity to the distal links. A large percentage of the motions that are measured at the elbow are the result of trunk and shoulder rotation and proximal arm muscular activity. This proximal input is very important because the musculature around the elbow joint is not capable of generating the rotational torques and velocities necessary in throwing and hitting motions. In the baseball throw, the tennis serve, or the tennis forehand stroke, anterior shoulder strength, shoulder internal rotation, and trunk rotation are needed to propel the arm forward through the throwing or hitting zone. Similarly, in the backhand stroke in tennis, posterior shoulder musculature is the predominant motor for the arm through the hitting zone.

The ligaments are not capable of independently withstanding the varus or valgus torques placed on the lateral or medial sides of the elbow. Muscular activity is necessary to control these forces and decrease the amount of tensile strain placed on the ligamentous structures. Also, shoulder rotation provides arm accelerations that counterbalance angular forces developed at the elbow in throwing, serving, or hitting. Shoulder internal rotation provides varus acceleration to protect against valgus elbow loads, whereas shoulder external rotation protects against varus elbow loads.

Once forces are passed through the elbow, forearm pronation adds to the generated forces and passes the transmitted forces down to the hand and wrist. Forearm pronation, which confers rotational activity and angular momentum, is more efficient than wrist flexion, which confers only linear momentum, in generating force and making maximal power available to the hand and wrist.

Throwing, serving, or hitting activities require a large range of elbow flexion and extension motion, but most activities occur at some degree of flexion short of full extension. Full extension is necessary for follow-through but not for actual initiation of the activity. In weight-bearing sports such as gymnastics, range of motion is not as important as is stability conferred by the bony ball and socket.

PHYSIOLOGY

Muscle activity in the entire kinematic chain and locally around the elbow is critical for elbow function and prevention of injury. Proper trunk rotation, proper shoulder internal or external rotation, and proper muscle firing organization throughout the links are important to decrease the load on the elbow. Locally, many muscles are active at high levels of firing intensity throughout the cocking, acceleration, and follow-through phases. How they are organized depends on the demands of the particular throwing activity. For example, the tennis serve and the baseball pitch require active elbow extension coupled with biceps control in an excitation agonist-antagonist force couple. However, baseball hitting and the tennis groundstroke require cocontraction force couples to stabilize the elbow in one narrow range of motion and conduct maximum force down to the hand. Important force couples around the elbow are listed in Table 12–1.

Proximal muscle activity is critical at the elbow because in the distal links, the muscles are smaller and have less force generation capability. A "catch-up" situation is more difficult in the distal links because of the relatively small musculature and the relatively short time to ball impact. Therefore, many elbow problems result from some proximal biomechanical or physiologic deficit, and each patient with elbow problems should be evaluated with this in mind.

TREATMENT

Treatment should be addressed as both local and distant problems. Locally, the joint must be rendered stable in terms of bony constraints and ligamentous constraints. Surgical

Table 12–1 Force Couples around the Elbow

Motion	Muscles Used
Arm extension from flexion	Triceps/biceps
Forearm pronation from supination	Pronator teres, pronator quadratus/supinator
Wrist flexion from extension	FCR, FCU, FDC/ECRL, ECRB, EC
Elbow stabilization	Triceps/biceps, brachioradialis; pronator teres/supinator; FCR, FCU/ECRB, ECRL

FCR, flexor carpi radialis; FCU, flexor carpi ulnaris; FDC, flexor digitorum communis; ECRL, extensor carpi radialis longus; ECRB, extensor carpi radialis brevis; EC, extensor communis.

treatment is sometimes necessary to take care of osteochondral injuries, ligamentous injuries, or bony avulsions. Also, musculotendinous injuries must be anatomically corrected to allow for proper rehabilitation. Treatment involves either reduction of the pain and restoration of muscle force capabilities through rest, bracing, or rehabilitation, or surgery to remove the damaged musculotendinous area and to repair the tissue for stable bony attachment. Excessive loads on the anatomic structures should be reduced in these early healing stages by the judicious use of counter-force bracing, relative rest, and improvement in the mechanics of the stroking or hitting pattern.

Treatment should be instituted with specific goals and functions in mind. The tissue response to the treatment should guide all the steps in the treatment program. Most of the overload injuries around the elbow should respond by six weeks of specific physical therapy. Resolution of the problem may not be complete, but there should be a reasonable progression toward decreased symptoms, increased range of motion, and increased function. If after six weeks there has not been major improvement or there is a discernible change in the symptomatology, further evaluation and other possible treatments should be considered. In chronic tendinosis, sometimes the most conservative treatment is to perform a surgical resection of the damaged tissue and repair it if there has been very little response to a well-designed and applied rehabilitation program. This avoids the continuous vicious cycle of more overload, more subclinical adaptations, and more functional biomechanical deficits.

SPECIFIC INJURIES

Lateral Epicondylitis

Lateral epicondylitis is characterized by pain along the lateral extensor muscle mass near the insertion of the tendon into the bone or at the musculotendinous junction. In tennis players, older ages and less skilled mechanics seem to be predisposing factors. This injury is seen in many types of athletic activities other than tennis, including throwing sports and golf. This is a specific diagnosis and should have specific diagnostic criteria, including point tenderness anteriorly and distally to the lateral epicondyle over the extensor carpi radialis brevis and muscle weakness of the extensor muscles. The primary pathology on the lateral aspect involves a microtear of the origin of the extensor carpi radialis brevis and, less commonly, the extensor carpi radialis longus and the anterior portion of the extensor communis tendon, with formation of subsequent fibrosis and granulation tissue as a consequence of repetitive trauma.[6–8] Repetitive concentric contraction of these muscles, shortening as they maintain tension to stabilize the wrist, produces chronic overload, which results in the symptoms of lateral epicondylitis.[6]

- *Method of Presentation*—Usually a chronic overload situation presents as a result of athletic activity or change in activity. An acute traumatic episode will occasionally present after a fall or direct blow.
- *Clinical Symptom Complex*—Point tenderness over the extensor carpi radialis brevis, anterior and distal to the epicondylar area. Additional point tenderness may exist over the epicondylar ridge and over the annular ligament. This pain is worse during activities that require eccentric loading of the extensor muscle mass, such as using the backhand stroke in tennis, cocking the arm in golf, and performing handstands in gymnastics.
- *Tissue Injury Complex*—Extensor muscle mass, specifically, extensor carpi radialis brevis. Other involvement may include extensor carpi radialis longus, annular ligament, and epicondylar ridge. In longstanding cases, there may be actual involvement of the capsule. The injury may range from a tensile overload to actual avulsion of the tendon away from the bone.
- *Tissue Overload Complex*—Proximally, external rotators of the shoulder, mainly the posterior deltoid and infraspinatus. Locally, biceps, extensors of the wrist, and radial collateral ligament.
- *Functional Biomechanical Deficit Complex*—External rotation strength weakness at the shoulder, flexion contracture of the elbow, and supination contracture of the forearm.
- *Subclinical Adaptation Complex*—Leading with the elbow, using the triceps muscle to hit strokes, using more flexion in the stroking pattern or in the handstand pattern, and hitting with more supination or hitting behind the body.

Rehabilitation

Most lateral epicondylitis patients can be treated without surgery. Complete diagnosis is necessary, and treatment of the proximal force generators is important. Treatment of any mechanical problems with the tennis or golf strokes also helps decrease the load on the elbow.

Acute Phase

Initial treatment focuses on controlling inflammation, relieving pain, and educating the patient. Often, no true inflammmatory process is active, yet pain perception due to nocioceptive fiber activation still occurs. A decrease in abusive activity to the injured structures is needed, although absolute rest is usually counterproductive and can increase random cross-linking of collagen fibers while tissue repair is underway. Rarely, in the highly acute phase, the use of a cock-up wrist splint may be helpful for a few days to rest the extensor musculature. Identifying the person's activities in the home or recreationally that exacerbate the condition is extremely important. Bathing and lifting young children, cooking on a stovetop with iron cookware, and carrying a heavy attaché case can all produce wrist extensor muscle overload. Cryotherapy, elevation, medications, and therapeutic modalities should be instituted to minimize any harmful excesses of inflammatory exudation, hemorrhage, and diminished oxygen perfusion.[9,10] Cryotherapy may include local ice massage for 10- to 15-minute intervals 3–5 times daily during the acute period. CryoJobst dressings are commercially available and easy to use. Antiinflammatory medications may be helpful for inflammation and exudation, but in the absence of overt inflammatory cells, they probably still help because of their general analgesic properties. Therapeutic modalities can be quite helpful in decreasing pain via endorphin pathways or, theoretically, gate-control pain relief.[11] Therapeutic modalities include high-voltage electrical stimulation, interferential treatment, and transcutaneous electrical nerve stimulation.[12,13] Iontophoresis and phonophoresis effects on lateral epicondylitis are controversial.[14–17] Ultrasound, a deep-heating modality, does not appear to be very efficacious in lateral epicondylitis.[6] Regardless of which type of therapeutic modality is employed, the use of a passive, modality-oriented approach is not advocated for more than a few therapy sessions and should be used only as an adjunct so that the patient may tolerate a more aggressive, active therapy program.[18]

Effective patient education early in the rehabilitation process can allow the patient to avoid actions that exacerbate the symptoms, as well as to learn which activities or actions to avoid in the future to prevent injury recurrence. Offending activities include shaking hands, picking up a coffee cup, doing needlework, and turning a key. Using ratchet- or power-driven tools also reduces the amount of forceful pronation/supination necessary to turn screws or the amount of flexion/extension necessary to drive nails.

In summary, acute phase treatment includes relative rest with decreased activities, counter-force bracing to reduce the load on the elbow, modalities such as phonophoresis and electrogalvanic stimulation to promote healing of the tissue, and deep-tissue massage to reduce adhesive contractures between the muscle bellies.

Recovery Phase

Restoration of normal tissue function occurs following proper anatomic healing. Symptom resolution alone is inadequate. During the recovery phase, after pain has started to subside and inflammation is under control, the focus is on enhancing the proliferative invasion of vascular elements and fibroblasts, and proper collagen deposition and maturation.[10,19] This time frame usually occurs within one to two weeks for lateral epicondylitis. Prolonged immobilization adversely influences the orientation and mechanical properties of periarticular soft tissue.[20] Promotion of healing fol-

lowed by aggressive strengthening and elimination of biomechanical deficits then prevents further tissue overload and recurrent symptoms and pathology.

As the acute symptoms diminish, the therapeutic exercise program becomes the focus, the initial goal being restoration of full pain-free flexibility. Specific attention is given to the wrist and finger extensors and supinators. In more chronic cases, biomechanical deficits of extensor inflexibility are observed, often up to a 10- to 15-degree lack of passive wrist flexion, as compared with the asymptomatic side.[16] To improve wrist flexion mobility, which is often limited by the tight extensor musculature, the wrist extensors are placed on passive stretch with the elbow extended (Figure 12–1). The use of myofascial release techniques and joint mobilizations may be useful during this treatment stage, along with deep-heating modalities to improve collagen extensibility and muscle reeducation.[21,22]

As flexibility starts to approach normal, strength training is initiated. Initially, multiple-angle isometrics within the pain-free range, focusing on the wrist extensors, are begun. Recovery phase rehabilitation includes strengthening of the muscles, beginning with isometric strengthening exercises

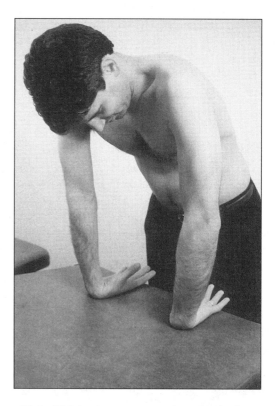

Figure 12–1 Wrist extensors on passive stretch. *Source:* Reprinted from *The Textbook of Military Medicine,* The Rehabilitation of the Injured Soldier, Borden Institute at Walter Reed Hospital.

and progressing to both isotonic and agonist-antagonist and cocontraction force couples. Progressive loading of the muscles can be accomplished as their strength and tolerance for this activity increase. Progression is made to limited motion arcs at submaximal intensity, progresssing to maximal intensity isometrics in the shortened, middle, and lengthened positions.[19,23] Isometric exercises are helpful early in the acute phase of rehabilitation because they can effectively decrease swelling (through the pumping action of the muscle), they do not irritate the joint as there is no motion, they prevent neural dissociation (the muscle contractions stimulate the mechanoreceptor system),[24,25] and they prevent further atrophy of muscle. A progressive resistance program is then incorporated, which may include free weights or Theraband (Figures 12–2 and 12–3). Strengthening of the muscles of pronation and supination can be accomplished by using a weighted rod (Figure 12–4). Weights are increased as guided by tolerance. The use of isokinetic devices may be helpful for the determination of strength imbalances. Triceps strengthening may be helpful because the more forceful supination becomes, the more the brachial biceps is activated, and the more the triceps muscle is needed to maintain a stable angle of elbow flexion.[26] As guided by symptoms,

more complex concentric-eccentric strengthening and endurance routines are initiated through the use of resistive tubing or a wrist roll (Figure 12–5).[27] Eccentric training is a critical component of the rehabilitation program because often the overload injury at the elbow occurred as a result of chronic eccentric stress on the wrist extensors, such as occurs with extensive keyboard use. Furthermore, eccentric exercises create less compressive force across a joint and may offer greater tendon loading.[24] Proprioceptive neuromuscular facilitation techniques to upgrade functional patterns, including push-ups, partial weight-bearing, and weight shifts, are also initiated at this time.[28] Liberal icing following exercise may be beneficial to control the inflammatory process.

If abnormal forces at the elbow cannot be controlled with adequate exercise or proper ergonomic modifications, control of force loads with bracing can be effective. Counterforce braces at the elbow can control intrinsic overload of the elbow by constraining key muscle groups while maintaining muscle balance.[10] Elbow counterforce bracing has been described by Groppel and Nirschl[29,30] to decrease elbow angular acceleration and to decrease electromyographic activity. Gradual weaning out of the counterforce

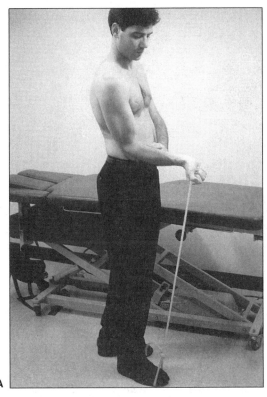 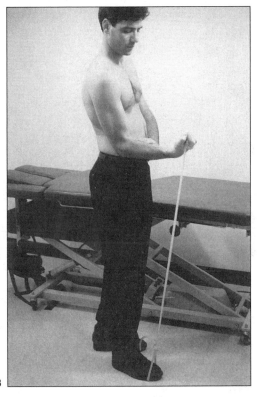

Figure 12–2 Isometric exercises. *Source:* Reprinted from *The Textbook of Military Medicine,* The Rehabilitation of the Injured Soldier, Borden Institute at Walter Reed Hospital.

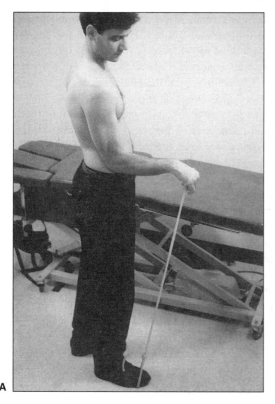
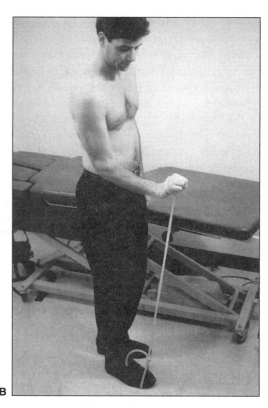

Figure 12–3 Progressive resistance exercises. *Source:* Reprinted from *The Textbook of Military Medicine,* The Rehabilitation of the Injured Soldier, Borden Institute at Walter Reed Hospital.

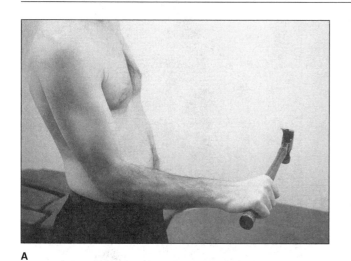
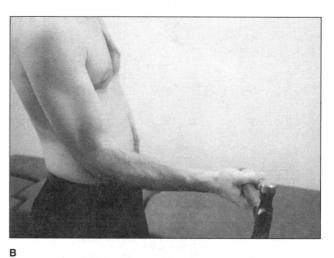

Figure 12–4 Strengthening using a weighted rod. (*A*) Pronation, (*B*) Supination. *Source:* Reprinted from *The Textbook of Military Medicine,* The Rehabilitation of the Injured Soldier, Borden Institute at Walter Reed Hospital.

brace should occur as full strength capabilities are present in the muscle.

During the recovery phase, anatomic and functional deficits along the kinetic chain must be addressed for complete rehabilitation. Attention must be directed specifically at any biomechanical limitations relating to the cervical, shoulder, and scapular stabilizing muscle functions. The cervical region and shoulder girdle provide a proximal base of support

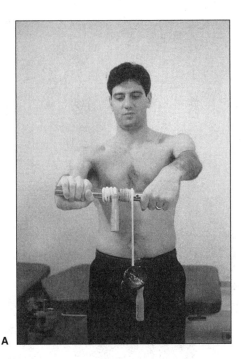

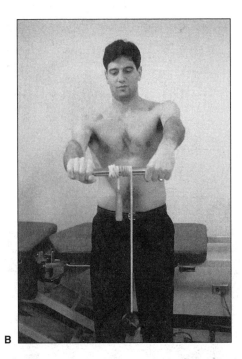

Figure 12–5 Strengthening exercises with wrist roll. *Source:* Reprinted from *The Textbook of Military Medicine,* The Rehabilitation of the Injured Soldier, Borden Institute at Walter Reed Hospital.

for elbow placement in space. Therefore, the effects of agonist-antagonist imbalances, which may involve limited cervical mobility, internal shoulder rotation inflexibility, and weakness of the posterior shoulder-scapular stabilizer muscles, transfer into abnormal compensatory overload patterns at the elbow.[1,31,32] For these reasons, scapular muscle strengthening, cervicothoracic extension training, and posture upgrading, e.g., chest-out, chin-tucked positioning, are critical components of a complete elbow rehabilitation program (Figure 12–6).

General body conditioning is another important component in the recovery phase of elbow rehabilitation. Advantages include: (1) central and peripheral aerobics provide increased regional perfusion; (2) neurophysiologic synergy and overflow provide neurologic stimulus to injured tissue; (3) weakness of adjacent uninjured tissue is minimized in the kinetic chain; and (4) negative psychologic effects are minimized.[10] The more the "general" conditioning exercise resembles the ultimate task, the more transferable the benefits of the conditioning exercise become. Therefore, use of an upper-body ergometer may be useful for cardiovascular conditioning; it is much more specific to upper-body work than is aerobic training by running, bicycling, or stair-climbing.

Continued use of the counterforce brace is appropriate, as is integration of the entire kinematic chain in the rehabilitation, starting from the hips and trunk and working out through the shoulder to the elbow and wrist. Complete functional range of motion should be obtained in the recovery phase with a special emphasis on forearm pronation and supination and elbow extension.

Maintenance Phase

Critical to the proper rehabilitation of any injured structure is a proper regime of flexibility and strengthening exercises to prevent recurrence of injury. Regular eccentric strengthening of the elbow extensors and maintenance of elbow flexion-extension and pronation-supination flexibility are important. Proper sports technique training is important as well. Functional phase rehabilitation should include using the racquet, the ball, or the club with full range of motion and normal strength activities integrating the kinematic chain into the wrist and elbow. Return to play may be started with decreased emphasis on power and length of time and play.

Local injection of corticosteroid may be considered in a patient who has failed aggressive rehabilitation after approximately three or four weeks. When used, an injection of corticosteroid, often combined with a local anesthetic, should be injected not into the tendon itself but at the point of maximal tenderness, which is commonly below the extensor brevis origin in the triangular recess formed by the medial slope of the lateral condyle and the brevis tendon.[33] Following injection, the patient is advised to avoid strenuous activities with the forearm for two weeks.[16] Most importantly, the use of injections should be only one component of a compre-

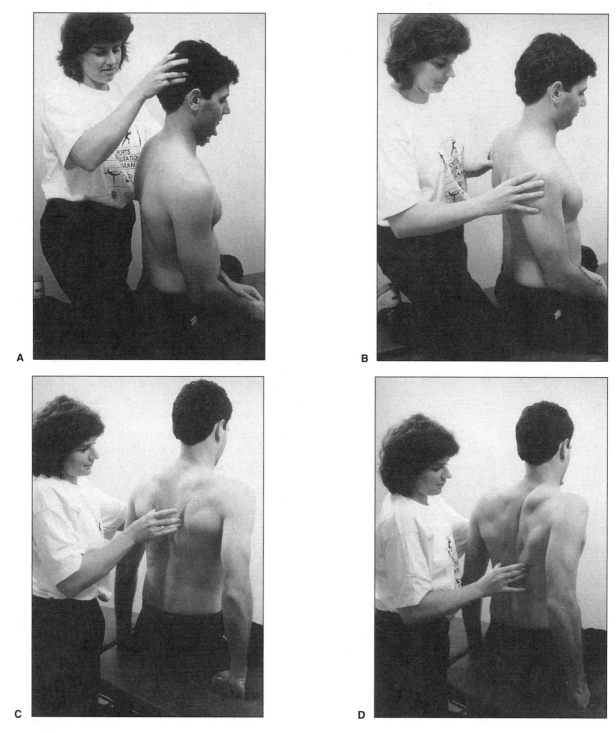

Figure 12–6 Posture exercise. *Source:* Reprinted from *The Textbook of Military Medicine,* The Rehabilitation of the Injured Soldier, Borden Institute at Walter Reed Hospital.

hensive rehabilitation program, and the injections should be spaced at least one month apart, with no more than three injections being administered to the same region within a one-year period.[34–35] Some clinical experiences have been re-

ported that indicate that patients who have had several corticosteroid injections are significantly more difficult to rehabilitate.[24] Furthermore, when encountering recalcitrant cases of conservatively treated lateral epicondylitis, the clinician must consider two other issues: (1) surgery may be necessary or (2) an incorrect initial diagnosis was made (i.e., failure to recognize posterior interosseus nerve entrapment, cervical radiculopathy, etc.). Injections are used only occasionally and are used for the specific purpose of reducing severe pain or inflammation. However, this is not very efficacious and does not usually control long-term symptoms. Injection should be used with a clear understanding of the deleterious effects of cortisone on an injured tendon.

Rehabilitation of Operative Cases

Initial rehabilitation of the operated and repaired lateral epicondyle should emphasize range of motion of the more proximal links of the kinematic chain and should emphasize strengthening of the scapular and posterior shoulder muscles. After complete healing of the repaired tissue, isometric contractions and range of motion can be started. At about four to six weeks, full range of motion and strengthening should be started, with the protection of a counterforce brace. Once complete healing of the repair has been achieved, the patient may return to the nonoperative rehabilitation protocol emphasizing range of motion and cocontraction activities of the muscles around the elbow.

Medial Epicondylitis

Medial epicondylitis is associated with pain along the medial side of the elbow in the tendon bone insertion or at the musculotendinous junction. It is usually associated with harder hit strokes or activities and is usually seen in more advanced and more skillful athletes. This is an absolute overload, compared with the relative overload of the lateral epicondylitis. Medial epicondylitis involves the pronator teres, flexor carpi radialis, and, occasionally, the flexor carpi ulnaris, all of which arise from the medial epicondyle of the humerus and from the fascia over it.[6] Differential diagnosis of medial and lateral epicondylitis includes cervical radiculopathy, nerve entrapment syndromes (particularly the radial nerve at the lateral elbow), and proximal radioulnar joint injuries.[6,19]

- *Method of Presentation*—Chronic overload with occasional acute exacerbation. Usually there is no history of acute trauma other than an occasional fall on the outstretched arm.
- *Clinical Symptom Complex*—Point tender pain along the medial epicondylar area just anterior and distal to the epicondyle at the insertion of the muscle, or in the muscle-tendon junction. This must be differentiated from the pain that exists on the posterior aspect of the elbow or in the ulnar collateral ligament. The pain is usually associated with the throwing motion in baseball, or the forehand or service motion in tennis, or the hand-

stand position in gymnastics. The pain is described as being a relatively sharp pain that occasionally will shoot down in the muscle area.
- *Tissue Injury Complex*—Flexor muscles of the forearm, most notably the flexor communis and the pronator teres. Occasionally, the flexor carpi radialis will also be involved.
- *Tissue Overload Complex*—The anterior shoulder musculature, the anterior capsule of the shoulder, the forearm flexors at the elbow, and the biceps muscle.
- *Functional Biomechanical Deficit Complex*—Shoulder instability, lack of shoulder internal rotation, pronator inflexibility at the elbow, or flexion contracture of the elbow.
- *Subclinical Adaptation Complex*—Short-arming the serve or throw, excessive wrist snap, excessive trunk rotation, and hitting behind the ball.

Rehabilitation

Just as in lateral epicondylitis, most medial epicondylitis problems can be effectively rehabilitated without surgery. Pain control should be attained at the elbow initially. Relative rest, control of excessive loads, and review of mechanics are also important.

Acute phase rehabilitation includes counter-force bracing to decrease the loads and adequate control of the shoulder instability or lack of shoulder internal rotation that may be present in the proximal links. Modalities with ultrasound or electrogalvanic stimulation will be beneficial to reduce the irritation and inflammation, and medications may be necessary on a short-term basis. Injections should be used with the same precautions and indications as listed for lateral epicondylitis. Full range of shoulder and elbow motion should be obtained early in the process of rehabilitation. Initially, extensive use of cryotherapy and judicious use of antiinflammatory medication are indicated, usually for the first two to three weeks.

In the recovery phase with epicondylar pain, the flexibility of the involved tight muscles can be improved by fully extending the elbow and by either palmar flexing or extending the wrist with increasing pressure against a table (Figure 12–7). Stretching should be done several times a day. Strengthening can initially be done isometrically, with resistance from the other hand at multiple angles of wrist flexion and extension. Progression can then be made to wrist strengthening with elastic bands or free weights. Ultimately, strengthening should be done both eccentrically and concentrically, such as with a weight tied to a piece of wood that is slowly raised up and lowered with wrist motion only.

Recovery phase rehabilitation includes further strengthening of the musculature, mainly in the cocontraction fashion, protection of the tissue as it is healing with a counterforce

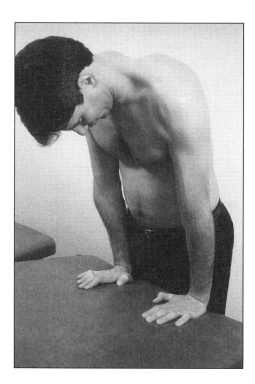

Figure 12–7 Flexibility exercises for wrist flexers. *Source:* Reprinted from *The Textbook of Military Medicine,* The Rehabilitation of the Injured Soldier, Borden Institute at Walter Reed Hospital.

brace, and further use of the hand and wrist in a graded muscle-strengthening fashion. Functional phase rehabilitation includes integration of the kinematic chain into the elbow motion, full range of motion of the elbow, and gradual weaning off of the counterforce brace.

Use of ultrasound or other heating modalities may provide some pain relief as well as loosen any scar tissue, allowing for better flexibility gains. Electrical stimulation modalities may also help with pain reduction and prevention of muscle atrophy. Counterforce braces may also be helpful by distributing the forces around the elbow over a greater surface area.[33] For lateral epicondylitis, the brace is applied firmly around the forearm over the wrist extensor muscle mass at the elbow. It is tightened enough so that when the patient contracts the wrist extensors, they do not obtain a full contraction of the muscle, which may relieve tension on the attachment of the extensor tendon.[6]

If during a period of 3–4 weeks, symptoms are not significantly reduced, a corticosteroid injection in the painful area may help. The steroid is mixed with a local anesthetic and injected into the subaponeurotic space at the point of maximal tenderness. Vigorous activity of the involved forearm should be avoided for two weeks after an injection. Injections may be repeated once if the patient receives some relief

but still has pain-limiting function. When conservative measures fail and the athlete is significantly disabled by epicondylitis, surgical treatment should be considered.

Operative treatment includes protection of the repaired site for 3–4 weeks. Acute phase rehabilitation should include the same type of proximal rehabilitation as recommended in nonoperative rehabilitation. At 3–4 weeks, the elbow brace should be removed, and full motion should be encouraged, both actively and passively. The patient should then be able to undertake the nonoperative rehabilitation program, with emphasis on full range of motion, integration of the kinematic chain, and cocontraction strengthening.

Valgus Overload Triad

This syndrome includes problems relating to the ulnar collateral ligament, the posterior medial joint, and the ulnar nerve, and is seen in repetitive activities of throwing and hitting. The medial aspect of the elbow is supported by the medial collateral ligament, the medial joint capsule, and the muscle mass. In overhead activities such as throwing, the elbow may be subject to intense valgus tension stress. Any of the structures on the medial aspect of the elbow may become injured. Tension on the medial aspect of the elbow is first resisted by the overlying flexor-pronator muscles. These muscles may tear or a partial avulsion of one of the tendons or muscle insertions may occur, with valgus overload injuries. Repetitive, violent stresses will involve the deeper capsule and ligament. Tension stress that the capsule and ligament put on the ulna and humerus can lead to spur formation and, ultimately, compression of the ulnar nerve. The differential diagnosis of medial capsuloligamentous injuries include ulnar neuropathies, radioulnar joint lesions, degenerative joint disorders of the elbow, cervical radiculopathy (especially C8 lesions), lower trunk brachial plexus lesions, and thoracic outlet syndrome.

- *Method of Presentation*—Most commonly a chronic overload problem with gradual onset of the symptoms. The first symptoms appear to indicate a tendinitis, but the other components of the syndrome then become apparent. Occasionally, a fall onto the outstretched arm will also cause an acute rupture of the ulnar collateral ligament with symptoms of the overload triad appearing shortly thereafter.
- *Clinical Symptom Complex*—Point-tender area over the ulnar collateral ligament, running just distally and inferiorly to the epicondyle down to the ulnar ridge. Pain along the ulnar nerve in the ulnar groove in zones 1, 2, or 3 proximally, midsubstance, or distally in the canal. Pain in the posteromedial aspect of the joint over the posterior aspect of the humerus and the posteromedial corner of the olecranon. This usually is in the cocking

position or the acceleration position of the baseball throw or at ball impact in tennis serve or forehand.

- *Tissue Injury Complex*—Ulnar collateral ligament, usually in midsubstance but also at either end. Ulnar nerve with compression due to scar tissue, or injury due to tensile stretch. Posteromedial joint with chondral or bony overgrowth with bone spur formation and/or chondral injury. Tendinitis problems may also coexist with the valgus overload syndrome.
- *Tissue Overload Complex*—Shoulder muscles with internal rotation weakness, biceps muscle, ulnar collateral ligament, and ulnar nerve.
- *Functional Biomechanical Deficit Complex*—Decreased range of motion of the shoulder, flexor contracture of the elbow, and pronation contracture of the forearm.
- *Subclinical Adaptation Complex*—Increased wrist snap, short-arming the ball, trunk rotation to improve shoulder rotation, and hitting behind the ball.

Rehabilitation

Milder forms of the valgus overload syndrome can be treated with the medial epicondylitis protocol, emphasizing proximal control of the scapula and shoulder, pain reduction around the inflamed tissues, emphasis on flexibility of the flexors and pronators, and cocontractions of the elbow musculature. Treatment begins with relative rest and judicious use of antiinflammatory medications. Symptoms should resolve in 7–14 days in most cases. Antiinflammatory modalities such as ultrasound and electrical stimulation are useful adjuncts to treatment early in the course. Therapy should be directed to stretching the flexor and pronator muscles of the forearm to improve range of motion. Maintaining and regaining a normal range of motion requires stretching in flexion, extension, pronation, and supination. Strengthening is also initiated, both concentrically and eccentrically. These types of strengthening exercises can be done as previously outlined with epicondylitis. Pronation and supination can be strengthened using a hammer or similar tool to produce torque throughout the full range of motion. Grip and shoulder exercises are also initiated. Rehabilitation programs for elbow problems should always address proximal stability at the shoulder to allow the elbow to be properly placed in space for appropriate function. Ice may be applied immediately after exercises.

Advanced cases will require surgical stabilization of the underlying ulnar collateral ligament instability and posterior medial bony impingement. This repair should be protected in a hinge brace to allow mild flexion without any extremes of flexion/extension or varus/valgus rotation. Range of motion may be allowed between 30 and 60 degrees of flexion for 10 days, then 0 degrees of extension to 60 degrees of flexion for 10 days, then 0–90 degrees of flexion for 10 days. Once the splint has been removed, typically between four and six weeks postinjury, active range of motion should be instituted, and further progression into the medial epicondylitis protocol is appropriate as healing continues.

REFERENCES

1. Dilorenzo CE, Parkes JC, Chmelar RD. The importance of shoulder and cervical dysfunction in the etiology and treatment of athletic elbow injuries. *J Orthop Sports Phys Ther.* 1990;11:402–409.
2. Weisner SL. Rehabilitation of elbow injuries in sports. *Phys Med Rehabil Clin North Am.* 1994;5:81–113.
3. Boone DC, Azen SP. Normal range of motion of joints in male subjects. *J Bone Joint Surg Am.* 1979;61:756–759.
4. Nirschl RP. Tennis injuries in the upper extremity. In: Nicholas JA, Hershman EB, eds. *Sports Medicine.* St Louis: CV Mosby Co; 1990: 827.
5. Nirschl RP, Morrey BF. Rehabilitation. In: Morrey BF, ed. *The Elbow and Its Disorders.* Philadelphia: WB Saunders Company; 1993: 173–180.
6. Leach RE, Miller JK. Lateral and medial epicondylitis of the elbow. *Clin Sports Med.* 1987;6:259.
7. Magee DJ. Elbow joints. In: *Orthopaedic Physical Assessment.* 2nd ed. Philadelphia: WB Saunders Company; 1992:143–167.
8. Roles NC, Mandsley RH. Radial tunnel syndrome: resistant tennis elbow as a nerve entrapment. *J Bone Joint Surg Br.* 1972;54:449–508.
9. Nirschl RP. Muscle and tendon trauma: tennis elbow. In: Morrey BF ed. *The Elbow and Its Disorders.* Philadelphia: WB Saunders Company; 1993:553–559.
10. Nirschl RP. Elbow tendinosis/tennis elbow. *Clin Sports Med.* 1992; 11:851.
11. Prentice WE. *Rehabilitation Techniques in Sports Medicine.* 2nd ed. St Louis: Mosby–Year Book; 1988.
12. Morrey BF, Regan WD. Tendinopathies about the elbow. In: Delee JC, Drez D, eds. *Orthopaedic Sports Medicine: Principles and Practice.* Philadelphia: WB Saunders Company; 1994:860.
13. Reid, DC. *Sports Injury Assessment and Rehabilitation.* New York: Churchill Livingstone; 1992:99.
14. Stratford PW, Levy DR, Gauldie S, et al. The evaluation of phonophoresis and friction massage for extensor carpi radialis tendinitis: a randomized controlled trial. *Physiotherapy Canada.* 1989;41:93–99.
15. Stratford PW, Levy DR, Gauldie S, et al. Extensor carpi radialis tendonitis: a validation of selected outcome measures. *Physiotherapy Canada.* 1987;39:250–55.
16. Halle JS, Franklin RJ, Karalfa BL. Comparison of four treatment approaches for lateral epicondylitis of the elbow. *J Orthop Sports Phys Ther.* 1986;8:62.
17. Fillion PL. Treatment of lateral epicondylitis. *Am J Occup Ther.* 1991;45:340–343.
18. LaFrenier JG. Tennis elbow—evaluation, treatment and prevention. *Phys Ther.* 1979;59:742–746.

19. Cyriax JH. The pathology and treatment of tennis elbow. *J Bone Joint Surg.* 1936;18:921.

20. Kushner S, Reid DC. Manipulation in the treatment of tennis elbow. *J Orthop Sports Phys Ther.* 1986;3:264.

21. Sobel J, Pettrone F, Nirschl R. Prevention and rehabilitation of racquet sports injuries in the upper extremity. In: Nicholas JA, Hershman EB, eds. *Sports Medicine.* St Louis: CV Mosby Co; 1990:843.

22. deAndrade JR et al. Joint distension and reflex muscle inhibition in the knee. *J Bone Joint Surg Am.* 1965;47:313.

23. Young JL, Press JM. The physiologic basis of sports rehabilitation. *Phys Med Rehabil Clin North Am.* 1994;5:9–36.

24. Basmajian JV, Deluca CJ. *Muscles Alive: Their Functions Revealed by Electromyography.* 5th ed. Baltimore: Williams & Wilkins, 1985.

25. Stanish WD, Rubinovich RM, Curwin S. Eccentric exercise in chronic tendinitis. *Clin Orthop.* 1986;208:65.

26. Knott M, Voss D. *Proprioceptive Neuromuscular Facilitation.* New York: Harper and Row, 1968.

27. Burton AK, Edwards VA. Electromyography and tennis elbow straps. *Br J Sports Med.* 1985;19:37.

28. Akeson WH, Amiel D, Woo SLY. Immobility effects on synovial joints: the pathomechanics of joint contracture. *Biorrheology.* 1980; 17–95.

29. Groppel JL, Nirschl RP. A mechanical and electromyographical analysis of the effects of various joint counterforce braces on the tennis player. *Am J Sports Med.* 1986;14:195.

30. Press JM, Herring SA, Kibler WB. Rehabilitation of musculoskeletal disorders. In: Dillingham T, ed. *The Textbook of Military Medicine.* Washington, DC: Borden Institute–United States Army. In press.

31. Cabrera JM, McCue FC. Nonosseous athletic injuries of the elbow, forearm and arm. *Clin Sports Med.* 1986;681–700.

32. Wells P. Cervical dysfunction and shoulder problems. *Physiotherapy.* 1983;68:66–71.

33. Jobe FW, Nuber G. Throwing injuries of the elbow. *Clin Sports Med.* 1986;5:621–636.

34. Leadbetter WB. Corticosteroid injection therapy in sports injuries in sports-induced inflammation. In: Leadbetter WB, Buckwalter JA, Gordin SL, eds. *Clinical and Basic Science Concepts.* Bethesda, MD: American Academy of Orthopedic Surgeons, 1989.

35. Parkes JC. Overuse of the elbow. In: Nicholas JA, Hershman EB, eds. *The Upper Extremity in Sports Medicine.* St. Louis: CV Mosby Co; 1990:335–346.

SUGGESTED READING

Kibler WB. Clinical biomechanics of the elbow. *Med Sci Sports Exerc.* 1994;26:1203–1207.

Kibler WB. Pathophysiology of overload injuries around the elbow. *Clin Sports Med.* 1995;14:447–459.

Plancher K. Medial and lateral epicondylitis in the athlete. *Clin Sports Med.* 1996;15:283–307.

Thomas DR. Prevention and rehabilitation of overuse injuries of the elbow. *Clin Sports Med.* 1995;14:459–479.

Wilk KE. Rehabilitation following elbow surgery in the throwing athlete. *Operative Techniques Sports Med.* 1996;4:114–132.

CHAPTER 13

Rehabilitation of the Wrist and Hand

W. Ben Kibler and Joel M. Press

GENERAL PRINCIPLES

The wrist and hand are very important in athletic activities because they represent the final link in the kinematic chain, and they represent the end point of all the directed forces and velocities. Also, the hand is what holds the implement to be thrown or struck, whether it be a baseball, golf club, or tennis racket. It is also the agent that meets with the ground or resistance as in gymnastics or swimming. A very large amount of diverse motions and positions has to be assumed by the wrist to achieve all of these different functions. The injuries to the wrist can be quite limiting in athletic function, both by causing pain and by limiting the athlete's ability to hold or grasp the object. Injuries can also be problematic because of the decreased motion that can occur with wrist problems. The wrist does not usually act on its own and must be considered a part of the linkage of the arm and trunk in the kinematic chain.

Biomechanics

Locally, the wrist is made up of several articulated linkages divided into two rows. These rows are geometrically and intrinsically unstable. Ligamentous stability is provided by a series of intrinsic and extrinsic ligaments that connect the individual bones and the rows. Muscular activity provides stability by providing concavity/compression between the curved articulating surfaces of each row.

From a functional standpoint, the wrist usually requires stabilization so that the hand and arm can perform the functions of hitting or striking. However, the wrist also has to assume the positions of dorsiflexion, palmar flexion, and ulnar and radial deviation, depending on the demands of the throwing or striking motion. In tennis, the wrist should be stabilized in extension at the moment of impact on the

ground strokes. In addition, the wrist assumes an ulnarly deviated position at impact in the serve and the forehand. It is in neutral deviation on the backhand.

The amount of actual wrist motion that is needed during active hitting for some athletic activities is surprisingly small. Only 40 degrees of total motion centered around neutral are necessary in the actual tennis serve and in tennis forehand and backhand. More motion than that is observed, but this occurs in follow-through after impact or ball release. Baseball throwing usually requires more range of motion in the cocking phase, as well as in the ball release phase, because the ball is actually being released out of the hand. The wrist, therefore, has to accept both proximally and distally based loads, which provide input in its motion. Proximally, the build-up of energy and force from the links of the kinematic chain moves the joint. Distally, the weight and velocity of the object held in the hand or the impact or position of the wrist on the ground will mandate certain positions of the joints. Full dorsiflexion must be obtained in a smooth pattern when the weight is borne on the hand, such as in gymnastics or in entering the water from a dive. The flexibility of the muscles and range of motion of the joints to achieve these positions are necessary for normal activity and injury prevention, as well as in injury rehabilitation.

Physiology

The muscles that actually move the wrist joint in dorsiflexion, palmar flexion, and radial and ulnar deviation are relatively small and cannot generate the velocities or forces that are seen in the throwing or striking motions. They work primarily to stabilize and concentrically load the carpal bones in a manner to confer stability to the wrist joint. Most of the velocity of the wrist joint is a result of the proximal kinematic chain and the inertial moment of the object held in the hand. The wrist muscles must also absorb a load in weight-bearing, such as gymnastics, swimming, or diving. The most important function of the muscles is a closed chain, cocontraction force couple activation.

Treatment

Because pain is such a major contributing factor in wrist injuries, efforts to reduce pain should be paramount. The wrist joint is a rather subcutaneous joint and many modalities, including cold, heat, ultrasound, and compression, can be quite effective as physical agents to reduce swelling, pain, inflammation, and edema to allow for more normal anatomic, physiologic, and biomechanical conditions in and around the joint. Treatment also must restore normal joint stability. Most of the time, this can be done by improving range of motion, allowing healing of the tissues and rehabilitation in cocontraction-stabilizing fashions. Surgical stabilization of the ligamentous or bony constraints may be necessary to achieve joint stability. Once joint stability has been established, work on mechanics of the strokes and on the kinematic chain can help to optimize the efficiency of the physiologic and biomechanical patterns across the wrist.

SPECIFIC INJURIES AND REHABILITATION PROTOCOLS

Wrist Tendinitis

Wrist tendinitis is a very common problem in athletics. Many of the wrist tendons can be involved, but the major involvement is from the extensor carpi radialis, extensor carpi ulnaris, flexor carpi radialis (FCR), the finger flexors, or the thumb extensors. In each situation, repetitive overload is the mechanism of injury. Usually, some transitional element, such as change in throwing or hitting pattern, excessive amount of work, or traumatic injury, is the inciting incident.

- *Method of Presentation*—Chronic overload tendinitis associated with gripping, striking, or hitting. Traumatic episodes of direct-blow injury or of indirect injury after a fall can also cause the tendinitis.
- *Clinical Symptom Complex*—Point tenderness over the tendon itself, usually in association with the extensor retinaculum or the flexor retinaculum. There is usually crepitus and soreness to direct pressure, with occasional snapping or locking of the tendon as it runs through the irritated area. Warmth, redness, and swelling may also be seen.
- *Tissue Injury Complex*—The tendon itself and the tendon sheath are the most commonly involved structures. There is very rarely a degenerative change in the tendon itself.

- *Tissue Overload Complex*—The muscle of the affected tendon is most commonly involved. Other problems include more proximal overloads, such as shoulder muscles, with consequent lack of internal rotation or shoulder abduction muscles with weakness.
- *Functional Biomechanical Deficit Complex*—Inflexibility of the wrist in dorsiflexion or palmar flexion, or in radial or ulnar deviation, and weakness of the muscles surrounding the wrist.
- *Subclinical Adaptation Complex*—More shoulder motion, striking the ball or throwing the ball from altered positions, or assuming altered positions upon weight-bearing in gymnastics.

Rehabilitation

Acute phase rehabilitation consists of relative rest, decrease in the overload activities, support of the wrist by taping, bracing, or casting in severe cases, and antiinflammatory modalities and medications. Surgical relief is necessary if there is a rupture or if there is enough crepitus and locking to give functional symptoms that do not improve with conservative treatment.

Initial treatment for tendinitis of the wrist and hand consists of rest, splinting, and use of cryotherapy and oral antiinflammatory agents. Injections are very rarely needed and can be quite deleterious in the acute situation. In chronic cases, soluble steroids such as dexamethasone are preferable to insoluble steroids, which tend to leave a deposit. Use of 0.5 mL of dexamethasone and 0.5 mL of 2% lidocaine is suggested.[1] Repeated injections, i.e., more than three, should be avoided.[2] In the initial phases of tendinitis, wrist and/or hand immobilization may be necessary for brief periods of time. In the management of de Quervain's disease, a wrist and thumb immobilization splint is fitted to relax the extensor pollicus brevis and the abductor pollicus longus. Appropriate positioning includes the wrist in approximately 15 degrees of dorsiflexion, the thumb carpometacarpal joint in 40 degrees of abduction, the metacarpophalangeal joint in 10 degrees of flexion, and the interphalangeal joint excluded. The appropriate splint for FCR tendinitis holds the wrist in 10 degrees of volar flexion and slight radial deviation to place the FCR in a shortened position.

Early range of motion of the wrist within a pain-free range of motion is important to avoid soft-tissue contracture and scarring. It has been shown that immobilization causes a loss of glycosaminoglycans, which are important in scar architecture.[3] An increase in muscle temperature helps facilitate metabolic processes, and a drop in muscle viscosity produces more rapid, forceful, and smooth contractions. Ultrasound treatment followed by stretching may be particularly helpful in chronic cases where extensive soft-tissue shortening has occurred. Tendon tensile strength has also been shown to decrease with immobilization and stress deprivation.[4] Increases in passive motion are best achieved through low-intensity, long-duration stretches. Strengthening should be started isometrically and progressed throughout the entire range of motion, concentrically and eccentrically, as tolerated.

Recovery phase rehabilitation includes early range of motion within the pain-free arcs, protected motion with wrist taping or wrist bracing, and early strengthening exercises, usually isometrics and cocontractions for the wrist muscles. Achievement of normal wrist positions and cocontractions with concavity compression of the joint surfaces confers the functional stability. In the recovery phase, proper mechanics of stroking, throwing, or landing are also emphasized so that proper loads are being transmitted through the wrist joint. Changes of technique in hitting or striking the ball and grip size of racquets should be considered at this time.

Functional phase rehabilitation includes full range of motion for the sport, complete muscle strength, and intact kinematic chain with normal mechanics of the stroking or hitting motions. Wrist braces are commonly used to support the wrist as the athlete returns to play. Most cases of wrist tendinitis should respond to appropriate treatment within 14–21 days. If conservative treatment fails or if the condition becomes chronic, surgical decompression may become necessary.[5]

Fractures

Fractures of the hand and wrist bones are rather common, due to the exposed position of the wrist and hand with both direct trauma due to external impact and indirect trauma due to loading in a fall. The most common fractures are of the distal radius, the metacarpals and phalanges, and the navicular bone.

Initial treatment of the fracture should confer stability to the fracture, whether by casting or by operative manipulation and internal fixation. During the acute phase, rehabilitation should maintain the other components of the kinematic chain. Running, jumping, and use of the upper extremity can be advocated while the involved extremity is in the cast or splint. Full range of motion of the distal phalanges should be emphasized in the cast as well. After the cast is removed, a variable period of time may be spent in a splint. This can be of the plaster variety or it may be made of other materials such as plastic or RTV-11. The fracture may be placed in these splints for most of the day and can be taken out of the splints for short periods of range of motion and strengthening rehabilitation. As soon as the fracture is stable, early range of motion rehabilitation should be instituted to minimize the joint stiffness, to improve range of motion of the fingers and wrists, and to allow early strengthening of the muscles. It is inevitable that some stiffness occur as a result of the treatment, whether it be casting or surgery, and this has

to be overcome to allow the physiologic motion for the specific sporting activity.

Recovery phase rehabilitation includes the same type of strengthening program that is prescribed for the tendinitis rehabilitation. Functional adaptations must be watched more carefully in this phase because of the restricted range of motion. Full range of motion of the wrist in the proper phase of throwing, striking, or hitting is necessary and should be advocated during this phase.

Functional rehabilitation activities include the same goals as for the tendinitis rehabilitation—full range of motion, good concentric stabilization, and full strength.

Ganglion Cysts

Ganglion cysts can be of two varieties: the external ganglion cyst that is evident on the dorsum of the wrist or the internal ganglion cyst, in which the cyst is actually intra-articular and in the depth of the wrist joint itself. The cysts can be treated symptomatically with rest, avoidance of activities, modalities for reduction of swelling, and antiinflammatory medications and injections. Symptomatic cysts that may recur or that interfere with range of motion may be considered for surgical treatment. There is usually a history of microtrauma or overt trauma as causative factors.

Nonoperative rehabilitation involves protective taping or splinting to avoid the extremes of motion or positions that cause symptoms. Judicious use of modalities may help reduce some of the symptoms. Icing after events can also help, and the athlete should be placed on cocontraction strengthening and avoidance of positions that are painful. Rehabilitation after surgical excision of the cyst involves protection of the wrist while the repair is healing. The patient is then advanced into the tendinitis protocol, with emphasis on range of motion, concentric stabilization, and strengthening.

Triangular Fibrocartilage Complex Injuries

Injuries to the triangular fibrocartilage complex (TFCC) can significantly impair wrist function, as the TFCC is a major stabilizer of the distal radioulnar joint and the ulnar side of the wrist. Proximal biomechanical abnormalities may trigger the onset of symptoms.

- *Method of Presentation*—They may present acutely after a fall on the supinated outstretched wrist or may present as a chronic overload after repetitive rotational loading.
- *Clinical Symptom Complex*—Point tenderness distal to ulnar styloid, pain with active ulnar deviation, or pain on passive supination and ulnar deviation.
- *Tissue Injury Complex*—TFCC with central or peripheral tears, ulnar collateral ligament, chondromalacia of the lunate or ulna.

- *Tissue Overload Complex*—Same as for the tissue injury, as well as wrist flexor muscles and shoulder internal rotator muscles.
- *Functional Biomechanical Deficit Complex*—Hypersupination on striking or hitting, kinematic chain breakage at elbow or wrist.
- *Subclinical Adaptation Complex*—Excessive wrist snap, forearm pronation, or swinging arms through larger arcs at the shoulder.

Initial treatment should be based on the stability of the distal radioulnar joint. If the joint is stable, casting or bracing may be sufficient to control the pathology. However, many symptomatic TFCC injuries will require open or arthroscopic debridement or repair to reduce the pain, remove the tear, or stabilize the joint and allow definitive rehabilitation.

Rehabilitation

Acute phase rehabilitation should emphasize proximal mechanics and muscle strengthening, even while the wrist is in the cast or splint. Often, poor proximal strength or power leads to a "catch-up" situation at the wrist. To achieve the extra velocity or acceleration necessary for catch-up, the wrist must be cocked in more ulnar deviation and extension. This will increase the pressure on the TFCC and cause injury.

After the splint is removed, recovery phase rehabilitation will first work on dorsiflexion/palmar flexion movements, followed by pronation/supination and radial/ulnar deviation. Muscle strengthening will emphasize cocontractions for wrist stability. Recovery phase rehabilitation will follow the same guidelines as for wrist tendinitis.

Ulnar Collateral Ligament of the Thumb

Injury to the ulnar collateral ligament of the thumb can be quite common. Abduction stress to the thumb while the metacarpophalangeal joint is near full extension can tear the ulnar collateral ligament. This type of injury is most often described in skiing.[6]

Early recognition and proper treatment are necessary to prevent instability and decreased functional use of the hand. Classification of injury is as follows: grade I and grade II lesions are degrees of partial disruptions of the ligament, and grade III lesions represent complete ligamentous disruptions. Joint stability is best evaluated by stress testing but should always be preceded by conventional roentgenograms,

when available, to determine whether a large, undisplaced intra-articular fracture is present. Injuries are classified by stress testing the metacarpophalangeal joint in slight flexion and in full extension to see whether any opening of the joint occurs. Comparison to the uninjured thumb is essential as there is a great variation in metacarpophalangeal range of motion from person to person. Differential diagnosis in chronic cases where no history of acute injury is present includes carpometacarpal arthritis of the first digit, carpal tunnel syndrome, adductor pollicis brevis or flexor pollicis brevis strain, and C6 radiculopathy.

- *Method of Presentation*—Acute injury.
- *Clinical Symptom Complex*—Pain and swelling in the medial aspect of the thumb.
- *Tissue Injury Complex*—Ulnar collateral ligament of the thumb, usually at the insertion point to the proximal interphalangeal joint.
- *Tissue Overload Complex*—Ulnar collateral ligament.
- *Functional Biomechanical Deficit Complex*—Loss of stability of the thumb.
- *Functional Adaptation Complex*—Decreased grip strength.

Rehabilitation

Treatment for partial first- or second-degree ligament injury in which there is no instability is immobilization in 20 degrees of flexion in a spica cast for 3–4 weeks.[7,8] The interphalangeal joint is left free to allow for active motion to prevent scarring of the extensor mechanism. A removable splint is fabricated after 3–4 weeks, and active exercises are allowed several times a day.[7] The splint may be removed at 6 weeks for normal activity. If there is severe swelling after the initial injury, a molded volar gutter splint may be used for the first weeks until the swelling subsides. This may be followed by the application of a thumb spica cast. Grip strength exercises will be important after a cast is removed and can be accomplished by squeezing a sponge or putty. Progression to a spring-loaded grip device can be made. Some devices provide for individual flexion of each finger. Surgery can be reserved for cases in which there is later disability or in which the diagnosis of instability is delayed for weeks after injury[9] or can be performed on any unstable joint.[8,10] Range of motion exercises will be important after immobilization for many weeks because of soft-tissue contracture.

REFERENCES

1. Kiefhaber TR, Stern PJ. Upper extremity tendinitis and overuse syndromes in the athlete. *Clin Sports Med.* 1992;11:39–55.
2. Shaw Wilgis EF, Yates AY Jr. Wrist pain. In: Nicholas JA, Hershman EB, eds. *The Upper Extremity in Sports Medicine.* St Louis: CV Mosby Co; 1990:483.
3. Jacobson MD. Evaluation of hand and wrist injuries in athletes. *Operative Techniques Sports Med.* 1996;4:210–227.
4. Osterman AL. Soft tissue injuries of the hand and wrist in racquet sports. *Clin Sports Med.* 1988;7:329–348.
5. Wood MB, Dobyns JH. Sports related extraarticular wrist syndromes. *Clin Orthop Rel Res.* 1986;202:93.
6. Engkvist O, Balkfors B, Lindsjo U. Thumb injuries in downhill skiing. *Int J Sports Med.* 1982;3:50.

7. Posner MA. Hand injuries. In: Nicholas JA, Hershman EB, eds. *The Upper Extremity in Sports Medicine*. St Louis: CV Mosby Co; 1990:495.

8. Kahler DM, McCue FC. Metacarpophalangeal and proximal interphalangeal joint injuries at the hand, including the thumb. *Clin Sports Med*. 1992;11:57–76.

9. Rettig AC. Wrist problems in the tennis player. *Med Sci Sports Exerc*. 1994;26:1208–1212.

10. Helm RH. Hand function after injuries to the collateral ligaments of the metacarpophalangeal joint of the thumb. *J Hand Surg*. 1982; 12B:252.

CHAPTER 14

Rehabilitation of Lumbar Spine Injuries

Matthew Kaul and Stanley A. Herring

INTRODUCTION

Wide variation exists in the diagnosis and treatment for back pain among different specialties. A review of the standard texts from orthopaedics, rheumatology, physiatry, internal medicine, neurology, neurosurgery, and osteopathy demonstrates some obvious overlap but also much variability in diagnostic categories.

Differences also exist in the use of diagnostic tests for low back pain (LBP) among different disciplines.[1] Physiatrists and neurologists were much more likely than other physicians to order electromyography (EMG). Discography was more likely to be ordered by orthopaedic surgeons than by neurosurgeons. Neurologists and neurosurgeons were most likely to order an imaging study for acute or chronic back pain without sciatica. For the patient with sciatica or chronic back pain, rheumatologists were the most likely specialists to order laboratory tests. Physiatrists were twice as likely to order a psychologic evaluation for the patient with chronic back pain.

Treatment is highly varied as well. Physiatrists belive modalities to be helpful more often than do rheumatologists.[2] Surgery rates for back pain have also been shown to vary significantly throughout the international community.[3] Regional variations in surgery rates within the United States have also been documented.[4] Back surgery rates increased almost linearly with per capita numbers of orthopaedic surgeons and neurosurgeons.

This chapter is meant to synthesize the literature from a number of relevant fields and to provide a basis for the rehabilitation of the LBP patient. Acuity and chronicity are considered where appropriate.

EPIDEMIOLOGY

Every year, at least one of every two adults in the United States experiences at least a day of back pain. Back pain is the second leading symptom culminating in physician visits. At some point in their lives, 80% of the population experiences back pain. Recovery after an episode of back pain occurs in 70% of cases within 3 weeks, in 90% within 3 months, and in 95% within 6 months. Recurrences occur within a year in about 12%. In 4%, back pain becomes chronic.[5,6] Up to 70% of patients have recurrent episodes of back pain.

Disc herniation occurs most commonly in middle age. This is probably due to the early effects of degeneration of the annulus fibrosis, combined with the high swelling pressure of the nucleus pulposus during middle age.[7] Patients with a proven lumbar herniated disc and surgical treatment have a 10 times higher risk of a subsequent herniated disc, compared with the general population.[8] The cumulative risk of having a second proven herniated disc during the next 20 years postoperatively is 8%.[8] Herniated discs are reported to be asymptomatic in 75% of conservatively treated patients at 6 months.[9] Although symptomatic improvement may occur readily, the high recurrence rate and the anatomic and functional changes known to occur in chronic back pain warrant maximizing rehabilitation of the spine.

Up to 70% of patients who undergo first-time surgery for intervertebral disc protrusion still complain of LBP years later.[10] Postoperative deficits have been documented and include deficits in lumbar extensor endurance.[11,12]

ANATOMY AND BIOMECHANICS

The reader requires a working knowledge of the functional anatomy and biomechanics of the lumbar spine as a basis for understanding the rehabilitative concepts presented later in this chapter. The optimum lumbar spine mechanism is an intrinsically stable yet physiologically mobile structure. The following has been previously reviewed by one of the authors (SAH).[13]

The Three-Joint Complex

The lumbar spine is comprised of a series of five articulated motion segments with the three-joint complex as the basic kinematic unit of the spine. Each motion segment consists of one intervertebral disc situated anteriorly between the endplates of two adjacent vertebral bodies and two posterior synovial facet joints formed by the articular processes of the superior and inferior vertebrae. Caudal vertebrae are larger, as is their contribution to load-bearing. The intervertebral disc is comprised of the central nucleus pulposus and the peripheral annulus fibrosis. The nucleus pulposus is a fibrogelatinous mass containing 80–90% water, collagen, and a mucopolysaccharide matrix. The annulus is formed by concentric lamellae of obliquely oriented cartilaginous fibers. Individual lumbar nerve roots exit bilaterally below the pedicle of each respective vertebra and travel laterally in the intervertebral foramen. The lateral recess is a semidistinct region within the spinal canal medial to the intervertebral foramen.

Innervation

Determination of clinically relevant pain generators in the lumbar spine is difficult. The outer one-third of the intervertebral disc is innervated but the remainder of the annulus and the nucleus pulposus are not. Both encapsulated and free nerve endings have been demonstrated, implying proprioceptive and nociceptive functions.[14] The greatest concentration of nerve receptors occurs at the lateral margin of the disc. The fewest number of nerve receptors occurs anteriorly, and an intermediate number occurs posteriorly. The posterior margin of the annulus and the posterior longitudinal ligament are supplied by the sinuvertebral nerve. This nerve is formed by a branch of the ventral rami (somatic) and from a branch of the grey ramus communicans (autonomic). Anteriorly—including the anterior longitudinal ligament—and laterally, the disc is innervated by grey ramus communicans and ventral rami. The significance of the sympathetic innervation of the disc is not clear.

The lumbar facet joints are richly innervated, receiving branches from up to three different segmental levels via the medial branches of the primary dorsal rami. Giles[15] has demonstrated free nerve endings in the synovium of the facet joints. In an animal model, the lumbar facet joints have been shown to contain both high-threshold afferents serving primarily as nociceptors, and low-threshold afferent fibers, which modulate proprioceptive feedback.[16,17] These nerve endings are located in the facet joint capsule, as well as in the border regions within the ligamentum flavum, muscles, and tendons. This implies that excessive tensile loading of the facet joint capsule may be the mechanism whereby "facet-mediated" nociception occurs. Finally, the musculoligamentous supporting structures of the lumbar spine are innervated by lateral, intermediate, and medial branches of the primary dorsal rami. The pain-producing areas of these muscles may be primarily at the musculotendinous junction, tendon-bone junction, and at sites of neurovascular bundles.[18,19]

Biomechanics

The cardinal planes of segmental motion include flexion, extension, torsion (axial or horizontal rotation and translation), and side bending. The inherent efficiency of lumbar segmental motion allows functional range of motion while protecting the three-joint complex from excessive forces.

Flexion and extension occur predominantly at the lower two lumbar segments, with up to 20 degrees occurring at each segment. This motion is defined by an instantaneous center of rotation (IAR). As with other joints, maintenance of IAR is important for proper joint stability. Through lumbar flexion and extension, a finite distribution of IAR points exist, known as a *centrode*. This centrode becomes more dispersed and random in an injured or degenerative segment.[19]

Pure lumbar flexion is tolerated well. Pain from a flexion injury can potentially result from a sprain of the interspinous ligaments or facet joint capsule, strain to the thoracolumbar fascia (TLF) or spinal extensor muscles. Following a hyperflexion injury, pain may result from a facet joint meniscoid structure, a fibroadipose tissue flap, or a redundant synovial that becomes trapped in the capsular recess. Annular tears are unlikely with flexion because the IAR lies close to the annulus, thus the lever arm is short, and the tensile force generated within the annular collagen fibers is not excessive. However, if the nucleus pulposus fragments and impinges, the annular fiber pain may occur. The acute "locked back syndrome" following pure flexion injury may result from a trapped facet meniscoid or nuclear fragmentation.

Compressive load to the normal lumbar spine is predominantly transmitted through the anterior vertebral endplates and annulus fibrosis. Pressure developing within the nucleus is evenly distributed to the annular fibers; therefore, annular disruption does not occur. Excessive loads place the vertebral endplate at risk for fracture. However, the above injury may lead to a secondary inflammatory cascade within the nucleus, with subsequent nuclear "degradation" and internal disc disruption. Ultimately, annular disruption and herniation may occur, although not acutely, following a compressive load.

Extension injury theoretically can result in spinous process impingement and periostitis. Impingement of the inferior facet joint capsule acts on the lamina of the vertebrae below. Ipsilateral bony limitation can result in torsional force to the segment and resultant strain to the contralateral facet joint.

Torsional stresses are relatively poorly tolerated. Farfan[20] assessed the relative contributions to resistance from individual structures of the motion segment. The ipsilateral (impacted) facet contributes 65% and the annulus 35% to torsion resistance. The orientation of the facets allows only 2–3 degrees of rotation, which protects the annulus. Beyond three degrees of rotation, facet impaction and fracture or pars interarticularis injury may occur. The IAR also moves posteriorly, which places the outer annulus at risk for circumferential tears and the contralateral facet joint at risk for strain.

Combined movements through the lumbar spine carry the highest injury potential. Forward flexion and rotation carry the greatest risk for disc injury. In flexion, the disc is preferentially loaded, which displaces the nucleus posteriorly. The posterior longitudinal ligament is thin posteriorly and is the area of least protection around the disc.

The five basic back support mechanisms have been reviewed[21] and are summarized below, as previously presented by the authors.

Intra-abdominal pressure (IAP) increases with heavy lifting when internal oblique and transverse abdominal muscles contract with the glottis closed. This may off-load the spine by transmitting increased forces through the abdominal cavity. Hemborg et al.[22] found that IAP did not improve with training. Increased IAP does increase tension in the TLF.

The *thoracolumbar fascia* has bony attachments to the spinous processes of the lumbar spine—the ribs superiorly, the illiac crest inferiorly—and the lateral margins blend with the internal oblique and the transverse abdominal muscles. The latissimus dorsi aponeurosis forms part of the TLF attaching to the iliac crest. During contraction of the latissimus dorsi, transverse abdominal, and internal oblique muscles, the TLF is actively engaged and creates an antiflexion moment through the lumbar spine. It is also engaged with contraction of the abdominal, hamstring, and gluteal muscles, which causes posterior pelvic tilt, thereby tensing the TLF. Passive engagement of the TLF occurs with lumbar flexion. The TLF provides important support during lifting in all postures. An increased antiflexion moment reduces the amount of intervertebral compression.

A *hydraulic amplifier mechanism* also adds tension to the TLF by contracting the erector spinae and transversospinalis within the inelastic envelope of the TLF. This provides a further antiflexion moment.

The *posterior ligamentous system* (supraspinous and interspinous ligaments) lies further posterior than the sacrospinalis muscles and, therefore, has a better lever arm for resisting flexion. Making use of the ligaments during lifting reduces the compressive forces through the lumbar spine.[23]

The *muscular support mechanism* of the spine is divided into intersegmental and polysegmental muscles. The intersegmental muscles are small and lie close to the axis of rotation. These muscles run between two adjacent vertebrae, and their function is to control flexion.

Polysegmental muscles are the the erector spinae, multifidi, longissimus, iliocastalis, and psoas. The erector spinae lie superficial to the multifidi and extend from the sacrum and the ilium to the thoracic region. The latter three muscles are short polysegmental muscles spanning between two and five vertebral levels. These muscles are variously involved in lumbar extension, side flexion, stabilization in axial rotation and lateral flexion, and motion in axial rotation. The psoas muscle has been shown to be active during unsupported sitting and in small amounts of lumbar flexion. This activity is thought to counteract the pull of the spinal extensor muscles. The psoas is thought to stabilize the spine in lateral flexion and rotation.

KINETIC CHAIN

The relationship of the pelvis to the spine is critical in understanding rehabilitation concepts in treating LBP. It also may have importance in the prevention of low back injuries. The pelvis may be tilted anteriorly or posteriorly in the saggital plane.

Anterior Pelvic Tilt

Anterior pelvic tilt increases lumbar lordosis and may be caused by weakness of abdominal muscles, tight iliopsoas, or thoracolumbar fascia. Hip flexors insert along the anterior portion of the lumbar vertebrae and exert a forward and downward pull on the vertebrae. Contracted or hypertonic hip flexors, therefore, may increase anterior pelvic tilt.

In anterior pelvic tilt, there is a relative lengthening of the hamstring and gluteal muscles, decreasing their advantage on the length–tension curve and allowing further pelvic tilt. Treatment consists of stretching the TLF and hip flexors while strengthening the abdominals, gluteus maximus, and hamstrings.

Posterior Pelvic Tilt

Posterior pelvic tilt decreases the lumbar lordosis and can result from weal paraspinal extensor muscles or tight gluteal and hamstring muscles. Hip flexors and back extensors in compensation are relatively elongated. Treatment is aimed at stretching the hamstrings, gluteus maximus, and abdominals with strengthening of hip flexors and back extensors.

BIOCHEMISTRY/NEUROPHYSIOLOGY

The following section is not meant to be an exhaustive review of the biochemistry or neurophysiology pertaining to lumbar pain or pain. Rather, it is meant to present information that has particular relevance to rehabilitation of the lumbar spine and the pathology discussed in the subsequent sections.

More Than Just Mechanical

Mechanical impingement of disc against nerve is unlikely to be a sufficient cause of symptoms. Numerous lines of evidence point to a multifactorial cause of pain related to disc herniation, including biochemical, neurochemical, immune, vascular, and mechanical. Multiple studies have demonstrated herniated discs in asymptomatic individuals.[24,25] Others have presented cases in which pain resolved, yet the anatomic disc herniation remained present.[26] A positive straight-leg-raising (SLR) test is not necessarily related to the size of a disc herniation, suggesting other than purely mechanical factors.[27] Hyperalgesia is induced and a pain signal may evolve when excessive mechanical stimulation occurs, but a reaction to injury appears to be necessary to cause symptoms. The reaction to injury may be mediated by neurogenic and nonneurogenic chemicals.

Nonneurogenic Pain Mediators

Endogenous chemicals are released from soft-tissue cells and cell membranes. Many of these have pain-producing capabilities. These include bradykinin, serotonin, histamine, acetylcholine, prostaglandins, and leukotrienes. Various mechanisms by which these chemicals mediate pain include enhancement of C and A nociceptors' response to nonnociceptive and nociceptive stimuli, and production of mechanical hyperalgesia.[28]

Neurogenic Pain Mediators/Dorsal Root Ganglion

Neuropeptides are produced within the dorsal root ganglion (DRG) in the cell bodies of primary afferent neurons and are delivered by axonal transport, both centrally and peripherally via neural architecture. Known neuropeptides include substance P, somatostatin, cholecystokinin-like substance, VIP, cacitonin gene-related peptide (CGRP), gastrin-releasing peptide, dynorphin, enkephalin, and galanin. These neuropeptides have been implicated as playing a role in neurotransmission and neuromodulation, and they are released from peripheral endings of nociceptive afferents in response to noxious chemical or mechanical stimulation.

Release of the above neuropeptides can increase blood flow and vascular permeability. They can also stimulate the release of leukotrienes and other leukotactic factors from mast cells; stimulate the synthesis of inflammatory factors (prostaglandin E_2); and stimulate the synthesis of degenerative enzymes.[28]

A number of studies has implicated the dorsal root ganglion as a source of LBP. Micro- and macroscopic changes in the DRG have been demonstrated in cadaveric studies of patients with disc herniation and nerve root compression.[29] Ultrastructural[30] and neurochemical changes[31] have been demonstrated in DRG of animals exposed to vibration. Ultrastructural changes included increased nuclear clefting and increased nuclear pores. Mitochondrial and lysosomal volumes were significantly increased, and subcellular structures were crowded in vibrated cells. Compression of the normal DRG produces prolonged bursts of nerve impulses.[32] Radicular pain can be induced by mild mechanical compression of the DRG with associated prolonged repetitive firing of the DRG.[33]

A model has been proposed by Weinstein that hypothesizes a causal link between environmental factors and functional spinal unit degeneration mediated by the discussed neurogenic and nonneurogenic mediators. The release of neuropeptides induced by environmental factors mediates the degenerative cascade by the proinflammatory effects of neuropeptides, by stimulating the synthesis of inflammatory agents and degradative enzymes.[28]

Immunochemistry

Nuclear material has been found to be antigenic and produces an autoimmune reaction in vitro. In patients with severe back pain with and without sciatica, serum antibodies have been shown to rise over several weeks after symptom onset.[34] An interesting parallel is seen in postcardiotomy syndrome, where more symptomatic patients demonstrate greater titers of heart-specific antibodies.

Skouen et al.[35] found elevated levels of cerebrospinal fluid (CSF) protein correlated with clinical parameters. Significantly higher levels of CSF:serum albumin and CSF:serum immunoglobulin G ratio were found in patients with positive SLR and paresis, compared with patients with no clinical findings.

Spiliopoulou et al.[36] assessed 10 patients undergoing back surgery for back pain and sciatica with computed tomography (CT) confirmed disc herniation with rate nephelometry and compared these patients to controls. They found increased values in the ratios of IgM (nucleus pulposus):IgM (serum) and IgM (CSF):IgM (serum) in patients with back pain and sciatica. These results were interpreted as a local inflammatory process at the nerve root exposed to nucleus pulposus.

Sensitization of Nociceptors

Peripheral Factors

Painful sensations from skeletal muscle and joints are mediated by slowly conducting thin myelinated and nonmyelinated fibers with free nerve ending receptors.[37] One of the first subjective symptoms of a pathologic alteration of a skeletal muscle or joint is tenderness. The most likely explanation of this phenomenon is that normally high mechanical threshold nociceptors change their receptive fields to respond to weak mechanical stimuli.[37,38] This lowered mechanical threshold of nociceptive endings is probably brought about by endogenous substances released from damaged muscle, joint, and/or polymodal primary afferent nociceptive fibers, depending on the structure. Alteration of the intra-articular environment or joint damage sensitizes joint receptors.[39–43] These substances include bradykinin, serotonin, histamine, galanin, bombesin, excitatory amino acids, neurokinin A, peptide histidine-isoleucine, and leukotrienes.[37,38] Direct local stimulation of the sensitized nerve terminals can also cause release of neurochemicals. The "sensory" fibers do have an efferent role.

Spinal Mechanisms

The DRG in animal experiments has been shown to receive inputs from deep tissue, including a large proportion of cells receiving input from skeletal muscle.[38] Many of the DRG cells had convergent input from deep tissues and skin. Tonic descending inhibitory influences are greater for skeletal muscles than for skin. A great deal of nociceptive information from skeletal muscle is likely suppressed under normal conditions.[38] The DRG is modulated not only by descending pathways but also by alterations of their receptive fields. Receptive field alteration can be seen with nociceptive input.[38]

Afferent fibers from a given muscle are distributed to many spinal segments and may account for the diffuse nature of muscle pain. Potential factors that may form the basis for referral of deep pain include the multiplicity of receptive fields of DRG neurons and convergence of input from muscle and skin onto the same cell.[38]

Sympathetic Activation

Muscle tension appears to be related to the sympathetic nervous system.[44–46] In animal studies, stimulation of the cervical sympathetic nerve produces an immediate increase in jaw tension, as measured by an isometric force transducer. This response to sympathetic stimulation was not blocked by curare but was totally blocked by the sympathetic alpha-blocker phentolamine. This indicates that this response is not due to alpha- or gamma-motoneuron activation of intrafusal muscle fibers. Modification of the sympathetic output is accompanied by changes in muscle tone. In clinical syndromes associated with muscle hypertonus (i.e., spasm), the peripheral sympathetic actions on muscle spindles could be responsible in part.

This effect has been supported in a study of patients with fibromyalgia where significant pain reduction was noted after sympathetic blockade with an accompanying reduction in the number of palpated tender points.[47] In an intriguing study, Hubbard and Berkoff found sustained spontaneous electrical activity localized to the 1- to 2-mm nidus of muscle tender points. They hypothesized that this activity was a reflection of sympathetically stimulated intrafusal contraction.[48]

Arthrogenous Muscle Inhibition

Arthrogenous muscle inhibition (AMI) describes a phenomenon seen in acute or chronic joint pathology where the pathology prevents full voluntary activation of muscles acting across the affected joint.[49] AMI is probably elicited by abnormal afferent information from the affected joint, resulting in decreased motor drive. Because AMI prevents full muscle activation, it may contribute to atrophy and weakness in muscles serving an affected joint.

Arthrogenous muscle inhibition may be part of the pathogenesis of degenerative joint diseases.[49] Perhaps these strength losses expose the joint to further structural damage. A well-known example of AMI can be seen in unilateral knee osteoarthritis. Multiple studies frequently have found the affected side's quadriceps muscle to be 40% weaker than the quadriceps of the unaffected side.[49]

NEUROMUSCULOSKELETAL CONSIDERATIONS

Acute/First-Time Back Injuries

Muscular Strength and Endurance

Short extension endurance time on the 240-sec over-the-table-edge test was predictive of first-time LBP in one study that used this assessment technique.[50] However, in other studies, other static or dynamic strength/endurance items did not have prognostic significance for first-time LBP.[51–53] Matching worker lifting capacity with job task in preemployment evaluation has been shown to reduce the incidence of LBP episodes.[54]

Hides et al.[55] assessed 26 patients with acute or subacute unilateral LBP with real-time ultrasound imaging. There were 51 controls. Multifidus cross-sectional area was measured from L2 to L5. The multifidus cross-sectional area was markedly asymmetrical in those with back injury. The muscle ipsilateral to symptoms was smaller. Interestingly, the wasting was confined to one vertebral level. The back injury patients' muscles were also of rounder shape than were those of control subjects. Because muscle wasting in acute unilateral back injury was unilateral and isolated to one level, disuse atrophy is unlikely to explain these findings. A long loop reflex preventing movement to protect structures at the level of pathology might be the explanation (i.e., AMI). Another important finding from this study was the lack of correlation between the severity of wasting and the clinical findings. Those thought to have relatively mild symptoms can have marked wasting, which can be missed in a routine clinical examination.

Not surprisingly, nonspecific strengthening exercises in a large randomized, placebo-controlled trial of exercise therapy in patients with acute LBP did not find any treatment effect.[56] Unfortunately, this study did not build on fairly well-established information that exercise therapy and physical therapy (PT) should be individualized.

Stankovic and Olof[57] assessed McKenzie treatment compared with "mini back school" in acute back pain patients. They found the McKenzie method of treatment for patients with acute LBP was superior at 3- and 52-week assessment. Donelson et al.[58] have also demonstrated that sagittal end-range spinal motion assessment before prescription of flexion-extension exercises is important. They found that end-range extension significantly decreased central and peripheral pain and resulted in centralization of pain, whereas flexion significantly increased mean central and peripheral pain. Forty percent preferred extension, and 7% preferred flexion. This study was a prospective, randomized, multicentered trial that included 145 subjects.

Delitto et al.[59] classified patients as to which series of motion tests induced symptoms, then randomized extension responders into one of two treatment groups: extension exercise/mobilization or flexion exercises. Investigators found that those randomized subjects treated with extension exercise/mobilization improved faster than those treated with a flexion exercise program. Intensive and active exercise appears to be a more effective treatment for acute low back injuries than are conventional community-based treatment methods.[60,61]

Flexibility

In prospective studies of lumbar flexibility, the only flexibility item found to be predictive of first-time LBP was *high* mobility of the lumbar spine, as measured by the modified Schober test.[62] Other range-of-motion (ROM) variables, including hamstring length and lumbar mobility in extension and lateral flexion, were not predictive of first-time LBP.

Any discussion of flexibility must include an understanding of generalized joint hypermobility and localized joint hypermobility. The "hypermobility syndrome" is characterized by generalized joint laxity and the occurrence of musculoskeletal symptoms in the absence of rheumatologic disease. Mobility for a given joint follows a Gaussian distribution, and, generally, those patients whose joint range is more than two standard deviations above the mean are those who suffer musculoskeletal symptoms.[63] Women's joints are more hypermobile than are men's and certain ethnic groups have higher rates of hypermobility. These patients present with a wide variety of common traumatic and overuse lesions of the spine and extremities. In the past, the commonly encountered arthralgia or myalgia had been difficult to explain. However, a strong association between hypermobility and fibromyalgia has been demonstrated more recently.[64] A postulated mechanism of pain in the hypermobility syndrome includes overstimulation of nociceptive nerve endings that are poorly supported by defective collagen fibrils.

Localized joint hypermobility has been found to be a risk factor in hip injuries in female athletes. Knapic et al.[65] found those with a 15% greater hip extensor ROM on the right side were 2.6 times more likely to be injured than were those with less than a 15% imbalance. Patients with left-sided flexibility imbalances were only 1.7 times as likely to be injured. Flexibility imbalances appear to be important in predisposing people to injury. (Localized joint hypermobility is also discussed in the "Examination" and "Specific Clinical Lesions" sections.)

Coordination

Effective functioning of the back requires coordination of the 24 vertebrae; the pelvis; and the muscles, fascia, and ligaments of the pelvic girdle and trunk. Coordination is task-specific and should be performed in a way that minimizes the stresses within the spine [Gracovetsky SM, 1985 #22]. Gracovetsky et al.[66] have used a mathematical model that predicts the existence of a relationship between pelvic tilt and the distribution of stresses within the spine. For every angle of flexion, there was a unique degree of lordosis that would minimize stresses within the spine. This was born out in EMG motion analysis with human subjects. It was found that a subject's most comfortable lordosis was associated with the lowest multifidus activity.[66]

Proprioception

Proprioception is decreased in hypermobility syndrome.[67] This may provide a link between the hypermobility syndrome and increased rates of many types of musculoskeletal injury. Decreased proprioception and increased joint play may lead to tissue injury from repetitive microtrauma or overstimulation of nociceptive nerve endings.

Poor scores in tests of generalized proprioception correlated with an increased incidence of back injury in one study.[68] In the ankle joint, those with superior proprioception had lower risk of athletic injury.[69]

Cardiovascular Fitness

Battie et al.[70] assessed whether maximal oxygen uptake was predictive of future back problems. Of those experiencing low back problems over the 4-year follow-up, maximal oxygen uptake was not predictive of injury.

Cady et al.[71] used a physical work capacity test to assess 1,652 firefighters. Three fitness groups were found (high, middle, and low). Subsequent back injuries were found in 7% of the least fit, 3% of the middle fit, and 1% of the most fit. Problems with the study include significant age differences between the highly fit group (mean age 31.8 years) and the least-fit group (mean age 46.3 years). Just one of the injuries in the highly fit group cost more than all 19 injuries in the least-fit group.

Cady et al.[72] also assessed a homogeneous age group. Those with the lowest physical work capacity had a higher proportion of all injury costs, compared with those with the highest physical work capacity.[72] With these conflicting studies, there is not conclusive evidence that high cardiovascular fitness protects against back injury.

Chronic or Recurrent Back Injuries

A committee of the National Academy of Sciences concerned with chronic pain of enigmatic origin concluded that the most reliable means to verify serious chronic pain and suffering was to identify decrements in the patient's function at all levels.[73] The following is a discussion of these decrements.

Muscular Strength and Endurance

Static and/or dynamic trunk flexion and extension strength/endurance showed some prognostic value in cases of recurrent LBP.

Although strength deficits have not been conclusively demonstrated in the back muscles of chronic back pain patients,[74,75] endurance deficits have been documented.[75] Using an EMG-derived spectral-variables fatigue index, LBP patients can be identified with an accuracy of 88–100%, and control subjects without LBP with an accuracy of 84–100%.[75,76] Those with LBP demonstrate a greater rate of spectral variables. Interestingly, investigators found that EMG spectral-variable measurements in fibromyalgia patients were not statistically different from measurements in pain-free controls, but both were statistically different than measurements in those with idiopathic LBP.[77]

Strength deficits have been demonstrated in the abdominal muscles of patients with LBP, compared with healthy controls.[78,79] It is unknown whether the weakness is the result of the back pain or is a risk factor for developing back pain. Strength deficits have been demonstrated in the postoperative discectomy patient extending to one-year follow-up.[74] Strength deficits in chronic LBP have been documented by some investigators[81] but not by others.[74] Differences in the results may be related to the many ways of assessing strength. For example, in the study of Mayer et al.,[81] subjects were tested in the standing position, whereas in the study by Shirado et al.,[74] subjects were tested in the semireclined posi-

tion. In standing, all muscles, such as quadriceps, hamstrings, and gluteals, are involved in addition to pure trunk muscles. The peak torque flexion:extension ratio has been used widely to assess differences between those with chronic LBP and healthy controls. Some investigators found extensors more affected than flexors in chronic LBP,[82] others found flexors were affected more significantly,[83] and still others found no significant differences.[84]

Multifidus and longissimus/iliocostalis magnetic resonance imaging (MRI) signal intensity differs at rest in chronic LBP patients compared with control subjects.[85] This may reflect residual injury and denervation. In chronic back pain, CT scan assessment was found to demonstrate generalized atrophy but a relative increase in multifidus cross-sectional area on the symptomatic side.[86] This finding is consistent with evidence of type I fiber hypertrophy and type II fiber atrophy,[87] and increased paraspinal muscle activation seen in chronic LBP.[88,89]

Up to 70% of patients who undergo first-time surgery for intervertebral disc protrusion still complain of LBP years later.[10] Postoperative deficits have been documented and include deficits in lumbar extensor endurance.[11,12] Manniche et al.[90] initially demonstrated that intensive back exercises of 30 sessions over 3 months significantly reduced LBP in chronic patients. However, in their study, the protocol included hyperextension exercises in addition to intensive back exercises. Manniche et al.[91] then assessed which component is more important in a subsequent study in which intensive dynamic exercises were performed in two groups: one with hyperextension and one without. Intensive dynamic back exercises in postdiscectomy patients with chronic back pain resulted in improvements in isometric endurance and decreased pain.[91] The added use of extension exercises did not confer any additional benefit to the intensive dynamic back exercises. Risch et al.[92] randomized 54 chronic LBP patients into a 10-week lumbar extensor exercise program and a control group. The treatment group significantly increased their strength (20–42%) and decreased pain levels. Psychologic distress remained high.

The presence of multifidus muscle changes associated with herniated discs includes segmental muscle atrophy, type 2 fiber atrophy, and internal structure abnormalities in type 1 fibers.[93] The significance of these changes has been demonstrated. Rantanen et al.[94] found clinical outcome correlated with multifidus muscle biopsy findings at 5-year follow-up assessment. Only in the positive outcome group did the type 2 fiber diameter expand, compared with the values obtained at the time of operation. In the negative outcome group, no expansion of the type 2 fiber diameter was seen. The negative outcome group also demonstrated a higher frequency of type 1 fiber internal structure abnormalities. These results were interpreted to indicate that the negative outcome group's muscle biopsy changes represented insufficient muscle exercise. However, an alternative explanation could be that joint pathology and associated AMI resulted in persistent symptoms and muscle atrophy.

Flexibility

Hamstring tightness showed prognostic value for recurrent back pain in four of five studies that assessed this parameter.[62] Lumbar extension ROM was predictive of recurrent LBP in one study. Lateral flexion range had prognostic value in one of two studies assessing this parameter. However, there was a wide overlap of scores between those who eventually had low back problems and those who did not.[62]

Kahlil et al.[163] assessed stretching in chronic LBP patients by randomizing a group of patients in a multidisciplinary pain program to back and leg stretch, with the controls receiving only the multidisciplinary back program. Those receiving stretch demonstrated a greater reduction in pain levels and a greater increase in back extensor strength gains.

Coordination

Soderberg and Barr[95] studied surface EMG activation of the trunk musculature in chronic back pain patients compared with controls. They found that subjects with chronic LBP did not activate abdominal musculature and extensor musculature during Valsalva as much as controls. Extensors were also not activated as much during sit-ups in LBP patients. In contrast, back extensor muscle activity was increased in chronic LBP patients when they performed toe touch and straight-leg lifts, compared with controls.

King et al.[96] applied a sudden external load to chronic LBP patients and controls monitored with EMG of the back extensors. Controls responded with a burst-quiet-tonic EMG pattern, whereas chronic LBP patients did not demonstrate this response.

Proprioception

Proprioception has been shown to be impaired in those with nonspecific chronic LBP when compared with healthy controls. Niles and Sinnott[97] found that those with back pain stand with their center of force (COF) posterior and have difficulty implementing a conservative strategy to maintain uprightness when their balance is challenged. This posterior COF causes the patient to flex the hips and back to move the COF instead of using ankle adjustments. Parkhurst and Burnett found back injuries correlated with proprioceptive deficits in the coronal and sagittal planes and in multiple planes.[98] Deficits in proprioception have also been demonstrated in those with chronic cervical pain.[99] Also, many other joints have been shown to have lower proprioception after injury.[98] This is probably a result of damage to afferent nerves from trauma[100] or due to a combined effect with AMI.

Some authors have cited evidence for cutaneous and muscle receptors being more important than joint receptors in proprioception.[101] Because there is widespread convergence of muscle, joint, and cutaneous receptors onto ascending tracts in the central nervous system, it appears that all play a role in proprioception.

Cardiovascular

When comparing subjects with treated or resolved herniated discs with age- and sex-matched controls, the groups differed in relationship to a single physiologic characteristic—maximal oxygen consumption.[102,103]

EXAMINATION

The basic neuromusculoskeletal examination is presumed to be part of the armamentarium of physicians rehabilitating the lumbar spine and its related disorders. A nice review is presented by Rodriguez and Gilbert.[104] In addition to strength, sensation, reflex, special tests (SLR, etc.), and ROM testing, passive joint mobility testing is advocated by a number of clinicians who are convinced of its reliability and clinical utility.[105–108]

Intervertebral motion segment disturbances consist of hypermobility and motion restriction (hypomobility). The clinical characteristics include changes in quantity and quality of movement. Restricted mobility in an extremity joint is easily assessed. It is more difficult to assess single motion segment abnormalities in the spine, however.

The most discussed exam finding on segmental spine assessment is lack of springing in the end position of a restricted joint (often termed *posteroanterior* [PA] displacement or mobilization). In a normal joint, the extreme range is not reached abruptly. Rather, a slight increase in pressure increases ROM (springing). In a joint with restricted mobility, springing is lost. Springing is a reflection of joint play when one joint surface shifts or slides, relative to another.

Even though a segment may be restricted, functional mobility may remain normal. These springing techniques are thought to be not only diagnostic but also the most effective way of restoring normal mobility. These techniques have been shown to result in increases in PA displacements.[109]

Restricted motion in a vertebral motor segment results in reflex changes at the same spinal segment. These reflex changes affect the dermatome and muscle, a process called *segmental facilitation* resulting in muscle hypertonus and decreased pain threshold. Motion segment restriction is probably ultimately an articular phenomenon, although many tissues contribute to the motion segment restriction. Muscle spasm usually is known to be a reflex response, with the stimulus for this response derived from the joint.

Hypomobilities can result from impairment of soft-tissue supporting structures such as muscles (decreased compliance or fascial restriction) or from intrinsic components of the three-joint complex. Adjacent hypomobile segments can cause increased stress on an injured segment. Hypermobility may result adjacent to hypomobile segments and may result in pain and tenderness at the hypermobile segment.

Evidence of the significance of this examination derives from a number of lines of reasoning and clinical evidence. Hides et al.[55] found in 92% of cases of unilateral LBP there were matches between physical therapists' assessments of symptomatic levels and the levels as determined by localized muscle atrophy detected by ultrasound. In another study, manual examination accuracy as assessed by physical therapists was tested against nerve or facet block.[110] There was a high level of sensitivity and specificity of manual examination in identifying the symptomatic level. A similar study comparing manual examination to discography in determination of symptomatic level found high sensitivity and specificity of the manual exam.[111] Maher and Adams[112] found segmental pain provocation tests to be highly reliable, whereas segmental stiffness assessment was not sufficiently reliable.

SPECIFIC CLINICAL LESIONS

Acute Muscle Strain/Contusion

Review

Muscle can be injured in a number of ways, including unaccustomed eccentric exercise, acute trauma, and acute muscle strain. Thus far, most studies of muscle injury involve the peripheral and not the axial musculature. The following discussion pertains to extremity muscle injury.

Delayed-onset muscle soreness (DOMS) generally follows repetitive eccentric exercise. Muscle strain damage is contingent on violent force against resistance. Both types of muscle injury tend to occur at the myotendinous junction (MTJ). Acute muscle strain occurs there exclusively. It is unknown how often muscle strain injury is the type of injury in what is generally considered mechanical or idiopathic LBP.

Acute muscle strain has been assessed radiographically and histologically. The strain injury is characterized by inflammation, edema, and hemorrhage. Radiographic imaging with CT and MRI have localized a strain injury to one muscle among a group of synergists, and the strain lesion occurs predictably at the MTJ.[113] Follow-up CT and MRI clearly demonstrate atrophy, fibrosis, and calcium deposition.[113] Histologic studies also demonstrate injury near the MTJ. Although muscle cells are syncytial and extend far into the muscle belly, the response to this injury is limited to a focal area near the MTJ.[114] In an animal model, experimental muscle strain injury acutely resulted in a contractile force generation, which was 33% of control values.[115] Peak tensile loads for the experimental muscle strain were 63% of controls'. These findings suggest that, even in severely injured muscle, there is enough structural strength for the

muscle to participate in functional rehabilitation with low-force exercises to prevent muscle atrophy, maintain tone, and maintain ROM with gentle stretch.[115] Because contractile force is reduced, the strained muscles have a functional deficit, which probably increases the risk of further muscle injury.

Delayed-onset muscle soreness typically occurs 24–48 hours after eccentric exercise, although it may occur to a lesser degree after concentric exercise. It has been assessed radiographically and histologically. Magnetic resonance imaging of DOMS demonstrates increased signal intensity in multiple muscles. A peripheral rim of increased signal intensity throughout the length of the muscle or a diffuse pattern of increased signal intensity is noted.[116] The initial response appears to be due to disruption of proteins within 48 hours, followed by inflammation about 5 days later.[117] Muscle and connective tissue damage occur after intense eccentric exercise, although this is not related to symptoms on a temporal basis. It may be that inflammation subsequent to damage is responsible for DOMS.[118]

Another described muscle injury pertaining to the spine is compartment syndrome of the lumbar paraspinal muscles. DeFazio et al.[119] described a case of severe LBP that began after prolonged skiing. The patient was found to have elevated creatinine phosphokinase, significantly elevated compartment pressures, abnormal erector spinae muscle signal intensity on MRI scans, and an otherwise negative workup. Symptoms were severe enough to continue hospitalization for six days, and the patient had mild symptoms persisting for some months. Acute compartment syndrome affecting the erector spinae muscles is uncommon and is not thought to require surgical decompression. One case of chronic compartment syndrome of the paravertebral muscles that responded to fasciotomy has been described.

- *Method of Presentation*—Acute traumatic injury. A tearing sensation while lifting or other traumatic event. Repetitive overload.
- *Tissue Injury Complex*—Muscle tissue or TLF. Myofibrilar damage involving the Z-band, sarcomere disruption, and localized contracted tissue.
- *Clinical Symptom Complex*—Localized lumbosacral discomfort.
- *Functional Biomechanical Deficit*—Segmental hypomobility of the three-joint complex secondary to muscle spasm and guarding. Delayed-onset muscle soreness after intense eccentric exercise has been shown to result in strength deficits that last at least 10 days. Regeneration takes longer than 10 days. Strength and ROM deficits have been shown to persist after pain has resolved.
- *Functional Adaptation Complex*—Loss of active and passive segmental and combined motions.
- *Tissue Overload Complex*—Muscle myofilament.

Rehabilitation

Strength training is commonly used in the rehabilitation of muscles affected by injury. Some studies suggest that strength training for isolated muscle groups may not be the most effective way to increase functional ability, and training may be better targeted to task-related training.[120] In an animal model following muscle injuries, immediate mobilization results in dense scar formation in the injury area, which prohibits muscle regeneration.[121] Immobilization for longer than one week results in marked atrophy of the injured muscle.

Initial treatment of muscle sprain should consist of limited periods of rest (less than three days). This should be followed by gentle activity and isometrics within the pain-free range, then a gradual increase in activities.

Modalities such as ice massage, cold packs, and electrical stimulation may be used for reduction of inflammation and muscle spasm. Treatment should then be directed to restoration of full strength, mobility, and posture. The first goal is to regain tissue flexibility and segmental motion. This is accomplished through a variety of techniques, including myofascial release, joint mobilization, stretching, and muscle energy techniques.

It is important to optimize function of the lumbar spine to maximize lower-extremity muscular flexibility. Gracovetsky and associates[23,66,122] have stressed the importance of balanced flexibility to optimize function of the lumbar spine. Poor flexibility will cause excessive stress to be transmitted to the lumbar motion segments and sacroiliac joints. (Typical inflexibility patterns are discussed in this chapter in the "Kinetic Chain" section). Tight hip flexors and quadriceps can cause extension and rotation hypermobilities in the lumbar spine. If the hip flexors are contracted, the pelvis is anteriorly tilted, which places the hip extensors at a mechanical disadvantage. Early recruitment of lumbar extensor muscles will then be necessary and results in excessive shear or torsion stress to the discs. Tight hip rotators influence the kinetic chain, causing increased stress to the sacroiliac joints, disc joints, and extensor muscular attachments.

Stretching techniques should be taught, the goal being to stretch with a neutral pelvic position to avoid excessive anterior or posterior tilt. After muscular flexibility is achieved, segmental lumbar motion should be assessed and treated. Assessment and treatment of hypomobile segments require precisely applied manual techniques.

Exercises to improve the function of the lumbar spinal muscles are generally referred to as *spine stabilization exercises*. Optimal strength can protect the spinal motion segment from acute dynamic overload and chronic repetitive shear stress. Spine-stabilizing exercises use force couple muscles acting in concert to provide a stable base, provide smooth motion, and produce efficient force transfer in the lumbar spine.[123] The five basic back support mechanisms include IAP, the TLF, the hydraulic amplifier mechanism, the posterior ligamentous system, and the muscular support system (see previous discussion). Intraabdominal pressure does not appear to improve with training.[22] Increased IAP does increase tension in the TLF. The TLF is actively engaged with contraction of the abdominal, hamstring, and gluteal muscles, which cause posterior pelvic tilt, thereby tensing the TLF. Passive engagement of the TLF occurs with lumbar flexion. The TLF provides important support during lifting in all postures. An increased antiflexion moment reduces the amount of intervertebral compression. A hydraulic amplifier mechanism also adds tension to the TLF by contracting the erector spinae and transversospinalis within the inelastic envelope of the TLF. This provides a further antiflexion moment. The posterior ligamentous system contributes to resistance of flexion. Making use of the ligaments during lifting reduces the compressive forces through the lumbar spine.[23] The muscular support mechanisms include the intersegmental muscles of the spine and the muscles that act on the pelvis and trunk,[124] as well as those that act through the TLF.

The intersegmental muscles act as tonic or postural stabilizers of the spine and tend to fatigue and atrophy first following injury. Initial stabilization exercises, therefore, are directed toward these muscles, which control individual segmental mobility. These exercises are typically manually resisted exercises of the trunk limited to short arcs. In addition, direct and indirect strengthening of muscle groups are performed at the midpoint between anterior and posterior pelvic tilt, a point termed *neutral*. Neutral spine position is a loosely packed position that is close to the center of reaction, allowing movement into flexion or extension readily. It also allows a more balanced force distribution between the discs and facets, provides the greatest functional stability with axial loading, and is generally the position of greatest comfort. After training in neutral spine and pelvic control, exercises of the extremities are added while maintaining neutral spine and pelvic control. Neutral spine techniques tend to strengthen the smaller postural stabilizers. Ultimately, strengthening is advanced to include abdominal muscles, erector spinae, lower extremity muscles, and trunk muscles. After strength training, cardiovascular conditioning is advised.

Delayed-onset muscle soreness has been the subject of multiple treatment trials. Ibuprofen has been shown in a small randomized study to be effective at reducing DOMS when given prior to exercise.[125] Ascorbic acid has also been shown to reduce DOMS in a double-blind randomized crossover study of 19 patients.[126] Other studies have shown cold application not helpful; ultrasound produced significant reductions in soreness; transcutaneous electrical nerve stimulator was studied without controls; topical analgesic antiinflammatory creams reduced DOMS; aspirin reduced DOMS; high-velocity isokinetic exercise in one study reduced DOMS, but soreness and strength loss were still present.[118]

Disc Herniation

Review

Sciatica is usually the first symptom leading to the suspicion of a herniated disc. The incidence of herniated disc is highest in young adults between the ages of 30 and 40 years. Typically, back pain occurs first, recurrences follow, then pain and paresthesia radiating to the leg indicate the onset of sciatica. Back pain may become less severe when leg pain develops.

Risk factors for disc herniation include: biomechanical factors such as repetitive rotational torsional stress;[127] acute or repetitive hyperflexion loading of the disc;[128,129] posture; occupation (sedentary, heavy manual labor, occupations requiring prolonged driving); obesity;[130] and cigarette smoking.[130]

Disc herniation may occur without symptoms. In a study of 98 patients, mean age of 42 years with no back or leg symptoms, 52% had a bulge at a minimum of one level; 27% had a protrusion, and 1% an extrusion. The prevalence of bulges increased with age, but the prevalence of protrusions did not.[25] In another study of asymptomatic subjects, the frequency of herniation increased with age, with herniations found in 20% in those under 60 years and 36% in those 60 years and older.[24] This reemphasizes the obvious: the clinical picture should be correlated with the MRI results. The presence of severe back pain and leg pain may occur without associated disc herniation. Although this knowledge has been available at least since 1956,[131] its republication appears to be thought significant. Symptoms that mimic a herniated disc without an anatomic herniation may occur, and it has been suggested that a chemical radiculitis may mimic discogenic radiculopathy without any imaging abnormalities. An animal model of this type of lumbar radiculopathy has recently been described.[132]

It is estimated that only 5–10% of patients with persistent sciatica will require surgery.[133] Spontaneous recovery occurs not only in leg pain but also in strength and sensory signs, although invasive treatments may accelerate their resolution. In a randomized trial that compared surgery with conservative treatment for herniated lumbar discs, the recovery of foot weakness was equivalent in the two treatment groups at 4-year follow-up.[9] The major advantage of surgery was more rapid pain relief and reduced relapse rate. Emergent surgery is required only for bowel and/or bladder incontinence.

More than 95% of lumbar disc herniations occur at L4–L5 or L5–S1. The natural history of herniated disc is for 75% to resolve spontaneously within 6 months. The cumulative risk of having a second proven herniated disc during the next 20 years postoperatively is 8%.[8]

Diagnosis includes exclusion of systemic disease as the cause of symptoms. The differential diagnosis of sciatica is broad and includes degenerative changes, spinal stenosis, spondylolisthesis, visceral disease (such as endometriosis), synovial cysts, congenital anomalies of the lumbar nerve roots, primary or metastatic cancer, and epidural abscesses.[130]

- *Method of Presentation*—Often acute injury occurring with flexion and rotation of the lumbar spine and history of previous episodes of LBP.
- *Tissue Injury Complex*—Annular fibers of the disc and chemical and/or mechanical irritation of the anterior and dorsal spinal root and/or posterior longitudinal ligament and other pain-sensitive intercanal and foraminal structures.
- *Clinical Symptom Complex*—Low back pain and leg pain, leg pain being usually much more pronounced than back pain when herniation of the disc occurs, versus more back symptoms when there is an annular tear without protrusion of the disc. Posterolateral herniations are the most common type of herniation, and symptoms are exacerbated by activities that increase intradiscal pressure. Disc herniation to the neuroforamina (far lateral disc) includes symptoms of leg pain in a radicular pattern with little or no back pain (there may or may not be neurologic involvement).[134] Exacerbants are typically standing, walking, lying down, and lumbar extension. Alleviants are sitting, lying in the fetal position, and knees to chest.
- *Functional Biomechanical Deficit*—Soft-tissue inflexibilities (muscle, fascia, ligament) due to spasm or tightness; segmental hypomobility. Segmental muscle atrophy, type 2 fiber atrophy, and internal structure abnormalities in type 1 fibers.[93]
- *Functional Adaptation Complex*—Loss of normal lumbopelvic rhythm, increased lumbar lordosis, increased loading of posterior elements, lateral pelvic shift.
- *Tissue Overload Complex*—Annulus fibrosis, nucleus pulposus, supporting paraspinal ligaments and musculature.

Rehabilitation

Education includes instruction in sitting (arm rests have been shown to decrease disc pressure up to 25%), standing posture (to maintain lordosis), and body mechanics. The goal is to protect injured structures and prevent further injury. Reviewing the specifics of activities of daily and nightly living is important, rather than simply discussing broad general concepts. Group education in patients with acute or chronic LBP does not appear to confer benefits at one-year follow-up.[135] However, it should not be concluded that education is unimportant in a comprehensive rehabilitation approach.

A short course of bedrest after an acute injury may be appropriate, although absolute bedrest longer than three days has not been demonstrated to be effective in reducing disability or dysfunction.[136] Note that this study assessed back pain and not radiculopathy.

Modalities can be effective during early stages in reducing pain and decreasing reflex muscle spasm. In the lumbar spine, cryotherapy and electrical stimulation do not reduce inflammation in the setting of disc herniation as neither can penetrate deep tissues. Therefore, even in the acute setting, it is irrelevant whether superficial heat or cold is used to reduce muscle spasm. However, ultrasound should be used cautiously in the setting of acute disc herniation as a number of reports have documented worsening of radiculopathy.[137]

Traction can be helpful in symptom management for acute discogenic LBP. Traction can be applied by manual, mechanical, inversion, and split table auto-traction techniques. Reduction of disc pressure by traction is only 20–30%. Traction may exert its effects by allowing vertebral body separation, decreasing compressive forces on nerve roots by increasing neuroforaminal size, improving blood flow to the nerve roots, and stretching spinal musculature. The force needed to adequately distract the vertebral bodies in a horizontal plane is 25–50% of body weight. Inversion traction carries a small risk of hypertension, headaches, gastrointestinal reflux, and ruptured berry aneurysm.

As discussed under the heading "Muscular Strength and Endurance," initial exercises are determined primarily by which motion produces less radicular and peripheral pain and does not significantly increase LBP. Back pain may increase as radicular symptoms become less peripheral. For acute disc injury, the activity that centralizes pain is typically extension, though flexion may be more appropriate in some cases.[58]

Lateral trunk shifts must be corrected before centralizing exercises begin. Patients often can be taught self-correction techniques. Usually, extension exercises are begun with the patient lying prone and supported under the stomach to maintain a neutral position. They are progressed (as tolerated) to the patient lying prone unsupported, to support under the chest, to prone on elbows, and then to press-ups. Repeated extension posturing in standing for use after sitting or flexion activities should be taught. Theoretically, extension exercises reduce pain by decreasing tension in nerve roots, reducing intradiscal pressure, promoting anterior migration of the nucleus pulposus, decreasing tension in the posterior

annular fibers, or increasing mechanoreceptor input activating the gate mechanism. Contraindications to extension exercises include segmental hypermobility, instability, large or uncontained herniation, increase in radicular sensory or motor deficits, bilateral sensory and/or motor signs, and significant increase in LBP unless associated with concomitant reduction in radicular pain. Exercises that increase pain should be avoided and other types of exercises prescribed.

If hypermobility exists at a segment adjacent to a disc herniation, manual therapy techniques may be helpful to avoid overstressing the hypermobile joint. Care must be taken to prevent secondary hypermobility at the thoracolumbar segment, which can occur if extension exercises are emphasized in a patient with lumbar segmental hypomobility.

Ultimately, neutral spine-strengthening exercises should be instituted, as discussed under the heading "Muscle Strain." After an acute disc injury, a transitional return to sport-specific activity may be required. Return to aerobic conditioning should be guided by those postures that centralize or diminish pain. For example, in an athlete who centralizes pain with extension exercises and whose symptoms increase with flexion, an appropriate regimen might be swimming, use of the cross-country ski machine, and walking.

A recent series of far lateral disc herniations found conservative therapy to be successful in 3 of 15 far lateral disc herniations.[134] Our success rate with conservative treatment of far lateral disc herniations is significantly higher than the described 20% success; however, we employ nerve root block in conjunction with comprehensive rehabilitation techniques. Extension exercises are inappropriate for these patients, due to extension typically being an exacerbant.

Acute Posterior Element Pain

Review

Acute posterior element pain is also known as *facet syndrome* or *dorsal compartment syndrome*. The diagnosis is usually based on the following common combination of clinical criteria: nearly continuous uni- or bilateral paravertebral pain, paravertebral tenderness, absence of objective neurologic signs, and pain provocation on hyperextension. Because these criteria are nonspecific, a positive diagnostic blockade must be added. Even a positive diagnostic block can give misleading information, however. Schwarzer et al.[143] found uncontrolled facet blocks performed on one occasion were associated with an unacceptably high rate of false-positive responses. Unfortunately, without specific and consistent criteria to diagnose facet syndrome, the incidence, natural history, and optimal treatment are impossible to know.

Revel et al.[144] found a discrete subpopulation of patients was identified based on response to facet injection and clinical variables. Their data suggested that facet joints are not commonly the single or primary cause of LBP. Interestingly, signs usually attributed to facet joint pathology, such as extension-rotation, were more frequent in patients who did not respond to the facet joint injections. A recent study by Schwarzer et al.[145] assessed 92 consecutive patients with discography and double blocks to the zygapophyseal joints at the most symptomatic level, based on palpation above and below this level. They found pain arising from the disc (36%) more common than pain arising from the facet joint (5%).

The diagnosis of facet syndrome has not been subject to randomized blinded trials among investigators to determine whether there is *interrater reliability of the diagnosis*. Nevertheless, facets are innervated by pain-sensitive fibers and remain a potential source of pain.

It does seem clear that the facet syndrome is not a common source of significant pain. Response to intraarticular injection does not correlate with or predict clinical results after solid posterior lumbar fusion, and it should not be used as a preoperative screening test.[146]

- *Method of Presentation*—Often acute injury occurring with extension and rotation of the lumbar spine, usually related to a torsional load on the spine.
- *Tissue Injury Complex*—Usually the zygapophyseal joints and surrounding synovium and joint capsule. Also the posterior longitudinal ligament of intraspinous and supraspinous ligaments may be involved.
- *Clinical Symptom Complex*—Nonradiating LBP or referred pain to the buttock or proximal thigh, rarely below the knee.
- *Functional Biomechanical Deficit*—Abnormal pelvic tilt and hip rotation secondary to tight hamstrings, hip rotators and quadratus, and weak erector spinae and hamstrings.
- *Functional Adaptation Complex*—If chronic, flattening or lumbar lordosis, rotation, or side bending at the sacroiliac or thoracolumbar area.
- *Tissue Overload Complex*—Initially synovium and capsule of zygapophyseal joints. When more chronic, articular cartilage of zygapophyseal joints.

Rehabilitation

The initial treatment stages for acute facet joint pain are similar to those for acute disc pain (education, relative rest, maintenance of positions that enhance comfort, cryotherapy, superficial heat, and exercises). In facet pain, flexion and neutral postures and exercises should be emphasized. Treatments that may reduce discomfort include hook lying and 90/90 traction. Important exercises include pelvic tilts to reduce the degree of lumbar lordosis. These should be performed in multiple positions (bent knees standing, straight-leg standing, sitting). Flexion exercises and pelvic tilts theoretically decrease facet joint compressive forces. Exercises that promote the above include stretch of hip flexors and lumbar extensors, and strengthening abdominal and gluteal muscles. Hamstring and hip internal and external rotator stretching is also essential.

Contraindications to flexion exercises are hypermobility or instability and increasing LBP or peripheralization of symptoms. Sustained or static traction should be avoided as this often exacerbates symptoms, probably from stretch of the facet joint capsule. Intermittent traction is preferable. The 90/90 position or inversion gravity traction may help unload the posterior elements, enhance joint lubrication and nutrition, and reduce pain through mechanoreceptor input.

Transition to increasing activities should emphasize stationary bicycling and use of stair climber machine and treadmill (at an incline). Prone lying should be avoided.

The role of facet injections in treatment has yet to be defined. Antiinflammatory medications and low-dose tricyclics may be useful adjunctive treatments.

Segmental Dysfunction/Somatic Dysfunction

Review

Potential sources of back pain include the ligaments, fascia, muscles of the lumbar spine, zygapophyseal joints, and intervertebral discs. Determination of which structure is the primary source of pain has been difficult. Some investigators endorse the concept of the three-joint complex, where pathology affects all three joints or some combination of the three joints. A recent study by Schwarzer et al.[145] assessed 92 consecutive patients with discography and double blocks to the zygapophyseal joints at the most symptomatic level, based on palpation above and below this level. They found that only 8% of the patients had both positive discograms and symptomatic zygapophyseal joint pain. Forty-nine percent suffered neither discogenic pain nor zygapophyseal joint pain. They found pain arising from the disc (36%) to be more common than pain arising from the facet joint (5%). Kuslich et al.[18] also found the disc to be the primary source of pain when various spinal structures were stimulated in patients undergoing spinal surgery for stenosis or herniated disc. Both the Kuslich and Schwarzer studies were done non–weight-bearing.

Segmental dysfunction denotes an injury to one or more components of the motion segments, which results in a series of compensatory changes that are identifiable and significant. These changes include lowered pain threshold, muscle hypertonus, segmental atrophy, reduced ROM, and "segmental facilitation." As discussed, there is growing evidence that validates the concept of segmental motion dysfunction, including the ability of physical therapists to predict the level of pathology, as confirmed by ultrasound of the multifidus[55] and as confirmed by selective injections.[108] Additionally, Denslow et al.[147] demonstrated a high degree of correlation between clinical palpatory examination and the motor reflex threshold determined by EMG. These segments with lowered motor reflex threshold have been termed *facilitated segments*. These muscles are predisposed to activity when other muscles are at rest; in a startle response, these muscles are the first to fire and the last to relax when compared with segments that do not have characteristics of "facilitation."[148] This latter response demonstrates the hyperresponsiveness of a facilitated segment to impulses reaching them from other sources of the body, including cerebral centers.

Segmental dysfunction is probably more appropriate as a diagnosis for the most common types of lumbar injury typically classified as "sprain." Most back injuries are not disc herniations, and facet pain is an uncommon source. Instead, segmental dysfunction encompasses a spectrum of injuries to one or more segment-related structures that can then result in a series of compensatory changes, including localized multifidus muscle atrophy,[55] decreased tissue compliance,[149] decreased pain threshold (tenderness),[148,149] altered segmental motion, muscular imbalances,[75,79] segmental facilitation,[148] and proprioceptive deficits.[97]

Theories proposed to explain the phenomenon of joint hypomobility include entrapment of synovial material or a synovial meniscoid between the joint; lack of congruence of articulating surfaces; altered physical and chemical properties of synovial fluid and synovial surfaces; altered tone and length of muscle (may be primary or secondary in the dysfunctional segment); and biochemical or biomechanical changes in motion segment structures.

Articular dysfunction is characterized by loss of joint "play" and/or normal mobility. Articular dysfunction causes musculoskeletal pain that is typically associated with a localized reduced pain threshold (tenderness) and reduced muscle compliance (increased tension or "spasm"). Joint dysfunction may be the initial cause or the perpetuator of myofascial pain, or vice versa. Dysfunctions in the vertebral column are considered single-level or group dysfunctions involving three or more vertebrae. Unfortunately, it is not known whether these two types of dysfunction have different natural histories.

- *Method of Presentation*—Often acute injury occurring with flexion and rotation of the lumbar spine with history of previous episodes of LBP that usually resolve unremarkably within three to five days.
- *Tissue Injury Complex*—Annular fibers of the disc and chemical and/or mechanical irritation of the anterior and dorsal spinal root and/or posterior longitudinal ligament and other facet and foraminal structures.
- *Clinical Symptom Complex*—Low back pain with a variable degree of regional referred pain.
- *Functional Biomechanical Deficit*—Soft-tissue inflexibilities (muscle, fascia, ligament) due to spasm or tightness, segmental hypomobility. Segmental muscle atrophy, type 2 fiber atrophy, and internal structure abnormalities in type 1 fibers.[93]
- *Functional Adaptation Complex*—Loss of normal lumbopelvic rhythm, increased lumbar lordosis, increased loading of posterior elements, lateral pelvic shift.
- *Tissue Overload Complex*—Annulus fibrosis, nucleus pulposus, supporting paraspinal ligaments and musculature.

Rehabilitation

Manual therapy techniques are appropriate for motion restrictions and hypomobility. Hypermobility should not be treated by manual techniques that attempt to increase mobility. The types of hypermobility are generalized hypermobility due to connective tissue disease, physiologic generalized hypermobility, localized joint hypermobility, and compensatory hypermobility due to hypomobility in adjacent areas of the spine. Often, the hypermobile segments become symptomatic because they compensate for adjacent motion segment restrictions.[150] These hypermobile segments then can become tender and painful. It is, therefore, important to treat the hypomobile segments to allow more uniform segmental motion and functional balance.[150] If significant hypermobility is suspected, flexion-extension X-rays are indicated to assess for instability.

Internal disc disruption/nonradicular back pain should be categorized as segmental dysfunction. A number of issues has clouded the universal acceptance of this diagnosis. Some authors have found that clinical results of fusion were related to the presence of bony union;[151] however, others have not found this association.[152–155] Advocates of the concept of internal disc disruption are advocates of the concepts of chemical, immunologic, and neural mediation of back pain.[156] The natural history, although poorly studied, has been thought to be one of ongoing chronic pain. However, a report of 36 patients who were considered confirmed surgical candidates by discography but who declined fusions assessed outcome to a mean of 4.9 years.[157] Sixty-eight percent were improved, 8% were unchanged, and 24% were worse. These outcomes are as good as those reported for surgery for this condition.

Treatment is extremely controversial, with some spine clinics rarely or never employing fusion for internally deranged discogenic back pain and some frequently employing fusion. Fischgrund and Montgomery reviewed fusion success and found that good outcome has varied from 30% to 90%. In another review, successful outcomes were noted in 16–95%.[158] They recommend patient selection criteria for fusion as disability for more than one year, failure of conservative treatment, and positive provocative discogram. The use of discograms in predicting fusion success is also controversial. We find fusion of limited value for our patients with internal disc disruption related to back pain.

Spondylolysis/Spondylolisthesis/Pars Interarticularis Injury

Review

Spondylolisthesis is categorized into multiple types: congenital, isthmic, traumatic, pathologic, and postsurgical.[159] Congenital subtypes are due to congenital anomalies of the lumbosacral junction or anomalies such as congenital kyphosis. The isthmic subtype is a fracture at the pars interarticularis. Lytic spondylolisthesis is due to pars stress injury or fracture and is rarely seen in people younger than five years of age. There is an increased incidence of spina bifida in the young athlete with fresh pars fractures. The degenerative subtype is due to long-standing segmental instability with remodeling of the articular processes at the affected level. The pathologic subtype is due to localized or generalized bone disease and is a rare type. The postsurgical type is due to removal of too much supporting structure.

The natural history of the congenital subtype with axial-oriented facets and often spina bifida is that early olisthesis appears, slip may be severe, severe hamstring spasm is present, and these patients probably need fusion more frequently than do other subtypes.[159] The congenital subtype with sagittal facet orientation less frequently demonstrates high-grade slip; iatrogenic stimulus is frequently leg pain, back spasm, hamstring spasm, and altered gait; cauda equina caudal to L5 may occur; and fusion may be needed.

Isthmic subtypes usually present in the first years of school. This subtype can occur into early adulthood in people participating in certain sports. Most high grades of slip develop during the age span of 10–14 years. High-grade slip is much more frequent in girls, but pars defects are more common in boys. The iatrogenic stimulus is frequently back and leg pain. When this subtype occurs in the absence of a dysplastic sacrum or elongation, this subtype is unlikely to progress during growth. Olisthesis up to 10% does not appear to increase the likelihood of back problems, but beyond 25%, it does increase the likelihood of low back symptoms, as does wedging of L5.[159]

Degenerative spondylolisthesis is common in the elderly, and women are more commonly affected than men. Pain includes a neurogenic claudication type and a sciatic type with unilateral leg pain. Slip rarely progresses beyond 33%. Foot drop may occur but sciatic tension signs are usually absent. Most patients can be treated nonoperatively but refractory symptoms may respond to surgery.

The following pertains to the more common pars stress reaction and isthmic spondylolysis/spondylolisthesis.

- *Method of Presentation*—Chronic overload injury.
- *Tissue Injury Complex*—Pars interarticularis, unilateral or bilateral, usually at L4 and L5, where maximum loading and shear occur. These pars lesions include pars stress reaction, isthmic spondylolysis, and spondylolisthesis. A pars stress reaction is a bony irritation to the pars interarticularis without a lytic lesion.[160] This lesion may progress to a true spondylolysis. Spondylolisthesis occurs if a spondylitic defect is bilateral and forward slippage of the superior vertebral body on the one below occurs.
- *Clinical Symptom Complex*—Localized lumbosacral discomfort, worse with extension and partially relieved with flexion. More commonly seen with activities of repetitive flexion, extension, and rotation. Neurologic examination is usually normal.
- *Functional Biomechanical Deficit*—Hamstring tightness.
- *Functional Adaptation Complex*—Loss of lumbar lordosis.
- *Tissue Overload Complex*—Pars interarticularis.

Rehabilitation

Multiple microfractures may progress to a bone defect. If a pars injury is suspected clinically, a radiographic workup is indicated that includes pain films and a single photon emission computed tomography (SPECT) scan. Even when plain X-ray demonstrates a pars defect, a bone scan can be helpful in documenting acuity. An X-ray may not reveal pars interarticularis injury, and if clinical suspicion is high, a SPECT scan should be considered (the gold standard for diagnosis).

Some controversy exists about management, ranging from rest to rigid immobilization. Micheli[161] recommends a rigid polypropylene brace (modified Boston Overlap Brace), constructed in zero degrees of lumbar flexion, prescribed for 23 hours per day for up to 6 months. Unilateral pars defects may have a greater chance of healing than do bilateral defects. The presence of a bilateral pars defect shown on plain X-ray may significantly decrease the chance for bony healing, even with immobilization. An abnormal SPECT scan with normal X-rays may indicate a greater chance of healing and warrants longer immobilization. If back pain persists despite bracing and rehabilitation, surgery may be considered. A report from one large series demonstrated that MRI grading of the spondylolysis was of prognostic significance for responding to conservative therapy.[162]

Most patients with isthmic spondylolysis/spondylolisthesis will benefit from initial nonsurgical treatment. In cases of symptomatic spondylolisthesis, one should rule out other causes of back pain, such as infection, herniated disc, and tumor, prior to considering treatment programs. Disc degeneration occurs more frequently in spondylolisthesis than in controls. Symptoms are usually minimal if the slip is less than 30% and conservative treatment consisting of restricted activities and temporary corset or brace can be instituted. Persistent symptoms, severe slip, and a high degree of slip angle require surgical consideration.

Sinaki et al.[163] assessed symptomatic patients with spondylolisthesis who were treated conservatively by either flexion or extension exercises. At three-year follow-up, only 19% of the flexion group had moderate or severe pain, whereas 67% of the extension group had moderate or severe pain. The above study makes sense from a biomechanical standpoint, where extension causes increased stresses to the posterior elements and therefore affects symptomatic spondylolisthesis.

Articular Dysfunction

Review

The role of the sacroiliac (SI) joint in LBP is speculative. The First Interdisciplinary World Congress on Low Back Pain and Its Relation to the Sacroiliac Joint was held in 1992. The mechanisms whereby the SI joint might cause pain are not known but speculation includes degenerative changes, strain of supporting ligaments, and joint subluxation. The SI joint is a diarthrodial joint with the highest coefficient of friction of any human joint. Innervation is via lateral branches of the posterior primary ramus from L4 to S3, which allows a perception of referred pain patterns in the distribution of these nerves. The joint is surrounded by dense ligamentous structures. The gluteus maximus and piriformis and a portion of the biceps femoris are continuous with sacral ligaments. Stressing the above muscles could, therefore, stress sacral structures. The erector spinae and multifidus connect to the posterior iliac ligaments via the TLF.

The SI joint moves an average of two degrees, with most motion created by hyperextension. Symptomatic joint sides in patients with presumed SI dysfunction showed no asymmetry in amount of motion radiographically.[164]

The suggested incidence of SI dysfunction in LBP varies from 8% to 98%.[142] The natural history is elusive, with this variation in incidence. Evaluation of the SI joint is evolving and will allow better definition of its incidence, natural history, and role in LBP. Tests for SI joint dysfunction that use palpation are considered unreliable.[142,165] A series of motion and provocation tests described by Laslett and Williams[165] appears to provide good interrater reliability in diagnosing SI joint dysfunction. SI joint injection may be the most precise manner with which to localize the source of SI pain, as SI pain is resistant to identification by historical and physical examination data.

- *Method of Presentation*—Acute onset, as with stepping off curb or lifting heavy object in twisted position.
- *Tissue Injury Complex*—Sacroiliac joint and/or supporting structures.
- *Clinical Symptom Complex*—Severe pain over the SI joint and sometimes groin pain.
- *Functional Biomechanical Deficit*—Abnormal lumbo-pelvic rhythm.
- *Functional Adaptation Complex*—Leg length discrepancy, soft-tissue inflexibilities.

Rehabilitation

A multifactorial approach should be considered, including strengthening those muscles influencing the SI joint, manipulation to produce reflex reduction in muscle tone, and hyperflexion self-mobilization of the hip to displace the ilium posteriorly, relative to the sacrum.[142,166]

Corticosteroids injected into the SI joint may be appropriate. In 72 patients who underwent SI injection for presumed SI dysfunction, satisfactory pain relief was achieved in 81% at 9-month follow-up.[167] Sacroiliac belts may affect the sacral-pelvic alignment and result in pain relief and reduced motion.

Coccydynia is defined as pain in and around the coccyx and should be defined as a symptom as the underlying pathophysiology is not understood.[168] Though the pathophysiology is unclear, this syndrome appears to best fit into the articular dysfunction rubric. Studies are unavailable as to frequency, natural history, and intra- and interrater reliability of diagnosis. Due to the very localized tenderness, interrater reliability is probably high. Rare causes include trauma and localized pathology (intra-osseous lipoma, chordoma, giant cell tumor, etc.). However, in the majority of cases, the etiology remains obscure, despite extensive assessment, including bone scan, CT scan, and psychologic evaluation[169]—all of which are typically normal. Hypotheses include pressure over an unusually prominent coccyx, ligamentous inflammation, referred pain from a lumbar disc, neuralgic state from irritated sacral nerves, and neurosis. The best-studied series was presented by Wray et al.[169] Their criteria for diagnosis was coccydynia as the main complaint, and they did not state whether pain was necessarily reproduced on palpation, although they do note that a nontender coccyx was most unusual. In our experience, a very-well-localized area of tenderness is demonstrable over the distal sacrum. Wray et al.[169] found in their treatment of 120 patients that injection and manipulation were significantly more effective than physiotherapy. Most patients responded to conservative therapy (85%), with the remainder responding with excellent results to coccygectomy.[21,23]

Bertolotti's syndrome is a pseudoarticulation of the L5 transverse process to the sacrum. In population-based studies, these lumbosacral segmentation abnormalities have not been associated with increased frequency of pain.[170] Nevertheless, in individual cases, their potential in causing symptoms should be considered. If symptoms improve with injection and fail to respond with placebo injection, resection can be considered.

Baastrup's disease is an uncommon cause of persistent LBP where impingement of adjacent spinous processes limits motion in extension. A periostitis may develop here with severe or repetitive trauma and is also known as *kissing spines*. Localized pain is noted over the interspinous ligament, with exacerbants being extension and alleviation with injection at this site but not at nearby paraspinous sites. In one large study, only 11 of 64 patients responded to surgical treatment,[171] so this condition either responds poorly to surgery or diagnosis and patient selection are difficult.

Myofascial Pain

Review

Myofascial pain syndrome (MPS) due to trigger points (TrPs) is complex, with as yet incompletely defined pathophysiology. The criteria for the diagnosis are currently the presence of five major criteria and at least one of three minor critera.[172] Major criteria are localized muscle pain; spontaneous pain or altered sensations in the expected referred pain area for a given TrP; taut, palpable band in an accessible muscle; exquisite, localized tenderness in a precise point along the taut band; and some degree of reduced ROM when measurable. Minor criteria are reproduction of spontaneously perceived pain and altered sensations by pressure on the tender point; elicitation of a local twitch response of muscular fibers by transverse "snapping" palpation or by needle insertion into the tender point; and pain relieved by muscle stretching or injection of the tender point.

Objective or semiobjective modifications at the site of the TrP have been defined at multiple tissue layers.[173] At the skin, there is increased temperature over the TrP on thermography, a prolonged ischemic phase of dermographism, and a decreased pain threshold to mechanical and electrical stimuli. In the subcutaneous tissue and muscle, there is a decrease in pain threshold to mechanical and electrical stimuli. In muscle, there is an increase in temperature for a maximal

duration of 60 seconds after the insertion of a needle thermocouple. These findings have been reproduced in healthy controls with experimental induction of a TrP in skeletal muscle.[174]

Questions have been raised regarding the reliability of aspects of the trigger point examination.[175,176] The distinction between fibromyalgia and MPS has been called into question, based on the similarity of findings in these two groups.[175] Reliability assessments of the diagnosis of MPS are required, as well as training to improve observer concordance. Active and/or latent trigger points are regarded by some as hypothetical concepts for which other explanations are possible, including pathogenesis by referred axial skeletal pain or neurogenic abnormality. Referred pain from these structures could account for muscle hyperesthesia.

The epidemiology of myofascial pain is difficult to know, due to the questions about reliability of diagnosis. Sola et al.[177] assessed 100 female and 100 male Air Force airmen and found 12.5% to have TrPs.

- *Method of Presentation*—Acute and/or chronic overload when skeletal muscle is the source of pain. The parietalization phenomena of visceral pain may result in apparent MPS.
- *Tissue Injury Complex*—Skeletal muscle or other.
- *Clinical Symptom Complex*—Localized lumbar spine pain with or without regional referral.
- *Functional Biomechanical Deficit*—Reduced ROM, increased tissue compliance, and sympathetic hyperactivity.
- *Functional Adaptation Complex*—Abnormal lumbopelvic rhythm.
- *Tissue Overload Complex*—Myofilament.

Rehabilitation

Myofascial pain syndromes are described in many texts. Diagnostic criteria are well described: Their diagnostic criteria have not been shown to be as reliable as, for example, criteria for fibromyalgia syndrome (FS). Also, opinions vary as to the frequency of MPS. Some authors note they are an uncommon cause of back pain, whereas others report their frequent occurrence.[178] Kirkaldy-Willis et al.[178] report that 50% of the lesions seen in cases of LBP over a 10-year period derive from myofascial syndromes, posterior facet joint syndrome, or SI joint syndrome.

The most commonly described myofascial syndromes include gluteus medius syndrome, piriformis syndrome, quadratus lumborum syndrome, gluteus maximus syndrome, tensor fasciae latae syndrome, and hamstring syndrome. Diagnostic criteria include pain and local tenderness in an area characteristic for each muscle. There is often referred pain in a characteristic distribution for each muscle. However, intra-

and interobserver reliability of these separate syndromes has not been established.

These syndromes may be confused with disc herniation or lateral stenosis. It is unknown how often these syndromes are referral pain patterns from articular dysfunction, disc herniation, etc., as opposed to distinct clinical entities. Injecting the tender site and abolishing symptoms can occur whether the pain is referred or muscle-based.

We have certainly seen cases similar to the series presented by Ingber,[179] where failure to recognize iliopsoas myofascial dysfunction results in "failed" LBP syndrome. As soon as treatment is directed to the iliopsoas, improvement is rapid. In this syndrome, it appears to be particularly important not to ignore the myofascial component, even though the syndrome is probably due to referral from lumbar spine segmental dysfunction.

A trigger point of the posterior iliac crest has been described by numerous authors, with various interpretations of its significance. It has been described as Mainge syndrome, iliac crest syndrome, multifidus triangle syndrome, and iliolumbar ligament syndrome. The syndrome has been characterized by localized tenderness—unilateral or bilateral—and normal neurologic exam. In a series of seven patients, Fairbank and O'Brien[180] described consistent response to local infiltration of anesthetic. Their criteria for diagnosis included the localizable tender point and normal neurologic exam, and their case had pain with all ranges of spinal motion. They hypothesize by correlating anatomy to the site of maximal tenderness that the underlying pathology is periosteal irritation at the origins of gluteus maximus and sacrospinalis muscles. Fairbank and O'Brien did not find thoracolumbar segmental dysfunction, as discussed by Maigne (see below). Bauwens and Coyer[181] described a similar group of 20 patients who responded to local injection. Other explanations of the significance of this tender point have included iliolumbar syndrome, described by Hackett.[182] He included pain on contralateral bending in the diagnosis. Maigne[183] hypothesized that pain at this site was referred from the thoracolumbar facets in the past with focal pain in the area of the dermatome corresponding to cutaneous dorsal rami of T12 or L1, maximal at the posterior iliac crest. Confirmation of painful facet at the thoracolumbar junction was by reproduction of pain to pressure over these facets, and anesthetic infiltration around the involved joint relieved the LBP. Maigne and Maigne[182] dissected 37 cadavers to examine the above painful site. The iliolumbar ligament was found to insert deep into the ventral margin of the iliac crest shielded by the crest dorsally. The crest was crossed by two or three lower thoracic or upper lumbar dorsal cutaneous rami often passing though an osseofibrous orifice, comprised of the TLF and the superior rim of the iliac crest. They found in two cases that this resulted in nerve compression. They postulate that this tender point derives either as referred pain from the thoracolumbar junction (making this syndrome a type of segmental dysfunction) or from local compression or irritation of the dorsal rami (a nerve compression syndrome).

Trigger point treatment includes treatment of perpetuating factors (postural dysfunction, segmental dysfunction) and treatment techniques that increase tissue compliance and ROM (mobilization, TrP injection, strengthening exercises, stretch, low-dose tricyclics, massage, modalities, and muscle energy techniques). Appropriate techniques include the previously discussed neutral spine-stabilization protocol.

Fibromyalgia

Review

Fibromyalgia syndrome is a subtype of chronic pain that has been scrutinized in a multicenter blinded controlled study.[184] The syndrome is characterized by generalized pain, sleep disturbance, fatigue, and stiffness, although the latter three symptoms are concurrently present in only 56% of patients. Interobserver reliability of the diagnosis has been shown to be excellent.[175] Underlying pathophysiology is unknown.

Population-based studies suggest that about 1% of randomly selected persons have FS, and 15–30% of patients presenting to rheumatology clinics have FS. Women are affected more commonly than are men, at a ratio of 5:1. The natural history of FS in three- to five-year follow-up studies is one of little to no improvement. Lumbar pain is present in FS in 79–92% of patients. In one large series of FS patients, 12% of patients had spine surgery performed inappropriately as the diagnosis of FS was not considered.[185]

The criteria for diagnosis are pain above and below the waist, pain on both sides of the body, axial pain, pain greater than three months of duration, and eleven or more tender points present at designated tender point sites. Blinded examiners were able to discriminate between those with FS and controls who were matched for age, sex, and disorders that could be confused with FS. This diagnosis should be reserved for those patients who meet accepted criteria.

Among the objections to the fibromyalgia construct has been the lack of "objective" abnormalities. To deal with this concern the above multicenter study used examiners who were blinded, trained, and unaware of the diagnosis or physical findings of the patients they were categorizing. The study also used dolorimetry, which has been validated as providing objective data.[186]

Fibromyalgia often occurs in association with other rheumatic disorders, so physicians must seek out the other potential associated conditions. The effective treatment of these conditions may influence the management of FS.

- *Method of Presentation*—Either acute after trauma or insidious idiopathic.
- *Tissue Injury Complex*—Central, peripheral, and autonomic nervous system imbalance. If associated with hypermobility syndrome, also periarticular supporting structures.
- *Clinical Symptom Complex*—Pain and/or stiffness widespread but may be isolated to neck and back.
- *Functional Biomechanical Deficit*—Widespread decreased tissue compliance. Often with superimposed asymmetrical regional decreased tissue compliance.
- *Functional Adaptation Complex*—Decreased maximal oxygen uptake.
- *Tissue Overload Complex*—Neuroendocrine system. Periarticular supporting structures.

Rehabilitation

Treatment of FS should be individualized, depending on the magnitude and spectrum of symptoms, balanced with their effect on the individual. Unaccustomed physical activity and stress are almost universal exacerbants. Targeting these exacerbants from multiple vantages is critical. Additionally, since fibromyalgia is a chronic pain syndrome, strategies useful in chronic pain management are frequently applied. Caution is prudent when discussing the benefits of treatment. For example, exercise reduces pain in only a subpopulation of FS patients, with the remainder either unchanged or worse.

Education is the first and most important facet of treatment. Education should encompass knowledge about fibromyalgia including: the high quality of research defining it; basic theories about underlying pathophysiology; its nondeforming and generally nonprogressive nature; the fact that it is not associated with long-term development of other pathologic conditions; and exacerbants and alleviants for pain.

Educate the patient about the protean symptoms associated with fibromyalgia. However, also instruct the patient not to assume that all symptoms that could be fibromyalgia symptoms are fibromyalgia symptoms. For example, although hand numbness may occur with fibromyalgia, FS and carpal tunnel syndrome may coexist.

Commonly, patients with FS have had extensive workups, including MRI scans, and symptoms may have been incorrectly attributed to an entity such as a degenerated or herniated disc. Patients need to be told that 20–30% of pain-free subjects have abnormal MRI scans.[24]

General health issues are important. Smoking should be discouraged, due to its association with higher frequencies of many types of musculoskeletal problems including rotator cuff tears, degenerative disc disease, back pain, and cumulative trauma disorders. At a minimum, alcohol screening questionnaires should be administered to screen for alcoholism as alcoholism is known to adversely affect sleep stages,

increase risk of depression, and interact with medications used in FS. Associated conditions such as irritable bowel syndrome should be evaluated and treated.

Sleep dysfunction is extremely common in FS, with sleep demonstrating a hyperarousal pattern. Sleep hygiene begins with improved habits. Patients should go to sleep and wake at the same time every night and morning; avoid caffeine, especially in the evening; use the bed for sleep, not television; ensure a quiet ambiance that may require use of ear plugs or moving to a quieter room. Soporific antidepressants may have a significant impact on hyperarousal states and may improve non-REM sleep. Drugs that commonly disrupt sleep include appetite suppressants, antiemetics, drugs that exacerbate sleep apnea (benzodiazepines), corticosteroids, and clonidine. Beta blockers have variable effects on sleep, with lipid-soluble drugs more likely to enter the brain and affect sleep.

Exercise has been found to have modest effects on some symptoms of fibromyalgia. Exercise did not affect pain scores, but global assessment ratings improved in those who exercised compared to a stretch control group. More of those in the exercise group noted a marked improvement in symptoms than in the stretch control group; however, this result did not reach statistical significance. Other support for the concept of exercise derives from studies in which fibromyalgia symptoms could be induced much more readily in unfit than in physically fit subjects.

Psychologic intervention may be helpful in patients who have severe symptoms or those with poor ability to cope or function and also those with anger and hostility. Pain management techniques may be indicated, as discussed under the heading "Chronic Pain Disability Syndrome."

As in chronic LBP, depression in FS occurs at a frequency two to three times that of the general population. Fibromyalgia patients tend to have an external locus of control rather than an internal locus of control. If repeated exacerbations occur without apparent cause, psychologic assessment should be considered to assist with identifying potential exacerbants.

Fibromyalgia patients whose symptoms develop after a specific traumatic event frequently feel that their plight is another person's fault. This belief needs to be identified and dealt with early. Because FS developing after a traumatic event (reactive fibromyalgia) is more likely to result in disability than is primary FS,[187] all patients with reactive FS should be identified early and multidisciplinary management instituted at the earliest sign of dysfunction in social, vocational, psychologic, or medical function.

Biofeedback has been assessed, and promising results include the fact that those receiving true biofeedback demonstrated significant improvements in symptoms, whereas those in the sham group did not show significant improvements. A significant benefit was still seen at six-month follow-up.

Hypnotherapy was assessed in a small group of patients with long-standing severe fibromyalgia by randomizing the patients into groups receiving either hypnotherapy or PT. At three months after hypnotherapy ceased, subjective measures (pain, stiffness, fatigue, sleep disturbance) in the hypnotherapy group were significantly better than in those receiving PT.

The most commonly used and best-studied medications are tricyclics (at doses lower than those effective in depression) and cyclobenzaprine (a muscle relaxer with a chemical structure similar to the tricyclics). The above studies are short-term, controlled trials that show meaningful clinical improvement in 25–45% of FS patients. Improvement in sleep occurs more frequently than does reduction in pain. Benefit is typically noted within days up to four weeks.

Vertebral Compression Fractures

Review

Vertebral compression fractures (VCFs) related to osteoporosis occur in about 25% of U.S. women older than age 50. They result in acute pain, loss of general health, decreased mobility, and a progressive decline in quality of life.[188]

Osteoporotic VCF and compression fractures related to significant trauma should be conceptualized differently. With significant trauma, VCF (involving only the anterior vertebral column) should be distinguished from a burst fracture (involving two or all three columns of the spine) because they require different treatment strategies. Either fracture with neurologic compromise will need assessment for less conservative treatment.

Burst fracture characteristics on plain films include loss of posterior vertebral body height, disrupted posterior superior vertebral body line, and increased interpedicular distance. Despite these criteria, a burst fracture may occur and not show any of these radiographic features. Ballock et al. assessed whether plain films can predict burst fractures. They studied consecutive patients with the above diagnosis, and all underwent CT scan. They found no statistically significant difference between burst and compression fractures for amount of anterior wedging. Interpedicular widening was not seen in 45% of burst fractures; no loss of posterior cortical height was seen in 41% of burst fractures; and neither was present in 14% of burst fractures. There was also poor correlation between amount of wedging and amount of canal compromise. The results demonstrated that when using plain radiographs to distinguish burst versus compression fractures, about 20% of patients with potentially unstable burst fractures would have been mistakenly diagnosed as having stable wedge compression fractures. Therefore, routine CT scans of the spine are warranted in all patients with acute traumatic compression fractures. Treatment of neurologi-

cally intact burst fractures remains controversial, but immobilization casting in extension is frequently performed.

A VCF may be a symptomatic clinical event or a radiographic finding. A commonly defined radiographic definition of VCF is 15–20% reduction of anterior, posterior, or central height.[189] About 80% of osteoporotic VCFs are symptomatic. The three types of VCF are anterior wedge, biconcave, and crush deformity. When a fracture is suspected, X-rays of the lumbar spine are indicated. If there is a question about whether the fracture is new, bone scan may be helpful. However, bone scans may not be positive for up to one week, and they may remain positive for a long time after VCF. Solitary wedge compression fractures rarely occur above the seventh thoracic vertebra and, if seen, infectious and metastatic causes should be suspected.

Osteoporotic VCF may be caused by relatively light compressive forces, such as opening a window, cough, or boat ride. Acute VCF often produces incapacitating pain for weeks, but the pain may be severe for up to months. Chronic pain persists due to deformity of the vertebrae, with altered joint articulation and accelerated degenerative joint changes. Radicular pain may occur. Potential associated complications such as urinary retention, ileus, and rare cord compression should be assessed. Signs of cord compression from a retropulsed bony fragment include bilateral leg pain, paresthesia, incontinence, and motor weakness. These signs may appear weeks after the initial injury, so close follow-up is required.

- *Method of Presentation*—Acute injury related to significant trauma or minimal compressive load applied to a weakened osteoporotic vertebra.
- *Tissue Injury Complex*—Vertebral body, annulus fibrosis, nucleus pulposis. May have associated mechanical irritation of spinal root.
- *Clinical Symptom Complex*—Localized thoracolumbar pain or lumbar pain. Tenderness to palpation is usually present. Step-off may be present.
- *Functional Biomechanical Deficit*—Altered joint articulation, accelerated disc degeneration with segmental hypomobility. Soft-tissue inflexibilities (muscle, fascia, ligament) due to spasm or tightness. Weakening of extensor musculature.
- *Functional Adaptation Complex*—Progressive kyphosis, increased lumbar lordosis, and cervical lordosis. Loss of normal lumbopelvic rhythm.
- *Tissue Overload Complex*—Vertebral body.

Rehabilitation

Short-term goals include pain control and prevention of complications associated with immobility (pneumonia-incentive inspirometry, venous thrombosis leg exercises in home physical therapy). Pain control may require bed rest, antiinflammatory medications, narcotic analgesics, local analgesia (ice, heat), and bracing. Narcotic side effects in the elderly may be significant and should be carefully scrutinized. Bracing for lower lumbar VCF is commonly achieved with a wide lumbar support and Velcro™ closures; for lower thoracic VCF, a cruciform brace; for thoracic VCF, a modified Taylor brace. If there is a burst fracture or neurologic compromise, the above bracing will be inadequate, and less conservative treatment may need to be considered. Calcitonin is frequently used in the acute setting for analgesia and appears to be effective.[190,191]

Long-term goals include prevention of further VCF, prevention of medical complications, and prevention of disability. Further VCF may be prevented by extension exercises,[192] estrogen therapy,[191] calcitonin therapy,[191] exercise such as a walking program, and optimized dietary calcium (1,000–1,500 mg/day) and vitamins.[191] Prevention of medical complications includes vigilance for weight loss caused by early satiety from reduced abdominal cavity size; diminished lung volume and restrictive pulmonary disease; sleep disturbance; and development of spinal stenosis. Progressive kyphotic deformity appears to be retarded by extension exercises,[193] and this may prevent functional problems related to loss of height and postural alignment.

Thorough evaluation of the patient with osteoporotic VCF must include basic lab work, including a complete blood cell count, chemistry profile, liver profile, alkaline phosphatase, proteins, and kidney profile.[191] If anemia is present, proteins are abnormal, or pain persists, a serum protein electrophoresis should be performed. All parameters should be normal except for alkaline phosphatase, which may be elevated for 2–3 months. If vitamin deficiency is suspected, serum 25-OH vitamin D should be checked.[191] Some advocate a more aggressive workup at presentation.[194]

Other Fractures

Facet fracture is an uncommon cause of persistent LBP. There usually is a persistent nonunion of the fragments with no callus formation. Treatment may require facet joint fusion to assuage persistent pain.

Transverse process fracture has been noted after massive muscle contraction and trauma. Traumatic transverse process fracture requires a tremendous amount of force. Some advocate overnight hospitalization of the patient for close monitoring, including careful assessment of internal organs. Nonunion is common and generally not considered to be a cause of ongoing chronic symptoms.

Spinal Stenosis

Review

Diagnosis of spinal stenosis is based on the clinical syndrome of neurogenic claudication. This is generally defined as radiating pain in the buttocks and lower extremities exacerbated by standing or walking and relieved by lumbar flexion. Radiologic evidence of cauda equina compression must accompany symptoms.

Controversy as it relates to spinal stenosis exists regarding its pathogenesis and its natural history. Katz[195] states that the natural history appears to consist of insidious progression of pain and disability. This previous understanding appears to be giving way to another view as studies become more complete. More recent studies of the natural history of spinal stenosis suggest that, in many cases, observation and conservative therapy are an acceptable alternative to surgery. Johnsson et al.[196] followed 32 patients with spinal stenosis for a mean time of 49 months. Investigators found that symptoms in 70% were unchanged, 15% improved, and 15% worsened. Walking capacity was improved in 37% and worse in 30%.

Neurogenic claudication is insufficiently explained by the mere presence of either central canal stenosis or root canal stenosis.[197] This fact has led to the theory that ischemia due to multilevel stenosis may be responsible for neurogenic claudication.[197] Ooi et al.[198] demonstrated dilatation and venous engorgement of the cauda equina vessels when spinal stenosis patients walked on a treadmill. This result did not occur in the control group. Yazaki et al.[199] showed that venous congestion of the cauda equina was relieved after spinal flexion, followed by improvement of claudication symptoms. Some studies support a combined mechanical and ischemic component to neurogenic claudication.[200]

According to Turner et al.[201] the scientific quality of the literature regarding surgery for spinal stenosis precludes analysis of outcome predictors for surgery. In a metanalysis of the literature, it was reported that 64% of patients treated surgically for lumbar spinal stenosis had good-to-excellent outcomes.[201]

- *Tissue Injury Complex*—Mechanical and/or ischemic compromise of the cauda equina.
- *Clinical Symptom Complex*—Back pain, buttock pain, radiating lower extremity pain or dysesthesia that worsens with standing and walking.
- *Functional Biomechanical Deficit*—Loss of lumbar lordosis, relative posterior tilt of pelvis.
- *Functional Adaptation Complex*—Loss of active and passive segmental and combined motions, particularly in extension.
- *Tissue Overload Complex*—Intrinsic arterial and venous systems, neural structures.

Rehabilitation

Although conservative treatment of spinal stenosis has not been systematically assessed, some logical recommendations can be made. As with spondylolistheisis, extension makes spinal stenosis worse. Prescription of a program of flexion exercises along with exercises to decrease the lumbar lordosis (see the section on kinetic chain) could induce a small amount of flexion and allow retraining into postures that would allow improved function.

Willner[202] found that subjects with spinal stenosis responded much more favorably than those with idiopathic LBP to bracing. In all groups, a predictor of effectiveness to bracing was noted when the patient had absence of pain when standing in flexion and lying supine. Patients were braced in flexion in this study. Hawkes and Roberts[203] found corset use appeared to result in remission in six of nine patients, although it was difficult to distinguish their improvement from the natural history.

Lumbar epidural injections are used in spinal stenosis, presumably to reduce inflammatory mediators. However, results in patient groups have not yet been published.[204]

Nerve Entrapment

Review

Piriformis syndrome is another controversial diagnosis with proponents who argue its frequency and others who argue against its existence. This syndrome can be difficult to distinguish from discogenic disease. The piriformis muscle originates from the ventrolateral aspect of the sacrum and inserts on the greater trochanter. The piriformis muscle is bisected by the sciatic nerve peroneal division in 10% of cadavers. In 1%, both tibial and peroneal portions bisect the piriformis. The piriformis is an external rotator of the hip. In hip flexion, it also contributes to abduction of the hip. A review of piriformis syndrome by Rich and McKeag[205] suggests clinical features, which include: reproduction of pain on palpation of the piriformis; reproduction of pain on stretching the piriformis with the supine patient by flexing, adducting, and internally rotating the hip; and Freiberg sign with pain on forced internal rotation of the extended thigh. Rectal exams may reveal piriformis tenderness; the patient may stand or lie with externally rotated hip; reflexes are typically normal but there may be weakness of hip external rotation or abduction; SLR test may be negative or equivocal.

Fishman and Zybert[206] recently reported electrophysiologic evidence of piriformis syndrome. Their inclusion criteria included positive SLR at 45 degrees (contrary to the Rich and McKeag criteria), sciatic notch tenderness, increased pain with piriformis stretch, and EMG-excluded neuropathy. H-reflexes were assessed in the standard prone position and then in the lateral decubitus position with flexion, adduction, and internal rotation at the hip of the upside. Controls included the contralateral asymptomatic extremity and asymptomatic volunteers. Delayed conduction was as-

sessed in the two positions, and investigators found statistically significant differences between symptomatic and asymptomatic legs. Therefore, they suggest a mechanical impingement of the sciatic nerve as causing piriformis syndrome.

In a series of five cases successfully treated by surgery with piriformis resection, Hughes et al.[207] found all patients to have positive provocation of pain with resisted active external rotation of the hip from a position of full passive internal rotation. Most of their patients demonstrated abnormal function of the inferior gluteal and peroneal nerves but normal function of superior gluteal nerve on electromyography.

- *Method of Presentation*—Sequela of acute traumatic event localized to piriformis region or idiopathic.
- *Tissue Injury Complex*—Inflammation, edema, and fibrosis, resulting in local entrapment of the nerve.
- *Clinical Symptom Complex*—Sciatic notch tenderness, hip and buttock pain with occasional thigh and calf pain, production of pain by resisted active external rotation of the hip from a position of full passive internal rotation.
- *Functional Biomechanical Deficit*—Soft-tissue inflexibilities (muscle, fascia, ligament) due to spasm or tightness. Possible gluteus maximus atrophy.
- *Functional Adaptation Complex*—Lateral pelvic shift, ipsilateral relative external rotation, altered lumbopelvic rhythm.
- *Tissue Overload Complex*—Neural and perineural strucutres.

Rehabilitation

Most reviews appear to agree that conservative treatment is usually successful with correction of leg length discrepancy; stretch in flexion, abduction, and internal rotation of the hip; stretch of hamstrings and hip extensors; local anesthetic injection; ultrasound; and nonsteroidal antiinflammatory drugs. Studies of the spinal canal, SI joints, and hips with bone scan, MRI, and X-ray are needed so that conditions that mimic sciatic pain may be excluded.

Lumbosacral tunnel syndrome has been described as a compression of the L5 nerve root after it leaves the intervertebral foramen and crosses over the sacral ala under the iliolumbar ligament. Information about this condition is scant but may need to be considered in L5 radiculopathies when other causes have been excluded.

Chronic Pain Disability Syndrome

Review

This section is not meant to present a comprehensive evaluation and treatment approach to chronic pain disability syndrome. However, it is important to be able to quickly identify the at-risk patients. Patients must be approached from the standpoint of medical issues, physical deactivation, behavioral and belief systems, vocational issues, and support systems.

Criteria for multidisciplinary pain treatment include medical stability, definable patient goals, and one or more patient behavioral issues that need to be addressed by the program. These include physical deactivation, medication dependency, somatic preoccupation, superstitious behavior, environmental factors, role disruption, and depression. Chronic pain subgroups based on combinations of physical, psychosocial, and behavioral subgroups appear to be definable and warrant different treatment strategies.[208–211]

Chronic pain and depression frequently occur together. Depression alone in the setting of chronic pain does not necessarily or automatically indicate the need for a pain clinic. Approximately 18% of the population with chronic pain were found to have depression in contrast to 8% of the population without chronic pain.[212] In patients with clinical levels of depression, serious consideration should be given to targeting and treating depressive symptomatology.[213]

CONCLUSIONS

Many studies have demonstrated the high risk of recurrence of LBP. In musculoskeletal rehabilitation, the importance of complete rehabilitation after trauma to reduce the risk of new trauma has been claimed by many authors.[214] The number of deficits present in acute and chronic pain indicates the importance of achieving functional rehabilitation to restore optimum strength, coordination, flexibility, and proprioception.

REFERENCES

1. Cherkin DC, Deyo RA, Wheeler K, et al. Physician variation in diagnostic testing for low back pain. *Arthritis Rheum.* 1994;37:15–22.

2. Rush PJ, Shore A. Physician perceptions of the value of physical modalities in the treatment of musculoskeletal disease. *Br J Rheumatol.* 1994;33:566–568.

3. Cherkin DC, Deyo RA, Loeser JD, et al. An international comparison of back surgery rates. *Spine.* 1994;19:1201–1206.

4. Taylor VM, Deyo RA, Cherkin DC, et al. Low back pain hospitalization. *Spine.* 1994;19:1207–1213.

5. Kelsey JL, White A. Epidemiology and impact of low back pain. *Spine.* 1980;5:133.

6. Roland M, Morris R. The natural history of low back pain. Development of guidelines for trials of treatment in primary care. *Spine.* 1983; 2:141.

7. Urban JPG, McMullin JF. Swelling pressure of the lumbar intervertebral discs: influence of age, spinal level, composition, and degeneration. *Spine.* 1988;13:179–187.

8. Bruske-Hohlfeld I, Merritt JL, Onofrio BM, et al. Incidence of lumbar disc surgery. A population-based study in Olmsted County, Minnesota, 1950–1979. *Spine.* 1990;15:31–35.

9. Weber H. Lumbar disc herniation. A controlled, prospective study with ten years of observation. *Spine.* 1983;8:131–139.

10. Dvorak J, Gauchat MH, Valach L. The outcome of surgery for lumbar disc herniation. *Spine.* 1988;13:1418–1422.

11. Kahanovitz N, Viola K, Gallagher M. Long-term strength assessment of postoperative discectomy patients. *Spine.* 1989;14:402–403.

12. Mayer TG, Mooney V, Gatchel RJ, et al. Quantifying postoperative deficits of physical function following spinal surgery. *Clin Orthop.* 1988;233:198–204.

13. Nicholas M. The value of medical history and physical exam in diagnosing sacroiliac joint pain. *Spine.* 1996;21:2594–2602.

14. Malinsky J. The ontogenetic development of nerve terminations in the intervertebral discs of man. *Acta Anat.* 1959;38:96.

15. Giles LGF, Taylor JR. Innervation of the lumbar zygapophyseal joint synovial folds. *Acta Orthop Scand.* 1987;58:43–46.

16. Avramov AI. The effects of controlled mechanical loading on group-II, III, and IV afferent units from the lumbar facet joint and surrounding tissue. An in vitro study. *J Bone Joint Surg Am.* 1992;74:1465.

17. Yamashita J. Mechanosensitive afferent units in the lumbar facet joint. *J Bone Joint Surg Am.* 1990;72:865.

18. Kuslich SD, Ulstrom CL, Michael CJ. The tissue origin of low back pain and sciatica: a report of pain response to tissue stimulation during operation on the lumbar spine using local anesthesia. *Orthop Clin North Am.* 1991;22:181.

19. Bogduk N, Twomey LT. The lumbar muscles and their fascia. *Clinical Anatomy of the Lumbar Spine.* 2nd ed. Melbourne: Churchill Livingstone, 1991.

20. Farfan HF. The effects of torsion on the lumbar intervertebral joints: the role of torsion in the production of disc degeneration. *J Bone Joint Surg Am.* 1970;52:468.

21. Sullivan MS, Jantzen W. Enhancing back support mechanisms through rehabilitation. *Crit Rev Phys Med Rehabil.* 1990;2:39–47.

22. Hemborg B, Moritz Q, Hamberg J, et al. Intra-abdominal pressure and trunk muscle activity during lifting—effects of abdominal muscle training in healthy subjects. *Scand J Rehabil Med.* 1983;15:183.

23. Gracovetsky S, Farfan H. The optimum spine. *Spine.* 1986;11:543.

24. Boden SD, Davis DO, Din. Abnormal magnetic resonance scans of the lumbar spine in asymptomatic subjects: a prospective investigation. *J Bone Joint Surg Am.* 1990;72:403–408.

25. Jensen MC, Brant-Zawadzki MN, Obuchowski N, et al. Magnetic resonance imaging of the lumbar spine in people without back pain. *N Engl J Med.* 1994;331:69–73.

26. Graffin SR, Rydevik BL, Brown RA. Compressive neuropathy of spinal nerve roots. A mechanical or biological problem? *Spine.* 1991;16: 162–166.

27. Thelander U, Fagerlund M, Friberg S, et al. Straight leg raising test versus radiologic size, shape, and position of lumbar disc hernias. *Spine.* 1992;17:395–399.

28. Weinstein JN. The role of neurogenic and non-neurogenic mediators as they relate to pain and the development of osteoarthritis. A clinical review. *Spine.* 1992;17:S356–S361.

29. Lindblom K, Rexed B. Spinal nerve injury in dorsolateral protrusions of lumbar disks. *J Neurosurg.* 1948:413–432.

30. McLain RF, Weinstein JN. Effects of whole body vibration on dorsal root ganglion neurons. Changes in neuronal nuclei. *Spine.* 1994;19: 1455–1461.

31. Wilder D, Frymoyer J, Pope M. The effect of vibration on the spine of the seated individual. *Automedica.* 1985;6:5–35.

32. Howe JF, Loeser JD, Calvin WH. Mechanosensitivity of dorsal root ganglia and chronically injured axons: a physiologic basis for the radicular pain of nerve root compression. *Pain.* 1977;3:25–41.

33. Howe JF. A neurophysiological basis for the radicular pain of nerve root compression. In: Bonica J, ed. *Advances in Pain Research and Therapy,* vol. 3. New York: Raven Press; 3:1979.

34. Marshall LL, Trethewie ER, Curtain CC. Chemical radiculitis. A clinical, physiological and immunological study. *Clin Orthop.* 1979; 129:61–67.

35. Skouen JS, Larsen JL, Vollset SE. Cerebrospinal fluid protein concentrations related to clinical findings in patients with sciatica caused by disk herniation. *J Spinal Disord.* 1994;7:12–18.

36. Spiliopoulou I, Korovessis P, Konstantinou D, et al. IgG and IgM concentration in the prolapsed human intervertebral disc and sciatica etiology. *Spine.* 1994;19:1320–1323.

37. Konttinen YT, Kemppinen P, Segerberg M, et al. Peripheral and spinal neural mechanisms in arthritis, with particular reference to treatment of inflammation and pain. *Arthritis Rheum.* 1994;37:965–982.

38. Mense S. Physiology of nociception in muscles. *J Manual Med.* 1991; 6:24–33.

39. Grubb BD, Birrel GJ, McQueen DS, et al. The role of PGE2 in the sensitization of mechanoreceptors in normal and inflamed ankle joint of the rat. *Exp Brain Res.* 1991;84:383–392.

40. Cervero F, Schailbe H-G, Schmidt RF. Tonic descending inhibition of spinal cord neurons driven by joint afferents in normal cats and in cats with an inflamed joint. *Exp Brain Res.* 1991;83:675–678.

41. Schauble H-G, Schmidt RF. Effects of an experimental arthritis on the sensory properties of fine articular afferent units. *J Neurophysiol.* 1985;54:1109–1122.

42. Guilbaud G, Iggo A, Tegner R. Sensory receptors in ankle joint capsules of normal and arthritic rats. *Exp Brain Res.* 1985;58:29–40.

43. Wall RD, Devor M. Sensory afferent impulses originate from dorsal root ganglia as well as from the periphery in normal and nerve injured rates. *Pain.* 1983;17:321–339.

44. Passatore M, Grassi C, Filippi G. Sympathetically induced development of tension in jaw muscles: the possible contraction of intrafusal muscle fibers. *Pflugers Arch.* 1985;405:279–304.

45. Passatore M, Filippi M, Grassi C. Cervical sympathetic nerve stimulation can induce an intrafusal muscle fiber contraction in the rabbit. In: Boyd I, Galdden M, eds. *The Muscle Spindle.* London: Macmillan; 1985;221–226.

46. Grassi C, Filippi G, Passatore M. Postsynaptic alpha 1 and alpha 2 adrenoceptors mediating the action of the sympathetic system on muscle spindles in the rabbit. *Pharm Res.* 1986;182:161–170.

47. Bengtsson A, Bengtsson M. Regional sympathetic blocks in primary fibromyalgia. *Pain.* 1988;33S:161–167.

48. Hubbard DR, Berkoff GM. Myofascial trigger points show spontaneous needle EMG activity. *Spine.* 1993;13:1803–1807.

49. Hurley MV, Newham DJ. The influence of arthrogenous muscle inhibition on quadriceps rehabilitation of patients with early, unilateral osteoarthritic knees. *Br J Rheumatol.* 1993;32:127–131.

50. Biering-Sorensen F. A one-year prospective study of low back trouble in a general population. *Dan Med Bull.* 1984a;31:362–375.

51. Leino PS, Aro S, Hasan J. Trunk muscle function and low back disorders: a ten year follow-up study. *J Chron Dis.* 1987;40:289–296.

52. Riihimaeki HG, Wickstrom K, Haenninen K, Luopajaervi T. Predictors of sciatic pain among concrete reinforcement workers and house painters—a five year follow-up. *Scand J Work Environ Health.* 1989; 15:415–423.

53. Troup JDG, Foreman TK, Baxter CE, Brown D. The perception of back pain and the role of psychophysical test of lifting capacity. *Spine.* 1987;12:645–657.

54. Chaffin KB, Herrin GD, Keyserling WM. Preemployment strength testing: an updated position. *J Occup Med.* 1978;20:403.

55. Hides JA, Stokes MJ, Saide M, et al. Evidence of lumbar multifidus muscle wasting ipsilateral to symptoms in patients with acute/subacute low back pain. *Spine.* 1994;19:165–172.

56. Faas A, Chavannes AW, van Eijk JThM, et al. A randomized, placebo-controlled trial of exercise therapy in patients with acute low back pain. *Spine.* 1993;18:1388–1395.

57. Stankovic R, Olof J. Conservative treatment of acute low back pain: McKenzie method of treatment versus patients education in "mini back school." *Spine.* 1990;15:120–123.

58. Donelson R, Grant W, Kamps C, et al. Pain response to sagittal end-range spinal motion: a prospective, randomized multicentered trial. *Spine.* 1991;16S:206–212.

59. Delitto A, Cibulka MT, Erhard R, et al. Evidence for use of an extension-mobilization category in acute low back syndrome: a predictive validation pilot study. *Phys Ther.* 1993;73:216–222.

60. Mitchell RI, Carmen G. Results of a multicenter trial using an intensive active exercise program for the treatment of acute soft tissue and back injuries. *Spine.* 1990;15:514–521.

61. Spratt KF, Lehmann TR, Weinstein JN, et al. A new approach to the low back physical examination: behavioral assessment of mechanical signs. *Spine.* 1990;15:96–102.

62. Plowman SA. Physical activity, physical fitness, and low back pain. *Exerc Sport Sci Rev.* 1992;20:221–242.

63. Grahame R. The hypermobility syndrome. *Ann Rheumatol.* 1990;49: 199–200.

64. Gedalia A, Press J, Klein M, et al. Joint hypermobility and fibromyalgia in schoolchildren. *Ann Rheum Dis.* 1993;52:494–496.

65. Knapic JJ, Bauman CL, Jones BH, et al. Preseason strength and flexibility imbalances associated with athletic injuries in female collegiate athletes. *Am J Sports Med.* 1991;19:76–81.

66. Gracovetsky S, Kary M, Pithcen I. The importance of pelvic tilt in reducing compressive stress in the spine during flexion-extension exercises. *Spine.* 1989;14:412–416.

67. Mallik AK, Ferrell WR, McDonald AG, Sturrock RD. Impaired proprioceptive acuity at the proximal interphalangeal joint in patients with the hypermobility syndrome. *Br J Rheumatol.* 1994;33:631–637.

68. Owen BD, Damron CF. Personal characteristics and back injury among hospital nursing personnel. *Res Nurs Health.* 1984;7:305–313.

69. Tropp H, McCloskey DI. Prevention of ankle sprains. *Am J Sports Med.* 1985;13:259–262.

70. Battie MC, Bigos SJ, Fisher LD, et al. A prospective study of the role of cardiovascular risk factors and fitness in industrial back pain complaints. *Spine.* 1989b;14:141–147.

71. Cady LD, Bischoff DP, O'Connell ER. Strength and fitness and subsequent back injuries in fire fighters. *J Occup Med.* 1979;21:269–272.

72. Cady LD, Thomas PC, Karwasky RJ. Program for increasing health and physical fitness of fire fighters. *J Occup Med.* 1985;27:110–114.

73. Medicine Io. *Pain and Disability: Clinical, Behavioral and Public Policy Perspectives.* Washington, DC: National Academy Press, 1987.

74. Shirado O, Kaneda K, Ito T. Trunk-muscle strength during concentric and eccentric contraction: a comparison between healthy subjects and patients with chronic low-back pain. *J Spinal Disord.* 1992;5: 175–182.

75. DeLuca CJ. Use of the surface EMG signal for performance evaluation of back muscles. *Muscle Nerve.* 1993;16:210–216.

76. Robinson ME, Cassisi JE, O'Connor PD, MacMillan M. Lumbar iEMG during isotonic exercise: chronic low back pain patients versus controls. *J Spinal Disord.* 1992;5:8–15.

77. Stokes MJ, Colter C, Klestov A, et al. Normal paraspinal muscle electromyographic fatigue characteristics in patients with primary fibromyalgia. *Br J Rheumatol.* 1993;32:711–716.

78. Hause M, Fujiwara M, Kikuchi S. A new method of quantitative measurement of abdominal and back muscle strength. *Spine.* 1980;5: 143–148.

79. Helewa A, Goldsmith CH, Smythe HA. Measuring abdominal muscle weakness in patients with low back pain and matched controls: a comparison of 3 devices. *J Rheumatol.* 1993;20:1539–1543.

80. Kahanovitz N, Viola K, Gallagher M. Long-term strength assessment of postoperative diskectomy patients. *Spine.* 1989:402–403.

81. Mayer TG, Smith SS, Keeley J, et al. Quantification of lumbar function. II: Sagittal plane trunk strength in chronic low-back pain patients. *Spine.* 1985;10:765–772.

82. Alston W, Carlson KE, Feldman DJ, et al. A quantitative study of muscle factors in the chronic low back syndrome. *J Am Geriatr Soc.* 1966;14:1041–1047.

83. Pope MH, Bevins T, Wilder DG, et al. The relationship between anthropometric, postural, muscular, and mobility characteristics of males ages 18–55. *Spine.* 1985;10:815–830.

84. Suzuki N, Endo S. A quantitative study of trunk muscle strength and fatigability in the low-back pain syndrome. *Spine.* 1983;8: 69–74.

85. Flicker PL, Fleckenstein JL, Ferry K, et al. Lumbar muscle usage in chronic low back pain. *Spine.* 1993;18:582–586.

86. Stokes MJ, Cooper RG, Jayson MIV. Selective changes in multifidus dimensions in patients with chronic low back pain. *Eur Spine J.* 1992; 1:38–42.

87. Fitzmaurice R, Cooper RG, Freemont AJ. A histo-morphometric comparison of muscle biopsies from normal subjects and patients with ankylosing spondylitis and severe mechanical low back pain. *J Pathol.* 1992;163:182A.

88. Cooper RG, Stokes MJ, Jayson MIV. Electro- and acoustic myographic changes during fatigue of the human paraspinal muscles in back pain patients. *J Physiol.* 1991;438:338P.

89. Sihvonen T, Partanen J, Hanninen O, et al. Electric behavior of low back muscles during lumbar pelvic rhythm in low back pain patients and healthy controls. *Arch Phys Med Rehabil.* 1991;72:1080–1087.

90. Manniche C, Hesselsoe G, Bentzen L, et al. Clinical trial of intensive muscle training for chronic low back pain. *Lancet.* 1988;2:1473–1476.

91. Manniche C, Asmussen K, Lauritsen B, et al. Intensive dynamic back exercises with or without hyperextension in chronic back pain after surgery for lumbar disc protrusion. A clinical trial. *Spine.* 1993;18: 560–567.

92. Risch SV, Norvell NK, Pollock ML, et al. Lumbar strengthening in chronic low back pain patients. *Spine.* 1993;18:232–238.

93. Mattila M, Hurme M, Alarantal H, et al. The multifidus muscle in patients with lumbar intervertebral disc herniation. *Spine.* 1986;11: 732–738.

94. Rantanen J, Hurme M, Falck B, et al. The lumbar multifidus muscle five years after surgery for a lumbar intervertebral disc herniation. *Spine.* 1993;18:568–574.

95. Soderberg GL, Barr JO. Muscular function in chronic low back dysfunction. *Spine.* 1983;8:79–85.

96. King JC, Lehmkuhl DL, French J, et al. Dynamic postural reflexes: comparison in normal subjects and patients with chronic low back pain. *Curr Concepts Rehabil Med.* 1988;4:7–11.

97. Niles N, Sinnott PL. Variations in balance and body sway in middle-aged adults. Subjects with healthy backs compared with subjects with low-back dysfunction. *Spine.* 1991;16:325–330.

98. Parkhurst TM, Burnett CN. Injury and proprioception in the lower back. *J Orthop Sport Ther.* 1994;19:282–295.

99. Revel M, Andre-Deshays C, Minguet M. Cervicocephalic kinesthetic sensibility in patients with cervical pain. *Arch Phys Med Rehabil.* 1991;72:288–291.

100. Freeman MAR, Dean MRE, Hanham IWF. The etiology and prevention of functional instability of the foot. *J Bone Joint Surg Br.* 1965; 47:678–685.

101. McCloskey DI. Kinaesthetic sensibility. *Physiol Rev.* 1978;58: 763–820.

102. Brennan GP, Ruhling RO, Hood RS, et al. Physical characteristics of patients with herniated intervertebral lumbar discs. *Spine.* 1987;12: 699–702.

103. Brennan GP, Shultz BB, Hood RS, et al. The effects of aerobic exercise after lumbar microdiscectomy. *Spine.* 1994;19:735–739.

104. Hochschuler SH, Cotler HB, Guyer RD. *Rehabilitation of the Spine.* St. Louis: Mosby; 1993.

105. Gonnella C, Paris SV, Kutner M. Reliability in evaluating passive intervertebral motion. *Phys Ther.* 1982;62:436–444.

106. Kaltenborn F, Lindahl O. Reproducibility of the results of manual mobility testing of specific intervertebral segments. *Swed Med J.* 1969;66:962–965.

107. Twomey LT, Taylor JR. Sagittal movements of the human lumbar vertebral column: a quantitative study of the role of the posterior vertebral elements. *Arch Phys Med Rehabil.* 1983;64:322–325.

108. Jull G, Bogduk N, Marsland A. The accuracy of manual diagnosis for cervical zygapophyseal joint pain syndromes. *Med J Aust.* 1988;148: 233–236.

109. Lee R, Evans J. Load-displacement-time characteristics of the spine under posteroanterior mobilisation. *Aust J Physiother.* 1992b;38: 115–123.

110. Jull G, Bogduk N, Marsland A. The accuracy of manual diagnosis for cervical zygapophyseal joint pain syndrome. *Med J Aust.* 1988;148: 233–236.

111. Janos SC, Ray CD. *Mechanical Examination of the Lumbar Spine and Mechanical Discography of the Facet Joint Injection.* Proceedings of the 5th International Conference International Federation of Orthopaedic Manipulative Therapists. 1992; 92.

112. Maher C, Adams R. Reliability of pain and stiffness assessments in clinical manual lumbar spine examination. *Phys Ther.* 1994;74: 801–811.

113. Speer KP, Lohnes J, Garrett WE. Radiographic imaging of muscle strain injury. *Am J Sports Med.* 1993;21:89–96.

114. Reddy AS, Reedy MK, Seaber AV, et al. Restriction of the injury response following an acute muscle strain. *Med Sci Sports Med.* 1993; 25:321–327.

115. Taylor DC, Dalton JD, Seaber AV, et al. Experimental muscle strain injury. Early functional and structural deficits and the increased risk for reinjury. *Am J Sports Med.* 1993;21:190–194.

116. Nurenberg P, Giddings CJ, Stray-Gundersen J, et al. MR imaging-guided muscle biopsy for correlation of increased signal intensity with ultrastructural change and delayed-onset muscle soreness after exercise. *Radiology.* 1992;84:865–869.

117. Jones DA, Newham DJ, Round JM, et al. Experimental human muscle damage: morphologic changes in relation to other indices of damage. *J Physiol.* 1986;375:435–448.

118. Cleak MJ, Eston RG. Delayed onset muscle soreness: mechanisms and management. *J Sports Sci.* 1992;10:325–341.

119. DeFazio FA, Barth RA, Frymoyer JW, et al. Acute lumbar paraspinal compartment syndrome. *J Bone Joint Surg Am.* 1991;73:1101–1103.

120. Rutherford OM. Muscular coordination and strength training. Implications for injury rehabilitation. *Sports Med.* 1988;5:196–202.

121. Jaevinen MJ, Lehto MUK. The effects of early mobilisation and immobilisation on the healing process following muscle injuries. *Sports Med.* 1993;15:78–89.

122. Gracovetsky S, Kary I, Pitchen S. The abdominal mechanism. *Spine.* 1985;10:317–324.

123. Morris JM, Lucas DB, Bresler B. Role of the trunk in the stability of the spine. *J Bone Joint Surg Am.* 1961;43:327–351.

124. McGill SM, Norwan RW. Partitioning of the L4-L5 dynamic moment into disc, ligaments, and muscular components during lifting. *Spine.* 1986;11:666–678.

125. Hasson SM, Daniels JC, Divine JG. Effect of ibuprofen use on muscle soreness, damage, and performance: a preliminary investigation. *Med Sci Sports Exerc.* 1993;25:9–17.

126. Kaminski M, Boal R. An effect of ascorbic acid on delayed onset muscle soreness. *Pain.* 1992;50:317–321.

127. Farfan FH, Cossette JW, Robertson GH, et al. The effects of torsion in the lumbar intervertebral joints: the role of torsion in the production of disc degeneration. *J Bone Joint Surg Am.* 1970;52:468.

128. Adams MA, Hutton WC. Prolapsed intervertebral disc: a hyperflexion injury. *Spine.* 1982;7:184.

129. Adams MA, Hutton WC. Gradual disc prolapse. *Spine.* 1985;10:524.

130. Deyo RA, Loeser JD, Bigos SJ. Herniated lumbar intervertebral disk. *Ann Intern Med.* 1990;112:598–603.

131. McRae DL. Asymptomatic intervertebral disc protrusions. *Acta Radiol.* 1956;46:9–27.

132. Kawakami M, Weinstein JN, Spratt KF, et al. Experimental lumbar radiculopathy. Immunohistochemical and quantitative demonstrations of pain induced by lumbar nerve root irritation of the rat. *Spine.* 1994;19:1780–1794.

133. Frymoyer JW. Back pain and sciatia. *N Engl J Med.* 1988;318:291–300.

134. Faust SE, Ducker TB, Van Hassent JA, et al. Lateral lumbar disc herniations. *J Spinal Dis.* 1992;5:97–102.

135. Cohen JE, Goel V, Frank JW, et al. Group education interventions for people with low back pain. An overview of the literature. *Spine.* 1994;19:1214–1222.

136. Deyo RA, Diehl AK, Rosenthal M, et al. How many days of bed rest for acute low back pain? A randomized clinical trial. *N Engl J Med.* 1986;315:1064–1970.

137. Gnatz SM. Increased radicular pain due to therapeutic ultrasound applied to the back. *Arch Phys Med Rehabil.* 1989;70:493–494.

138. Bogduk N, Marsland A. The cervical zygapophyseal joints as a source of neck pain. *Spine.* 1988;13:610–617.

139. Marks RC, Houston T, Thulbourne T. Facet joint injection and facet nerve block: a randomized comparison in 86 patients with chronic low back pain. *Pain.* 1992;49:325–328.

140. Stolker RJ, Vervest ACM, Ramos LMP, et al. Percutaneous facet denervation in chronic thoracic spinal pain. *Acta Neurochir.* 1993;122:82–90.

141. Hove B, Gyldensted C. Cervical facet joint arthrography. *Neuroradiology.* 1990;32:456–459.

142. Mooney V, Robertson J. The facet syndrome. *Clin Orthop.* 1976;115:149–156.

143. Schwarzer AC, Aprill CN, Fortin J, et al. The false-positive rate of uncontrolled diagnostic blocks of the lumbar zygapophyseal joints. *Pain.* 1994;58:195–200.

144. Revel ME, Listrat VM, Chevalier XJ, et al. Facet joint block for low back pain: identifying predictors of a good response. *Arch Phys Med Rehabil.* 1992;73:824–827.

145. Schwarzer AC, Aprill CN, Derby R, et al. The relative contributions of the disc and zygapophyseal joint in chronic low back pain. *Spine.* 1994;19:801–806.

146. Jackson RP. The facet syndrome. *Clin Orthop Rel Res.* 1992;279:110–121.

147. Denslow JS, Korr IM, Krems AD. Quantitative studies of chronic facilitation in human motoneuron pools. *Am J Physiol.* 1945;150:229–238.

148. Korr IM. Proprioceptors and somatic dysfunction. *J Am Osteopath Assoc.* 1975;74:123–134.

149. Grarges G, Littlejohn G. Pressure pain threshold in pain-free subjects, in patients with chronic regional pain syndromes, and in patients with fibromyalgia syndrome. *Arthritis Rheum.* 1993;36:642–646.

150. Greenman PE. *Concepts of Vertebral Motion Dysfunction. Principles of Manual Medicine.* Baltimore: Williams & Wilkins.

151. Stauffer RN, Coventry MB. Posterolateral lumbar-spine fusion. *J Bone Joint Surg Am.* 1972;54:1195.

152. Freebody D, Bendall R, Taylor RD. Anterior transperitoneal lumbar fusion. *J Bone Joint Surg Br.* 1971;53:617.

153. Flynn JC, Hoque MA. Anterior fusion of the lumbar spine. *J Bone Joint Surg Am.* 1979;61:1143.

154. Greenough CG, Taylor LJ, Fraser RD. Anterior lumbar fusion. A comparison of noncompensation patients with compensation patients. *Clin Orthop Rel Res.* 1994;300:30–37.

155. O'Beirne J, O'Neill D, Gallagher J, et al. Spinal fusion for back pain: a clinical and radiological review. *J Spinal Dis.* 1992;5:32–38.

156. Crock HV. Internal disc disruption. A challenge to disc prolapse fifty years on. *Spine.* 1986;11:650–653.

157. Rhyne AL, Smith SE, Wood KE, et al. Outcome of unoperated discogram positive for low back pain. NASS, 9th Annual Meeting. October 19–22, 1994; Minneapolis.

158. Turner JA, Herron L, Deyo RA. Meta-analysis of the results of lumbar spine fusion. *Acta Orthop Scand.* 1993;64(suppl 251):120–122.

159. Wiltse LL, Rothman SLG. Spondylolisthesis: classification, diagnosis, and natural history. *Semin Spine Surg.* 1989;1:78–94.

160. Jackson DW, Wiltse LL, Dingemann RD, et al. Stress reactions involving the pars interarticularis in young athletes. *Am J Sports Med.* 1981;9:304–312.

161. Micheli LJ. Back injuries in gymnastics. *Clin Sports Med.* 1985;4:85–94.

162. Morita T, Ikata T, Katoh S, et al. *Pathogenesis of Spondylolysis and Spondylolisthesis in Young Athletes.* NASS-JSRS Spine across the Sea. April 19, 1994; Maui, HI.

163. Sinaki M, Lutness MP, Ilstrup DM, et al. Lumbar spondylolisthesis: retrospective comparison and three-year follow-up of two conservative treatment programs. *Arch Phys Med Rehabil.* 1989;70:594–597.

164. Mooney V. Understanding, examining for, and treating sacroiliac pain. *J Musculoskel Med.* 1993;10:37–49.

165. Laslett M, Williams M. The reliability of selected pain provocation tests for sacroiliac joint pathology. *Spine.* 1994;19:1243–1249.

166. Donigny RL. Anterior dysfunction of the sacroiliac joint as a major factor in the etiology of idiopathic low back pain. *Phys Ther.* 1990;70:250–265.

167. Bernard TN, Kirkaldy-Willis WH. Recognizing specific characteristics of nonspecific low back pain. *Clin Orthop.* 1987;217:266–280.

168. Traycoff RB, Crayton H, Dodson R. Sacrococcygeal pain syndromes: diagnosis and treatment. *Orthopedics.* 1989;12:1373–1377.

169. Wray CC, Easom S, Hoskinson J. Coccydynia. *J Bone Joint Surg Br.* 1991;73:335–338.

170. Elster AD. Bertolotti's syndrome revisited: transitional vertebrae of the lumbar spine. *Spine.* 1989;14:1373–1377.

171. Bogduk N, Twomey LT. *Clinical Anatomy of the Lumbar Spine.* 2nd ed. Melbourne: Churchill Livingstone, 1991.

172. Simons DG. Muscular pain syndromes. In: Friction JR, Awad E, eds. *Adv Pain Res Ther.* 1990;17:1–41.

173. Vecchiet L, Giamberardine MA, Saggini R. Myofascial pain syndromes: clinical and pathophysiological aspects. *Clin J Pain.* 1991;7 (suppl 1):S16–S22.

174. Vecchiet L, Galletti R, Giamberardino MA, et al. Modifications of cutaneous, subcutaneous and muscular sensory and pain thresholds after the induction of an experimental algogenic focus in the skeletal muscle. *Clin J Pain.* 1988;4:55–59.

175. Wolfe F, Simons DG, Fricton J, et al. The fibromyalgia and myofascial pain syndromes: a preliminary study of tender points and trigger points in persons with fibromyalgia, myofascial pain syndrome and no disease. *J Rheumatol.* 1992;19:944–951.

176. Nice DA, Riddle DL, Lamb RL, et al. Intertester reliability of judgments of the presence of trigger points in patients with low back pain. *Arch Phys Med Rehabil.* 1992;73:893–898.

177. Sola AE, Rodenberger ML, Gettys BB. Incidence of hypersensitive areas in posterior shoulder muscles. *Am J Phys Med.* 1955;34:585–590.

178. Kirkaldy-Willis WH, Burton CV. *Managing Low Back Pain.* 3rd ed. New York, Edinburgh, London, Melbourne, Tokyo: Churchill Livingstone; 1992:126–130.

179. Ingber RS. Iliopsoas myofascial dysfunction: a treatable cause of "failed" low back syndrome. *Arch Phys Med Rehabil.* 1989;70:382–386.

180. Fairbank JCT, O'Brien JP. The iliac crest syndrome. *Spine.* 1983;8:220–224.

181. Bauwens P, Coyer AB. The "multifidus triangle" syndrome as a cause of recurrent low back pain. *Br J Med.* 1955;2:1306–1307.

182. Maigne J-Y, Maigne R. Trigger point of the posterior iliac crest: painful ligament insertion or cutaneous dorsal ramus pain? An anatomic study. *Arch Phys Med Rehabil.* 1991;72:734–737.

183. Maigne R. Low back pain of thoracolumbar origin. *Arch Phys Med Rehabil.* 1980;61:389–395.

184. Wolfe F, Smythe HA, Yunus MB, et al. The American College of Rheumatology 1990 criteria for the classification of fibromyalgia. *Arthritis Rheum.* 1990;33:160–172.

185. Wolfe F. Fibrositis, fibromyalgia and musculoskeletal disease: the current status of the fibrositis syndrome. *Arch Phys Med Rehabil.* 1988;69:527–531.

186. Campbell SM, Clark S, Tindall EA, et al. Clinical characteristics of fibrositis. I. A "blinded," controlled study of symptoms and tender points. *Arthritis Rheum.* 1983;26:817–824.

187. Greenfield S, Fitzcharles MA, Esdaile JM. Reactive fibromyalgia syndrome. *Arthritis Rheum.* 1992;35:678–681.

188. Linnel PW, Hermansen SE, Elias MF, et al. Quality of life in osteoporotic women. *J Bone Miner Res.* 1991;6S:S106.

189. Eastell R, Cedel SL, Wahner HW, et al. Classification of vertebral fractures. *J Bone Miner Res.* 1991;6:207–215.

190. Levernieux J, Julien D, Caulin F. The effect of calcitonin on bone pain and acute resorption related to recent osteoporotic crush fractures. Result of a double blind and an open study. In: Cecchetin M, Segre G, Elsevir BV, eds. *Calciotropic Hormones and Calcium Metabolism.* Amsterdam: Excerpta Medica; 1986:171–178.

191. Lukert BP. Vertebral compression fractures: how to manage pain, avoid disability. *Geriatrics.* 1994;49:22–26.

192. Sinaki M, Mikkelsen BA. Postmenopausal spinal osteoporosis: flexion versus extension exercises. *Arch Phys Med Rehabil.* 1984;65:593–596.

193. Lukert BP, Ball JM, VanderVeen DK. Effect of extension exercise on posture in women ages 50–60. *Proc Am Soc Gerentol.* 1991;44S.

194. Hughes RA, Costello C, Keat ACS. Vertebral osteoporosis—the importance of serum and urine electrophoresis. *Ann Rheum Dis.* 1994;53:147–148.

195. Katz JN. The assessment and management of low back pain: a critical review. *Arthritis Care Res.* 1993;6:104–114.

196. Johnsson K-E, Rosen I, Uden A. The natural course of lumbar spinal stenosis. *Clin Orthop Rel Res.* 1992;279:82–86.

197. Porter RW, Ward D. Cauda equina dysfunction. The significance of two-level pathology. *Spine.* 1992;17:9–15.

198. Ooi Y, Mita KF, Satoh Y. Myeloscopic study on lumbar spinal canal stenosis with special reference to intermittent claudication. *Spine.* 1990;15:544–549.

199. Yazaki S, Muramatsu T, Yoneda M, et al. Venous pressure in the vertebral venous plexus and its role in cauda equina claudication. *J Jpn Orthop Assoc.* 1988;62:733–745.

200. Hiraizumi Y, Transfeldt EE, Fujimaki E, et al. Electrophysiologic evaluation of intermittent sacral nerve dysfunction in lumbar spinal canal stenosis. *Spine.* 1993;18:1355–1360.

201. Turner JA, Ersek M, Herron L, et al. Surgery for lumbar spinal stenosis. Attempted meta-analysis of the literature. *Spine.* 1992;17:1–7.

202. Willner S. Effect of a rigid brace on back pain. *Acta Orthop Scand.* 1985;56:40–42.

203. Hawkes CH, Roberts GM. Lumbar canal stenosis. *Br J Hosp Med.* 1980;23:498.

204. Stolker RJ, Vervest ACM, Groen GJ. The management of chronic spinal pain by blockades: a review. *Pain.* 1994;58:1–20.

205. Rich BSE, McKeag D. When sciatica is not disk disease. *Phys Sports Med.* 1992;20:105–115.

206. Fishman LM, Zybert PA. Electrophysiologic evidence of piriformis syndrome. *Arch Phys Med Rehabil.* 1992;73:359–364.

207. Hughes SS, Goldstein MN, Hicks DG, et al. Extrapelvic compression of the sciatic nerve. *J Bone Joint Surg Am.* 1992;74:1553–1548.

208. Keefe FJ, Bradley LA, Crisson JE. Behavioral assessment of low back pain: identification of pain behavior subgroups. *Pain.* 1990;40:153–160.

209. Deyo RA, Bass JE, Walsh NE, et al. Prognostic variability among chronic pain patients: implications for study design, interpretation, and reporting. *Arch Phys Med Rehabil.* 1988;69:174–178.

210. Turk DC. Customizing treatment for chronic pain patients: who, what, and why. *Clin J Pain.* 1990;6:255–270.

211. Barnes D, Smith D, Gatcel RJ, et al. Psychosocioeconomic predictors of treatment success/failure in chronic low-back pain patients. *Spine.* 1989;14:427–430.

212. Magni G, Caldeiron C, Rigatti-Luchini S, et al. Chronic musculoskeletal pain and depressive symptoms in the general population. An analysis of the 1st National Health and Nutrition Examination Survey data. *Pain.* 1990;43:299–307.

213. Sullivan MJL, Reesor K, Mikail S, et al. The treatment of depression in chronic low back pain: review and recommendations. *Pain.* 1992; 50:5–13.

214. Renstroem P, Johnson RJ. Overuse injuries in sports. A review. *Sports Med.* 1985;2:316–333.

CHAPTER 15

Rehabilitation of the Hip, Pelvis, and Thigh

Michael C. Geraci, Jr.

INTRODUCTION

Sports injuries to the hip, pelvis, and thigh may not be as common as other injuries, such as those to the shoulder, knee, and ankle. However, injuries to this region can disable an athlete for an entire season. This is best exemplified in the "simple" adductor strain, which can be difficult to manage or resolve in a reasonable period of time. Dysfunctions of the pelvis and sacroiliac joints have all too often been overlooked or poorly understood as competent producing causes of athletic injuries, although with an understanding of the biomechanics and functional anatomy of these regions, more specific diagnoses and, therefore, more specific treatments can be rendered. The incidence of injuries to the hip, pelvis, and thigh have been reported at approximately 5% of all athletic injuries.[1] However, when utilizing a biomechanical approach and understanding the concept of muscle imbalances, the incidence can rise to 21% of all athletic injuries, as reported in a review of all sports injuries to a general sports medicine center.[2]

All too often, injuries to the athlete have been treated using an approach that focuses on a particular joint or muscle condition. Overuse injuries, especially, should be approached from a more global understanding of muscle imbalances and the influence of other biomechanical factors and their relationships to the entire lower extremity kinetic chain, including the lumbar spine and pelvis. In fact, in one report, overuse injuries accounted for 82.4% of injuries to the hip and pelvis region, whereas trauma accounted for the remaining 17.6%.[3] The most common bone injuries from this study were reported as sacroiliitis, pelvic and femoral neck stress fractures, and osteitis pubis. The diagnoses of sacroiliitis and osteitis pubis in the biomechanical model should be thought of less frequently as primary inflammatory conditions and more commonly as the result of muscle imbalances and joint dysfunctions that may predispose to inflammatory processes at these joints if they are not identified and are left untreated. These investigators go on to state that the three most common soft-tissue injuries are gluteus medius (G Med) strain/tendinitis, trochanteric bursitis, and hamstring (HS) strain. To further illuminate on the concept of muscle imbalances, it is necessary to understand that the G Med muscle has a tendency to become inhibited and to develop weakness. This type of muscle is more likely to develop tendinitis and trigger points. It is common to find these muscles as antagonists to muscles that have a tendency to develop tightness (in this case in particular, the adductors). The sports medicine practitioner should not chase the pain or provide treatment initially only to the muscle that appears to be involved, such as the G Med in this example. Treatment should be started by first stretching the tight adductors so that they neurologically can release their inhibition on the G Med. A retraining program may then be introduced to facilitate the G Med and eventually incorporate this into closed-chained kinetics, balance, coordination retraining, and stabilization training to maintain correction and proper balance.

FUNCTIONAL ANATOMY AND BIOMECHANICS

The pelvis is the link between the trunk and the lower extremities. Primary compression and tension trabecula of the femoral neck and hip carry on through to the pelvis, iliac crest, and lumbar spine. The multiaxial ball and socket joint of the hip has three degrees of freedom. This allows for approximately 120 degrees of flexion, 20 degrees of extension, 40 degrees of abduction, and 25 degrees of adduction. Internal and external rotation are approximately 45 degrees each. The acetabular triangular fibrocartilage adds more congruency to the articular surfaces, providing greater stability. Through the attachments of the muscles, fascia, and ligaments, one can appreciate the relationship between the hip, pelvis, thigh, and lumbar spine. The strong capsule is reinforced by the iliofemoral, ischiofemoral, and pubofemoral intrinsic ligaments. Interconnections between these regions are again exemplified by the femoral, obturator, and sciatic nerves, all of which contribute to the innervation of the hip region. The extracapsular blood supply includes the profunda femoris artery, as well as the lateral and medial circumflex branches. The intracapsular blood supply is from the medial circumflex femoral artery and its superior and inferior retinacula vessels, along with the obturator artery via the artery of the ligamentum teres.

The biomechanics of the neck-shaft angle, which is approximately 120–130 degrees, with an average of 14 degrees of anteversion, allows for a unique arrangement. This permits angular movements of the thigh to be converted to rotatory hip motion. The resting position of the hip is considered to be 30 degrees of flexion and 30 degrees of abduction. The capsular pattern seen commonly with joint dysfunction is that flexion is lost more than is abduction, and internal rotation is decreased. The closely packed position of the hip is at full extension, with internal rotation and abduction. Peak focal pressures average 1,000 psi and reach 3,000 psi from a sitting to standing position.

The relationships to the hips, pelvis, and thigh are easily seen again when considering the muscles and fascia of the thigh. The biceps femoris, gluteus maximus (G Max), and piriformis all have attachments to the sacrotuberous ligaments and lumbodorsal fascia. The nerve and blood supplies are similar to those of the hip joint, with the femoral and obturator arteries supplying blood and the femoral and sciatic nerves innervating the anterior and posterior compartments, while the obturator nerve supplies the medial compartment of the thigh.

The functional anatomy and biomechanics of the pelvis and sacroiliac joints must be thoroughly reviewed as there has been considerable controversy and misunderstanding regarding this important region. The pelvis is comprised of three bones, the right and left innominates, which function as lower extremity bones, and the sacrum, which functions as part of the spine. These three bones form three joints, which should be thought of as functioning together but capable of having their own independent dysfunctions. The symphysis pubis and the sacroiliac joints are the three joints comprising the pelvis. The sacral articular surface is composed of hyaline cartilage and, in the adult life, is 1.5 times thicker than the ilial side, which is fibrocartilage.[4] The sacroiliac joint is an atypical synovial joint that, in most cases, is patent throughout life. Fusion can occur, however, by either synostosis or fibrosis.

The relationship between the form and the function of the sacroiliac joint is exemplified by the ridges and depressions. These ridges and depressions are clearly visible at the mac-

roscopic level. They appear to involve both the cartilage and the underlying bone, as well as to be complementary on both sides of the joint. In women, there appear to be less pronounced ridges and depressions. Radiographically, the visible osteophytes may, in fact, represent cartilage-covered ridges that are not pathologic. The amount of friction between the articular surfaces of the sacroiliac joints relates to the degree of macroscopic roughening. High-friction coefficients are seen in the sacroiliac joints with coarse texture and ridges and depressions. Theoretically, when the sacroiliac joints are forced into a new position where the ridges and depressions are no longer complementary, they may be regarded as a dysfunctional, or blocked, joint.[5,6] To add to the complexity of this region, it would appear that no two sacroiliac joints are the same, neither within an individual nor across specimens.[7]

The ligamentous relationships of the pelvis include the iliolumbar ligament which attaches to the L5 and, at times, to the L4 transverse process, linking the lower lumbar segments to the pelvis. The thinner anterior sacroiliac joint ligaments are relatively weaker and form a sling under the inferior surface of the sacroiliac joints. There are multilevel short posterior ligaments, as well as long posterior sacrotuberous and sacrospinous ligaments. The innervation of the sacroiliac joints is generally considered to be from levels of L2 through S2. In particular, the majority of the posterior aspect of the joint is innervated by L5, S1, and S2. Some of the important muscular relationships in the pelvic, hip, and thigh region are between the abdominals and adductors. Their imbalance can lead to symphysis pubis dysfunction as the abdominals attach to the symphysis from above and the adductors from below. Other relationships, such as inhibition or weakness of the G Med may be as a result of tight adductors, leading to abnormal lateral pelvic tilt and piriformis overuse as it tries to substitute for the inhibited hip abductors. Tightness of the iliopsoas (IP) muscle or other hip flexors, such as the tensor fascia latae (TFL) and rectus femoris (RF), can lead to inhibition of the G Max, allowing for an anterior pelvic tilt. The piriformis is probably the most important muscle in recurrent sacroiliac dysfunctions, because it crosses the joint anteriorly, attaching to the sacrum, and when tight, can cause torsional movements. The pelvis and genitourinary diaphragms also play an important role in supporting the pelvis and, when dysfunctional, in leading to pain generation.

The sacroiliac joint is an important link through which loads are transmitted from the lower extremities to the spine, and vice versa. For the sacroiliac joint to remain stable, there must be a self-bracing mechanism that relies on proper functioning of the spine, pelvis, and lower extremities. In fact, the sacrotuberous ligaments are an important structure in the kinematic chain between the pelvis and vertebral column.[8] Muscle attachments to these ligaments include the G Max in all specimens studied and, in some cases, the piriformis and long head of the biceps femoris. The sacrotuberous ligament, when tensed by straight-leg raising and more so in the presence of muscle shortening, can influence the tension in this ligament that bridges the sacroiliac joint; therefore, the position of the sacrum may be changed. Kinematically, asymmetrical pull on the pelvis can rotate the innominates in relationship to the sacrum. The iliolumbar ligament is then stretched and can act on the lower lumbar vertebrae. With maximum hip extension during G Max activation, stability results in the sacroiliac joints through either direct muscle action or the pull on the sacrotuberous ligament. The G Max is oriented approximately perpendicular to the anterior and medial aspect of the sacroiliac joint. Therefore, strong muscle contraction can compress the sacroiliac joint and increase the perpendicular force. It can be speculated that the training of the G Max can influence rotation of the sacroiliac joints secondary to direct connections with the sacrum and sacrotuberous ligament.

Although motion of the sacroiliac joints has remained controversial over the years, the anatomic and biomechanical research studies document motion within the sacroiliac joint throughout life. However, only a small amount of rotation and translation occurs,[9–12] rotation averaging only 2.5 degrees, with a range from 0.8 to 3.9 degrees. The translation averages 0.7 mm, with a range from 0.1 to 1.6 mm. Of note is that the motion analysis during relaxing influence yields an increase in sacroiliac joint motion by 25%. The motions of the sacroiliac joints and pelvis are best described by using a biomechanical model; the understanding of their various dysfunctions is extremely important.[7] The best-known motion is that of nutation (flexion) and counternutation (extension) of the sacrum. This motion occurs primarily across a transverse (x) axis. A translatory movement—primarily cephalic to caudad—that accompanies nutation and counternutation has been described. A coupled motion of side-bending and rotation of the sacrum between innominates that is polyaxial in nature occurs around an oblique axis. This small amount of motion is coupled to opposite sides. From the clinical perspective, the innominates function as lower-extremity bones. Movement of the innominates appears to be primarily that of rotation anteriorly and posteriorly around another transverse (x) axis. The symphysis pubis has a superior-to-inferior translatory movement that occurs with one-legged standing. Its primary movement is rotation around a transverse axis.

Abnormal pelvic mechanics can adversely affect the entire kinetic chain. The most common abnormalities are excessive anterior pelvic tilt, excessive lateral tilt, and asymmetric pelvic movements.[13] The excessive anterior pelvic tilt is due to the tightness of the hip flexors and inhibited or weak glutei muscles—in particular, the G Max. This leads to increased lordosis and stress on the lower two lumbar discs,

facet joints, and sacroiliac joints. Knee flexion is greater than normal at heel strike and midstance. Eccentric load increases across the extensor mechanism of the knee and may contribute to patellar tendon injury. With increased knee flexion, patellar compressive forces against the femur are greater and may predispose to patellofemoral problems. Excessive lateral pelvic tilt is usually seen with tight adductors and weak or inhibited contractions of the hip abductors—in particular, the G Med and gluteus minimus (G Min). This usually leads to overuse of the tensor fascia latae, thereby tightening the lateral knee structures. Finally, asymmetrical pelvic movements are due to the large number of muscles that attach to the pelvis. The resultant asymmetry is secondary to imbalances of the tight muscles and their antagonist inhibited muscles, as well as to structural abnormalities such as leg length discrepancy and scoliosis. Asymmetry may also represent an adaptation to a previous injury. These asymmetries often are exacerbated by running, prolonged walking, or use of a cross-country ski machine and can subsequently lead to osteitis pubis, sacroiliitis, and overuse injuries to the lower extremities.

METHOD OF PRESENTATION

Several conditions are discussed in this section; in the next section, a more complete differential diagnosis is discussed. When considering soft tissue injury to the thigh region, tendinitis, strains, tears, and ruptures are common. Most commonly, the HS, quadriceps, G Med, IP, TFL, and short adductors are involved. Tendinitis, in particular, is more common in the inhibited and weak muscles such as the G Med and quadriceps. Muscles that have a tendency to develop tightness, such as the IP, TFL, short adductors, and HS, have a tendency for strains, tears, and ruptures. Gluteus medius strain and tendinitis were the most common soft-tissue injuries in a series of 200 hip and pelvic injuries.[3] This condition may be difficult to differentiate from trochanteric bursitis. The patient presents with lateral hip and thigh pain that is exacerbated by prolonged walking (especially on hard surfaces) or with running activities. The condition usually results from chronic, repetitive stress to the inhibited or weak G Med and lateral pelvis and thigh structures. The patient presenting with symptoms may be young—in high school or college—or may be a recreational runner or a senior tennis player. The patient often has associated adductor or groin pain.

The physical examination generally reveals on ambulation-excessive lateral tilting of the pelvis. During the stance phase of the involved side, a tilting will occur away from the weak or inhibited G Med. The modified Thomas test position (Figure 15–1) reveals tightness of the adductors, in particular, the short adductors. Inhibition or weakness of the G Med and TFL overuse on side-lying hip abduction is observed.

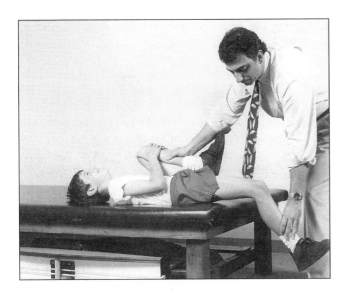

Figure 15–1 Modified Thomas test position.

Trigger points in the G Med, as well as tenderness over the trochanteric region, are also common.

Trauma to the quadriceps muscle represents a spectrum of injury that can range from mild bruising to severe tearing with development of localized hematoma or myositis ossificans. It is most often seen in sports such as football, rugby, soccer, basketball, and hockey. The most common site of injury is the anterior and lateral thigh, with resultant disability depending on severity of bleeding and amount of muscle injury. The athlete can usually localize the site of pain in the case of a contusion. It can be differentiated from muscle strains, which usually occur at the midbelly, as compared with contusions that can occur anywhere in the quadriceps muscles. The mechanism of injury may also help in differentiating the two conditions. The muscle strain usually occurs when the athlete strives for increased speed or extra distance, such as in a kicking motion in soccer. A contusion results from a direct blow. Factors that help determine the severity of the contusion are level of function and degree of swelling; however, disability is usually underestimated.

Generally, the most consistent finding is restriction in knee flexion or worsening pain on active contraction of the quadriceps. In severe cases, marked swelling and difficulty in ambulation are also noted. Symptoms on occasion should be reproduced by having the patient stand or ambulate, or even demonstrate a functional activity that may bring on the pain.

Trauma to the muscle will cause damage to the myofibrils and fascia, as well as to blood vessels. It is the localized bleeding that causes the inflammatory response with swelling. Regional anoxia can then develop, with resultant secondary tissue damage. Contusions that occur in the lower third of the thigh are of particular concern as bleeding may track down to the knee and result in irritation of the patellofemoral joint.[13]

Myositis ossificans is thought of with any increased hardness of the hematoma or when pain with decreased range of motion occurs over two or more treatment sessions. Radiographic signs are present at three to six weeks, and bone scanning may be positive one week prior to the plain films.

Dysfunctions of the pelvis and sacroiliac joint are a relatively common—however overlooked—and, at times, poorly understood etiology in producing pain in the hip, pelvic, and thigh regions. The precipitating event can be a fall on the buttocks or repetitive running on uneven surfaces. The patient complains of buttock and posterior thigh pain; however, it is not uncommon for groin and lower back pain to be the presenting symptom. Symptoms are common in athletes who perform running as either the main or a major activity of their sport.

The physical examination generally will start with documentation of the side of sacroiliac joint restriction. The Gillet's test, as well as standing and sitting forward flexion tests[7] (Figures 15–2 through 15–4), all have been used to identify restriction. The standing forward flexion test corresponds to restriction of the ilium on the sacrum or so-called iliosacral movement. The seated forward flexion test is generally used to identify the side of the restricted sacral motion in relationship to the stable ilium when in the seated position. The most common of the 14 different dysfunctions of the sacroiliac joints and pelvis in athletes, as well as in nonathletes, is the right innominate anterior rotation. These patients have certain muscle imbalances that also represent the most commonly seen pattern of the lumbopelvic imbalances. There is tightness of the ipsilateral adductors, rectus

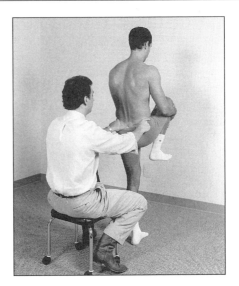

Figure 15–2 Gillet's test.

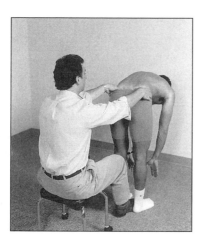

Figure 15–3 Standing forward flexion test.

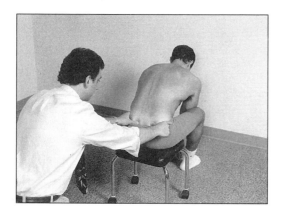

Figure 15–4 Seated forward flexion test.

femoris, IP, and quadratus lumborum (QL), along with the contralateral TFL. Ipsilaterally inhibited and weak muscles include the G Max, G Med, and G Min, as well as the lumbosacral paraspinals. This results in increases in the lumbar lordosis and anterior pelvic tilt. In the supine position, the anterior superior iliac spine is inferior on the right, and the right lower extremity appears longer when measuring the medial malleoli. It should be pointed out here that the side of the sacroiliac joint restriction does not necessarily correlate with the side of the symptoms. For example, if the right sacroiliac joint is restricted, symptoms can occur on the contralateral side, due to relative hypermobility that develops in a compensatory manner.

DIFFERENTIAL DIAGNOSIS

The differential diagnosis can be divided into four major groups consisting of specific soft tissue injuries, primary joint and bone pain, referred pain, and radicular pain. The soft-tissue injuries (Exhibit 15–1) are divided into seven sub-

categories, the first of which includes tendinitis, strains, tears, and ruptures, as previously discussed. The second subcategory is related to bursitis, of which IP, subtrochanteric, and ischiogluteal bursitis are the most common. It is essential to differentiate bursitis from tendinitis, which at times can be difficult and may coexist. With tendinitis, resisted motions are usually more painful, whereas exquisite tenderness is elicited on palpation of an inflamed bursa. The third subcategory consists of contusions and myositis ossificans, also previously discussed. The snapping (clicking) hip is the fourth subcategory, the hip joint suction phenomenon being its most common cause. Less common is subluxation, loose body, or osteochondromatosis. The psoas tendon, iliotibial band, or biceps femoris snapping over bony prominences is also common. Symphysis pubis dysfunction—whether posttraumatic, postpartum, or as seen with generalized ligamentous laxity—is a less common cause. The fifth subcategory involves meralgia paresthetica and other nerve entrapments. The lateral femoral cutaneous nerve of the thigh may be entrapped in the pelvis adjacent to the anterosuperior iliac spine. There can be fibrous or fibro-osseous tunnels, through which emerge either single or multiple branches. The obese athlete, such as a football player, is at risk, especially when restrictive equipment is worn. Electrodiagnostic testing is useful in confirming the diagnosis, and dermatomal-evoked potentials are quite helpful when standard electrodiagnostic testing is technically difficult. Muscle imbalances account for the sixth subcategory and can be divided into the pelvic crossed syndrome—exhibited by tight hip flexors and HS, and inhibited glutei and lumbar erector spinae—piriformis syndrome, and hip impingement syndromes. The pelvic crossed syndrome is quickly recognized when the athlete is in a partial bridge position with one-legged support. The HS is seen to cramp on the supported side within a few seconds, indicating overuse of the HS and inhibited or weak G Max activity. Lumbopelvic muscle tightness patterns are easily identified in the modified Thomas test position (see Figure 15–1). The IP versus rectus femoris tightness (Figure 15–5), short adductors (Figure 15–6), and TFL tightness (Figure 15–7) can be observed. On prone hip extension, the sequence of firing involves ipsilateral HS, G Max, then contralateral lumbosacral paraspinals, ipsilateral lumbosacral paraspinals, and, finally, the contralateral thoracolumbar and ipsilateral thoracolumbar paraspinals.[14] A common abnormal firing pattern occurs when the G Max is inhibited and fires late in the sequence or not at all.

The piriformis syndrome may involve little or no lower back pain with predominate symptoms in the ipsilateral buttock; varying degrees of thigh and lower extremity paresthesia are common. Tightness below 90 degrees of hip flexion can be identified in the supine position, with 60 degrees of hip flexion, slight adduction, then the introduction of internal rotation (Figure 15–8). Flexion of the hip at greater than 90

Exhibit 15–1 Differential Diagnosis

A. Specific Soft-Tissue Injuries
   1. Tendinitis, strains, tears, and ruptures
   2. Bursitis
   3. Contusions and myositis ossificans
   4. Snapping (clicking hip)
      a) hip joint
         1) Most common: suction phenomenon
         2) Less common: subluxation, loose body, or osteochondromatosis
      b) psoas tendon, iliotibial band, biceps femoris—over bony prominences
      c) symphysis pubis dysfunction
         1) posttraumatic, postpartum, or with generalized ligamentous laxity
   5. Meralgia paresthetica and other nerve entrapments
   6. Muscle imbalances
      a) pelvic crossed syndrome
      b) piriformis syndrome
      c) impingement syndrome
         1) anteromedial impingement
         2) anterolateral impingement
         3) proximal impingement
   7. Myofascial pain syndromes
B. Primary Joint and Bone Pain
   1. Dysfunctions of the pelvis and sacroiliac joints
      a) symphysis pubis
         1) superior
         2) inferior
      b) sacroiliac
         1) bilateral anterior nutation
         2) bilateral posterior nutation
         3) unilateral anterior nutation (flexion)
         4) unilateral posterior nutation (extension)
         5) anterior torsion (left-on-left or right-on-right)
         6) posterior torsion (right-on-left or left-on-right)
      c) iliosacral
         1) anterior rotation
         2) posterior rotation
         3) superior shear (upslip)
         4) inferior shear (upslip)
         5) medial rotation (inflare)
         6) lateral rotation (outflare)
   2. Joint inflammation and bony pathology
      a) spondyloarthropathy, sacroiliitis, and osteitis pubis
      b) stress fractures, avascular necrosis, and slipped capital femoral epiphysis
      c) contusions, apophysitis, avulsion fractures, enthesopathy, and coccydynia
      d) osteoarthritis, synovitis, and rheumatologic disorders affecting the hip
      e) subluxations and dislocations of the hip
      f) tumors
C. Referred Pain
   1. Lumbar degenerative disc disease, internal disc disruption, spondylolysis, pars stress reaction, stenosis with neurogenic claudication, and lumbar facet dysfunctions
   2. Nonmusculoskeletal disorders
      a) bowel and bladder dysfunction; testicular, renal, abdominal, rectal, and lymph node etiologies
D. Radicular Pain
   1. Lumbar herniated nucleus pulposus with radiculopathy
   2. Spondylolisthesis with radiculopathy
   3. Lateral recess/foraminal stenosis with radiculopathy

Source: Reprinted with permission from M.C. Geraci, Rehabilitation of Pelvis, Hip, and Thigh Injuries in Sports, in J.M. Press, ed., *Physical Medicine and Rehabilitation Clinics of North America*, pp. 161–162, © 1994, W.B. Saunders Company.

degrees with full external rotation and some adduction (Figure 15–9) allows for detection of tightness of the piriformis above 90 degrees of hip flexion. The rectal exam is essential and can identify a tight and tender piriformis. The piriformis is often overloaded and tight as it tries to substitute, as on hip abductor, for an inhibited G Med. The hip impingement syndromes[15] include anteromedial, anterolateral, and proximal impingements. In the anteromedial impingement, groin pain on hip flexion or posterior pain during loaded weight-bearing is the primary complaint, such as with jogging or dancing. On knee-to-chest, there is anteromedial displacement of the greater trochanter. On extension, HS muscles predominate over G Max; tightness of the tensor fascia latae is also noted. In the anterolateral impingement, pain with loaded weight-bearing will increase external rotation of the lower extremity in standing. External rotators and HS are tight. The proximal impingement syndrome is noted by complaints of deep hip pain, pain just lateral to the muscle belly of the TFL, or pain along the inner thigh region. This impingement syndrome is often associated with osteoarthritis. The athlete complains of discomfort and/or stiffness in the morning, with activity worsening the symptoms. The capsular pattern of decreased hip flexion and internal rotation is seen. The associated muscle imbalances are tightness of the iliopsoas, rectus femoris, and tensor fascia latae.

The final subcategory of soft-tissue injuries is the myofascial pain syndrome. Trigger points and tendinitis develop in muscles with a tendency for inhibition or weakness. Classic examples have been discussed previously, such as those

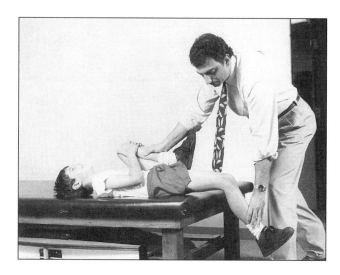

Figure 15–5 Modified Thomas test position. Tightness of the rectus femoris does not allow the normal resting position of the knee to be at 90 degrees.

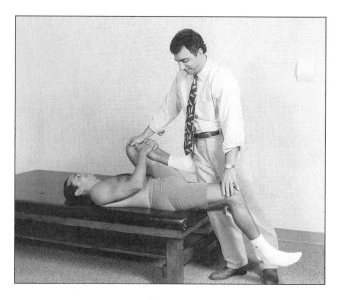

Figure 15–7 Modified Thomas test position. Tightness of the TFL does not allow for the normal 30 degrees of adduction at the hip.

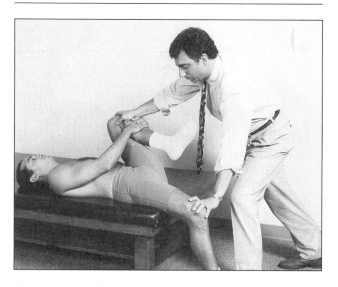

Figure 15–6 Modified Thomas test position. Tightness of the short adductors does not allow for the normal 30 degrees of abduction at the hip.

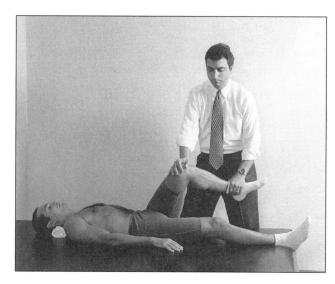

Figure 15–8 Piriformis test. For detection of tightness at less than 90 degrees of hip flexion.

involving the G Med and G Min, as well as the vasti of the quadriceps, especially the vastus medialis. Needling of a trigger point is sometimes necessary to help in its deactivation and to allow for proper stretching of the involved segment. However, to go on a search-and-destroy mission of attacking numerous trigger points with needling techniques would be chasing the pain instead of identifying biomechanical precipitating factors. A study concluded that dry needling of trigger points appears to be equally as effective as needling with local anesthetic and/or steroid.[16] Pelvic floor myalgias, especially in the female athlete, are most often associated with tautness of the sacrotuberous ligament and its surrounding fascia, as well as with coccydynia. In fact, most coccydynia is referred to the coccyx and not primarily an injury such as a fracture. When female athletes have stress incontinence, the pelvic floor muscles and related structures should be thoroughly evaluated. Physical therapists experienced in vaginal and rectal exams of the pelvic floor muscles, as well as the rehabilitation of these structures, can be extremely helpful to the athlete.

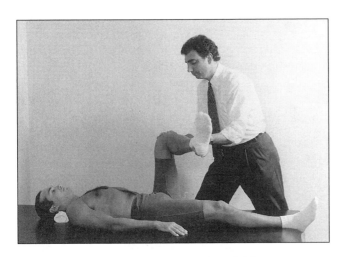

Figure 15–9 Piriformis test. For detection of tightness at greater than 90 degrees of hip flexion.

The second category of differential diagnosis is primary joint and bone pain (see Exhibit 15–1). Dysfunctions of the pelvis and sacroiliac joints are among the most common. There are 14 different dysfunctions of the pelvis and sacroiliac joints[7] (see Exhibit 15–1). From a general sports medicine center, 195 consecutive cases showed that approximately 21% of the injuries were to the pelvis, hip, and thigh, with the most common pelvic dysfunctions involving a right innominate anterior rotation or right inferior pubic rami, followed by right innominate posterior rotation.[2] All 14 of the different pelvic and sacroiliac dysfunctions were noted, but with decreasing frequency.

The second subcategory of primary joint and bone pain involves joint inflammation and other bony pathology such as seen in spondyloarthropathy, sacroiliitis, and osteitis pubis. Suspicion from history and physical examination leads to requesting of radiographic examinations and, usually, a bone scan. If spondyloarthropathy is suspected, rheumatologic workup would be appropriate. Sacroiliitis and osteitis pubis are still less frequent than are dysfunctions in these joints related to fascial and muscle imbalances. Stress fractures, avascular necrosis, and slipped capital femoral epiphysis are also listed in this subcategory. Avascular necrosis from Legg-Perthes disease is common between the ages of 2 and 8 years, unless posttraumatic disruption of the blood supply to the femoral head has occurred. The slipped epiphysis is common between 10 and 14 years of age, especially in overweight males. Stress fractures and synovitis are common between 15 and 25 years of age. Between 20 and 40 years of age, rheumatoid arthritis involving the hip, synovitis, and avascular necrosis is common. It is essential that early detection of stress fractures is documented and treated to prevent these fractures from becoming complete and/or

displaced fractures. Inguinal or anterior groin pain is a common presenting symptom, aggravated by activity such as single-leg standing and hopping. A consistent finding is that extremes of hip rotation reproduce the pain. Pelvic stress fractures most commonly involve the inferior pubic ramus. The superior pubic ramus and ischial areas are less common sites. Palpation over the pubic rami may produce intense local pain.

Avascular necrosis in the athlete is usually due to traumatic causes involving femoral neck fractures, hip dislocation, blood vessel damage, or use of steroids. In ages up to 8 years, transient synovitis of the hip may also be an etiology. Magnetic resonance imaging is very helpful in confirming the diagnosis. The slipped capital femoral epiphysis presents with symptoms of hip pain worsening particularly with rotation; it should be noted that 20–25% of symptoms are bilateral. In the young athlete between the ages of 8 and 12 years, knee discomfort without effusion makes this diagnosis suspect. Physical examination reveals on passive hip flexion that the hip moves into external rotation and slight abduction. Radiographic evaluation reveals widening of the epiphyseal line and defines the degree of slip.

Contusions, apophysitis, avulsion fractures, and enthesopathy—as well as coccydynia—are all part of the differential diagnosis. Iliac crest contusion (hip pointer) is caused by a direct blow to the iliac crest, such as seen in football, hockey, or volleyball. Apophysitis and avulsion fractures are seen less commonly. These result from active muscle contractions during forced muscle stretching. Apophysitis is caused from traction applied to the attaching tendon, with resultant inflammation at the apophyseal growth plate. Avulsion fracture results if the force applied to the apophysis is too great, seen particularly in muscles with a tendency to shorten, i.e., the HS muscles, rectus femoris, and sartorius. These happen to be the sites of most avulsion fractures in the pelvis—the ischial tuberosity at the HS attachment, the anterior inferior iliac spine at the rectus femoris attachment, and the anterior superior iliac spine at the sartorius attachment. Enthesopathy can occur at any tendon or ligament attachment to bone and is frequent at the iliac crest. The patient usually complains of intense pain along the iliac crest that worsens with walking or running activities. Radiographic examinations usually reveal a spur formation. Coccydynia most often results from referred pain to the coccyx and not from primary injury, such as fracture, to this area. Often, rectal palpation of the sacrococcygeal joint with traction, rotation, and anterior and posterior gliding is helpful in assessment and treatment.

Also as subcategories of primary joint and bone pain are osteoarthritis, synovitis, and rheumatologic disorders affecting the hip. Osteoarthritis and synovitis of the hip present in middle-aged to older athletes. The capsular pattern of pain on flexion and internal rotation is very helpful when present, if this diagnosis is suspected. Radiographic changes may or may not be present at the time of the initial presentation. If imaging studies are negative but clinical suspicions are high, a local injection of anesthetic under fluoroscopic guidance can be done for diagnostic purposes. Treatment also consists of mobilization of the anterior and posterior hip joint capsule, along with reduction of impact loading through muscle rebalancing. Other rheumatologic disorders of the hip should be kept in mind, especially as presentation of rheumatoid arthritis and/or connective tissue disease can present initially with hip pain and arthritis. Subluxations and dislocations of the hip are much less common than in the shoulder region. Approximately 90% are posterior when related to sporting injuries. Symptoms and signs involve severe pain and a slightly flexed, adducted, and internally rotated hip position present at the time of injury. Anterior dislocation results in slight hip flexion, abduction, and external rotation. The history of high-speed sporting injury or heavy contact on a flexed and adducted hip is often the presenting mechanism of injury. Tumors must be included in the differential diagnosis as the femur is a common site in young individuals. Benign tumors such as giant cell, aneurysmal bone, fibrous dysplasia, and fibrous cortical defects may all produce pain. Osteochondroma may produce bursitis or tenderness, as well. Osteosarcoma should always be considered in the young adult, especially if pain is unremitting and deep in nature. In these cases, radiographic examination should always be done.

Lumbar degenerative disc disease, internal disc disruption, spondylolysis, pars stress reaction, stenosis with neurogenic claudication, and dysfunction of the lumbar facets are also included in the differential diagnoses of referred pain. Nonmusculoskeletal disorders such as bowel and bladder dysfunction or testicular, renal, abdominal, rectal, and lymph node etiologies are all possible sources of referred pain.

The fourth category of radicular pain (see Exhibit 15–1) includes radiculopathy secondary to lumbar herniated nucleus pulposus, spondylolisthesis, and lateral recess/foraminal stenosis. The presence of dural root tension signs, such as seen on slump testing[17] (Figure 15–10), as well as classic straight-leg raising signs, are often helpful in making the diagnosis. It is not uncommon for S1 and, to a lesser extent, L5 radiculopathies to present as posterior thigh pain without back or buttock symptoms; these must be considered when a hamstring injury fails to respond to adequate treatment.

COMPLETE AND ACCURATE DIAGNOSIS

Several different entities are discussed in detail here using the vicious cycle complexes.

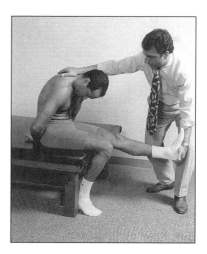

Figure 15–10 The slump test.

Sacroiliac and Pelvic Dysfunctions—Innominate Anterior Rotation

Sacroiliac and pelvic dysfunction is the first area for discussion; the innominate anterior rotation will be used, as this is the most common dysfunction seen in the athletic population.

The *Tissue Injury Complex* involves the sacroiliac joint, including the sacral hyaline and the ilial fibrocartilage, supporting ligaments, and joint capsule. In particular, the anterior sacroiliac joint capsule can show diverticulae or tears, as outlined quite well on sacroiliac joint arthrography. Also, the iliolumbar ligaments are part of the *Tissue Injury Complex,* due to their attachments.

The *Clinical Symptom Complex* generally involves the patient's primary complaints of buttock and posterior thigh paresthesia, along with groin and lower back pain to a lesser extent.[18,19]

The *Functional Biomechanical Deficits* are demonstrated by tight ipsilateral adductors, RF, IP, QL, and latissimus dorsi (LD). The contralateral or ipsilateral TFL also is tight. The inhibited and/or weak muscles are primarily the G Max, G Med, and G Min on the ipsilateral side, as well as the lumbosacral paraspinals and abdominals, and, in particular, the lower abdominals on the ipsilateral side.

The *Functional Adaptation Complex* reveals increase in the lumbar lordosis and an anterior pelvic tilt. There can also be relative hypermobility of the contralateral sacroiliac joint. Compensatory changes are also seen in the lumbar spine, which will go into ipsilateral side-bending and contralateral rotation of the lower segments. This is due, in part, to tension from the iliolumbar ligaments and from the IP and QL tightness on the ipsilateral side—these are side-benders and rotators of the lumbar segments to the opposite sides. Hip external rotators become tight and try to compensate for a loss of pelvic stability from reduced activity of the gluteal muscles. An inferior pubic rami usually accompanies an innominate anterior rotation ipsilaterally.

The *Tissue Overload Complex* is exhibited by increased stress across the L4–L5 and L5–S1 discs and zygapophyseal joints, as well as the contralateral sacroiliac joint. The hip joints also receive considerable impact loading, due to the muscle imbalances described above. Distal along the kinetic chain, the anterior pelvic tilt yields knee flexion greater than normal at foot flat in midstance, thus increasing the eccentric load across the extensor mechanism of the knee, which may contribute to patellar tendon injury as well as predisposing to patellofemoral problems. As knee flexion becomes greater, so do the compressive forces of the patella on the femur. With these changes in pelvic as well as lower extremity mechanics at the knee, the overall kinetic chain is disrupted and can lead to overload of the shoulder joint in throwing athletes as there are decreased ground reaction and spinal forces imparted to the shoulder.

Muscle Strains—Adductors

The next example concentrates on muscle strains—in particular, the adductors. These muscles are commonly injured in sporting activities, especially those involving sudden change in direction. Recurrent adductor muscle strains are very common and are due mainly to inadequate rehabilitation after the initial injury. In particular, balance must be restored between the ipsilateral lower abdominals and the adductors, along with the lateral pelvis and thigh structures.

The *Tissue Injury Complex* involves the adductors, usually the adductor longus at the proximal musculotendinous junction, tendo-osseus insertion to the inferior pubic ramius, or the muscle belly itself.

The *Clinical Symptom Complex* presents primarily as groin and inner thigh pain. Also commonly seen is ipsilateral pelvic and hip pain, worse with walking or running activity.

The *Functional Biomechanical Deficits* include tightness of the ipsilateral ADD and contralateral TFL. The inhibited and/or weak muscles are the ipsilateral G Med and G Min, as well as lower abdominals.

The *Functional Adaptation Complex* is demonstrated by increase in lateral tilt of the pelvis, where the contralateral pelvis drops in the swing phase of gait. There is usually an inferior pubic ramius on the ipsilateral side, as well as compensatory lumbar side-bending to the ipsilateral side and rotation to the contralateral side. The ipsilateral piriformis substitutes as an abductor for the inhibited G Med and G Min. This results in ipsilateral hip external rotation.

The *Tissue Overload Complex* is exhibited by excessive strain and inflammation of the lateral pelvis and hip structures, including the G Med and G Min, as well as the trochanteric bursa. Also, the TFL and iliotibial band and lateral knee structures, as well as the lumbar spine, have increased overload. The ADD inhibit the contraction of the glutei after the propulsion phase of running. The distal kinetic structures—in particular, the knee—are overloaded; the shoulder has potential overload due to altered pelvic stability. The abdominals are considerably overloaded due to the inferior pubic ramius, which causes the abdominals to be on stretch and relatively increases their length, placing the throwing athlete at risk for tears in this muscle group. The ipsilateral piriformis is overloaded, causing the entire lower limb to rotate externally, interfering with running and normal walking.

Muscle Strains—Hamstring

Hamstring injuries are similar to injuries of the adductors, in that they tend to be chronic or recurrent in nature and can disable the athlete for an indefinite period of time. In particular, runners involved in sprinting, long-jumping, or hurdles are more susceptible to HS injury; however, it is not uncommon in long-distance runners. It is probably the most frequently strained muscle in the body. Two theories as to why this muscle is so susceptible to injury are based on its role of eccentric contraction as the knee comes to full extension at heel strike. Higher forces are produced with eccentric muscle contraction, which places the musculotendinous junction at greater risk. This is especially true at high velocities. The other possible etiology is an injury resulting from a violent stretch or rapid contraction of the muscle. We feel very strongly that chronic HS overload is the result of an inhibited G Max that cannot work synergistically with the G Max and, therefore, places chronic overload on the HS. This muscle imbalance pattern is commonly seen when the IP muscle is tight and leads to reciprocal inhibition of the G Max, with resultant overuse of the HS.

The *Tissue Injury Complex* involves injury to the muscle at its junction with the aponeurosis proximally. This is the most common site of hamstring injury; however, the muscle may tear at the common tendon insertional to the ischium or in the muscle belly itself.

The *Clinical Symptom Complex* presents with pain in the posterior thigh region, usually in the proximal or middle third.

The *Functional Biomechanical Deficits* include tightness of the IP and hamstrings, as well as adverse mechanical tension that develops in the sciatic nerve distribution. The major inhibited muscle is the G Max, which is synergistic to the HS but has a tendency for inhibition that may lead to chronic hamstring overuse. The adverse mechanical tension in the sciatic nerve does not allow for proper stretching of the HS and, in this author's experience, is the most common reason that HS muscles are still tight after apparent adequate stretching by the athlete for months or even years. This adverse mechanical tension that develops in the sciatic nerve distribution must be stretched using neuromobilization techniques before the HS muscles can be adequately stretched.

Other *Functional Biomechanical Deficits* may include eccentric HS weakness—even though the muscle has a tendency for tightness, it may not be able to develop the proper eccentric contraction necessary during running—and imbalance between the quadriceps and HS strength. The HS should be capable of producing 60% of the muscle strength generated by the quadriceps. When this ratio is imbalanced, there is an increased frequency of HS injury. Any anterior tilting of the pelvis resultant from G Max inhibition or sacroiliac dysfunctions, such as an innominate anterior rotation, may also place the hamstring at risk, due to abnormal length.

The *Functional Adaptation Complex* is seen when the pelvis cannot anteriorly rotate secondary to HS tightness. The anterior rotation is necessary at push-off. If the HS muscles are too tight, they may keep the innominate posteriorly rotated, causing a flexion moment at the knee, increasing patellofemoral forces and leading to knee pain and possible patellofemoral dysfunction.

The *Tissue Overload Complex* is not only on the HS muscles themselves but also on the quadriceps—in particular, the vasti, which become inhibited due to HS tightness. The patellofemoral joint again can become overloaded, as can the sacroiliac joints, which are overloaded due to the posterior rotation of the innominate from HS tightness. Due to the high frequency of injury of HS muscles, it is essential that the athlete learn proper stretching techniques. Most importantly, stretching should be done immediately after running, or at least with an adequate warm-up of 10–15 minutes of the running activity itself. This author's preference is for athletes to stretch after a run; neuromobilization techniques should be taught prior to attempting to stretch the HS muscles, for reasons mentioned above. Proper muscle balance must be restored to the IP due to its inhibitory effects on the G Max. The G Max must also be re-educated to fire and unload the HS muscles.

In the early phases of treatment after an HS injury, the guidelines for initial treatment, as mentioned earlier, should be followed. When 75% range of motion is reached, resisted exercises may be started. Light running activities may resume when the strength is 70% of normal. More ballistic-type work requires approximately 80% of baseline strength. Eventually, it is essential to incorporate high-speed eccentric exercises in the final phase of rehabilitation.

Quadriceps Contusion/Myositis Ossificans

The final example is the quadriceps contusion, with or without myositis ossificans. The severity is usually underestimated, and suspicion should be high after direct trauma in sports.

The *Tissue Injury Complex* involves direct injury to myofibrils, fascia, and blood vessels. Subsequently, osteoblasts can replace fibroblasts in myositis ossificans within the healing hematoma one week after injury.

The *Clinical Symptom Complex* involves a history of direct blow to the anterior or lateral thigh, with resultant tenderness and swelling. Worsening of symptoms is seen on active contraction of the quadriceps or on passive stretching.

The *Functional Biomechanical Deficits* evolve around preexisting tightness of the HS muscles, gastrocsoleus (GS), and, in particular, the RF. The weak and/or inhibited muscles are generally the vasti of the quadriceps.

The *Functional Adaptation Complex* may demonstrate ipsilateral anterior pelvic tilt in an attempt to slacken the fascia of the quadriceps and the RF. The knee is generally held in an extended position, resulting in compensatory hip circumduction and premature plantar flexion of the ankle at heel strike.

The *Tissue Overload Complex* directly involves the patellofemoral joint, especially if the contusion is in the distal third of the quadriceps. This is secondary to irritation when blood tracks down the fascia planes to the knee. Overload is also on the lateral pelvis and hip, as well as on knee structures, due to the anterior pelvic tilt, knee extension, and premature plantar flexion.

REHABILITATION

Any rehabilitation program for the injured athlete with hip, pelvic, and thigh pain must deal effectively with the relationship between these three regions and the lumbar spine and lower extremity kinetic chain, as a minimum. The biomechanical approach to this region and the identification of *Functional Biomechanical Deficits*, muscle imbalances, joint dysfunctions, and their relationship as predisposing factors to soft-tissue injuries must be emphasized. Long-term outcome, success, and the prevention of reinjury will be more likely if the focus is on functional restoration of the hip, pelvic, and thigh region, and its relationship to the entire kinetic chain, rather than on pain alleviation.

The concept of muscle imbalances is reviewed here to give a thorough understanding of this as the basis for functional rehabilitation.[14,15,20] Theoretical causes of muscle imbalances are listed in Exhibit 15–2.

Muscle imbalances develop in adolescence, between the ages of 8 and 16 years old.[21] The incidence of short muscles

Exhibit 15–2 Theoretical Causes of Muscle Imbalances

1. Postural adaptation to gravity
2. Neuroreflexive due to joint blockage
3. Central nervous system malregulation (impaired programming)
4. Response to painful or noxious stimuli
5. Response to physical demands
6. Lack of variety of movement patterns (habitual)
7. Psychologic influences
8. Histochemical differences

Source: Data from: Syllabus—exercise prescription as an adjunct to manual medicine. In: Bookhout MR, Greenman PE, eds. *Continuing Medical Education Course.* Michigan State University: College of Osteopathic Medicine, September 30–October 2, 1994.

in 115 school-aged children revealed that 21% had significant muscle imbalances. Two follow-up periods at ages 12 and 16 showed that incidence of muscle tightness increased, then remained constant. Without treatment, these imbalances were not seen to spontaneously correct. In young athletes, the development of muscle tightness is seen as early as 6 or 7 years of age.[2] A tight muscle has a profound influence on the entire motor program. In cortical regulation, a tight muscle yields peripheral receptor stimulation, leading into the cerebellum, then postcentral sensory cortex, which is essential for creation of movement. Information is then carried to the precentral motor cortex, which acts as an effector or transmitter of the finished program. Finally, information is transmitted back to the periphery and striated muscle. Critical, but often overlooked, areas in this motor control are at the levels of the parietal lobe and the afferent system. The entire mechanism depends on proprioceptive input from these peripheral structures. Cortical regulation provides an advantage of new movements and new programming being available. The disadvantage is that this process is too fatiguing.

Subcortical regulation, however, has the advantage of being nonfatiguing. The disadvantage is that, once a movement becomes established, it is very difficult to change. In this stage of motor learning, at the subcortical or reflex level, information is transmitted from the proprioceptor to the cerebellum, then to subcortical areas, before being transmitted back to the periphery and, finally, to the striated muscle. It must be understood that no biomechanical lesion remains localized. Vertical generalization implies that a lesion at any particular site in a neuromuscular apparatus may eventually lead to dysfunction in other areas.[14] Horizontal generalization deals with the lesion, such as a muscle imbalance or

joint dysfunction, that does not remain localized and has an effect on other muscles and joint dysfunctions if left untreated. It should be noted that most joint dysfunctions are painless unless muscle dysfunction (spasm) develops.[14] Tissue texture abnormality and asymmetry, along with changes in range of motion, are very helpful in identifying a painful joint dysfunction.

Certain muscles have the tendency to develop tightness, and these in the lumbopelvic region include IP, RF, TFL, short ADD, HS, QL, LD, and the thoracolumbar erector spinae. In addition, the piriformis and gastrocsoleus muscle groups have a tendency for tightness. Other muscles have a tendency for developing inhibition and/or weakness, including the lumbosacral erector spinae, all glutei muscles, tibialis anterior, and the peronei. The abdominals and vasti of the quadriceps, especially the vastus medialis, are also included. A general guide to the treatment sequence of injuries to the hip, pelvis, and thigh is discussed at this point (Exhibit 15–3). Initially, most joint dysfunctions correct with proper muscle rebalancing, using postisometric relaxation stretching of the tight muscles, as well as myofascial stretching. Correction of somatic joint dysfunctions remaining after muscle rebalancing, using muscle energy techniques, myofascial release, and other manual techniques, is useful. There is also a limited role for modalities in this phase. Self-

Exhibit 15–3 A General Guide to Treatment Sequence

A. Muscle rebalancing
   1. Postisometric relaxation stretching of tight muscles (especially those interfering with the quality of movement)
   2. Myofascial stretching
   3. Self-stretching—proper isolation and contraction of antagonist, emphasizing proper biomechanical alignment
B. Correction of somatic joint dysfunctions remaining after muscle rebalancing, with muscle energy techniques, myofascial release, and manual treatment. Also, limited use of modalities is appropriate.
C. Sensorimotor stimulation through balance and coordination training may be more important than strengthening. Reeducate movement pattern preventing undesirable overactivation or substitution patterns.
D. Strength, endurance, and cardiovascular training
E. Sport-specific skills

Source: Reprinted with permission from M.C. Geraci, Rehabilitation of Pelvis, Hip, and Thigh Injuries in Sports, in J.M. Press, ed., *Physical Medicine and Rehabilitation Clinics of North America,* pp. 170–171, © 1994, W.B. Saunders.

stretching with proper isolation and contraction of the antagonist, using biomechanically correct alignment, is taught to the patient at this point to prevent compensatory movements. The next phase involves sensorimotor stimulation through balance and coordination retraining; stimulating the subcortical pathways would allow for better protection. This phase may be more important than strengthening as muscles can become facilitated, thus decreasing the need for additional strengthening in many cases. Strength, endurance, and cardiovascular conditioning can usually be done safely at this point without risking perpetuation of muscle imbalances. Cardiovascular conditioning can be done throughout the entire rehabilitation program, providing that it does not involve activities that would serve only to perpetuate the pre-existing functional and biomechanical deficits and muscle imbalances. The final phase is developing a sports-specific skills program with attention to the proper biomechanics of that sport.

A guide to proper self-stretching is included in Exhibit 15–4. Demonstrations of proper self-stretching techniques for patients are clearly shown (Figures 15–11 through 15–19). Specific rehabilitation programs for the several conditions outlined earlier follow.

Sacroiliac and Pelvic Dysfunctions: Innominate Anterior Rotation

Acute Phase (First 48 Hours)

Acute phases of rehabilitation for innominate anterior rotations focus on treatment of the *Tissue Injury Complex* and

---

Exhibit 15–4 A Guide to Proper Self-Stretching

A. Patient holds stretch for 30 seconds and may repeat three times on the tighter side, compared to two times on the opposite side.
B. Activation of antagonist helps to inhibit the reciprocal tight muscle, allowing for better stretch.
C. Stretching is usually best accomplished after 5–10 minutes of warm-up of the actual sporting activity at a mild to moderate intensity.
D. If possible, avoid stretching and sports in the first two hours after rising. The neuromuscular system is not as prepared to receive maximum benefit from the stretching, and there is increased risk of injury.

Source: Reprinted with permission from M.C. Geraci, Rehabilitation of Pelvis, Hip, and Thigh Injuries in Sports, in J.M. Press, ed., *Physical Medicine and Rehabilitation Clinics of North America*, pp. 170–171, © 1994, W.B. Saunders.

Clinical Symptom Complex. In most cases, however, the onset is insidious in nature, and an acute traumatic event may occur several weeks, months, or even years before the onset of symptoms. It may be only after the athlete performs the sport—in particular, walking and running movements—for a prolonged period of time before actual symptoms develop. There may still be acute presentation, with pain either on the ipsilateral or often on the contralateral side to the dysfunction. Under these circumstances, ice applied every hour or a minimum of four times per day for 20 minutes, along with limited use of antiinflammatory medications for several days to two weeks, would be appropriate. Relative rest, such as avoiding activities stressful to the sacroiliac joints, as with prolonged walking or running, should be practiced.

In most cases, an attempt can be made to correct the dysfunction using muscle energy techniques (MET) or myofascial release (MFR). Several different positions are available to treat the dysfunction when using muscle energy techniques (Figure 15–20). The practitioner positions the patient so that an intrinsic activating force by the patient helps to reposition the dysfunctional joint into its proper alignment. Treating the innominate anterior rotation with MFR, the supine position is best suited (Figure 15–21). At this stage, it is also beneficial to instruct the patient in self-correction techniques (Figure 15–22). However, the symphysis pubis should always be treated first (Figure 15–23), as this is the center of rotation for pelvic movements.

Recovery Phase (7 Days to 8 Weeks)

The *Functional Biomechanical Deficits* and *Tissue Overload Complex* are treated in this phase of rehabilitation. Because the innominate anterior rotation is an iliosacral dysfunction and the innominate bone is considered to be part of the lower extremity, the imbalances of muscle length and strength in the lower extremity must be addressed as they will have significant influence on iliosacral dysfunction.[20] It is essential to first stretch the muscles having a tendency for developing tightness and representing part of a pattern seen with an innominate anterior rotation. This should be followed by facilitation and reeducation techniques to the muscles that have a tendency to become inhibited and/or weak. Following this, closed-chain kinetics will be used beginning with facilitation of the inhibited and/or weak muscles. Pelvic stabilization training follows this. The patient is moved into functional exercises, and sport-specific skills are next addressed. The stretching program to the lumbopelvic musculature is essential for correction of biomechanical deficits. In particular, the IP, RF, TFL, ADD, QL, and LD muscles are the most important (see Figures 15–11, 15–17, and 15–19). The adductors have a pull on the inferior pubic rami, tending to draw it downward. The hip flexors, including TFL, RF, and iliacus of the IP, have a ten-

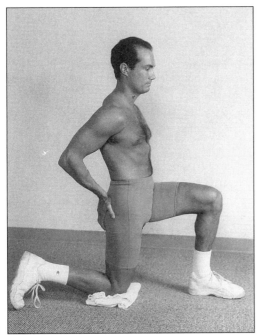

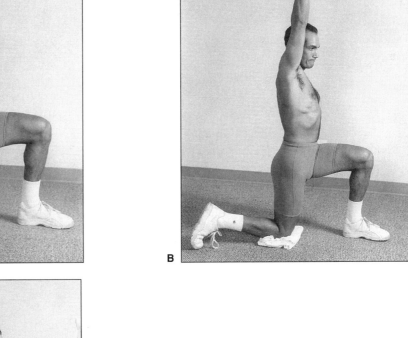

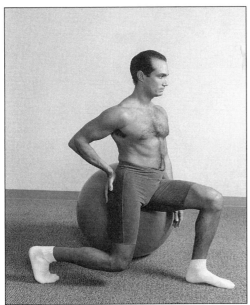

Figure 15–11 Iliopsoas stretch. (*A*) A posterior pelvic tilt, along with hip internal rotation and activation of the gluteus maximus, allows for proper isolation; (*B*) advanced stretch with addition of myofascial stretching from above; (*C*) advanced stretch with dynamic stretch introduced by using an exercise ball.

dency to rotate the innominate anteriorly. The QL and LD add to the increase in anterior pelvic tilt. Self-correction techniques are taught at the same time, and the patient should be performing these stretches two times per day with 3–5 repetitions. Before beginning a facilitation program to the inhibited and/or weak muscles, proper stretching should be carried for 2–3 weeks. Often, the inhibited muscles, in particular, can be retested and found to be firing normally at this point, due simply to the release of the inhibitory effects from their antagonistic muscles, which were tight.

The inhibited and weak muscles—in particular, the G Max, G Med, and G Min—are facilitated next. A figure-of-four position helps to decrease the activity of the ipsilateral hamstring and, with attempt at raising the knee off of the table or floor, facilitation is provided to the glutei muscles (Figure 15–24). Once the patient is able to facilitate the glutei muscles, instruction is begun in closed-chain kinetic facilitation techniques. Standing on the leg of the inhibited and/or weak glutei while the other leg is flexed with the knee up against the wall, the patient is instructed to rotate the thigh

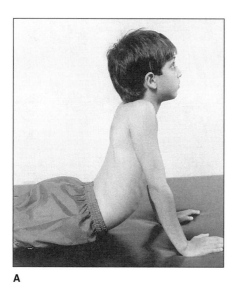

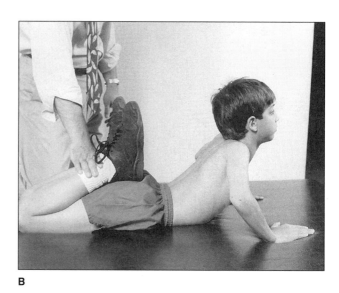

A   **B**

Figure 15–12 Iliopsoas stretch. (*A*) Bilateral, a press-up position with active gluteal contractions allows for symmetric iliopsoas stretching; (*B*) advanced bilateral with full knee flexion shortening the myofascial structures, making the stretch more difficult.

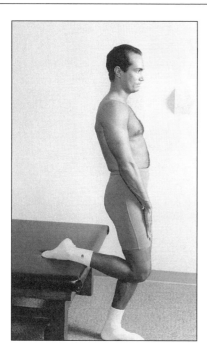

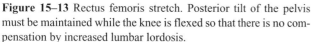

Figure 15–13 Rectus femoris stretch. Posterior tilt of the pelvis must be maintained while the knee is flexed so that there is no compensation by increased lumbar lordosis.

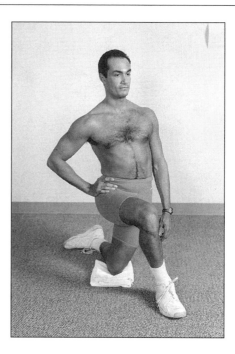

Figure 15–14 Tensor fascia latae stretch–left. A posterior pelvic tilt is maintained while the left hip is placed in slight external rotation and the right lower extremity is crossed over the left. Translation of the pelvis from right to left is then introduced.

in a counterclockwise direction for the left lower extremity and clockwise for the right lower extremity. This can be done only with active contraction of the glutei muscles, and the patient is reminded to keep the shoulders and trunk, as well as the foot, facing forward (Figure 15–25). Following this, standing on one leg introducing flexion of the knee to 20–30 degrees and asking the patient to extend the knee by

using active contractions of the glutei muscles is then attempted. With increasing difficulty, and helping to restore subcortical reflexes through balance and coordination activity, the glutei muscles will begin to fire more on a reflex basis. Using a small trampoline (Figure 15–26A), wobble board (Figure 15–26B), or balance beam will be ideal for

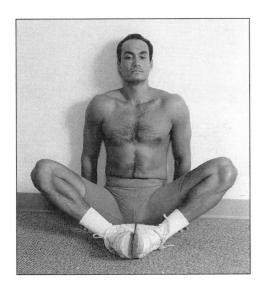

Figure 15–15 Short adductor stretch–bilateral. An anterior pelvic tilt is introduced while active contractions of the abductors try to bring the knees to the floor.

these activities. Increasing difficulty to these activities is added by crossing the arms on the chest, then closing the eyes and having the therapist introduce forces from many different directions as the patient advances through this phase or by adding arm movements with weights (Figure 15–26C). Lumbopelvic stability training can be achieved by using a sliding board, fitter (Figure 15–27A, B), and/or a standing bike exercise (Figure 15–27C) and cross-country ski machine (Figure 15–27D). All of these activities are done in the closed-chain kinetic fashion and will stimulate the lumbopelvic musculature considerably more than in an open-chain fashion.

At times, specific injection into the sacroiliac joint can be helpful in differentiating pain generation and has the potential to be of therapeutic benefit. This technique basically involves using a 25-gauge spinal needle passed into the posterior inferior position of the sacroiliac joint.[22] Pain referral maps have been demonstrated, and, in general, referred pain from the sacroiliac joints includes buttock and posterior thigh regions.[18,19]

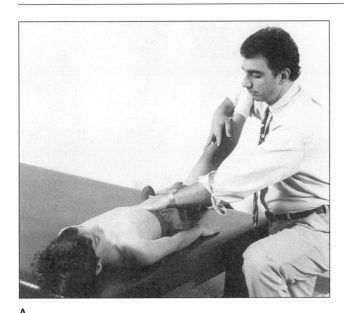

A

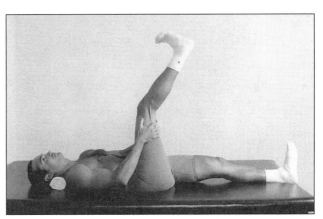

B

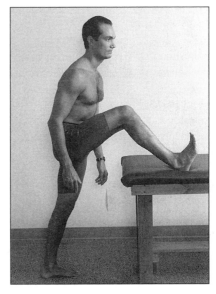

C

Figure 15–16 Hamstring length assessment. (*A*) The right knee is maintained in an extended position, and the lower extremity is held in neutral by cradling the heel. Monitoring over the contralateral anterior superior iliac spine allows for notation of pelvic tilt and degree of hamstring tightness. (*B*) The hip and knee are held at ninety degrees while the quadriceps activates knee extension, allowing for reciprocal inhibition of the hamstring being stretched. (*C*) Upper hamstring stretch.

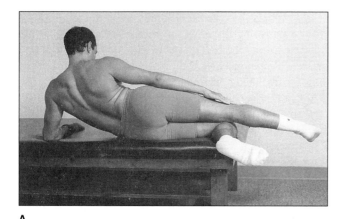

A

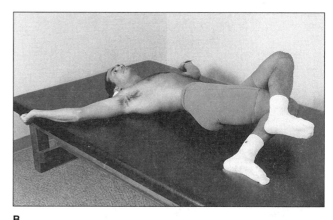

B

Figure 15–17 Quadratus lumborum stretch. (*A*) The pelvis is maintained on the table while right side-bending is introduced. (*B*) Rotation component.

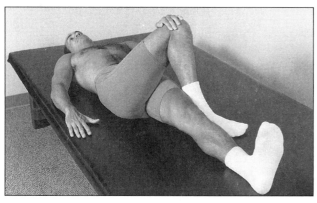

A

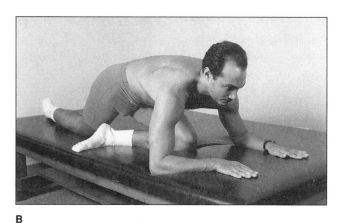

B

Figure 15–18 Piriformis stretch. (*A*) Used when tightness exists below 90 degrees of hip flexion. (*B*) Used when tightness exists at greater than 90 degrees of hip flexion.

The criteria to advance to the maintenance phase include absence of pain and inflammation, no joint dysfunction of the innominate and accompanying pelvic joints, and at least 75% of strength and flexibility regained and able to be maintained during normal activities, especially with walking.

Sacroiliac belts or pelvic stabilization orthoses can be particularly useful in innominate shear dysfunctions; in an innominate anterior rotation, they can also be helpful in providing proprioceptive feedback. Wearing these devices for approximately six weeks after correction can allow time for ligamentous healing. Properly positioned, these belts can significantly limit sacroiliac motion.[23]

Maintenance Phase

In this phase of rehabilitation, continual work is spent on correcting *Functional Biomechanical Deficits* and addressing the *Functional Adaptation Complex*. A complete under-

standing of the stabilization concept of the pelvis and sacroiliac joints is necessary. Several individual muscles, such as the glutei (including the maximus and medius), the iliopsoas, and, in particular, the iliacus and piriformis, all would appear to have very important roles. In anterior innominate rotations, the G Max serves to stabilize the pelvis in the posterior position, due mainly to its attachment to the ilium and sacrotuberous ligaments. Concurrently, if the innominate is allowed to rotate anteriorly, due partly to inhibited and/or weak contractions of the G Max, then a stretch is placed on the iliolumbar ligament that can act on the lower lumbar vertebra, influencing this as part of the *Functional Adaptation Complex*. It is essential that lumbar dysfunctions be corrected before treatment is directed toward the innominates. The G Max is oriented approximately perpendicular to the anterior and medial aspect of the sacroiliac joint. Therefore, strong muscular contraction can compress the sacroiliac

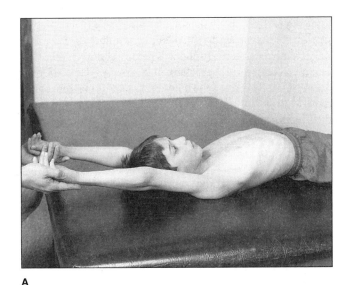

A

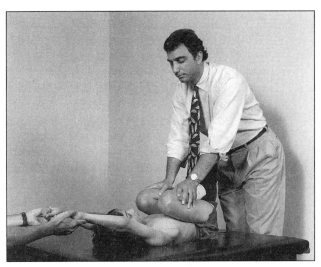

B

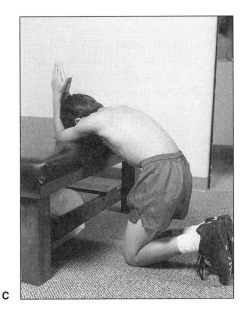

C

Figure 15–19 Latissimus dorsi assessment. (*A*) Tightness is seen when the arms do not reach the table and a compensatory increase in lumbar lordosis occurs. (*B*) Bilateral latissimus dorsi stretch. The knees are brought to the chest to stretch the muscle from below by decreasing the lumbar lordosis with a posterior pelvic tilt. (*C*) The prayer stretch. This allows self-stretching of the muscle bilaterally while introducing posterior pelvic tilt. The arms are touching at the elbows to introduce external rotation while the patient sits back on the heels.

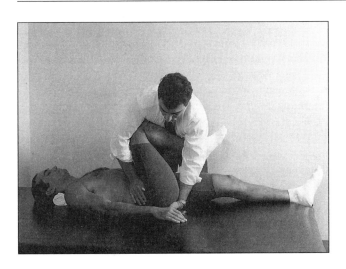

Figure 15–20 Muscle energy technique, correction of anterior innominate rotation. Hand placement allows for monitoring and facilitation of posterior rotation of the innominate while the patient performs isometric hip extension.

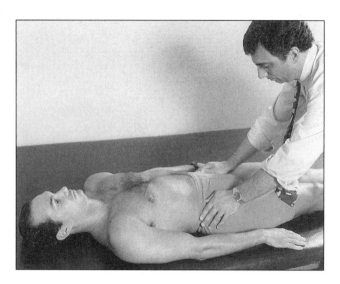

Figure 15–21 Myofascial release technique, right innominate anterior rotation.

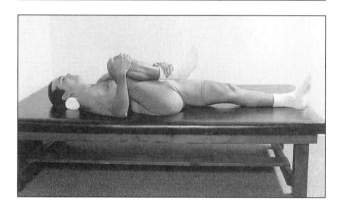

Figure 15–22 Self-correction technique, right innominate anterior rotation.

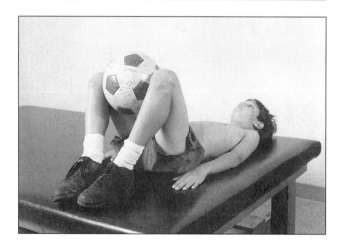

Figure 15–23 Self-correction technique, symphysis pubis dysfunction.

joint and increase the perpendicular force. The IP and, in particular, the iliacus, with its tendency for tightness, can rotate the innominate anteriorly and will require continual monitoring to maintain its proper length in this phase. The piriformis muscle directly crosses the anterior surface of the joint and is thought to be the culprit most often in recurrent sacroiliac dysfunctions. This muscle must be checked for tightness above and below 90 degrees of hip flexion (see Figures 15–8 and 15–9) and must be stretched in both positions if found to be tight.

In the maintenance phase, the role of these individual muscles as mentioned above is very important; however, stabilization of the pelvis and sacroiliac joints through a mass-action effect of numerous muscles is more important. Also during this phase, functional activities are directed toward maintaining flexibilities of those muscles having a tendency for tightness. These activities include stabilization exercises, strength training, advanced proprioceptive and balance retraining, pyelometrics, and sports-specific skills. In anterior innominate rotations, functional agility drills are important, especially in soccer and tennis players. Running as a major component of any sport must be addressed in the maintenance phase in tolerance to normal walking activities without recurrence of anterior innominate dysfunction. Therefore, in the first 5–7 days of the maintenance phase, walking is introduced on a treadmill, making sure that the athlete provides reciprocal trunk and pelvic motions with full upper and lower extremity swing. If this is tolerated without recurrence of anterior innominate dysfunction, which should be monitored before and after these activities by checking the position of the anterior superior iliac spine and medial malleoli in the supine position, advancement can be undertaken. This should be continued, working up to 3 miles over the first 5–7 days in the maintenance phase. Following that, running activities on a treadmill may be started again over a 5- to 7-day period, working up to 3 miles. With no recurrent dysfunctions of anterior innominate rotation noted, the athlete may resume running on level surfaces and, finally, on the actual sport surface.

Because certain muscles that are major stabilizers of the sacroiliac joint have a tendency to become inhibited and/or weak, maintenance of proper reflex activity of these muscles is paramount. In the advanced proprioceptive and balance retraining, a simple maintenance program while using a balance shoe will usually maintain glutei muscle reflex activity.[24] Finally, sports-specific skills are introduced during the maintenance phase, again making sure that the athlete is checked before and after these activities for recurrence of the anterior innominate rotation.

Criteria for Return to Play

As may be expected, each athlete is treated on an individual basis; only guidelines are given here. The athlete

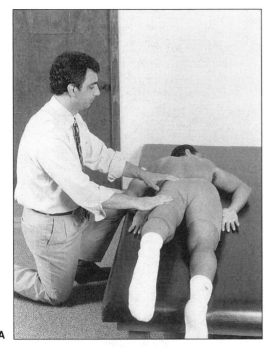
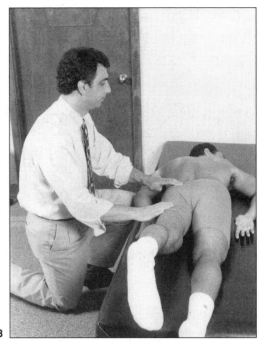

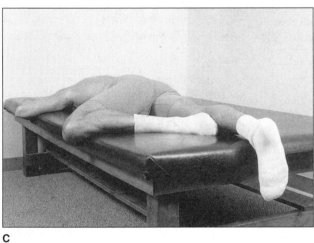
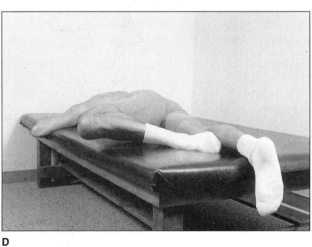

Figure 15–24 Prone hip extension assessment. (*A*) Firing patterns are monitored by hand placement over the hamstring and gluteus maximus while visual observation of the lumbar paraspinals simultaneously occurs. (*B*) Abnormal firing pattern. The gluteus maximus contracts after lumbar paraspinal muscles, rather than before. (*C*) Glutei facilitation technique. Starting position with knee flexed in a figure-of-four position to decrease hamstring activity. (*D*) Glutei facilitation technique. Facilitation occurs when the patient elevates the left knee while trying to maintain the pelvis on the table.

should be off all pain medication and relatively pain free, without return of symptoms during sports-specific activities. The joint dysfunctions should be resolved, and muscles should be rebalanced for length and strength—especially for strength ratios of antagonistic muscles. Proprioceptive balance and coordination should be restored in a limited period of approximately 1–2 weeks, depending on how long the athlete has been off the sport. These should be per-

formed without increase in symptoms or recurrence of dysfunctions.

Muscle Strains—Adductors: Rehabilitation

Acute Phase (0–48 Hours)

The Tissue Injury Complex in this phase involves injury to the adductor longus, usually at its proximal musculotendi-

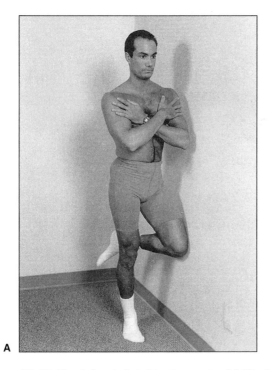
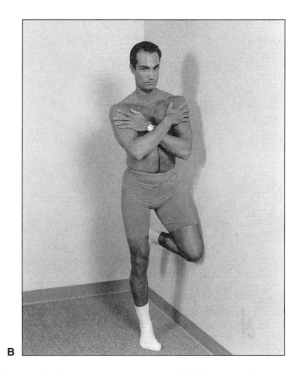

Figure 15–25 Glutei closed-chain kinetic exercise. (*A*) The femur is rotated externally by using glutei muscles. (*B*) After external rotation of the femur, the second step is to introduce knee flexion to approximately 20–30 degrees. Then the knee is extended, using the glutei muscles.

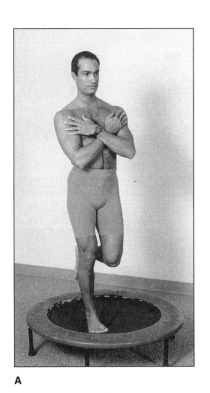
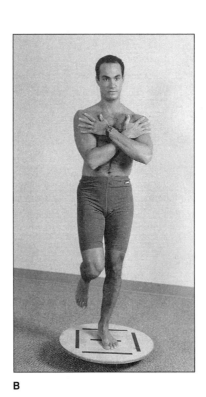
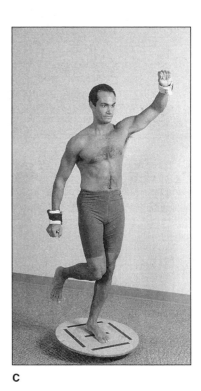

Figure 15–26 Sensorimotor stimulation. (*A*) Minitrampoline, (*B*) wobbleboard, (*C*) advanced.

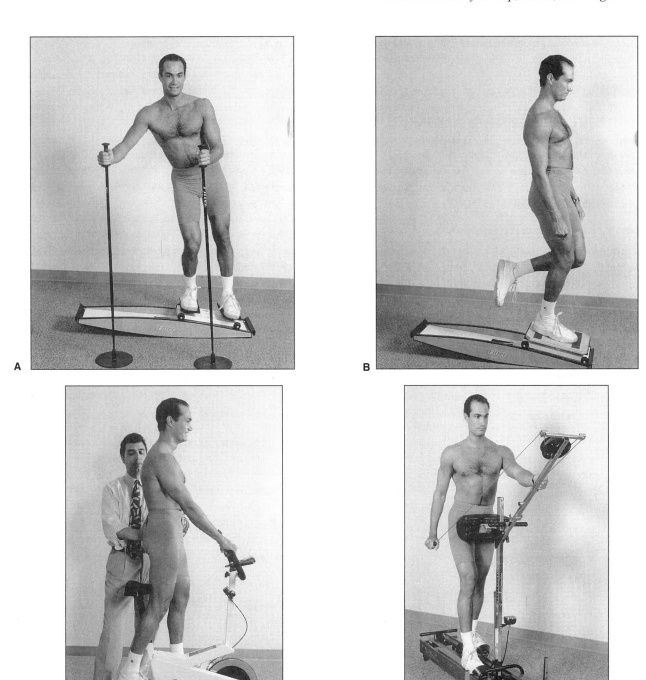

Figure 15–27 Lumbopelvic stability exercise. (*A*) Poles are used in the early stages of retraining. (*B*) Using one leg without poles provides an advanced degree of difficulty. (*C*) Standing bike—a posterior pelvic tilt is maintained while pedaling a bike in the standing position, stimulating cocontraction of lumbopelvic musculature in a dynamic fashion. (*D*) Cross-country ski machine allows for reciprocal trunk and pelvic movements.

nous junction, tendo-osseus insertion into the inferior pubic rami, or the muscle belly itself. Actual muscle strain or tendinitis also may occur. The *Clinical Symptom Complex* is usually one of acute onset of pain, which strongly suggests

that muscle injury can be very well localized or poorly defined. When tendinitis is present, the pain is usually worse after exercise, especially on the following day, and gradually lessens during exercise. Exam findings usually will localize the site of injury with palpation. Pain on passive abduction or resisted adduction generally clue the examiner to focus on the adductors.

In the acute phase, relative rest, ice, and compression are indicated. This should reduce the bleeding and local swelling that are likely to occur. Decreased weight-bearing, which may necessitate the use of crutches if pain-free ambulation is not possible, may be required. Gentle stretches to the onset of pain, along with active range of motion exercises in the pain-free range, are begun. Electrotherapeutic modalities to reduce swelling may be started in this phase.

Recovery Phase (3–7 Days to 4–6 Weeks)

Treatment evolves around addressing the *Functional Biomechanical Deficits* and *Tissue Overload Complex*. From 3 to 7 days, modalities such as electrotherapy and passive as well as active range of motion in the pain-free range are continued, and myofascial release is helpful. In the first through the third weeks, progressive stretching of the adductors is accomplished. This can be accomplished by the physician or therapist providing prolonged 30-second stretch or utilizing postisometric relaxation stretching (Figure 15–28). It is important to instruct the patient during this phase in self-stretches utilizing the seated butterfly position, anterior pelvic tilt, and active contraction of the antagonistic abductors, providing for reciprocal inhibition of the adductors during the stretch (see Figure 15–15). Modalities such as hot packs, ultrasound, or other deep-heating modalities can help in blood resorption and are introduced in this phase if necessary. Nonsteroidal antiinflammatory medications can also be

introduced at this time if a component of tendinitis is suspected. Progressive strengthening using isometrics in the pain-free range, proprioceptive neuromuscular facilitation patterns, as well as adduction and flexion against resistance using rubber tubing, pulleys, and light weights, may also be started.

It is important to evaluate the symphysis pubis as, generally, on the ipsilateral side of the tightness and injury, there is an inferior translatory position noted. A bilateral isometric contraction of the adductors will serve to gap the joint and allow for proper realignment (Figure 15–29). Myofascial release and/or muscle energy techniques are well tolerated and suited for the symphysis pubis dysfunction.[7] It is advisable at this time to evaluate the hip abduction muscle firing sequence. As mentioned earlier, the hip abductors, in particular the gluteus medius, is inhibited and/or weak on the ipsilateral side of the tight adductors. The patient lies on the contralateral side with the bottom knee flexed and the top knee fully extended. The examiner then observes and palpates the firing pattern, which usually will show G Med to fire first, followed by TFL in the normal pattern (Figure 15–30A). However, the common substitution pattern is for the TFL to fire first and, when the G Med is inhibited and/or weak, this produces flexion and internal rotation of the hip that can be noted during active hip abduction by the heel leading the abduction movement (Figure 15–30B). It is important to reestablish a normal firing pattern in hip abduction and to have the G Med and G Min uninhibited. Better balance must be gained between the weak lower abdominals and the tight hip adductors (Figure 15–31). Retraining for this is accomplished by the patient lying in the supine position with knees bent and feet flat on the table or floor while performing a posterior pelvic tilt. Then the patient slowly abducts the

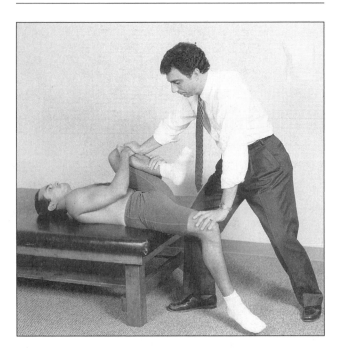

Figure 15–28 Adductor stretch—right.

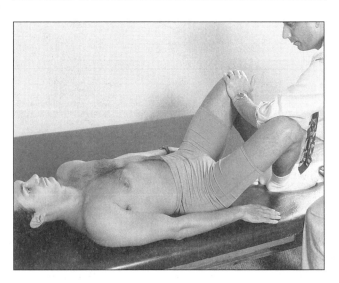

Figure 15–29 Symphysis pubis dysfunction correction—muscle energy technique.

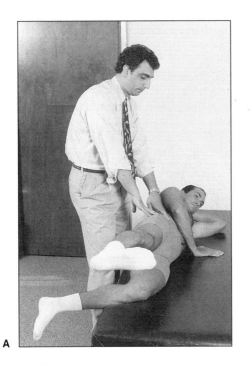 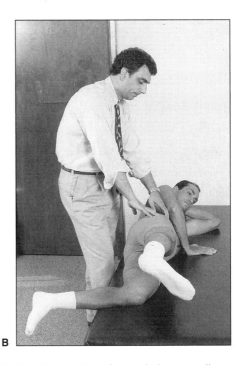

A   B

Figure 15–30 Hip abduction assessment. (*A*) Monitoring with the hands should allow for detection of normal gluteus medius contraction, followed by that of tensor fascia latae. (*B*) Hip abduction firing pattern—abnormal firing pattern is observed when the tensor fascia latae contracts before the gluteus medius, introducing slight hip flexion and internal rotation.

thighs while maintaining a posterior pelvic tilt. When an imbalance of weak abdominals and tight adductors exists, the posterior pelvic tilt cannot be maintained, and the pelvis will rotate anteriorly on the ipsilateral side. This is an excellent evaluation test as well as a self-retraining technique. Stabilization training is begun in a closed-chain kinetic fashion, as previously discussed with innominate anterior rotation dysfunction. These dysfunctions of the inferior pubic rami and abnormal hip abduction firing sequence are a part of the *Functional Adaptation Complex* treatment.

Advancement criteria to the maintenance phase include that pain is no longer present and that inflammation is adequately controlled. Range of motion should be equal to the uninvolved side, and active motion should be pain free. Strength is difficult to assess because most forms of testing are done in open-chain kinetics and do not reliably predict more functional closed-chain kinetic strength. The patient should be able to perform normal walking and daily activities without pain, and no recurrent symphysis pubis dysfunction should be noted.

Maintenance Phase

The *Functional Biomechanical Deficits* continue to be treated in this phase, mainly through self-stretching by the patient. Special attention in this phase is aimed at the *Tissue Overload Complex,* which can be thought of as avoiding ex-

cessive strain and inflammation of lateral hip and pelvic structures. Continued retraining and stabilization exercises are recommended while avoiding overuse of the TFL. Also, the lateral knee structures and the lumbar spine are not to be forgotten—even distal kinetic chain structures such as shoulder mechanics should be evaluated to make sure they are not being overloaded. Continual work on abdominal retraining is essential to maintain balance between the adductors and their effect on the symphysis pubis. Stabilization training, as described with innominate anterior rotation, would be appropriate in the treatment of adductor strain as well. Stabilization exercises using functional movements and proprioceptive neuromuscular facilitation patterns with rubber tubing, pulleys, and weights may be advanced in this phase. However, before weight machines for hip abduction and adduction are used, the firing sequence on hip abduction must be normal. Otherwise, it will serve only to strengthen the TFL, and the inhibited and/or weak abductors will remain so.

Progression through walking and running, as well as through advanced proprioceptive and balance retraining, is the same as discussed in the previous section with innominate anterior rotation. The proper mechanics of kicking are essential and should be reviewed as the adductors are very active in this motion. Specific skills such as agility drills, along with running, jumping, kicking, and pyelometrics, round out the maintenance phase.

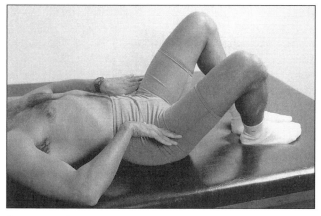

A

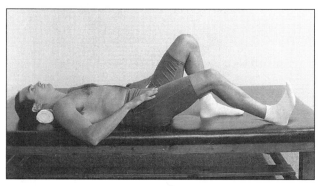

B

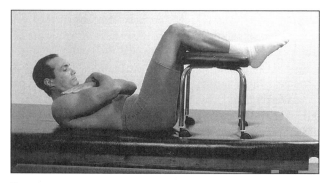

C

Figure 15–31 Lumbopelvic retraining. (*A*) The hips fall into external rotation and abduction while maintaining a posterior pelvic tilt. This improves muscle balance between the weak lower abdominals and tight adductors. (*B*) A posterior pelvic tilt is maintained while sliding each heel out so that the lower extremity is fully extended. This helps to balance the weak lower abdominals with a tighter iliopsoas. (*C*) Finally, the abdominals are isolated by decreasing activity to the iliopsoas. Plantar flexion and activation of hamstrings, along with gluteal squeezes, inhibit the iliopsoas muscles.

Criteria for Return to Play

The criteria for return to play are as discussed in the previous section and must include, as a minimum, that the athlete is off all pain medication and is relatively pain free. There should be full range of motion and normal strength as well as balance between agonist and antagonist muscles. Proper mechanics with sports-specific progression of skills should have been evaluated and fully treated.

Quadriceps Contusion/Myositis Ossificans

Acute Phase (0–48 Hours)

Contusions to the quadriceps muscles represent a spectrum of injury that can range from mild bruising to severe tearing with development of localized hematoma. This most commonly occurs in such sports as football, rugby, soccer, basketball, and hockey. The most common site of injury is the anterior and lateral thigh, where a resultant disability depends on severity of bleeding and amount of muscle injury. History suggesting a direct blow to the anterior or lateral thigh and an examination can confirm the tenderness and swelling, which usually worsen on active contraction or passive stretching. These represent the *Clinical Symptom Complex,* which can often underestimate the severity of injury present. During the first 24–48 hours, treatment consists of ice up to 20 minutes every hour, compression dressing, crutches with limited or no weight-bearing, and gentle active range of motion in the pain-free range only. The first 24 hours following the injury are the most critical period, and the athlete should be removed from the field of play. Along with the above-mentioned methods of treatment, elevation should also be instituted immediately. The athlete must be cautioned not to aggravate the injury—which would certainly worsen any bleeding—by excessive activity, alcohol ingestion, or the application of heat. The soft-tissue therapies, such as massage and myofascial release, are contraindicated in the first 48 hours.

A grading system may be helpful and may also decrease the chances for minimizing the severity of the injury.[13] A mild quadriceps contusion generally represents restriction of full range of motion between 5% and 20%. Often, the athlete may or may not remember the incident and usually continues activity. In a moderate degree, the athlete usually remembers the incident and continues activity despite stiffening occurring with rest. Moderate restriction of range of motion at 20–50% is noted. When a severe injury is present, the athlete usually remembers the incident and may not be able to control the rapid onset of swelling and/or bleeding. Severe loss of movement at 50% or greater is noted. There is difficulty with full weight-bearing as well.

Recovery Phase (2–5 Days to 3–4 Weeks)

In this phase, the *Functional Biomechanical Deficits* of tight hamstrings, gastrocsoleus, and rectus femoris are dealt with. Generally, the quadriceps and, in particular, the vasti are inhibited and/or weak. Within 2 to 5 days, active range of motion, as well as proprioceptive neuromuscular facilitation and reciprocal relaxation patterns, is introduced. Modalities such as hot packs, ultrasound, and deep heating can be helpful in blood resorption but should be used with caution. Nonsteroidal antiinflammatory medications may be introduced in this phase but generally can be avoided. In the next several weeks, crutches may be discontinued and increased resisted quadriceps exercises using rubber tubing and pulleys, as well as cycling, can be started. Radiographs at three weeks to rule out myositis ossificans are advisable, especially if clinically indicated in the presence of a firm, unresolving hematoma. It should be noted that isometrics and concentric strengthening in the pain-free range are started before eccentric exercises are permitted (Figure 15–32). Pool walking, swimming, and kicking can also be started at this time. Soft-tissue therapy, such as massage or myofascial release, must be light and should produce no pain, with the aim of promoting lymphatic drainage in the early phase.

Stretching of the RF, HS, and GS (Figure 15–33) is done first by the physician or physical therapist; in this phase, self-stretching is also taught (see Figures 15–13 and 15–16). The vasti and, in particular, the vastus medialis oblique, have a tendency for inhibition, especially if any blood or swelling is present. The vasti are best stimulated in a closed-chain ki-netic fashion while standing on one leg and introducing 20 to 30 degrees of knee flexion, then asking the athlete to extend the knee using the glutei muscles and quadriceps, noting that it is essential for glutei contractions to facilitate the quadriceps. Isokinetic measurements will serve only to frustrate the athlete as there is little change noted in strength in this open-chain testing; yet, functional gains can be remarkable in the closed-chain kinetic patterns (see Figure 15–25).

The *Functional Adaptation Complex* also is treated in this phase, and there is usually an ipsilateral anterior pelvic tilt that slackens the quadriceps and its fascia. As previously discussed with innominate anterior rotation, MET and MFR are used here, should these dysfunctions be present. The patient is also resistant to flex the knee and holds it in extension. In the terminal end range, this can be accomplished by HS and in a closed-chain fashion through the GS muscle groups, which must be stretched properly in this phase. Knee extension results in premature plantar flexion at heel strike. This

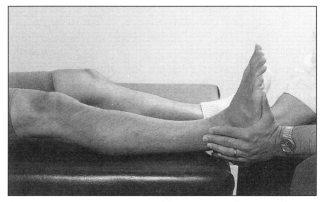

A

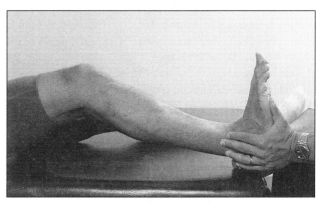

B

Figure 15–33 Heel cord length assessment. (*A*) Dorsiflexion is introduced, and the degree of shortening is noted by lack of motion past neutral. (*B*) Knee flexion helps to differentiate between gastrocnemius and soleus tightness.

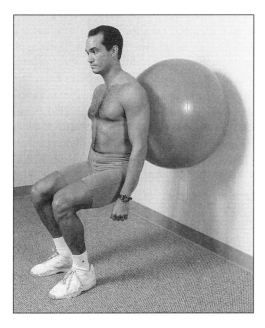

Figure 15–32 Quadriceps exercise—exercise ball. Provides not only eccentric loading but a dynamic component.

can be easily evaluated on a treadmill, and correction of this adaptation can be dealt with at that time.

Before moving on to the maintenance phase, it is essential to rule out myositis ossificans. As mentioned earlier, at 3–6 weeks, a plain radiographic examination can be done with concentration on the soft tissues. Should suspicion still be high and the radiographs be negative, bone scanning may be positive as early as one week prior to the plain films showing soft-tissue calcification. Nonsteroidal antiinflammatory medications, along with reduced activities and reassessment in 7–10 days, are advised if myositis ossificans is present. If the condition has not worsened, rehabilitation may restart slowly. If no improvement is noted, a 10-day tapering course of prednisone or etidronate disodium can be tried in high-risk cases. Surgical excision is considered if the bone mass is limiting range of motion. Optimum timing for the surgery is usually 6–12 months, when there is marked reduction in bone scan activity.

Maintenance Phase

After 3–4 weeks, maintenance activities, including walking, running, starting, and stopping, as well as sprinting, can be considered. Also, more sports-specific activities are introduced. This is also an excellent time for adjustments to equipment; additional padding is advisable before return to sport. Other stabilization activities, as mentioned in the two previous sections, are also appropriate. More specific to the quadriceps contusion injury are wall squats (see Figure 15–32), step downs, and hopping. It is important to introduce jumping activities at this time. Resisted motion that was previously done underwater may now be accomplished with rubber tubing and pulleys; use of multidirectional activities is essential. Agility drills such as figure-of-eight patterns, pyelometrics, and graduated specific sporting activities are added. Balance and proprioceptive retraining is critical and is almost always significantly lost with this type of injury. Using the same techniques as described in the previous two sections would be appropriate.

The *Tissue Overload Complex,* in particular, evolves around evaluation of the patellofemoral joint, especially when irritation secondary to bleeding tracking down in the fascial planes due to a lower thigh contusion has occurred. Stretching of the lateral retinaculum and TFL, with continued neuromuscular facilitation to the vastus medialis oblique, is essential. This is discussed in this text under a separate chapter in detail.

The criteria to return to sport are the same as outlined in the previous two sections. Emphasis should be placed on the prevention of quadriceps contusion. Protection may help prevent recurrence for those high-risk sports such as wearing thigh padding routinely. Certain athletes are susceptible to sustaining a series of minor contusions during the course of a game. Therefore, a cumulative effect may result in impaired performance toward the end of a game. Protective padding helps to minimize this effect.

In conclusion, the athlete who presents with pain in the hip, pelvic, and thigh region is a challenge to the sports medicine practitioner. It is important to keep in mind the relationship between the hip, pelvis, and thigh, as well as that of the lower lumbar spine and lower extremity, in the approach to injuries in this area. Emphasis should be placed on the biomechanical approach to the entire region, as well as on the identification of mechanisms of lumbopelvic and lower extremity muscle imbalances and joint dysfunctions—especially their role as predisposing factors to soft-tissue injury. A comprehensive differential diagnosis should always be considered. This will lead to a more specific diagnosis and, therefore, more specific treatment. The successful long-term outcome and prevention of reinjury are more likely if the goal of rehabilitation is functional restoration of the hip, pelvic, and thigh region, rather than on pain alleviation. The nonoperative sports medicine specialist is in an excellent position to integrate muscle imbalances and biomechanical evaluation into the rehabilitation of the injured athlete. Training, however, is not always adequate, and the practitioner is encouraged to seek additional training in these areas. Nonoperative sports medicine practitioners must also familiarize themselves with the roles, knowledge, and expertise of the sports medicine physical therapist, athletic trainer, and orthopedist. The athlete is best taken care of in a setting where these different specialists are available and work well as a team. No one specialist can or should provide the athlete with total care for all injuries.

REFERENCES

1. Clement DB, Taunton JE, Smart GW, et al. A survey of overuse running injuries. *Phys Sports Med.* 1991;9:47–58.

2. Geraci MC. Rehabilitation of pelvis, hip and thigh injuries in sports. In: Press JM, ed. *Physical Medicine and Rehabilitation Clinics of North America.* Philadelphia: WB Saunders Company; 1994: 157–173.

3. Lloyd-Smith R, Clement DB, McKenzie DC, et al. A survey of overuse and traumatic hip and pelvis injuries in athletes. *Phys Sports Med.* 1995;13:131–141.

4. Bowen V, Cassidy JD. Macroscopic and microscopic anatomy of the sacroiliac joint from embryonic life until the eighth decade. *Spine.* 1981;6:620–628.

5. Vleeming A, Stoeckart R, Volkers ACW, et al. Relationship between form and function in the sacroiliac joint. I: Clinical anatomical aspects. *Spine.* 1990;15:130–132.

6. Vleeming A, Stoeckart R, Volkers ACW, et al. Relationship between form and function in the sacroiliac joint. II: Biomechanical aspects. *Spine.* 1990;15:133–135.

7. Greenman PE. Principles of diagnosis and treatment of pelvic girdle dysfunction. In: Greenman PE, ed. *Principles of Manual Medicine.* Baltimore: Williams & Wilkins; 1989:225–230.

8. Vleeming A, Stoeckart R, Snijders CJ. The sacrotuberous ligament: a conceptual approach to its dynamic role in stabilizing the sacroiliac joint. *Clin Biomech.* 1989;4:201–203.

9. Colachis SC, Worden RE, Bechtol CO, Strohm BR. Movements of the sacroiliac joint in the adult male. *Arch Phys Med Rehabil.* 1963; 44:490–498.

10. Egund N, Olsson TH, Schmid H, Selvik G. Movements in the sacroiliac joints demonstrated with roentgen stereophotogrammetry. *Acta Radiol.* 1978;19:833–846.

11. Sturesson B, Slevik G, Uden A. Movements of the sacroiliac joints: a roentgen stereophotogrammetric analysis. *Spine.* 1989;14:162–165.

12. Weisl H. The movements of the sacroiliac joints. *Acta Anat.* 1955; 23:80–91.

13. Brukner P, Khan K. Hip and groin pain. In: Brukner P, Khan K, eds. *Clinical Sports Medicine.* New York: McGraw-Hill; 1993:302–315.

14. Jull GA, Janda V. Muscles and motor control in low back pain: assessment and management. In: Twomey LT, Taylor JR, eds. *Physical Therapy of the Low Back, Clinics in Physical Therapy.* New York: Churchill Livingstone; 1987:253–278.

15. Sahrmann SA. A program for identification and correction of muscular and mechanical imbalance: principles and methods. *Clin Manage.* 1983;3:23–28.

16. Lewit K. The needle effect in the relief of myofascial pain. *Pain.* 1979;6:83.

17. Butler DS. Mobilization of the nervous system. Melbourne: Churchill Livingstone; 1991:139–145.

18. Fortin JD, Dwyer AP, West S, Pier J. Sacroiliac joint: pain referral maps upon applying a new injection/arthrography technique. I: Asymptomatic volunteers. *Spine.* 1994;19:1475–1482.

19. Fortin JD, Aprill CN, Ponthieux B, Pier J. Sacroiliac joint: pain referral maps. II: Clinical evaluation. *Spine.* 1994;19:1483–1489.

20. Bookhout MR. Examination and treatment of muscle imbalances. In: Bourdillon JF, Day EA, Bookhout MR, eds. *Spinal Manipulation.* Oxford: Butterworth-Heinemann Ltd; 1992:313–333.

21. Mackova J, Janda V, Macek M, et al. Impaired muscle function in children and adolescents. *J Manual Med.* 1989;4:157–160.

22. Aprill CN. The role of anatomically specific injections into the sacroiliac joint. In: Vleming A, Mooney V, Snijders C, Dorman T, eds. *Low Back Pain and Its Relationship to the Sacroiliac Joint.* Congress Proceedings of the First Interdisciplinary World Congress on Low Back Pain and Its Relationship to the Sacroiliac Joint. San Diego, CA; 1992:373–380.

23. Buyruk HM. Effect of pelvic belt application on sacroiliac joint mobility. In: Vleeming A, Snijders CJ, Stoeckart R, eds. *Progress in Vertebral Column Research.* First International Symposium on the Sacroiliac Joint: Its Role in Posture and Locomotion. Rotterdam, Netherlands; 1991:94–95.

24. Bullock-Saxton JE, et al. Reflex activation of gluteal muscles in walking. An approach to restoration of muscle function for patients with low-back pain. *Spine.* 1993;18:704–708.

CHAPTER 16

Rehabilitation of Knee Injuries

David B. Richards and W. Ben Kibler

INTRODUCTION

The knee is arguably the most common site of sport-related injury in the lower extremity. It obviously plays a vital role in running and jumping sports, and it is also a critical component of the kinetic chain of linked joint activities.

The knee is part of the stable base of the legs, necessary for most sports. Stability of the knee is critical as the large muscles around the knee generate considerable force for most athletic activity. The knee is also a vital link in the kinetic chain, responsible for transferring the ground reactive force and force generated in the legs up to the hip and trunk. The knee also absorbs and regulates forces in the lower extremities during running, landing, cutting, and stopping. Normal knee function, therefore, is essential, not only for its local action, but for normal functioning of the kinetic chain as well.

ANATOMY AND BIOMECHANICS

The knee is the largest joint of the body and may be the most complex. It is situated between two long, very muscular lever arms (the femur and the tibia) that are capable of generating and transferring considerable force to the knee. Consideration of the knee is usually oversimplified; it is often viewed as a simple hinge joint capable of only flexion and extension. In actuality, the knee is capable of clinically significant motion within six degrees of freedom (three rotational and three translational)[1]. This complex interaction of translational and rotational forces is referred to as *coupled motion* and most accurately describes knee kinematics.[2]

The knee joint is composed of three separate articulations: the patellofemoral joint and the medial and lateral tibiofemoral joints. Injuries to the knee may involve one or more of these articulations, with the net result of total knee dysfunction. Stability of the knee is dependent on the tight investing joint capsule, the collateral ligaments (medial and lateral), the posteromedial and posterolateral ligament complexes, the cruciate ligaments, and the extensor mechanism. Injuries to any of these structures may render the knee relatively unstable and disrupt the normal knee function.

The important intra-articular components of the knee are the medial and lateral menisci and the anterior and posterior cruciate ligaments (ACL/PCL). The menisci are C-shaped fibrocartilage discs that play vital roles in knee stability and in load transmission across the joint. As much as 50% of the compressive load across the knee is transmitted through the menisci, and this increases with knee flexion.[3–5] Any injury resulting in loss of part or all of the meniscus reduces the weight-bearing contact area in the knee, resulting in a dramatic rise in the load per unit area borne by the articular cartilage and thereby placing the articular cartilage at risk for failure and subsequent degenerative changes.[6,7] The menisci contribute to knee stability by increasing the depth and congruity of the tibiofemoral articulations. Studies have shown small increases in varus-valgus and anteroposterior laxity in postmeniscectomy knees. This effect is even greater in postmeniscectomy knees with deficient ACLs (Figure 16–1).[8–10]

It is apparent that complete or perhaps even partial loss of the meniscus places the knee at considerable risk for further damage through alteration in normal joint stability and exposure of the articular cartilage to supraphysiologic loads. In addition, it has been suggested that the menisci may play some role in normal knee proprioception. This, too, may be altered in the postmeniscectomy knee.[11,12]

The primary function of knee ligaments is to allow normal physiologic motion of the knee while stabilizing the knee

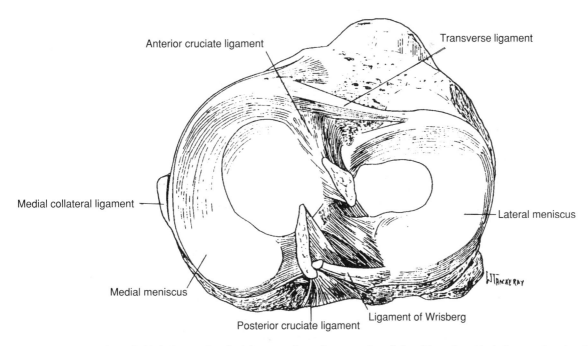

Figure 16–1 Drawing of tibial plateau showing shapes and attachments of medial and lateral menisci. *Source:* Reprinted with permission from J.A. Nicholas and E.B. Hershman, *The Lower Extremity and Spine in Sports Medicine,* 2nd edition, Vol. 1, p. 592, © 1995, Mosby Year-Book Inc.

against abnormal translational and rotational forces that may result in injury. Ligaments are composed primarily of parallel bundles of collagen oriented along the axis of motion of the joint. Ideally, they allow motion in the direction of their collagen bundles and provide tensile stress to prevent motion outside of that plane.

These ligaments include the ACL, the PCL, and the medial (MCL) and lateral (LCL) collateral ligaments. Each of these functions as both a primary and a secondary stabilizer to knee motion, which becomes very important when one or more of the ligaments is injured.

INJURIES

Injury to the collateral ligaments is usually graded from 1 to 3, based on pathologic joint laxity. Up to 5 mm of increased laxity to varus or valgus stress is a grade 1 injury; 5–10 mm with a discernible end point on exam defines a grade 2 injury; and greater than 1 cm increased laxity without a firm end point characterizes a grade 3 injury or complete collateral ligament tear.

The MCL is the primary restraint to valgus stress and is a primary restraint to internal tibial rotation (Figure 16–2A). It provides secondary restraint to anterior tibial translation as well, which is of clinical importance in the ACL-deficient knee. The most common mechanism of injury is a blow to the lateral aspect of the knee or leg with the foot planted.

Method of Presentation—Acute Macrotrauma Injury from Valgus Stress

- Clinical Symptoms Complex: Tenderness along medial collateral ligament, swelling and/or bruising, pain upon cutting or twisting
- Tissue Injury Complex: MCL, posteromedial ligament, occasionally medial meniscus
- Tissue Overload Complex: Same
- Functional Biomechanical Deficit Complex: None in acute injuries; shortened stride, decreased quadriceps strength in chronic injuries
- Subclinical Adaptation Complex: None

The vast majority of MCL injuries is now treated nonoperatively. The notable exception may be the grade 3 injury in the ACL-deficient knee. Grade 1 injuries usually respond to rest, ice, protected weight-bearing, and appropriate rehabilitation. Grade 2 injuries may require bracing for support but are then managed essentially as grade 1 injuries. Grade 3 injuries are usually braced with a hinged knee brace and allowed protected range of motion and weight-bearing. An appropriate rehabilitation program is essential for management of these injuries.

The LCL is the primary restraint to varus stress. In full extension, the posterior capsule and posterolateral corner (arcuate ligament complex and popliteal tendon) also contribute to varus stability (Figure 16–2A, B). Isolated LCL in-

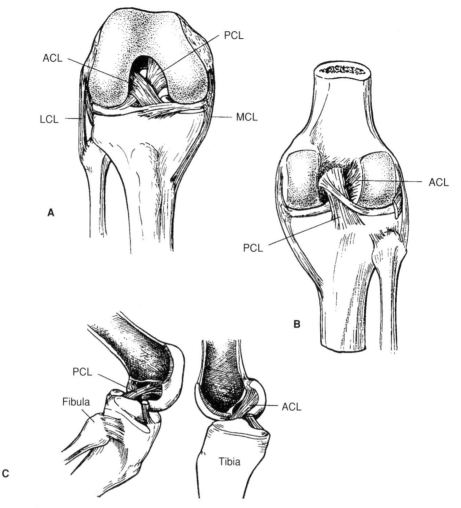

Figure 16–2 (*A*) Anterior view of anterior and posterior ligaments. (*B*) Posterior view of anterior and posterior cruciate ligaments. (*C*) Lateral views of anterior and posterior cruciate ligaments. *Source:* Reprinted with permission from F. Fu and D. Stone, *Sports Injuries: Mechanisms, Prevention, and Treatment,* p. 952, © 1994, Williams & Wilkins.

juries with or without injury to the posterolateral corner are relatively uncommon and generally result from a blow to the medial or anteromedial aspect of the knee.

Method of Presentation—Acute macrotrauma injury from varus stress
- Clinical Symptom Complex: Tenderness along lateral collateral ligament, swelling and/or bruising, pain upon cutting or twisting
- Tissue Injury Complex: LCL, posterolateral arcuate ligamentous complex, occasionally lateral meniscus or peroneal nerve
- Tissue Overload Complex: Same
- Functional Biomechanical Deficit Complex: None
- Subclinical Adaptation Complex: None

Injuries to the LCL are graded in the same fashion as are MCL injuries, and treatment is essentially the same with rest, protected weight-bearing, bracing, and rehabilitation.

The ACL is arguably the most important stabilizing structure in the knee (Figure 16–2C). Injuries are common and can produce considerable morbidity, depending on the age, lifestyle, and occupation of the patients. The significance of this injury on normal knee function is illustrated by the fact that attempts at surgical repair of the ACL date back to as early as 1917. Our understanding of this injury has since evolved to the point that surgical reconstruction is now the gold standard for symptomatic ACL-deficient patients who want to continue with relatively high-demand activities, whether recreational or professional. Nonoperative management is also appropriate in select patients.

Method of Presentation—Acute Microtrauma Injury from Contact and Rotation, or Indirect Stress from Noncontact Deceleration

- Clinical Symptom Complex: POP, pain, swelling, decreased range of motion, giving way with rotation or deceleration
- Tissue Injury Complex: ACL, MCL or LCL, medial or lateral menisci
- Tissue Overload Complex: Same plus quadriceps and/or hamstrings
- Functional Biomechanical Deficit Complex: None in acute injuries; shortened stride, quadriceps weakness, hamstrings overactivity (quadriceps avoidance gait pattern) in chronic cases
- Subclinical Adaptation Complex: Quadriceps avoidance gait pattern

Ruptures of the ACL may occur as a result of a direct blow to the knee with the foot planted. Much more often, however, they are the result of a noncontact twisting injury associated with a hyperextension or varus or valgus stress on a weight-bearing leg. Patients will frequently, but not always, describe a pop in the knee at the time of injury, followed by acute pain. An effusion is very common within 24 hours of the injury. It is critical to remember that associated injuries (meniscal and ligamentous) are common with ACL injuries and must be carefully looked for on physical exam.

The ACL serves as the primary restraint to anterior tibial translation and as a secondary restraint to tibial rotation. It also acts as a minor secondary restraint to varus-valgus stress at full knee extension. The ACL-deficient knee is characterized by abnormal anterior tibial translation, relative to the femur, as well as increased internal tibial rotation in full extension. Loss of the ACL as a secondary stabilizer also explains why grade 3 MCL injuries in the ACL-deficient knee are particularly devastating.[13]

The PCL is the primary restraint to posterior tibial displacement. It also serves as a major secondary restraint to external tibial rotation, particularly at 90 degrees of knee flexion (Figure 16–2C).[5] Posterior cruciate injuries are far less common than are ACL injuries and are generally much less disabling.

Method of Presentation: Acute Microtrauma Injury, with Direct Blow to Flexed Knee or Hyperextension to Knee

- Clinical Symptom Complex: Pain, POP, swelling, decreased motion
- Tissue Injury Complex: PCL, posteromedial or posterolateral ligaments
- Tissue Overload Complex: Same
- Functional Biomechanical Deficit Complex: None in acute injury; lack of quadriceps strength and increased patellofemoral contact stress in chronic injuries
- Subclinical Adaptation Complex: None

The majority of PCL injuries results from a direct blow to the flexed knee. Hyperflexion and hyperextension injuries have also been shown to result in PCL ruptures. As a general rule, isolated PCL injuries tend to be less disabling than do ACL injuries; however, combined injuries to the PCL and posterolateral corner can be particularly troublesome and frequently require operative repair.

Isolated PCL-deficient knees are characterized by straight posterior laxity. This is most easily demonstrated at 70–90 degrees of flexion. Injuries to the PCL and posterolateral corner result in straight posterior laxity as well as posterolateral rotary instability. The latter condition can be particularly disabling.[14]

Meniscal tears usually result from a twisting injury on a weight-bearing knee.[15,16] Tears through the vascular zone in the periphery of the meniscus are usually repaired and can be expected to heal reliably. Tears in the avascular "central" portion of the meniscus usually can be managed arthroscopically by performing a subtotal meniscectomy, leaving as much stable meniscus as possible in the knee.

Method of Presentation: Acute Macrotrauma Injury Following Hyperflexion or Twisting Rotational Trauma; or Chronic Microtrauma Injury Due to Running or Jumping Stress

- Clinical Symptom Complex: Point tender along medial or lateral joint line, slight swelling, popping, clicking, or locking with rotation, pain upon running
- Tissue Injury Complex: Medial or lateral meniscus, femoral articular cartilage
- Tissue Overload Complex: Same
- Functional Biomechanical Deficit Complex: None in acute injuries; decreased stride, quadriceps weakness in chronic injuries
- Subclinical Adaptation Complex: None

REHABILITATION

Effective rehabilitation of the knee should be based on a thorough understanding of the anatomy of the knee as well as the biomechanics of the kinetic chain of the lower extremity. In addition, the pathophysiology of the injury and the healing process must be clearly understood.

We have developed a functional rehabilitation program based on the factors described above. The general framework of the rehabilitation program is applicable to essentially all patients, regardless of the injury. In addition, the goal of the treatment plan is always to reestablish normal joint or extremity function and for the athlete to resume his or her activities at the preinjury level. Lastly, education about future injury prevention utilizing sport-specific training techniques remains a critical component of our rehabilitation program.

The functional rehabilitation program is divided into three phases through which the athlete must progress before returning to play (Exhibits 16–1 through 16–4). Progression through the program is dependent on completion of phase-specific goals and on meeting the criteria for advancement into the next phase. Completion of the program includes not

Exhibit 16–1   ACL Rehabilitation

ACUTE PHASE

Week 1
Goals
1. PROM 20–70 degrees
2. Control of inflammation and effusion
3. Prevention of adhesion of PF joint
4. WBAT
5. Quadricep set with patella movement

Evaluation
1. Pain
2. Hemarthrosis
3. Patellar mobility and ROM
4. Quadriceps contraction

Treatment
1. Pain management and control of hemarthrosis with ice, EGS, elevation, ankle pumps 5'/hr for circulation
2. Mobilization of patella for 5 minutes 4 ×/day
3. ROM exercises; heel slides, prone curl
4. Muscle reeducation: quad set, hamstring set, 10 sec × 10, SLR in supine, electrical stimulation/biofeedback as needed for VMO reeducation
5. CPM: progress to 0–90 degrees
6. ROM brace 0–90 degrees

Weeks 2–3
Goals
1. PROM 0–125 degrees
2. Quadriceps muscle control
3. Control of inflammation and effusion to prevent scarring
4. WBAT with crutches
5. Normal patella mobility
6. Prevention of quadricep atrophy

Evaluation
1. Pain and effusion
2. Patellar mobility
3. ROM
4. Muscle control

Treatment
1. Continuation pain management and effusion control with ice, EGS, elevation, continuation of ankle pumps
2. Continuation of patella mobility
3. ROM: heel slides, AAROM on bike with no resistance, continuation of CPM until achievement of 0–120 degrees
4. Continuation of electrical stimulation/ biofeedback for VMO until good quad set with full patella movement

5. Strengthening exercises:
   • 4-way SLR, beginning with weight proximal-distal when patient has good knee control
   • prone curl
   • sitting hip flex, weight proximal
   • pillow squeezes (adduction)
6. Weight-bearing exercises begun when 50% WB
   • toe raise
   • mini squats
   • balance training in bilateral stance
7. Continuation of ROM brace 0–120 degrees

CRITERIA FOR PROGRESSION FROM ACUTE PHASE TO RECOVERY PHASE
1. Pain and effusion control
2. ROM 5–115 degrees
3. Quadriceps control, ability to lift 8–10 lb for SLR
4. Ambulation: single crutch to independent

RECOVERY PHASE

Weeks 4–8
Goals
1. ROM 0–135 degrees with normal patella mobility
2. 100% FWB with a normal gait
3. Improvement of muscular endurance and control
4. Control of inflammation and effusion
5. Fit with functional brace

Evaluation
1. Pain and effusion
2. Patellar mobility and ROM
3. Complete extension
4. Gait
5. Muscle control

Treatment
1. Continuation of pain management/effusion control
2. ROM, flexibility (quads, hams, gastroc, iliopsoas)
3. Strengthening/endurance training: closed chain, isotonic, bike
4. Balance training—bilateral stance activities progressing to single stance
5. Addressing of gait abnormalities
6. Functional brace

continues

Exhibit 16–1 continued

CRITERIA FOR PROGRESSION FROM RECOVERY
PHASE TO FUNCTIONAL PHASE
1. Absence of effusion
2. Joint stability
3. FWB with normal gait
4. Performance of ADL without pain
5. Knee ROM 0–135 degrees

MAINTENANCE PHASE

Weeks 8–24+
Goals
1. Increase in strength and endurance so that
   there is no fatigue with ADLs
2. Preparation for return to sports activity
3. Sport-specific training to full return to athletic
   activity

Evaluation
1. Swelling
2. PF mobility and crepitus
3. Ligament stability

Treatment
1. Increase in isotonic exercise: periodization or
   daily adjustable progressive resistive exercise
   (DAPRE); initiation of isokinetics midrange
   velocity Q/H; initiation of quads isotonic
   90–30 degrees with care for PF symptoms
2. Aerobic conditioning: low-impact bike,
   StairMaster™, treadmill, swimming
3. Proprioceptive training: progress to closed-
   chain rehabilitation exercise
4. Progression to jogging when medically cleared
5. Progression in sport-specific activity
6. Maintenance and improvement in neuromuscular strength

CRITERIA FOR PROGRESSION FROM STAGE III TO
RETURN TO SPORTS
1. Absence of pain
2. Isokinetic test 80% of uninvolved leg
3. Satisfactory clinical exam by physician
4. Normal performance of sport-specific exercises

Exhibit 16–2 Meniscus Repair—Rehabilitation

I. ACUTE PHASE 1–3 WEEKS
   A. Goals
      1. Reduction of pain and inflammation
      2. Retardation of muscle atrophy of entire lower
         extremity
      3. Neuromuscular control of the patella
      4. Maintenance of components of fitness
   B. Pain and Inflammation
      1. NSAIDs 48–96 hours
      2. Modalities 2–3 weeks
      3. Patellar mobilization
      4. Joint protection (splint/non–weight-bearing) ROM
         20–70 degrees
   C. Muscle Atrophy/Neuromuscular Control
      1. Local
         a. isometrics
         b. straight-leg raises (avoidance of adduction/
            abduction 2 weeks)
         c. biofeedback—patellar control
      2. Distant
         a. open chain—nonpathologic areas (ankle, hip)
            1. concentrics
            2. eccentrics
   D. Maintenance of Components of Fitness
      1. Aerobic endurance
      2. Anaerobic endurance

   E. Criteria for Advancement
      1. Elimination of most swelling
      2. Level II pain
      3. Healing of injured tissue to allow mild tensile
         stress, ROM, weight-bearing
      4. Straight-leg raises, 8 pounds
II. RECOVERY PHASE 3–8 WEEKS
   A. Goals
      1. Reestablishment of nonpainful active and passive
         ROM
      2. Regain and improvement in lower extremity
         muscle strength
      3. Improvement in lower extremity neuromuscular
         control
      4. Normal arthrokinematics in single plane of motion
   B. Range of Motion
      1. Dependent
         a. patellar mobilization
         b. manual capsular stretch and cross-friction
            massage
      2. Independent
         a. knee flexion/extension active/passive
         b. heel wall slides
         c. bike/rowing machine
         d. stretching—quad/hamstring/IT band/hip
            flexor/gastrocsoleus

continues

Exhibit 16–2   continued

C. Strengthening
   1. Dependent
      a. PNF
   2. Independent single planes
       (avoidance of aggressive hamstring work with
       post horn tear)
      a. open chain
         1. concentric/eccentric isotonics
         2. isokinetics
         3. tubing/free weights
      b. closed chain
         1. Nautilus™/StairMaster™
         2. life line/tubing
         3. free weights
D. Neuromuscular Control
   1. Balance board
   2. BAPS
   3. Fitter/slide board
   4. Minitramp
   5. Life line
E. Arthrokinematics
   1. Joint mobilization
   2. Kinetic chain movement patterns (sport- or
       activity-specific)
F. Criteria for Advancement
   1. Nearly full active/passive nonpainful ROM equal
       to other side
   2. Quad/hamstring ratio 66% and strength 75% of
       noninvolved
   3. Static balance on one leg for 1 minute
   4. Normal/smooth arthrokinematics with single-
       plane motion
III. FUNCTIONAL PHASE 8–12 WEEKS
A. Goals
   1. Increase in power and endurance in lower
       extremity
   2. Increase in normal multiple-plane neuromuscular
       control
   3. Sport-specific and activity-specific activities
B. Power and Endurance (avoidance of compressive/
    shear loads for 6–8 weeks)
   1. Multiple-plane motions
      a. side lunges
      b. change of direction motions
   2. Pyelometrics
   3. Conditioning based on periodization
C. Neuromuscular Control, Multiple Planes
   1. Agility drills
   2. Footwork drills
D. Sport-Specific Training Functional Progression—
    Tennis and Baseball

Stage I
1. Standing on one foot
2. Jumping on two legs (forward, backward, sides)
3. Jumping on a minitrampoline
4. Jumping from stool, 40 cm (1 ft)
5. Rope skipping on both feet
6. Balance board with both feet (forward, side/side,
    45-degree angle)
7. Balance board with both feet (catch tennis ball or
    baseball)
Stage II
1. Rope skipping on one foot
2. Jumping from stool, 40 cm, landing one foot
3. Jumping from stool, 80 cm, landing two feet
4. Hopping one foot (forward, backward, sides)
5. Jogging in place
6. Jogging around court, field
7. Jog figure eight (large-small)
8. Jog figure eight backward
9. Balance board with one foot (forward, side to
    side)
Stage III
1. Running with direction changes
2. Carioca running
3. Running 1–1.5 miles
4. Jumping: two-footed takeoff, landing one foot
5. Balance board with one foot (catch tennis ball or
    baseball)
6. Balance board with one foot (45-degree angle)
Stage IV
1. Sprint start—slow stop
2. Sprint start—fast stop
3. Sprint with cutting on demand
4. Jumping two feet—landing one foot, cutting on
    demand
5. Sport-specific training
   a. Tennis
      • Five-dot drill
      • Hexagon drills
      • Spider drills
   b. Baseball
      • Crow hop to on the mound
      • Crow hop from mound to half wind-up to
         full wind-up
IV. CRITERIA FOR RETURN TO PLAY
A. Normal Arthrokinematics in Multiple Plane
B. Normal ROM/Flexibility Equal to Opposite Side
C. Isokinetic Strength 90% of Normal Side
D. Passing of Functional Exam—Hop Test
E. Negative Clinical Exam
F. Completion of Sport-Specific Exercises

Exhibit 16–3 MCL Rehabilitation

ACUTE PHASE

Weeks 1–2

Goals
1. Full PROM
2. Control of inflammation and effusion
3. Prevention of adhesion of PF joint
4. NWB → TDWB with crutches → full WB when tolerated
5. Quadriceps set with patella movement
6. Quadriceps muscle control

Evaluation
1. Pain
2. Hemarthrosis
3. Patellar mobility and ROM
4. Quadriceps contraction

Treatment
1. Pain management/control of hemarthrosis with ice, EGS, evaluation, ankle pumps 5'/hr for circulation
2. Mobilization of patella 5 minutes 4 ×/day
3. ROM exercises: heel slides, prone curl, wall slides
4. Muscle reeducation: quad set, hamstring set, 10 sec × 10, SLR in supine, electrical stimulation/biofeedback as needed for VMO reeducation
5. ROM brace 0–90 degrees only for grade 3 injuries
6. Stationary bike
7. Mini squats
8. Balance training

CRITERIA FOR PROGRESSION FROM ACUTE PHASE TO RECOVERY PHASE
1. Pain and effusion control
2. ROM 5–115 degrees
3. Quadriceps control, ability to lift 8–10 lb for SLR
4. Ambulation: single crutch to independent

RECOVERY PHASE

Weeks 3–4

Goals
1. ROM 0–135 degrees with normal patella mobility
2. 100% FWB with a normal gait
3. Improvement of muscular endurance and control
4. Control of inflammation and effusion
5. ROM brace 0–135 degrees grade 3 only

Evaluation
1. Pain and effusion
2. Patellar mobility and ROM
3. Complete extension
4. Gait
5. Muscle control

Treatment
1. Continuation of pain management/effusion control
2. ROM, flexibility (quads, hams, gastroc, iliopsoas)
3. Strengthening/endurance training: closed chain, isotonic, bike
4. Balance training—bilateral stance activities progressing to single stance
5. Addressing of gait abnormalities
6. Functional exercises
7. Jogging, light running

CRITERIA FOR PROGRESSION FROM RECOVERY PHASE TO FUNCTIONAL PHASE
1. Absence of effusion
2. Joint stability
3. FWB with normal gait
4. Performance of ADL without pain
5. Knee ROM 0–135 degrees

FUNCTIONAL PHASE

Weeks 4–6

Goals
1. Increase in strength and endurance so that there is no fatigue with ADLs
2. Preparation for return to sports activity

Evaluate
1. Swelling
2. PF mobility and crepitus
3. Ligament stability

Treatment
1. Increase of isotonic exercise: periodization or DAPRE; initiation of isokinetics midrange velocity Q/H, initiation of quads isotonic 90–30 degrees with care for PF symptoms
2. Aerobic conditioning: low-impact bike, StairMaster™, treadmill, swimming
3. Proprioceptive training: progress to closed-chain rehabilitation exercise
4. Progress to full-speed running
5. Sport-specific skills and exercises
6. Progressive return to sports

Exhibit 16–4   PCL Rehabilitation

PCL rehabilitation closely follows ACL rehabilitation protocol, with a few notable exceptions:

- No isolated hamstring exercises are performed during the first 6–8 weeks
- Closed-chain exercises are emphasized, allowing for hamstring strengthening but protecting against posterior tibial translation through the quadriceps hamstring force couple and compressive forces across the joint.

The recovery process proceeds essentially the same as the ACL rehabilitation program.

only returning to play but also an ongoing participation in a sport-specific "prehabilitation" program designed to maximize future performance and to minimize future injury.

The acute phase of the program actually begins at the time of the injury, with the onset of clinical symptoms. A timely and accurate diagnosis allows prompt and appropriate treatment, which creates the environment for healing. The goals of the acute phase are to: (1) reduce pain and swelling; (2) minimize muscle atrophy/weakness; (3) attain early neuromuscular control; and (4) maintain general fitness.

Pain and swelling are potent inhibitors of normal muscle function. Early control of these problems is essential to progressing through the program. This allows early neuromuscular training and minimizes muscle weakness. Relative rest, ice, compression, and elevation are initiated as soon as possible. Control of pain with analgesics and nonsteroidal antiinflammatory drugs (NSAIDs), as well as with physical therapy modalities, is critical. Brief, intermittent immobilization may be beneficial during the acute phase.

This is then followed with early, controlled range of motion exercises and further bracing, if necessary, for protection of the knee. Isometric exercises, including straight-leg raises and quad sets, are begun to minimize muscle weakness. Gentle, closed-chain exercises and patella mobilization techniques are begun as well. Criteria for progression are reduced swelling and pain, healing of injured tissue, and early weight-bearing.

The recovery phase of the program is usually the longest and most complex phase of the rehabilitation program. During this phase, any tissue overload problems and functional biomechanical deficits are addressed. Injured tissues must be sufficiently healed so as to allow loading in tension and compression in order to restore normal strength and flexibility. The goals of the recovery phase include achievement of full

range of motion, improvement in muscular strength and neuromuscular control, restoration of normal force couple patterns and normal single-plane joint kinematics.

Range of motion is addressed through patella mobilization, cross-friction massage, flexion/extension exercises, and stationary bike exercises. Wall slides and stretching and flexibility of the quads, hamstrings, IT band hip flexors, and gastrocsoleus are also stressed.

Both open- and closed-chain exercises are utilized to build strength and to restore neuromuscular firing patterns such as cocontractions. Further neuromuscular training includes using the biomechanical ankle platform system (BAPS), balance board, slide board, minitrampoline, and life line. Kinetic chain movement patterns are used, as well, to help restore joint biomechanics and neuromuscular firing patterns.

Criteria for progression to the maintenance phase include: (1) full range of motion equal to the opposite knee; (2) quad/hamstring strength ratio of 2:3 and equal to 75% or greater of the opposite leg; (3) ability to perform one-leg squat for 10–15 repetitions; and (4) normal single-plane kinematics.

The maintenance or functional phase addresses any remaining functional biomechanical deficits, corrects any subclinical adaptations, and prepares the athlete for return to play. Specific goals include increased power and endurance, restoration of multiplane neuromuscular control, and completion of sport-specific activities.

Power and endurance are increased through the use of isokinetic and isotonic exercise, and stair climber and stationary bike exercise.

Side lunges, slide board exercises, pyelometrics, and agility and footwork drills are used to develop neuromuscular skills. Sport-specific exercises and drills are added late in the functional phase as the athlete approaches return to play.

Successful completion of the functional phase requires normal range of motion of the injured extremity, strength equal to 90% or greater of the opposite side, and a normal physical exam.

A well-designed rehabilitation program begun as soon as possible is essential to achieve optimum results following a significant knee injury. Our rehabilitation program is a functionally based program designed to safely restore range of motion as soon as possible and to allow early strengthening using closed-chain exercises. The goal for all patients is to restore normal function to the injured extremity and to return to the preinjury level of activity. We also emphasize a year-round program of sport-specific exercises to maintain flexibility, strength, aerobic fitness, and sport-specific neuromuscular skills throughout the year. This "prehabilitation" program is a key element in improving performance and in minimizing future injuries.

REFERENCES

1. Kibler WB, ed. *ACSM Handbook for the Team Physician.* Baltimore: Williams & Wilkins; 1996:311–332.

2. Delee JC, Drez D Jr. *Orthopedic Sports Medicine.* Philadelphia: WB Saunders Company; 1994;2:1113–1162.

3. Ahmed AM, Burke DL. In vivo measurement of static pressure distribution in synovial joints. Tibial surface of the knee. *J Biomech Eng.* 1983;105:201–209.

4. Ahmed AM. The load bearing role of the knee meniscio. In: Mow VC, Arnoczky SP, Jackson DW, eds. *Knee Meniscus: Basic and Clinical Foundations.* New York: Raven Press; 1992:59–73.

5. Shrive NG, O'Connor JJ, Goodfellow JW. Load bearing in the knee joint. *CORR.* 1978;131:279–287.

6. Baratz ME, Fu FH, Mengato R. Meniscal tears: the effect of meniscectomy and repair on intra-articular contact areas and stresses in the human knee. *Am J Sports Med.* 1986;14:270–275.

7. Seedholm BB, Hargreaves DJ. Transmission of the load in the knee joint with special reference to the role of the menisci. *Eng Med.* 1979;8:220–228.

8. Levy IM, Torzilli PA, Warren RF. The effect of medial meniscectomy on anterior-posterior motion of the knee. *JBVS.* 1982;64A:883–888.

9. Johnson RJ, Kettelkamp DB, Clark W, Leaverton P. Factors affecting late meniscectomy results. *JBJS.* 1974;56A:719–729.

10. Tapper EM, Hoover NW. Late results after meniscectomy. *JBJS.* 1969;51A:517.

11. Wilson AS, Legg PG, McNeur JC. Studies on the innervation of the medial meniscus in the human knee joint. *Anat Rec.* 1969;165:485–492.

12. Zimny ML, Albright DL, Dabeziew E. Mechanoreceptors in the human medial meniscus. *Acta Anat.* 1988;133:35–40.

13. Daniel D, Akeson W, O'Connor J. *Knee Ligaments Structure, Function, Injury and Repair.* New York: Raven Press, 1990.

14. Grood ES, Stowers SF, Noyes FR. Limits of motion in the human knee. Effect of sectioning the posterior cruciate ligament and posterolateral structures. *JBJS.* 1988;70A:88–97.

15. Baker BE, Peckham AC, Pupparo F, Sanborn JC. Review of meniscal injury and associated sports. *Am J Sports Med.* 1985;13:1–4.

16. Daniel D, Daniels E, Aronson D. The diagnosis of meniscus pathology. *Clin Orthop.* 1982;163:218–224.

17. Griffin, Letha Y. *Rehabilitation of the Injured Knee.* St. Louis, MO: Mosby–Year Book; 1995.

CHAPTER 17

Rehabilitation of Patellofemoral Pain Syndrome

Joel M. Press and Jeffrey Young

INTRODUCTION

Patellofemoral pain syndrome is one of the most common musculoskeletal injuries seen in the athletic population. Anterior knee pain, often termed *patellofemoral pain syndrome,* probably represents a spectrum of specific clinical entities that relate to abnormal motion of the patella in the trochlear groove. This spectrum ranges from patellar tendinitis to malalignment problems, frank patellar subluxation, and dislocation to chondromalacia.[1,2] Patellofemoral pain may be due to local factors or factors proximal or distal to the knee joint along the kinetic chain. Local factors include abnormalities of patellar position (patella alta, baja, infera), local muscle imbalances (i.e., vastus medialis to vastus lateralis ratios, hamstrings to quadriceps ratios), soft-tissue restraints (i.e., tight lateral retinacula and retinacular stress).[1,3–8] Proximal factors that can predispose to patellofemoral pain include increased lordosis of the lumbar spine, femoral anteversion, and inflexibility in hip flexors, hamstrings, iliotibial band, hip abductors, and medial or lateral hip rotators. Distal factors in the kinetic chain that may predispose or cause patellofemoral pain include internal tibial torsion, tight Achilles tendon, increased pronation, and a rigid cavus foot.

ANATOMY AND BIOMECHANICS

The extensor mechanism of the knee consists locally of the quadriceps femoris, quadriceps tendon, patella, and patellar tendon.[9] The posteriorly located hamstrings are important structures in dynamic control of flexion and extension of the knee as an antagonistic muscle group to the quadriceps. The vastus medialis is recognized as the only primary medial dynamic stabilizer of the extensor mechanism and patellar alignment.[10] The dynamic stabilizing forces of the vastus medialis obliquus (VMO) are assisted by the adductor magnus, whose tendon provides the insertion for most of the VMO fibers.[11] The lateral dynamic forces acting on the patella are the iliotibial band, the lateral retinaculum, and the vastus lateralis.[11] The patella is the centerpiece of all the stabilizing forces. Ficat and Hungerford[12] have shown that throughout the range of motion of the knee, the patella increases the effective extension force by as much as 50%. As these stabilizing forces act through the patella, a patellofemoral joint reactive force (PFJRF) is created by compression of the patella against the femur.[13] The greater the tension generated by the knee extensor muscles (quadriceps), the greater will be the resultant PFJRF. Furthermore, the patella transmits force to subchondral bone.[12] The PFJRF increases significantly with increased knee flexion such that at 15 degrees of flexion it is 1 × body weight; at 30 degrees, 2 × body weight; at 45 degrees, 3 × body weight; and at 75 degrees, 6 × body weight.[14] Normal walking creates a PFJRF of about 0.5 × body weight, ascending stairs 3.3 × body weight, and squatting 6–7 × body weight.[12,15] Limitation of knee extension or resistance to knee extension necessitates development of greater tension within the quadriceps, thereby increasing the PFJRF. It is easy to see why decreasing effective knee flexion (e.g., stretching tight hamstrings, gastrocnemius, and iliotibial band muscles) is a cornerstone of patellofemoral rehabilitation.

Knee flexion is not the only consideration in determining at what angle of knee range of motion to perform patellofemoral exercises. Patellofemoral contact areas determine what percentage of the undersurface of the patella articulates with the trochlear groove throughout knee flexion. Patellofemoral joint reaction stress (PFJRS) refers to the PFJRF per unit of contact area. A large PFJRF distributed over a large contact area yields a relatively lesser degree of articular stress. A large PFJRF over a small area of contact yields very high articular stresses and a greater chance of chondral degenerative changes. From 20 degrees of flexion to full extension, little patellofemoral contact occurs.[16] After 90 degrees of flexion, the center or the patella again does not articulate significantly with the trochlear groove. In this range of motion, more contact occurs over the odd facet and laterally on the patella. It is primarily in the mid ranges, from 30 to 90 degrees of flexion, where the patellofemoral contact areas are the greatest.

An appreciation of the biomechanics of open kinetic chain (OKC) and closed kinetic chain (CKC) exercises is critical in the treatment of patients with patellofemoral pain. If, during knee flexion or extension, the foot is allowed to move freely through space, the system is called *open*. In an OKC system, the hamstrings are predominant in flexion while extension is dominated by the quadriceps. Therefore, these types of exercises that place a greater load on the patellofemoral joint should be avoided, particularly early in patellofemoral rehabilitation.[14] They also are less physiologic for most sports activities, except for sports where kicking is an open-chain movement until contacting the ball. During CKC exercises for the lower limbs, the foot is kept immobile or maintains contact with a ground reactive force, and there is the creation of a multiarticular "closed chain." Rather than the near isolation of the large muscle groups seen during OKC exercises, performance of CKC knee flexion and extension results in "co-activation" of both hamstrings and quadriceps groups.[17,18] Examples of CKC exercises are leg presses or partial squats. These types of exercises strengthen agonist and antagonist muscles simultaneously via cocontraction and are more physiologic for lower extremity sporting activities (i.e., running). Examples of OKC exercises are straight-leg raises and knee extensions while wearing ankle weights.

Steinkamp et al.[19] looked at the effects on PFJRF and PFJRS values in patients who performed leg presses (CKC) versus knee extensions (OKC). They found that the resultant PFJRF and, most important, PFJRS were different for leg presses when compared with leg extension exercises, depending on the angle of flexion. At angles of flexion less than about 45 degrees, PFJRF and PFJRS were less with leg presses than with leg extensions. This is clinically relevant when one considers that the functional range of motion for most activities of daily living, as well as sports, is in the lower end of the knee flexion range and that strengthening with leg extensions in this range of motion subjects the patellofemoral joint to significant amounts of stress.[14,15,18–20] In contrast, leg press maneuvers place minimal stress on the patellofemoral joint in the functional range of motion.[14,15,19,20]

The important anatomy and biomechanics of patellofemoral pain syndrome also include functional anatomy and biomechanics of all kinetic chain structures that may affect patellofemoral motion (e.g., the lumbar spine, the hips, the thigh, the leg, the foot, and the ankle). Proximal hip mechanics are important in patellofemoral motion. Increased femoral internal rotation creates a disruption of normal patellofemoral mechanics, inducing obligate external tibial rotation because of the shape and dynamics of the semilunar cartilage at the knee. Internal femoral rotation may be due to femoral anteversion, tight tensor fascia lata (TFL), imbalance of internal and external rotators of the hip (e.g., tight TFL), and relatively weak gluteus maximus and piriformis muscles.[8,21] Regardless of the cause of internal femoral rotation, the end result will be increased torsion at the patellofemoral joint.

Tight hip flexor muscles also adversely affect the patellofemoral joint by increasing the flexion moment at the knee to maintain the center of gravity posterior to the knee joint.[8] Tight hamstrings, with their insertions distal to the knee joint, further increase knee flexion and PFJRF. An inflexible iliotibial band (ITB) will also lead to increased lateral patellar tracking because distal ITB fibers insert into the lateral retinaculum of the knee.

Distally, increased pronation at the foot is associated with increased tibial internal rotation, which can increase the torsion at the patellofemoral joint. A tight Achilles tendon can increase PFJRF through increased knee flexion because of the insertion of the gastrocnemius muscle proximal to the knee joint. Also, tight gastrocnemius muscles can increase obligate foot pronation.[22] Increased pronation at the foot increases the valgus vector force at the knee, increasing patellofemoral shear forces. A rigid cavus foot will have less shock absorption at the foot and ankle, with footstrike during gait causing increased force to be passed up the kinetic chain to the knee.

METHOD OF PRESENTATION

Patellofemoral pain syndrome usually presents as a chronic overload injury. The problem is usually one of chronic, repetitive overload to musculoskeletal structures from long-standing inefficiency of altered biomechanical loading. The pain usually emanates from one of two places, either the subchondral bone or the synovial/capsular and retinacular soft tissues. The onset is insidious except in cases where a direct precipitating trauma has occurred. The typical patient is a young, active person, often female, with retropatellar and peripatellar pain. Often, the pain location is quite vague, and swelling of the knee may be only minimal. The patient will have symptoms with most activities that increase patellofemoral loading (i.e., knee flexion). Difficulty will arise when getting into a squat position, sitting for prolonged periods (the positive "theater sign"), and while descending stairs. Pain with descending stairs rather than ascending stairs occurs because during stair descent, the knee flexion angle is greater (approximately 118 degrees versus 87 degrees for ascending),[23,24] and eccentric contractions are greater as the back leg lowers the body to the next lowest step. Pain with knee extension should alert the clinician to the possibility of infrapatellar fat pad impingement between the inferior pole of the patella and the femoral condyle.

The physical examination may be fairly unspectacular. Peripatellar pain with gliding of the patella may be seen. Patellofemoral compression may cause pain. If symptoms are more severe or if chondromalacia exists, pain may be present even when the patient does an isometric quadriceps contraction. Patella alta or baja may be present. Manual gliding and tilting of the patella and assessment of patellar rotation and anteroposterior position of the patella should be done to help evaluate patellofemoral tracking.[25] Hip abductor/external rotator weakness is common, as are hamstring, ITB, and gastrocsoleus tightness. Excessive callus beneath the first metatarsophalangeal joint and development of a hallux valgus may be subtle indicators of excessive pronation and hip muscle weakness as well. The athlete with suspected fat pad impingement syndrome should also be examined for genu recurvatum, an inferior tilting patella, and antetilting of the pelvis.

An important point to clarify in the patient with patellofemoral pain is the kinetic chain injury history. Previous injuries to other joints or musculoskeletal structures in the kinetic chain can have very significant implications and consequences at the knee. An unstable ankle due to multiple inversion injuries may increase torsion stresses at the knee. Previous hip or pelvis injuries may alter proximal muscle balance at the hip, which has direct implications to patellofemoral motion. Contralateral hip or knee problems may have increased ipsilateral loading of the entire lower limb with gait activities. Similarly, a kinetic chain physical examination should include inspection, range of motion testing, and muscle strength testing of proximal and distal joints. Quite often with patellofemoral pain, as well as with musculoskeletal disorders in general, radiographic, laboratory, or electrophysiologic tests do not give the diagnosis, and relative symmetries in flexibility and strength will be the key to proper diagnosis and rehabilitation.

DIFFERENTIAL DIAGNOSIS

Patients with patellofemoral pain should respond to treatment measures in a predictable manner if complete and accurate anatomic and biomechanical diagnoses are made. When patients fail to respond to treatment, it must be determined whether therapeutic measures were prescribed adequately, performed properly by the patient, and done on a regular basis. If these issues are addressed and the patient is still not improving, the diagnosis of patellofemoral pain must be reassessed and other potential problems must be considered. The differential diagnosis of patellofemoral pain includes referred pain from the hip and low back, osteochondritis dessicans of the femur or patella, Osgood-Schlatter disease, bone tumors (especially in cases of unilateral symptoms), osteoarthritis, inflammatory joint disease, meniscus pathology, and a synovial plica. Other potential etiology includes saphenous neuropathy and neuroma formation, particularly in patients who have had previous surgery.[26]

COMPLETE AND ACCURATE DIAGNOSIS

The *tissue injury complex* (Exhibit 17–1) is the area of actual tissue disruption and is often the main pain generator. In patellofemoral pain syndrome, it is most often the patellar cartilage, synovium, and the tendon insertion into the patella.[12,26]

The *functional biomechanical deficits* are those inflexibilities and/or muscle strength imbalances that create abnormal mechanics. In patellofemoral pain syndrome, they are insufficiency of medial quadriceps musculature, inflexibility of the iliotibial band, lateral retinaculum, hamstrings, and gastrocnemius muscles (all of which either increase knee flexion or cause lateral tracking of the patella), hamstring muscle weakness, hip abductor and external rotator weaknesses (which lead to increased medial rotation of the femur and further stress on the patellofemoral joint), imbalance of internal and external rotators at the hip (leading to increased

---

Exhibit 17–1 Components of a Complete and Accurate Diagnosis

Tissue Injury Complex
    Patellar cartilage and synovium
    Patellar tendon
Clinical Symptom Complex
    Peripatellar pain
    Positive "theater" sign
    Pain descending stairs
Functional Biomechanical Deficit Complex
    Insufficiency of the medial quadriceps
    Inflexible ITB
    Tight lateral retinaculum
    Tight hamstrings and gastrocsoleus
    Hamstring weakness
    Hip abductor and external rotator weakness
    Excessive pronation
Functional Adaptation Complex
    Knee flexion contracture
    Lateral patellar tracking
    Jumping off the contralateral leg
Tissue Overload Complex
    Lateral retinaculum
    Patellar tendon
    Hip external rotators
    Medial longitudinal arch of foot

torque at the knee), and excessive pronation. Sometimes, the functional biomechanical deficit may be the cause of the problem, other times it is the result of the problem, and still other times it is both. Again, it is important to look for these deficits locally at the knee, proximally, and distally.

The *functional adaptation complex* is the substitution pattern used by an athlete to try to maintain performance. In patellofemoral pain syndrome, this includes knee flexion contracture (loss of terminal knee extension), lateral patellar tracking, increased pain with running (often associated with a decreased stride length) and axial loading of the knee, and jumping off the opposite leg to avoid full loading of the involved knee. All of these adaptations will lead to inefficiencies in performance of sports, as well as to tissue overload of other structures in the kinetic chain.

The *tissue overload complex* involves those tissues subject to eccentric and tensile overloads. In patellofemoral pain syndrome, tissue overloads occur both locally and distally along the kinetic chain. Locally, the lateral retinaculum and patellar tendon are overloaded. These structures are the same as the tissue injury complexes in this syndrome. Other tissues that can be overloaded at a distant location include the hip external rotators. Because the hip external rotators may not be strong enough to balance the internal hip rotators, increased medial femoral rotation occurs, and increased patellofemoral shear results.

REHABILITATION

Acute Phase (0–7 Days with Emphasis on the First 48 Hours)

Acute phases of rehabilitation of patellofemoral disorders focus on treating the tissue injury complex and the clinical symptom complex (Exhibit 17–2). In most patellofemoral pain syndromes, the actual symptoms are not the result of an acute inflammatory reaction or of tendinitis, but rather the result of a chronic repetitive overload problem resulting in cellular damage and degeneration, with scar formation of the patellar tendon and lateral retinaculum. Still, there will be an acute, painful presentation of the problem with a lesser degree, if any, of inflammation. Under these conditions, it is unlikely that more than 24–48 hours of acute treatment are necessary. If there has been true subluxation or dislocation of the patella, a much greater period may be necessary to control swelling and inflammation. Symptomatic treatment may start with judicious use of antiinflammatory and pain medications and modalities. Intra-articular corticosteroid injection is rarely, if ever, indicated for patellofemoral symptoms. Therapeutic activities include relative rest (i.e., avoiding abusive or stressful activity to the knee but maintaining some motion to the injured part) and conditioning of other parts of the kinetic chain (i.e., stationary bike exercise using arms

Exhibit 17–2 Acute Phase of Rehabilitation

> Complexes Involved
>   Tissue injury
>   Clinical symptom
> Therapeutic Activities
>   Relative rest
>   Conditioning opposite leg, proximal and distal leg
>   musculature
>   Aerobic conditioning (i.e., arm ergometer, etc.)
>   NSAIDs and antiinflammatory modalities
>   Protected range of motion—avoiding excessive closed-
>   chain flexion (>50 degrees)
>   Isometric quad sets
> Criteria for Advancement
>   Resolution of swelling and inflammation
>   Decreased pain—level 2
>   Full range of motion with minimal pain

and the uninvolved leg, arm ergometers, and hip musculature strengthening). Cryotherapy is useful to decrease any joint effusion that may be present due to the inhibitory effect of an effusion on quadriceps function.[27,28] Protected range of motion is critical to avoid soft-tissue contracture. Initial muscle activity includes isometric exercise, often at multiple angles, avoiding painful arcs.[29] Criteria for advancement to the recovery phase include resolution of edema, improved range of motion, and pain decreased to level 2.

Recovery Phase (5–7 Days to 5–7 Weeks)

The complexes involved in this phase are the tissue overload complex and the functional biomechanical deficits (Exhibit 17–3). Therapeutic activities will include regaining lost flexibility, appropriate loading, resistive exercises, and kinetic chain and functional exercises aimed at improving patellar tracking.

Flexibility exercises must focus on many lower extremity muscles, in particular, the ITB, rectus femoris, gastrocnemius, and hamstrings.[30] The ITB is important because of its insertion into the lateral aspect of the patella and laterally deviating forces on the patella.[31–33] It is critical to stabilize the patella, often manually in a medially oriented direction, while stretching the ITB to avoid stressing the medial retinaculum; it is also essential to add shear stress on the patellofemoral joint by stretching the ITB and patella instead of the ITB alone as it inserts into the patella (Figure 17–1). The hamstrings and gastrocnemius, because of their propensity to shorten and increase the PFJRF with increasing flexion of the knee, must be stretched properly (Figures 17–2 and 17–3). Gastrocnemius-soleus inflexibility causes compensatory pronation of the foot, resulting in increased tibial rotation and additional patellofemoral stress.[25] Manual medial

Exhibit 17–3 Recovery Phase of Rehabilitation

Complex Involved
    Tissue Overload
    Functional Biomechanical Deficit
Therapeutic Activities
    Flexibility exercises for hip rotators, ITB, hamstrings,
        quads, gastrocsoleus
    Resistive exercises at spine, hip, ankle, as well as
        locally at knee
    Progress to eccentric and closed-chain quadriceps
        loading
    Weight-bearing activities
    Functional activities (i.e., partial squats, step-ups, and
        step-downs)
    Proprioceptive training
    Therapeutic taping
Criteria for Advancement
    No pain
    Range of motion equal to that on opposite side
    Strength at least 75% of opposite side

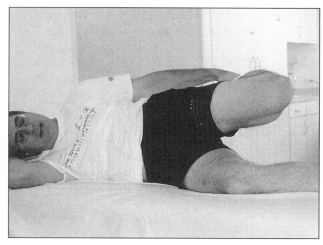

A

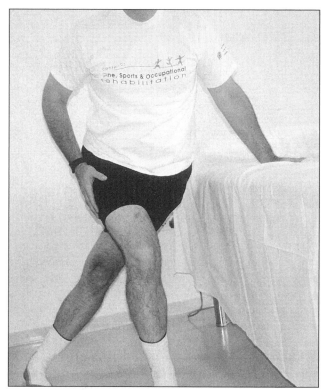

A

Figure 17–1 ITB stretch with patella manually stabilized.

glide and tilt of the patella may be employed to stretch the tight lateral retinaculum, specifically (Figure 17–4).[3] The rectus femoris, if tight, affects patellar movement during knee flexion.[25] A tight rectus femoris creates a patella alta. This is most prominent during hip flexion, when the rectus femoris functions as a hip flexor as well as a knee extensor. Patellar taping, as described by McConnell,[25] can be used to correct patellar glide, tilt, and rotation[21] (Figure 17–5).

Lower extremity malalignment problems (i.e., genu varum, tibia vara, hindfoot varus, and forefoot pronation [which can cause a compensatory subtalar joint pronation and obligatory internal tibial rotation]), if present, must be corrected. Strengthening exercises of the supinators of the foot can also be instituted (i.e., posterior tibialis, inverters of the ankle) to decrease pronation (Figure 17–6). Strengthening of the hip external rotators to correct hip internal/external rotation imbalance and tendency toward an internal rotated femur is also essential. Often, resolution of the tight ITB through aggressive stretching alone will not alleviate symptoms because the external rotators of the hip are still relatively weak. Orthotics may occasionally be necessary, although they should not be seen as an immediate solution to any weaknesses or imbalances.

All strengthening programs for patellofemoral pain must consider not only quadriceps strength but also what effect knee flexion angle and type of exercise (OKC versus CKC) have on PFJRF. The goals of patellofemoral rehabilitation are to maximize quadricep strengthening while minimizing PFJRF and PFJRS. Strengthening of the quadriceps and hip flexors is typically done via short-arc (–30 degrees of extension to 0 degree of extension) quadriceps exercises, although

the selectivity in strengthening only the VMO is debatable.[34,35] Selective VMO strengthening can possibly be enhanced by hip adduction exercises.[36] Besides strengthening the VMO, hip adductor strengthening may also serve to give the VMO a stable origin from which to contract. Hanten and Schulthies[36] have shown that during hip adduction, the electrical activity of the VMO was significantly greater

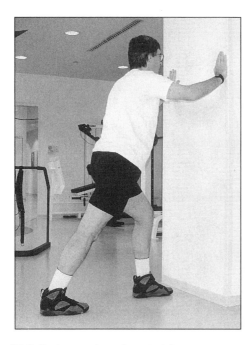

Figure 17–2 Gastrocnemius-soleus stretch.

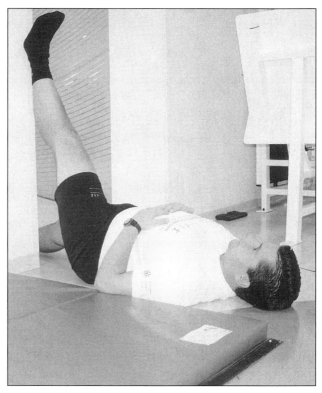

A

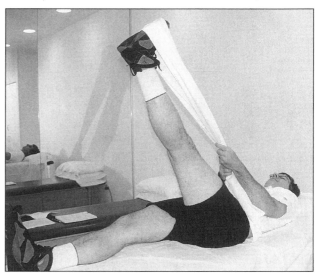

B

Figure 17–3 Hamstring stretches.

than that of the vastus lateralis. Therefore, the use of hip adductor contraction in conjunction with quadricep sets and straight-leg raises is recommended to facilitate VMO strengthening.

Often, isometric contractions can strengthen the quadriceps muscles without the significant increase in PFJRF seen with isotonic exercises. It is also important to keep in mind that articular cartilage is adversely affected by shear forces (which are theoretically minimized with isometrics) and may actually derive its nutrition through diffusion that occurs with intermittently applied compression.[34] Specifically, isometric contraction at 90 degrees of flexion, where compression is maximized and shear minimized, has been shown in some studies to increase VMO activity relative to vastus lateralis activity, compared with 15 degrees of knee flexion.[34,37] Kannus and Niittymaki[38] showed that 70% of patients with patellofemoral pain symptoms of greater than two months' duration had complete recovery of symptoms, with their only strengthening exercises being intense isometric quadriceps exercises in full extension. Wild et al.[39] emphasized the importance of doing isometric contractions in full knee extension as 10 degrees of flexion of the knee reduced the effective muscle effort in the vasti group to an average of one-fourth of the muscle effort demonstrated in full extension of the knee.

Emphasis should be placed on strengthening lower extremity muscles in the ranges where the PFJRF and PFJRS are lowest. During CKC exercises (leg presses) in lower knee flexion ranges (<45 degrees of flexion), consistently

less PFJRS is generated than during OKC (leg extension) exercises. As discussed earlier, when increased knee flexion angles are used (> 50 degrees of flexion), OKC (leg extension) activities show less PFJRF and PFJRS than do CKC (leg presses) exercises.[19] Therefore, a biomechanically

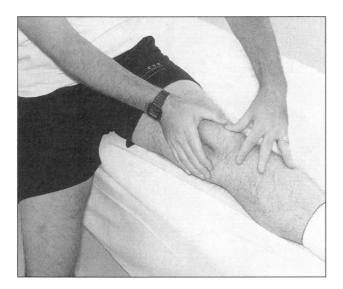

Figure 17–4 Manual medial glide of the patella.

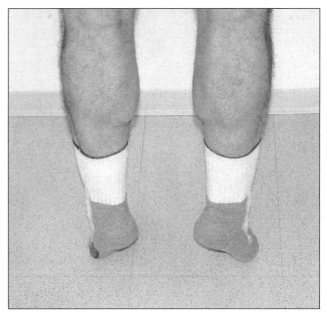

A

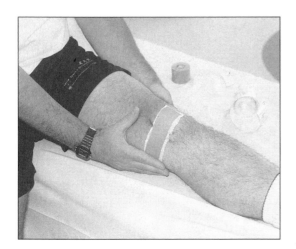

Figure 17–5 McConnell taping technique.

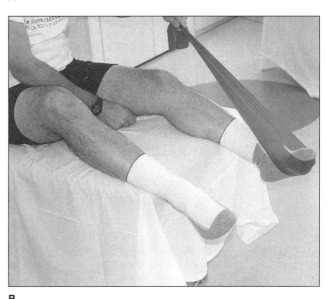

B

Figure 17–6 Strengthening foot supinators/inverters.

sound rehabilitation program, at least in terms of isometric strengthening, should consist of CKC exercises near terminal extension (Figure 17–7) and OKC exercises between 60 degrees and 90 degrees of flexion (Figure 17–8).

Strengthening must be done as soon as possible in weight-bearing activities also, as these are more physiologic. Closed-chain kinetic exercises, with cocontraction of quadriceps, hamstrings, and gastrocsoleus muscles are important to reduce excessive forces across the patella.[12,14,20] The same degree of force generation to maintain any degree of knee flexion is shared by two major muscle groups instead of one. Therefore, quadriceps tension necessary to generate a given

position of knee flexion is less with consequently less PFJRF. Furthermore, partial squats (one-fourth of a full squat) will also eccentrically load the knee, which will be more physiologic in nature. Training in an eccentric mode, which is the mode in which most overload injuries occur, is essential for proper patellofemoral rehabilitation. Later, progression of strengthening exercises, especially those for the VMO muscle, with sports-specific activities, is done.

The position of the femur during knee extensor strengthening is also important to consider. When the femur is inter-

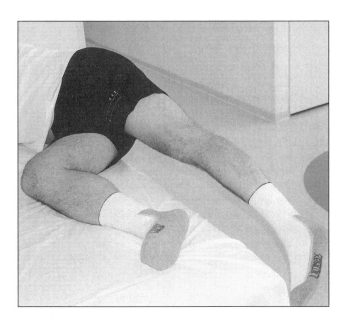

Figure 17–7 Strengthening external rotators of the hip and subsequently stretching ITB.

nally rotated, knee extension is assisted by the TFL muscle through its attachment into the iliotibial band.[40] This increases the lateral pull on the patella and, thus, decreases the effectiveness of the VMO.[25,31]

Muscular imbalances between the medial and lateral rotators and adductors, and the abductors of the hip must be addressed because they may lead to excessive medial rotation and adduction of the hip during stance phase of gait, with an associated increased valgus vector at the patellofemoral joint.[3,25] Strengthening the external rotators with the leg slightly extended and adducted can accomplish appropriate strengthening of the external rotators at the same time that the ITB is stretched (Figure 17–9). Distally, a weak tibialis anterior muscle can also reduce foot control at heel strike and cause increased stress at the knee.[41] Strengthening the anterior tibialis, as well as addressing footwear problems or other factors that increase stress at the ankle, may need to be part of a patellofemoral pain syndrome rehabilitation program.

Some controversy exists regarding the effects of patellofemoral taping and "selective VMO training" for improving patellofemoral tracking in the treatment of patellofemoral pain. McConnell[25] has claimed improvement rates of better than 90% in patellofemoral patients with taping and a neuromuscular reeducation program.[21] Selective training of the vastus medialis muscle using electromyographic biofeedback or combining biofeedback with a graded exercise program has also been shown to be beneficial.[42–44] However, the clinical benefits of taping have yet to be conclusively borne out by laboratory investigation. Bockrath, Wooden, Worrell, Ingersoll, and Farr[45] reported that patellofemoral taping caused no change in patellofemoral congruency or rotational

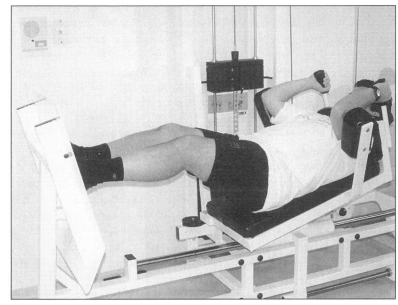

A

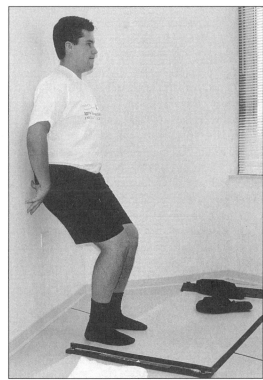

B

Figure 17–8 Partial squat exercise—closed kinetic chain exercise in weight-bearing.

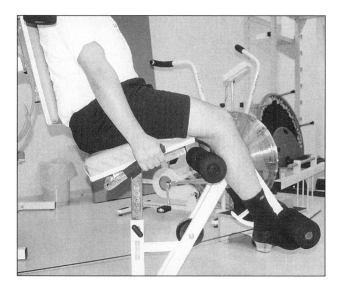

Figure 17–9 Open kinetic chain strengthening between 60 and 90 degrees of flexion.

Exhibit 17–4 Maintenance Phase of Rehabilitation

Complexes Involved
    Functional biomechanical deficit
    Subclinical adaptations
Therapeutic Activities
    Quad/hamstring balance
    ITB, hip rotator flexibility
    Hip internal/external rotator balance
    Functional progressions—running, kicking, cutting
    Pyelometrics
    Therapeutic taping/bracing as appropriate
Criteria for Return to Play
    Essential full ROM
    Normal strength and balance
    Sports-specific activities achieved—cross-cutting,
       figure-of-eight, cariocas

angles, as measured by Merchant views on X-rays. These measurements were done statically at one specific flexion angle, and no measures of dynamic motion were addressed. Nevertheless, they did notice a 50% reduction in pain on visual analogue scales with patellofemoral taping. Grabiner et al.[35] in their extensive review of patellar neuromechanics, were unable to conclude that selective VMO strengthening is possible. Rather, they suggested that a generalized quadriceps strengthening effect is the outcome of these rehabilitation programs and that it is perhaps the achievement of a "threshold" for absolute VMO strength that leads to reacquisition of normal tracking.[35] Under any circumstance, the problem with all of these studies is that full kinetic chain assessment was not performed. Dynamically, patients may be improving by these techniques because control at the level of the hip, the knee, or the ankle may be stabilizing the entire kinetic chain system. Examination of one joint in isolation is inadequate. Using electromyographic biofeedback to facilitate VMO control of the patella has also been described and may be of benefit in patellofemoral rehabilitation.[25,46]

Criteria for advancement to the maintenance phase include absence of pain or inflammation, range of motion equal to that of the opposite side, and strength at greater than 75% of normal smooth kinetic motion.

MAINTENANCE PHASE

The complexes involved in the maintenance phase of a patellofemoral rehabilitation program include the functional biomechanical deficit complex and the subclinical adaptation complex (Exhibit 17–4). Therapeutic activities are geared toward optimizing strength and flexibility, proprio-

ception retraining, balance, pyelometrics, and sports-specific activities. Agility drills, running, jumping, and kicking are stressed. Use of a balance board to provide a basic proprioceptive stimulus to the knee could also ease the transition into more functional activities and could serve to improve the kinesthetic sense in the knee.[30]

In most cases, athletes are able to resume activity without knee bracing. However, the use of a knee sleeve with fenestration for the patella has also been occasionally helpful.[47] Knee sleeves may work by simply providing some proprioception to the knee or by simply warming the soft tissues of the knee. It is important to restrict the wearing of the knee brace in competitive or high-demand situations. The more "supportive" a brace is, the more likely it is to promote muscular atrophy, particularly if it is worn on a constant basis. Infrapatellar straps may also help decrease patellofemoral symptoms by increasing the area for force dissipation of the patellar tendon.

Thorough evaluation of sports-specific demands on the knee will be necessary during the maintenance phase of rehabilitation. The athlete must demonstrate the ability to assume proper limb placement and coordinated patterns of muscle firing to prevent further patellofemoral overload. It is during this phase that more definitive equipment modifications may take place, as well. For example, the runner who continues to pronate excessively may be encouraged to purchase shoes with greater rear foot control and a straight last. Analysis of a cyclist often reveals the need to adjust the bicycle seat height slightly higher or to alter the cam type.[35] A beginning power lifter may need reminders to maintain a "toes-out," hips externally rotated position when performing squats.

Criteria for return to play include essentially full range of motion, normal strength and balance, normal techniques, and evidence that a sports-specific progression has occurred.

REFERENCES

1. Insall J. Current concepts review patellar pain. *J Bone Joint Surg Am.* 1982;46:147–152.

2. Fulkerson J, Hungerford D. *Disorders of the Patellofemoral Joint.* Baltimore: Williams & Wilkins; 1990.

3. Beckman M, Craig R, Lehman RC. Rehabilitation of patellofemoral dysfunction in the athlete. *Clin Sports Med.* 1989;8:841.

4. Bourne MH, Hazel WA, Scott SG, Sim FH. Anterior knee pain. *Mayo Clin Proc.* 1988;63:482–491.

5. Fulkerson JP, Tennant R, Jaivin JS, et al. Histologic evidence of retinacular nerve injury associated with patellofemoral malalignment. *Clin Orthop.* 1985;197:196–208.

6. Krammer PG. Patella malalignment syndrome: rationale to reduce excessive lateral pressure. *J Orthop Sports Phys Ther.* 1986;8: 306–308.

7. Radin EL. A rational approach to the treatment of patellofemoral pain. *Clin Orthop.* 1979;144:107–109.

8. Sommer HM. Patellar chondropathy and apicitis, and muscle imbalances of the lower extremity in competitive sports. *Sports Med.* 1988;5:381.

9. Moller BN, Jurik AG, Tidemand-Dal C, Kribs, Airis K. The quadriceps function in patellofemoral disorders: a radiographic and electromyographic study. *Arch Orthop Trauma Surg.* 1987;106:195–198.

10. Lieb FJ, Perry J. Quadriceps function: an anatomical and mechanical study using amputated limbs, *J Bone Joint Surg Am.* 1968;50: 1535–1548.

11. Bose KI, Kanagasuntherman R, Osman MBH. Vastus medialis oblique: an anatomic and physiologic study. *Orthopedics.* 1980;3: 880–883.

12. Ficat RP, Hungerford DS. *Disorders of the Patellofemoral Joint.* Baltimore: Williams & Wilkins; 1977.

13. Brunet ME, Stewart GW. Patellofemoral rehabilitation. *Clinics Sports Med.* 1989;8:319–329.

14. Hungerford DS, Barry M. Biomechanics of the patellofemoral joint. *Clin Orthop.* 1979;144:9–15.

15. Hungerford DS, Lennox DW. Rehabilitation of the knee and disorders of patellofemoral joint relevant biomechanics. *Orthop Clin North Am.* 1983;14:397.

16. Goodfellow J, Hungerford DS, Zindel M. Patellofemoral joint mechanics and pathology. 1. Functional anatomy of the patellofemoral joint. *J Bone Joint Surg Br.* 1976;58:287–290.

17. Draganich LF, Jaeger RJ, Kralj R. Coactivation of the hamstrings and quadriceps during extension of the knee. *J Bone Joint Surg Am.* 1989;71:1075–1081.

18. Palmitier RA, An KN, Scott SG, et al. Kinetic chain exercises in knee rehabilitation. *Sports Med.* 1991;11:402–413.

19. Steinkamp LA, Dillingham MF, Markel MD, Hill JA, Kautmann KR. Biomechanical considerations in patellofemoral joint rehabilitation. *Am J Sports Med.* 1993;21:438–444.

20. Reilly DJ, Martens M. Experimental analysis of quadriceps muscle force and patellofemoral joint reaction force for various activities. *Acta Orthop Scand.* 1972;43:126–137.

21. Hilyard A. Recent developments in the management of patellofemoral pain, the McConnell programme. *Physiotherapy.* 1990;76:559–565.

22. Root M, Orien W, Weed J. *Clinical biomechanics.* Vol. 2. Los Angeles: Clinical Biomechanics Corporation; 1977.

23. Post WR, Fulkerson J. Knee pain diagrams: correlation with physical examination findings in patients with anterior knee pain. 1994;10: 618–623.

24. Inman VT, Ralston HJ, Todd F. *Human Walking.* Baltimore: Williams & Wilkins; 1981:125.

25. McConnell J. The management of chondromalacia: a long term solution. *Aust J Physiother.* 1986;32:215–233.

26. Fulkerson JP, Kalenak A, Rosenberg TD, Cox JS. Patellofemoral pain. American Academy of Orthopedic Surgery Instructional Lectures, 1993.

27. Spencer J, Hayesk, Alexander I. Knee joint effusion and quadriceps inhibition in man. *Arch Phys Med Rehabil.* 1984;65:171–177.

28. Fahrer H, Reutsch HU, Gerber NJ, Beyerler C, Hess CW, Grunig B. Knee effusion and reflex inhibition of the quadriceps. *J Bone Joint Surg Br.* 1988;70:635–638.

29. O'Neill DB, Micheli LJ, Warner JP. Patellofemoral stress: a prospective analysis of exercise treatment in adolescents and adults. *Am J Sports Med.* 1992;20:151–156.

30. Shelton GL, Thigpen LK. Rehabilitation of patellofemoral dysfunction: a review of literature. *J Orthop Sports Phys Ther.* 1991; 14:243–248.

31. McNichol K. Iliotibial tract friction syndrome in athletes. *Can J Appl Sports Sci.* 1981;6(2):76–80.

32. Noble C. Iliotibial band friction syndrome in runners. *Am J Sports Med.* 1980;8:232–234.

33. Punicello MS. Iliotibial band tightness and medial patellar glide in patients with patellofemoral dysfunction. *J Orthop Sports Phys Ther.* 1993;17:144–148.

34. Boucher JP, King MA, Lefebvre R, Pepin A. Quadriceps femoris activity in patellofemoral pain syndrome. *Am J Sports Med.* 1992; 20:527–532.

35. Grabiner MD, Koh TJ, Draganich LF. Neuromechanics of the patellofemoral joint. *Med Sci Sports Exerc.* 1994;261:10–21.

36. Hanten WP, Schulthies SS. Exercise effect on electromyographic activity of the vastus medialis oblique and vastus lateralis muscles. *Phys Ther.* 1990;70:561–565.

37. Stoles M, Young A. Investigations of quadriceps inhibition: implications for clinical practice. *Physiotherapy.* 1984;70:425–428.

38. Kannus P, Niittymaki S. Which factors predict outcome in the nonoperative treatment of patellofemoral pain syndrome? A prospective follow up study. *Med Sci Sports Exerc.* 1994;26:289–296.

39. Wild JJ, Franklin TD, Woods GW. Patellar pain and quadriceps rehabilitation: an EMG study. *Am J Sports Med.* 1982;10:12–15.

40. Kaplan ED. The iliotibial tract. *J Bone Joint Surg Am.* 1958;40: 817–832.

41. Black JE, Alten SR. How I manage infrapatellar tendinitis. *Phys Sports Med.* 1984;12:86–92.

42. Ingersoll CD, Knight KL. Patellar location changes following EMG biofeedback or progressive resistive exercise. *Med Sports Exerc.* 1991;23:1122–1127.

43. LeVeau BF, Rogers C. Selective training of the vastus medialis muscle using EMG biofeedback. *Phys Ther.* 1980;60:1410–1415.

44. Wise HH, Fiebert IM, Kates JL. EMG biofeedback as treatment for patellofemoral pain syndrome. *J Orthop Sports Phys Ther.* 1984; 6:95–103.

45. Bockrath K, Wooden C, Worrell T, Ingersoll CD, Farr J. Effects of patella taping on patella position and perceived pain, *Med Sci Sports Exerc*. 1993;25:989–992.

46. Felder CR, Leeson MA. The use of electromyographic biofeedback for training the vastus medialis obliquus in patients with patello-femoral pain. Clinical protocol. Montreal, Canada: Though Technology Ltd. 1990.

47. Kowall MG, Kolk G, Nuber GW, Cassisi JE, Stern SH. Patellar taping in the treatment of patellofemoral: A prospective randomized study. *Am J Sports Med*. 1996;24:63.

SUGGESTED READING

Cerney K. Vastus medialis oblique/vastus lateralis muscle activity ratios for selected exercises in persons with and without patellofemoral pain syndrome. *Phys Ther*. 1995;75:672–683.

Doucette SA, Goble EM. The effect of exercise on patellar tracking in lateral patellar compression syndrome. *Am J Sports Med*. 1992;20: 434–440.

Flynn TW, Soutas-Little RW. Patellofemoral joint compressive forces in forward and backward running. *J Orthop Sports Phys Ther*. 1995; 21:277–282.

Fulkerson JP. The etiology of patellofemoral pain in young active patients. A prospective study. *Clin Orthop*. 1983;179:129–133.

Luessenhop S, Behrens P, Bruns J, Rehder U. Bilateral osteochondritis dissecans of the medial trochlea femoris: an unusual case of patellofemoral pain. *Knee Surg, Sports Traumatol Arthroscopy*. 1993; 1:187–188.

Mori Y, Kubo M, Shimokoube J, Kuroki Y. Osteochondritis dissecans of the patellofemoral groove in athletes: unusual cases of patellofemoral pain. 1994;2:242–244.

Muneta T, Yamamoto H, Ishibashi R, Asahina S, Furuya K. Computerized tomographic analysis of tibial tubercle position in the painful female patellofemoral joint. *Am J Sports Med*. 1994;22:67–71.

Powers CM, Maffucci R, Hampton S. Rearfoot posture in subjects with patellofemoral pain. *J Orthop Sports Phys Ther*. 1995;22:155–160.

Winslow J, Yoder E. Patellofemoral pain in female ballet dancers: correlation with iliotibial band tightness and tibial external rotation. *J Orthop Sports Phys Ther*. 1995;22:18–21.

CHAPTER 18

Overuse Injuries of the Leg

Robert E. Windsor and Krystal Chambers

INTRODUCTION

Participation in athletics has reached an unprecedented level of popularity in recent years. Sports provide entertainment, health benefits, relaxation, prestige, and, for some, a source of income. As the number of individuals participating in athletics increases, so does the number of injuries.

Lower extremity pain is commonly associated with athletic activity. Injury occurs when the cumulative forces exceed the tissue's ability to withstand them. This may be as a result of macrotrauma or repeated microtrauma. Often, specific biomechanical or physiologic factors predispose an individual to injury. Identification and correction of these conditions are key to treatment of overuse injuries of the lower extremity. This chapter addresses overuse injuries of the leg.

MEDIAL TIBIAL STRESS SYNDROME

Pain in the distal third of the posteromedial aspect of the tibia is a common affliction of the runner, the dancer, and other athletes who regularly engage in ballistic activities.[1] Although classified by its symptoms for decades, the exact etiology of medial leg pain remains controversial. In 1974, Puranan[2] coined the term *medial tibial stress syndrome* and proposed that the etiology of medial leg pain was an ischemic posterior compartment syndrome.[2–4] However, only one of the athletes in his series had visible ischemic changes demonstrated by fasciotomy.

Also in 1974, Clement[5] named the condition *tibial stress syndrome* and thought the symptoms arose from a painful periostitis due to muscle fatigue that allowed for increased force transmission to bone. Clement postulated that the pain then led to subsequent muscle weakness that allowed for additional muscle stress transmission to bone, with the eventual development of a stress fracture. In 1982, Mubarak et al[6] coined the term *medial tibial syndrome* and recommended that it be reserved for the athlete suffering from tibial periostitis.

In 1985, Michael and Holder[7] provided additional insight into the etiology of medial tibial stress syndrome when they demonstrated that the area of abnormal uptake on bone scan correlated with the origin of the soleus muscle (Figure 18–1). Biopsy subsequently confirmed an intense inflammation of the periosteum of the tibial origin of the soleus muscle. In cases where the bone scan was unremarkable, Michael and Holder proposed that an inflammatory response of the fascia adjacent to the soleus accounted for the symptoms. Detmer[8] has reported on a series of patients with chronic medial tibial stress syndrome with normal bone scans. He hypothesized that these patients had detached the involved periosteum; in fact, he found avulsed periosteum with interposed adipose tissue at the time of surgery.

Detmer[8] also proposed that medial tibial stress syndrome be categorized by etiology. Type 1 includes local stress fractures, type 2 describes those patients with medial tibial pain due to periostitis and periostalgia, and type 3 is reserved for those with pain due to deep posterior compartment syndrome.

Presently, medial tibial stress syndrome is based on finding an area of point tenderness on the posteromedial tibia, with an area of diffuse tenderness over the posteromedial aspect of the distal third of the tibia. In mild cases, pain is relieved by rest but in more severe cases, pain is present even at rest. The third phase of a three-phase bone scan typically becomes positive as the severity of symptoms increases.[1,9–11] When performed, biopsies usually reveal inflammatory change of the periosteum and fascia. Eventually, periosteal thickening may become evident on plain radiograph.

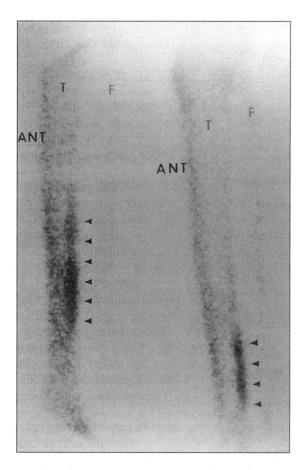

Figure 18–1 Bone scan with increased uptake at the attachment site of the soleus muscle. *Source:* Reprinted with permission from *Imaging of Athletic Injuries,* p. 56, © 1992, The McGraw-Hill Companies.

Although there are no pathognomonic signs or symptoms of medial tibial stress syndrome, a number of predisposing factors have been identified. Increased valgus forces on the rear foot result in increased eccentric contraction of the soleus and posterior tibial muscles, and is often the underlying cause. Etiologies for increased valgus forces on the rear foot include leaning too far into a curve, running on a track with tight corners, increasing external rotation of the hip (e.g., femoral anteversion), genu varum, and a large "Q" angle.[1]

In addition to mechanical problems, a common training error leading to overuse injuries of the leg is inadequate footwear.[12] Running shoes must be well made, with a properly aligned heel counter, a well-designed last, good arch support, and a heel without excessive flare. Footwear should be regularly inspected and replaced as shock absorption deteriorates. Other predisposing training errors include inadequate warm-up, running on uneven terrain, advancing training too rapidly, running on hard surfaces, running in cold weather, and low calcium intake.[1,12]

Excessive pronation, pes planus, pes cavus, a tarsal coalition, and lower extremity length and muscle imbalance adversely affect lower extremity mechanics and may lead to medial tibial stress syndrome.[13,14] Lower extremity length and muscle imbalance may also predispose to this condition.[5,15]

Treatment of medial tibial stress syndrome is relatively generic and may be generalized to many other lower extremity overuse syndromes. Prevention, adequate relative rest of the involved area, antiinflammatory medication, physical modalities, modification of training technique, strapping, orthotic prescription, and improvement of footwear are the cornerstones for treating lower extremity overuse syndromes.[16,17]

Prevention is obviously the best treatment of all. This includes appropriate rest, proper warm-up activities before a training session, and gradual introduction of a new workout or training surface. In addition, attention must be paid to alignment, technique, flexibility, muscle balance, and footwear.

Once an athlete has become symptomatic, early recognition and therapeutic intervention are important to a successful outcome. Initial treatment should include relative rest, gentle stretching activities, ice massage, and antiinflammatory medication. Physical modalities such as ultrasound and interferential stimulation should be used to increase influx of nutrients and efflux of metabolic by-products, to promote analgesia, and to decrease the viscosity of the involved area.[18] Although relative rest is very important, it should apply only to the involved area and not to the entire body. Cessation of regular training activities may induce significant psychologic alterations that may be manifested as sleep disturbance, irritability, mood swings, memory disturbance, depression, and appetite change.[19,20] Such changes may be seen as soon as 72 hours after the abrupt discontinuation of a training regimen. It is almost always possible to "work around" an injured area, thus maintaining overall physical and psychologic health.

The degree of relative rest depends on the athlete's symptoms. Mild exercise-induced leg pain without pain at rest may require only a temporary reduction in training intensity. If the athlete is experiencing severe pain, a total, temporary cessation of all forceful loading of the lower extremity should be considered. If the athlete continues to be severely symptomatic over the course of the ensuing week, a non–weight-bearing status with or without bracing may be appropriate.

In addition to rest, oral antiinflammatory medication should be started at the initiation of treatment unless there are contraindications such as pregnancy, peptic ulcers, or allergy. As a group, athletes are known for noncompliance with the usage of medication. As a result, it is very important to reinforce the importance of these medications and to emphasize their antiinflammatory potential, aside from their analgesic properties. It is also important to point out to the athlete that the medication should not be considered a failure unless it has been taken as prescribed for at least 10 days without eliciting the intended results. If the antiinflammatory medicine is being well tolerated and is achieving adequate reduction in pain and swelling, it is acceptable to continue the medication for up to six weeks. If the medication is required longer than six weeks, it is necessary to obtain baseline serum studies, including a complete blood count, liver function tests, urine analysis, SMA-6, and creatinine. If the athlete develops any laboratory or clinical evidence for end organ dysfunction, the medications should be discontinued.

Once symptoms begin to subside, athletes should be gradually returned to their premorbid activities. The rate of return will depend on a host of factors, including the severity and chronicity of the condition, the degree to which biomechanical dysfunction played a role in creating the condition (e.g., isolated muscles weakness, muscle imbalance, leg length discrepancy, equinous deformity), and the premorbid functional level of the athlete. Other, less important factors include the age, sex, and psychologic makeup of the individual.

The initiation of rehabilitative activities of a severe injury begins once the athlete's symptoms begin to subside. This process begins with the slow, sustained stretch of the involved region, as well as isometric exercises of all injured muscles at various degrees of length. Other relevant muscles may be gently exercised in a concentric and eccentric manner as long the injured region is not unduly taxed. During this phase, the athlete should maintain cardiovascular conditioning with open-chain or low-impact activities such as stationary bike exercise or swimming. Once the athlete has regained a normal, painless range of motion of the injured area and at least 90% of the strength of the contralateral side, a gradual return to premorbid activities is indicated. Strict attention should be paid to proper lower extremity alignment, muscle length and strength balance, footwear, warm-up, technique, and—if running is involved—terrain.

STRESS FRACTURES

Stress fractures are microfractures that usually occur as the result of repetitive loading of the lower extremity, such as that seen in running, jumping, and dancing.[21] They are the result of localized bone resorption exceeding bone deposition.[1] This injury is best viewed as ranging from diffuse stress reaction to macrofracture. Factors that increase ground reactive forces tend to aggravate this condition. Poor lower extremity alignment, inadequate footwear, improper training surface, decreased flexibility, and accelerated training programs contribute to the development of stress fractures.[22]

The area of stress fracture appears to be highly related to activity.[23] In one study of military recruits, 40% developed metatarsal stress fractures, 30% developed os calcis stress fractures, and 20% developed tibial stress fractures.[24,25] In athletes, 30–50% of stress fractures occur in the tibia, and 12–25% occur in the fibula.[15,26,27]

Stress fractures tend to occur at the origin of powerful lower extremity muscles. It is not clear whether this is due to repetitive forceful contraction of these powerful muscles or to muscle fatigue that allows for greater force transmission to bone. It is clear, however, that the bony origin of these powerful muscles is subjected to greater forces and is, consequently, the area of greatest local stress reaction.[1,28]

Clinically, patients with stress fractures present with a history of gradually increasing activity-related pain.[1,22] The pain surrounds the area of stress reaction or stress fracture. It is aggravated by repetitive, forceful loading of the lower extremity and is improved by rest.

Proximal tibial stress fractures are often misdiagnosed or overlooked as nonspecific knee pain (Figure 18–2). The pos-

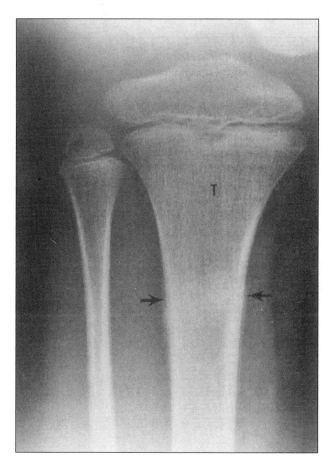

Figure 18–2 Proximal tibial stress fracture with periosteal reaction. *Source:* Reprinted with permission from *Imaging of Athletic Injuries,* p. 57, © 1992, The McGraw-Hill Companies.

teromedial aspect of the tibia, approximately 12–15 m proximal to the medial malleolus, is most commonly involved.[25] Midshaft tibial stress fractures tend to heal most slowly because bending moments are highest in this area and because blood supply may be marginal due to the vascular "watershed" zone.[29–31]

Diagnosing stress fractures is occasionally difficult, because diagnostic tests may be normal or equivocal in certain phases of injury.[32] Stress fractures are difficult to see early on routine radiographs unless they are viewed in perfect silhouette (Figures 18–3 and 18–4). Fifty percent of stress fractures may be missed on routine radiographs for the first two to four weeks postinjury, when reactive sclerosis becomes prominent.[1]

Treatment includes placing the athlete on relative rest status, applying ice for 15–20 minutes 3–4 times per day for the first 2–3 days following diagnosis and judiciously using anti-inflammatory agents. After two to three days, it is acceptable to begin using modalities such as superficial heat and interferential stimulation.

Relative rest entails maintaining cardiovascular fitness through minimally stressful activities such as stationary bicycling, swimming, using a cross-country ski machine, or running in a water vest. The athlete should stretch all lower extremity muscles, strengthen all relatively weak lower extremity muscles to expedite muscle balance, and continue regular strengthening activities of all musculature unrelated to the stress fracture.

In injured muscles, strengthening should begin in an isometric manner and should progress through eccentric to concentric conditioning. It is also in this phase of treatment that alignment and footwear should be addressed. Taping and orthotics should be prescribed as indicated.

Once strength and flexibility have been restored and the athlete is pain free with activities of daily living, conditioning activities may be advanced. This usually involves jogging on a minitramp or in the shallow end of a pool, or some comparable activity. Eventually, the athlete is advanced to activities such as treadmill running, jumping rope, or shuttle walking. Running on familiar terrain and cutting or jumping are added last.

Only severe cases or those not healing promptly should be immobilized. If immobilization is necessary, an air cast is usually all that is needed. Immobilization should be limited

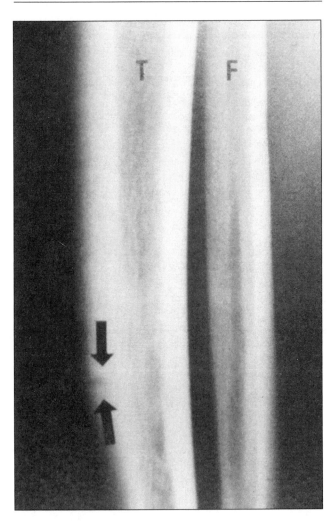

Figure 18–3 Anterior tibial stress fracture. *Source:* Reprinted with permission from *Imaging of Athletic Injuries,* p. 61, © 1992, The McGraw-Hill Companies.

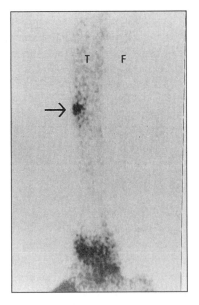

Figure 18–4 Bone scan of the same tibia in Figure 18–3, demonstrating increased uptake at the site of the stress fracture. *Source:* Reprinted with permission from *Imaging of Athletic Injuries,* p. 61, © 1992, The McGraw-Hill Companies.

to the time necessary to achieve clinical improvement. Midshaft tibial stress fractures tend to develop delayed nonunions and should be immobilized from the time of recognition. If the condition is becoming chronic, an external bone growth stimulator may be recommended.[33] Depending on the athlete's sport, career goals, and clinical status, an open bone grafting procedure may be considered. Decreased bone scan activity in the absence of healing may also prompt bone grafting.[1]

COMPARTMENT SYNDROME

A compartment syndrome occurs when increased intramuscular pressure inhibits the blood flow and function within an osteofascial compartment.[34] Acute and chronic compartment syndromes usually have different etiologies, natural histories, and treatments. An acute compartment syndrome is usually the result of macrotrauma and may be a medical and surgical emergency. A chronic compartment syndrome usually occurs in athletic activities that involve the repetitive dorisflexion and plantar flexion of the ankle, as in running and walking.[35]

Although the exact etiology of a chronic compartment syndrome is not known, several theories have been proposed. The prevailing theory is that repetition microtrauma injures the microcirculation, lymphatics, and musculature.[33] This promotes the buildup of interstitial fluid by increasing the vascular permeability and inducing myositis. The net effect is an increase in compartment pressures during rest and exercise.

Normal resting compartmental pressures range from 5 to 15 mm Hg.[36–38] Exercising compartmental pressures usually rise to 25–30 mm Hg, with dips between contractions to 15–25 mm Hg.[22,39] Elevated compartment pressures usually return to normal within 5–10 minutes.[4]

In a compartment syndrome, resting pressures may be as high as 20–30 mm Hg, and exercising pressures rise as high as 80–120 mm Hg. In addition, postexercise pressures remain elevated above normal values for over 10 minutes and occasionally as long as 20–25 minutes. Prolonged postexercise pressure elevation is probably the most important single diagnostic parameter.[4,38,40–43]

Clinically, the diagnosis of compartment syndrome is suspected when pain in a particular muscle group occurs only with athletic activity, often at a particular point in the regimen. Pain occurs along the muscle involved and may be associated with numbness or tingling in the distribution of a nerve traversing the compartment.[1] Symptoms generally resolve rapidly upon cessation of the activity, as long as it is stopped shortly after the pain begins. If the athlete attempts to "push through the pain," muscle weakness and prolonged pain may occur. If the athlete continues to push frequently, pain may occur with normal walking or jogging.

CHRONIC COMPARTMENT SYNDROMES

Chronic compartment syndromes have been recognized in all five fascial compartments of the leg. The anterior compartment is most frequently involved.[44,45]

Anterior Compartment Syndrome

Anterior compartment syndrome is common in race walkers, joggers, and soccer players.[36,46,47] The pain is located in the anterolateral, middle third of the leg. Athletes who persist in training may report that the pain occurs at a specific mileage. In more severe cases, numbness in the first web space and a foot drop may occur.[1]

In anterior compartment syndrome, muscular herniations may be found (Figure 18–5).[48,49] They generally occur between the anterior and lateral compartment at the junction of the distal and middle third of the leg.[50] Branches of the superficial peroneal nerve usually pass through these defects; thus, no attempt should be made to pass a needle through or to surgically close the defect because this may precipitate an acute compartment syndrome.

Deep Posterior Compartment Syndrome

In deep posterior compartment syndrome (Detmer's medial tibial stress syndrome, type 3), athletes usually describe

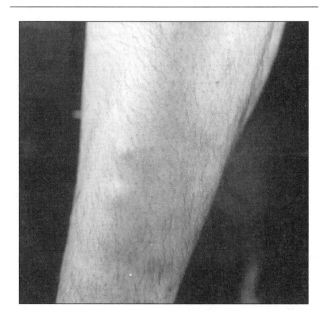

Figure 18–5 Muscular herniations in the anterior compartment to chronic compartment syndrome.

an aching pain in the posteromedial border of the tibia that may be very difficult to separate from other causes of posteromedial leg pain.[2,8] It is usually precipitated by a dramatic increase in training intensity. This condition is often bilateral and may progress to include paresthesia in the instep and, less frequently, in the toes. In addition, weakness in the toe flexors and ankle invertors may be demonstrated if the athlete is examined immediately after a training session. If paresthesia is present in the instep, the posterior tibial muscle is weak, and there is a diminished pulse in the posterior tibial pulse, then an acute compartment syndrome is likely.

Superficial Posterior Compartment Syndrome

The superficial posterior compartment contains the soleus and gastrocnemius muscles. It is rarely involved in a chronic compartment syndrome, although it is occasionally involved acutely.[51,52] The typical presentation of a chronic compartment syndrome is a feeling of tightness and discomfort involving the upper part of the posterior leg after exercising. If compartmental pressures become too high, the sural nerve and plantar flexors may become involved, causing the athlete to experience numbness or tingling on the lateral border of the foot and weakness with plantar flexion.

Isolated Posterior Tibialis Compartment Syndromes

Isolated posterior tibialis and lateral compartment syndromes are very rare. In the isolated posterior tibialis compartment syndrome, the posterior tibialis compartment syndrome is separated from the rest of the deep posterior compartment musculature by an all-enveloping fascial sheath.[53] This sheath may be the reason for a failed fasciotomy of the deep posterior compartment and may require its own fasciotomy. In this syndrome, pain is worst on push-off, located along the posteromedial border of the tibia, and may radiate into the arch. There are no sensory changes in this syndrome.

Lateral Compartment Syndrome

The lateral compartment syndrome is very rare and must be distinguished from tenosynovitis of the tibialis anterior and flexor hallucis longus, fibular stress fracture, and lateral gastrocnemius strain. There is tenderness along the proximal half of the leg, and the lateral compartment may be found to be edematous and tense. There may be associated numbness over the dorsum of the foot as a result of compression of the superficial peroneal nerve.[34,50,52,54]

An accurate diagnosis is paramount to proper treatment. Diagnosing a lateral compartment syndrome requires a high degree of suspicion and should be established as soon as possible because conservative care is less successful in this con-dition, compared with other lower extremity overuse syndromes.

Conservative care begins with relative rest, education, and evaluation for underlying etiologies. Lower extremity malalignment, muscle imbalances in both strength and/or length, training errors such as alterations in terrain or intensity, inadequate footwear, and poor technique are all recognized causes of chronic compartment syndrome.

If the symptoms are relatively mild, a short course of relative rest, education, and antiinflammatory agents is all that may be required. If symptoms are more severe, complete cessation from repetitive loading of the lower extremity may be required. If this is required, aerobic conditioning should be maintained via an open-chain or extremely low-impact activity such as water vest running or stationary bicycling. In addition, gentle stretching of tight muscles, strengthening of weak muscles, and correction of training errors should be introduced at appropriate intervals in the rehabilitation program.

If conservative care does not succeed in relieving the athlete's symptoms, an open fasciotomy should be performed via a limited incision with a subcutaneous division of the fascial sheath along its entire length.[39] Care must be taken to prevent injury to sensory nerves traversing the compartment. Success rates of limited fasciotomy for refractory compartment syndromes approach 90% in most series.[1,55] Failures include those patients who had been symptomatic for long periods of time and had sustained damage to intracompartmental structures, those who had inadequate fasciotomies, those with an improper diagnosis, and those who had the wrong compartment released.

ACUTE COMPARTMENT SYNDROME

An acute compartment syndrome is a medical and surgical emergency, and it is extremely important to distinguish it from its chronic counterpart.[56,57] It is usually the result of acute macrotrauma, such as a crush injury, fracture, or acute vascular occlusion.[58,59] Occasionally, an acute compartment will result from a contusion in an athlete taking antiinflammatory agents or in an athlete engaging in extreme activities that are unfamiliar.[1,60]

Acute compartment syndromes may present with extreme pain that appears out of proportion to the obvious abnormality. Over the course of several hours to a day, the athlete may complain of sensory abnormalities or weakness. Increasing pain while at rest is a ubiquitous characteristic of the condition. Pulses are usually diminished if a large vessel passes through the compartment, but the presence of normal pulses does not rule out the condition. It is important to note that total obliteration of one or more pulses is a late sign.

If clinical suspicion for the condition exists, compartment pressures should be measured.[61] Pressures less than 30 mm

Hg are acceptable, 30–50 mm Hg is borderline, and anything greater than 50 mm Hg constitutes a surgical emergency.[1] The use of ice during the first 2–4 hours after onset of symptoms is recommended but beyond this point is controversial. The involved extremity should not be elevated as this will decrease the local arterial pressure without decreasing venous pressure. All bandages should be removed so the extremity can be easily evaluated.

If surgery is necessary, decompression should be complete, and the wounds should be left open.[1] Healing by secondary intension or skin grafting is acceptable practice. During surgery, no tourniquet should be used. If extensive muscle damage has occurred or if the condition has been present for an extended period of time, renal and metabolic function should be monitored closely.

Compartment pressures rising over a short period of time have the potential for causing irreversible changes sooner than do the same pressures that developed over a longer period of time. The compartment pressure required to cause an acute compartment syndrome is dependent on the duration of increased pressure, the rate of pressure rise, metabolic rate of the tissues, vascular tone, and local blood pressure.[1]

Peripheral nerves will exhibit microscopic changes after 30 minutes of ischemia and irreversible changes after 12–24 hours.[62] Muscles will exhibit functional changes within 2–4 hours and permanent changes shortly thereafter. Myoglobinuria occurs after 4 hours of ischemia and may become worse after the restoration of adequate circulation.[1]

If treated within 12 hours, the prognosis of acute compartment syndrome is generally very favorable, with a complication rate of 10–15%. If an acute compartment syndrome is allowed to go on beyond 12 hours, the prognosis for recovery is much worse. The amputation rate may be as high as 40%, and permanent functional impairment may occur in as many as 80% of cases.[1]

CONCLUSION

Overuse injuries are prevalent with athletic endeavors. They are generally easily treated but occasionally require surgery to improve. Left untreated and pursuing the training philosophy of "no pain, no gain," they will generally become chronic conditions. However, with knowledge of normal and abnormal biomechanics, pathomechanics of each specific overuse injury, and proper rehabilitation philosophy, most overuse injuries can be effectively treated, and the athlete can be kept on the field rather than on the sidelines.

REFERENCES

1. Reid DC. Exercise induced leg pain. In: Reid DC. *Sports Injury Assessment and Rehabilitation*. New York: Churchill Livingstone; 1992:269.

2. Puranen J. The medial tibial syndrome: exercise ischemia in the medial fascial compartment of the leg. *J Bone Joint Surg Br.* 1974; 56:712.

3. Byrk E, Grantham SA. Shin splints—a chronic deep posterior ischemic compartmental syndrome of the leg? *Orthop Rev.* 1983; 12:29.

4. Wallenstein R, Eriksson E. Intramuscular pressures in exercise induced lower leg pain. *Int J Sports Med.* 1984;5:31.

5. Clement DB. Tibial stress syndrome in athletes. *J Sports Med.* 1974;2:81.

6. Mubarak SJ, Gould RN, Lee YF, et al. The medial tibial syndrome: a cause of shin splints. *Am J Sports Med.* 1982;10:201.

7. Michael RH, Holder LE. The soleus syndrome: a cause of medial tibial stress (shin splints). *Am J Sports Med.* 1985;13:87.

8. Detmer DE. Chronic shin splints: classification and management of medial tibial stress syndrome. *Sports Med.* 1986;3:436.

9. Allen MJ, O'Dwyer FG, Barnes MR, Belton IP, Finlay DB. The value of 99Tcm-MDP bone scans in young patients with exercise-induced lower leg pain. *Nucl Med Commun.* 1995;16(2):88.

10. Piffanelli A, Giganti M, Cittanti C, Colamussi P. Nuclear medicine in the integrated diagnosis of fatigue fractures. *Radiol Med.* May 1993;85(suppl 1):272–275.

11. Samuelson DR, Cram RL. The three phase bone scan and exercise induced lower-leg pain. The tibial stress test. *Clin Nucl Med.* 1996; 21:89–93.

12. Myburgh KH, Srobler N, Noskes TD. Factors associated with shin soreness in athletes. *Phys Sports Med.* 1983;11:125.

13. Sommer HM, Vallentyne SW. Effect of foot posture on the incidence of medial tibial stress syndrome. *Med Sci Sports Exerc.* 1995;27: 800–804.

14. Viita Sala JT, Kuist M. Some biomechanical aspects of the foot and ankle in athletes with and without shin splints. *Am J Sports Med.* 1983;11:125.

15. Clement DB, Tauton JE, Smart GW, et al. A survey of overuse running injuries. *Phys Sports Med.* 1981;9:47–58.

16. Andrish JT, Bergerfield JA, Walhein J. A prospective study on the management of shin splints. *J Bone Joint Surg Am.* 1974;56:1697.

17. Jackson SW, Bailey D. Shin splints in the young athlete—a nonspecific diagnosis. *Phys Sports Med.* 1975;3:45.

18. Windsor R, Lester J, Herring S. Electrical stimulation in clinical practice. *Phys Sports Med.* 1993;21:85.

19. Snyder RB, Lipscomb AB, Johnston RK. The relationship of tarsal coalition to ankle sprains in athletes. *Am J Sports Med.* 1981;9:313.

20. Walsh WM. Exercise for stress management. *Postgrad Med.* 1983; 74:245.

21. Fanciullo JJ, Bell CL. Stress fractures of the sacrum and lower extremity. *Curr Opin Rheumatol.* 1996;8(2):158.

22. Sullivan D. Stress fractures in 51 runners. *Clin Orthop.* 1984;187:188.

23. Brukner P, Bradshaw C, Khan KM, White S, Crossley K. Stress fractures: a review of 180 cases. *Clin J Sports Med.* 1996;6(2):85.

24. Gilbert RS, Johnson HS. Stress fractures in military recruits—a review of 12 years experience. *Milit Med.* 1966;131:716.

14. Viita Sala JT, Kuist M. Some biomechanical aspects of the foot and ankle in athletes with and without shin splints. *Am J Sports Med.* 1983;11:125.

15. Clement DB, Tauton JE, Smart GW, et al. A survey of overuse running injuries. *Phys Sports Med.* 1981;9:47–58.

16. Andrish JT, Bergerfield JA, Walhein J. A prospective study on the management of shin splints. *J Bone Joint Surg Am.* 1974;56:1697.

17. Jackson SW, Bailey D. Shin splints in the young athlete—a nonspecific diagnosis. *Phys Sports Med.* 1975;3:45.

18. Windsor R, Lester J, Herring S. Electrical stimulation in clinical practice. *Phys Sports Med.* 1993;21:85.

19. Snyder RB, Lipscomb AB, Johnston RK. The relationship of tarsal coalition to ankle sprains in athletes. *Am J Sports Med.* 1981;9:313.

20. Walsh WM. Exercise for stress management. *Postgrad Med.* 1983; 74:245.

21. Fanciullo JJ, Bell CL. Stress fractures of the sacrum and lower extremity. *Curr Opin Rheumatol.* 1996;8(2):158.

22. Sullivan D. Stress fractures in 51 runners. *Clin Orthop.* 1984;187:188.

23. Brukner P, Bradshaw C, Khan KM, White S, Crossley K. Stress fractures: a review of 180 cases. *Clin J Sports Med.* 1996;6(2):85.

24. Gilbert RS, Johnson HS. Stress fractures in military recruits—a review of 12 years experience. *Milit Med.* 1966;131:716.

25. McBride AM. Stress fractures in athletes. *J Am Sports Med.* 1976; 3:212.

26. Hansson CJ. On insufficiency fractures of femur and tibia. *Acta Radiol.* 1938;19:554.

27. Hulko A, Orava S. Stress fractures in athletes. *Int J Sports Med.* 1987;8:221.

28. Markey KL. Stress fractures. *Clin Sports Med.* 1987;405.

29. Blank S. Transverse tibial stress fractures: a special problem. *Am J Sports Med.* 1987;25:597.

30. Green NE, Rogers NA, Lipcomb AB. Nonunions of stress fractures in the tibia. *Am J Sports Med.* 1985;13:171.

31. Orava B. Stress fractures. *Br J Sports Med.* 1984;14:40.

32. Martheson GO, Clement DB, McKenzie DC, et al. Stress fractures in athletes, a study of 320 cases. *Am J Sports Med.* 1987;15:46.

33. Rettig AC, Shelbourne DK, McCarroll JR, et al. The natural history and treatment of delayed unions of stress fractures of the anterior cortex of the tibia. *Am J Sports Med.* 1988;16:250.

34. Styf JR. Chronic exercise-induced pain in the anterior aspect of their lower leg: an overview of diagnosis. *Sports Med.* 1989;7:331.

35. McDermott AGP, Marble RH, Yabsley RH, et al. Monitoring anterior compartment pressure during exercise: a new technique using the STIC catheter. *Am J Sports Med.* 1982;19:83.

36. Lawson S. *Compartment Pressures in Nordic Skiers.* Edmonton, Alberta, Canada; University of Alberta: 1989. Thesis.

37. Logan JG, Rorabeck CH, Castle GSP. The measurement of dynamic compartment pressures during exercise. *Am J Sports Med.* 1983; 11:220.

38. Styf JR, Korner LM. Microcapillary infusion technique for measurement of intramuscular pressure during exercise. CORR. 1986; 207:253.

39. Styf JR, Korner LM. Chronic anterior compartment syndrome of the leg: results of treatment by fasciotomy. *J Bone Joint Surg Am.* 1986; 68:1338.

40. Delacerda FG. Iontophoresis for treatment of shin splints. *J Orthop Sports Phys Ther.* 1982;3:183.

41. Puranen J, Alavaiko A. Intracompartment pressure increase on exertion in patients with chronic compartment syndrome in the leg. *J Bone Joint Surg Am.* 1981;63:1304.

42. Schepsis A, Martini D, Corbett M. Surgical management of exertional compartment syndrome of the lower leg: long term follow up. *Am J Sports Med.* 1994;121:811.

43. Styf JR, Korner LM. Diagnosis of chronic anterior compartment syndrome in the lower leg. *Acta Orthop Scand.* 1987;58:139.

44. Ross DG. Chronic compartment syndrome. *Orthop Nurs.* 1996; 15(3):23.

45. Schepsis AA, Lynch G. Exertional compartment syndromes of the lower extremity. *Curr Opin Rheumatol.* 1996;8:143.

46. Sanzen L, Forsberg A, Westlin N. Anterior tibial compartment pressures during race walking. *Am J Sports Med.* 1986;14:136.

47. Veith RG, Matsen FA, Newell SG. Recurrent anterior compartment syndromes. *Phys Sports Med.* 1980;8:80.

48. Fronek J, Murabak SJ, Hargens AR, et al. Management of chronic exertional anterior compartment syndrome of the lower extremity. *CORR.* 1987;220:217.

49. Pedowitz RA, Hargens AR, Murabek SJ, Gershuni DJ. Modified criteria for the objective diagnosis of chronic compartment syndrome of the leg. *Am J Sports Med.* 1990;18(1):35.

50. Styf JR. Diagnosis of exercise induced pain in the anterior aspect of the lower leg. *Am J Sports Med.* 1988;16:165.

51. Stack C. Superficial posterior compartment syndrome of the leg with deep venous compromise. *Clin Orthop.* 1987;220:233.

52. Wiley JP, Clement DB, Doyle DL, et al. A primary care perspective of chronic compartment syndrome of the leg. *Phys Sports Med.* 1987; 15:111.

53. Davey JR, Rorabeck CH, Fowler PJ. The tibialis posterior muscle compartment: an unrecognized cause of exertional compartment syndrome. *Am J Sports Med.* 1984;12:391.

54. Styf J. Entrapment of the superficial peroneal nerve: diagnosis and results of decompression. *J Bone Joint Surg Br.* 1989;71:131.

55. Detmer DE, Sharpe K, Sufit RL, Firdley FM. Chronic compartment syndrome: diagnosis, management, and outcome. *Am J Sports Med.* 1985;13(3):162.

56. Gerow G, Matthews B, Jahn W, Gerow R. Compartment syndrome and shin splints of the lower leg. *J Manipulative Physiol Ther.* 1993;16:225.

57. McConnell EA. Myths and facts . . . about acute compartment syndrome. *Nursing.* 1996;26(2):30.

58. Mabee JR. Compartment syndrome: a complication of acute extremity trauma. *J Emerg Med.* 1994;12:651.

59. Mabee JR, Bostwick TL. Pathophysiology and mechanisms of compartment syndrome. *Orthop Rev.* 1993;22:175.

60. Bealle S, Garner T, Oxley D. Anterolateral compartment syndrome related to drug induced bleeding: a case report. *Am J Sports Med.* 1983;11:454.

61. Gulli B, Templeman D. Compartment syndrome of the lower extremity. *Orthop Clin North Am.* 1994;25:677–684.

62. Finkelstein JA, Hunter GA, Hu RW. Lower limb compartment syndrome: course after delayed fasciotomy. *J Trauma.* 1996;40:342.

Rehabilitation of the Ankle and Foot

W. Ben Kibler

INTRODUCTION

The ankle and foot, although anatomically comprised of many different bones, ligaments, and muscles, often function as a unit to stabilize the leg and body, absorb loads, and provide propulsion for the athlete. Individual injuries of the foot and ankle should be evaluated and rehabilitated from both standpoints.

Identification of all of the specific anatomic structures that are affected in each injury is important. Treatment and rehabilitation of these structures must be implemented, but rehabilitation must also proceed to restore all of the functions of the ankle and foot unit.

These functions include: (1) acting as a shock absorber for the applied loads as the foot strikes the ground on running or jumping, or strikes an object in kicking; (2) storing energy while the foot is on the ground by foot positioning and ligament tensioning, releasing this upward in jumping or forward in running; (3) accommodating to uneven surfaces, due to the different alignment of the bones and geometric angles of the joint; (4) accommodating to different positions of the foot and ankle in cutting, jumping, starting, and stopping; and (5) creating a stable platform to allow muscles to generate appropriate force.

REHABILITATION PROTOCOL

Due to the integrated nature of the foot and ankle in functional activities, rehabilitation can be organized around a common framework for most foot and ankle problems. This common framework can then be altered for specific injuries, especially in the acute phase. As rehabilitation progresses to recovery and functional phases, the protocols merge toward functional restoration. (See Exhibit 19–1 and Figures 19–1 through 19–11.)

SPECIFIC INJURIES

Acute Lateral Ankle Sprain

Lateral ankle sprain is the most common athletic injury. Accurate diagnosis of all involved structures is a prelude to proper rehabilitation.

Method of Presentation—Acute injury due to sudden inversion of the ankle, often accompanied by some degree of plantar flexion. There may be an audible pop.

Clinical Symptom Complex—Point-tender pain to palpation over the affected ligaments (Figure 19–12). There is usually mild to moderate swelling in the grade I or II injuries, with more swelling in grade III injuries. There is usually athletic dysfunction, with limping and inability to run or jump.

Tissue Injury Complex—The anterior talofibular ligament is invariably involved. The fibulocalcaneal, anterior tibiofibular, and posterior talofibular ligaments may also be involved in decreasing order of frequency. The talar dome may be involved, either as a chondral or osteochondral injury.

Tissue Overload Complex—Peroneal muscles.

Functional Biomechanical Deficit Complex—If the ankle is immobilized, generalized ankle stiffness and inflexibility will be present, along with immobilization-induced muscle weakness. There will be some proprioceptive deficit, depending on the degree of injury and type and length of immobilization.

Subclinical Adaptation Complex—Pain-induced limping will create alterations in stride length, stride cadence, and time of weight-bearing.

Treatment Considerations—Acute ankle sprains, especially first-time or severe injuries, must be treated aggressively to promote maximum tissue healing with minimal proprioceptive and muscular deficits. Most sprains will do well without rigid immobilization, with its complications of

Exhibit 19–1 Rehabilitation Protocols

I. ACUTE PHASE
  A. GOALS
    1. Decrease pain and inflammation
    2. Reestablish nonpainful range of motion (ROM)
    3. Retard muscle atrophy of the entire lower extremity complex
    4. Increase neuromuscular control in non–weight-bearing to partial weight-bearing of the ankle complex
  B. PROGRESSIONS IN THE ACUTE PHASE
    1. Pain and inflammation
      a. Compression
      b. Support (air cast or brace)
      c. Modalities
      d. Joint mobilization
    2. Range of motion
      a. Dependent
        1. Grades I and II mobilization of the talocrural, subtalar, and midtarsal joints
        2. Manual capsular stretching
        3. Proprioceptive neuromuscular facilitation (PNF)
      b. Independent
        1. Towel stretches (Figure 19–1)
        2. Alphabet exercises
        3. Biomechanical ankle platform system (BAPS)/ball rolling (Figure 19–2)
        4. Active and passive flexibility exercises
    3. Muscle atrophy/neuromuscular control
      a. Isometrics
      b. Closed-chain exercises in sitting (Figure 19–3)
      c. Open-chain isotonics
        1. Concentrics
        2. Eccentrics
  C. CRITERIA FOR PROGRESSION FROM THE ACUTE PHASE TO THE RECOVERY PHASE
    1. Minimal pain and tenderness
    2. Full nonpainful passive ROM
    3. Manual muscle test (MMT) strength of the ankle complex grade IV/V
II. RECOVERY PHASE
  A. GOALS:
    1. Regain and improve lower extremity strength and endurance
    2. Improve neuromuscular control of the lower extremity complex in a full weight-bearing posture to unstable postures
    3. Normal arthrokinematics in single planes and triplanar motion of the ankle
  B. PROGRESSIONS IN THE RECOVERY PHASE
    1. Motion—active
      a. Single plane
      b. Multiple

    2. Strengthening
      a. Dependent
        1. PNF
        2. Manual resistance
      b. Independent
        1. Single planes
          a. Isotonics—concentric, eccentric
          b. Isokinetics
          c. Tubing exercises (Figure 19–4)
        2. Multiple planes
    3. Neuromuscular control
      a. Proprioception
        1. Wobble board (Figure 19–5)
        2. Writing the alphabet
        3. PNF (Figure 19–6)
      b. Closed kinetic chain (bilateral activities)
        1. Walking
        2. Loading
      c. Open chain
    4. Arthrokinematics
      a. Joint mobilization
      b. Gait activities
  C. CRITERIA FOR PROGRESSION FROM THE RECOVERY PHASE TO THE FUNCTIONAL PHASE
    1. Full nonpainful active and passive ROM
    2. No pain or tenderness
    3. Strength of the plantar flexors, dorsiflexors, invertors, and evertors 75–80% of the uninvolved side
    4. Balance on one leg for 30 seconds with eyes closed
III. FUNCTIONAL PHASE
  A. GOALS
    1. Increase power of the lower extremity complex
    2. Increase neuromuscular control in multiple planes of motion
    3. Utilize sport-specific training for full return to sport
    4. Achieve muscular control of lower extremity posture
  B. PROGRESSIONS IN THE FUNCTIONAL PHASE
    1. Power
      a. Pyelometrics
        1. Double-leg jumping to single leg jumping (Figure 19–7)
        2. Running to cutting progressions (Figure 19–8)
      b. Periodization training program
    2. Neuromuscular control
      a. Open chain
      b. Closed kinetic chain (single leg) (Figure 19–9)
      c. Closed kinetic chain (double leg)
    3. Control of entire leg
      a. Hip and knee strengthening (Figure 19–10)
      b. One-legged stance
      c. Agility drills (Figure 19–11)

continues

Exhibit 19–1 continued

4. Sport-specific functional progressions
   a. Jumping
   b. Cutting
   c. Kicking
C. CRITERIA FOR RETURN TO PLAY
   1. Normal arthrokinematics in multiple-plane activities

2. Strength 90% of the other side
3. Satisfactory clinical exam by the physician
4. Pass the functional exam

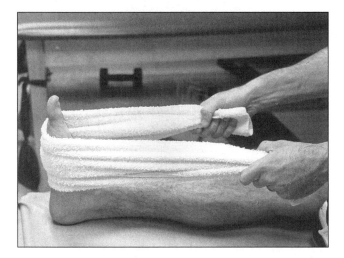

Figure 19–1 Towel stretches.

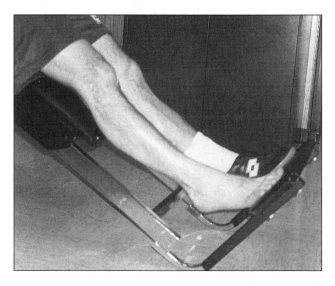

Figure 19–3 Closed-chain exercises with minimal loads in sitting.

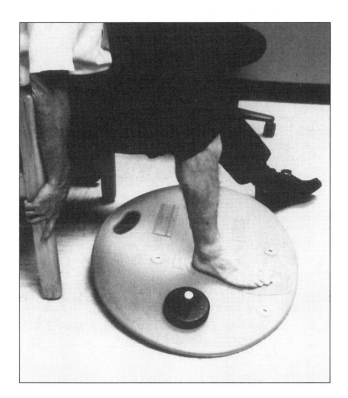

Figure 19–2 Use of BAPS board for range of motion exercises.

stiffness, weakness, and proprioceptive loss. A combination of early compression, ice, and a protective device such as a plastic and Velcro cast brace or an air splint is adequate to allow healing while allowing access to the joint for other modalities of rehabilitation. For mild sprains, protection is used continuously for 4–5 days. For more severe sprains, protection may be necessary for 7–21 days. Continuous protection should be employed until the swelling is minimal, there is little pain at the injury site, and plantar/dorsiflexion is smooth.

Rehabilitation

The rehabilitation program may follow the general ankle rehabilitation protocol.

Acute Phase Rehabilitation—Continuous protection as noted above. Contrast baths may be used within the first 1–2 days. Electrogalvanic stimulation may have some benefit to reduce pain. Passive and active assisted range of motion exercises in plantar flexion and dorsiflexion may be started as pain allows.

Recovery Phase Rehabilitation—Active ankle motion should be started and may be done in multiple planes—inversion/eversion and plantar flexion/dorsiflexion. Weight-

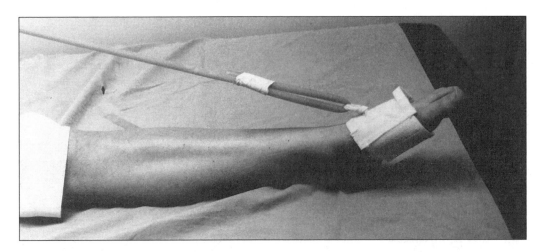

Figure 19–4 Tubing used in multiple planes.

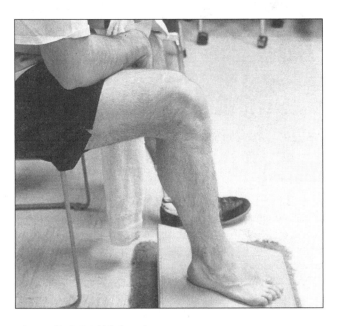

Figure 19–5 Wobble board.

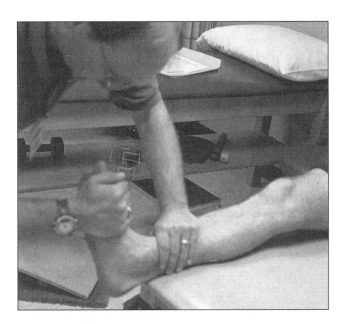

Figure 19–6 PNF patterns for proprioception.

bearing with the protective brace will allow protected loading in safe positions (Figure 19–13). Proprioceptive exercises include "writing the alphabet," walking on the side of the foot, walking on tiptoe and heel, and one-legged standing. Muscle strengthening should start with isometrics and proceed to closed-chain loading, such as squats and toe raises, and open-chain loading, such as plantar flexion and dorsiflexion against rubber tubing.

Functional Phase Rehabilitation—Emphasis should be placed on full range of motion in all positions of the foot and ankle. Muscles should be prepared for jumping and running by continued closed- and open-chain exercises. Power

should be developed by pyelometric activities such as hopping and depth jumping. Agility activities such as five-dot drill (see Figure 19–11), line jumping (Figure 19–14), jump rope, and agility runs can prepare the ankle and foot.

Criteria for Return to Play—Stable ankle, full range of motion, balanced muscle strength, completed progressions for running, jumping, or kicking.

Ankle Instability (Chronic Ankle Strain)

Chronic ankle instability is usually a sequel to repeated ankle sprains or incompletely treated acute ankle sprains.

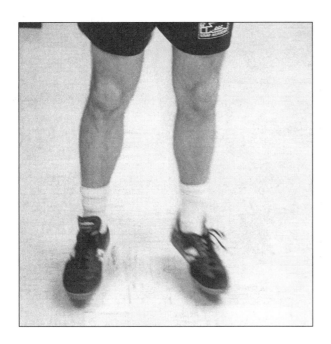

Figure 19–7 Double-leg jumping and loading.

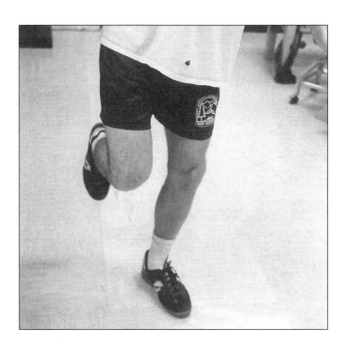

Figure 19–9 Closed-chain single-leg stance strengthening.

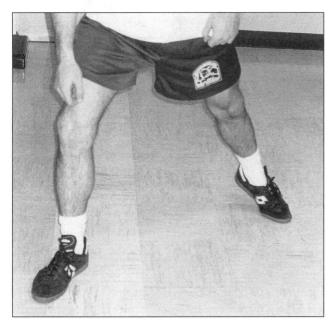

Figure 19–8 Cutting may be done at 90-degree and 45-degree angles.

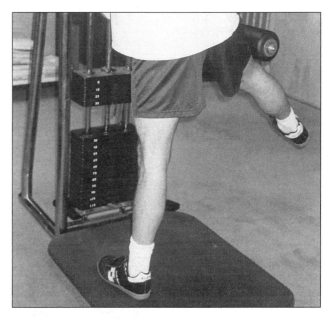

Figure 19–10 Hip strengthening using the total hip machine. Both hips are utilized in each exercise.

The symptoms of instability result from failure of the constraint mechanisms in the face of athletic demands.

Method of Presentation—Chronic injury, resulting from ligamentous stretch and incompetence. This is usually due to one major sprain, followed by many similar episodes. Occasionally, it will occur in patients with multiple joint laxity.

Clinical Symptom Complex—Repeated episodes of ankle "giving way," with pain, swelling, and athletic disability.

There may be point tenderness over the affected ligaments, but usually there is a generalized soreness over the joint. Joint instability tests, such as talar tilt and anterior drawer, are positive, and there is a positive anterior lateral rotary instability test (Figure 19–15). There may be signs of internal derangement of the ankle joint if there are interposed synovial tissue folds, loose bodies, or bone spurs.

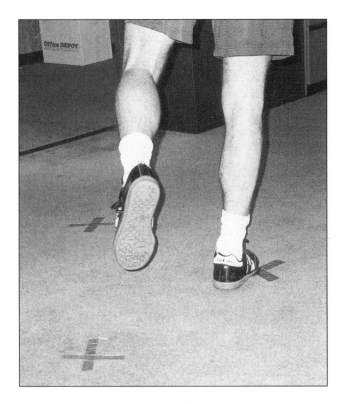

Figure 19–11 Five-dot drill for agility.

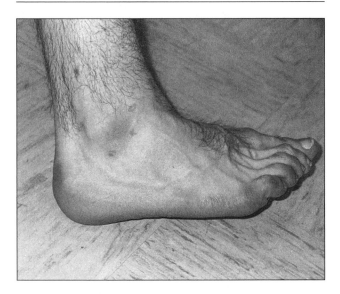

Figure 19–12 Ankle ligament locations. +, Anterior talofibular; O, anterior tibiofibular; •, fibulocalcaneal.

Tissue Injury Complex—Lateral ligaments, usually anterior talofibular and fibulocalcaneal. There may be chondral or osseus lesions along the joint margins and hyperplasia of the synovium. In some cases, there may be injury to the posteromedial deltoid ligament.

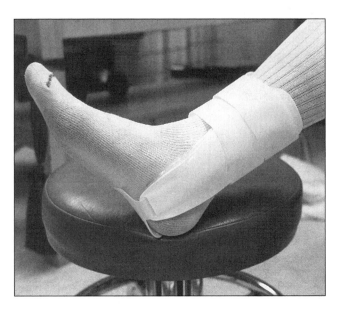

Figure 19–13 Air cast protection for early recovery activities.

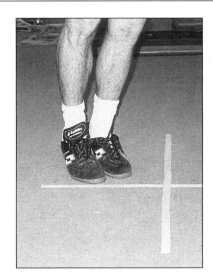

Figure 19–14 Line jumping.

Tissue Overload Complex—Peroneal muscles, with weakness of eversion. Gastrocnemius and soleus muscles, with weakness of plantar flexion.

Functional Biomechanical Deficit Complex—Plantar flexion and eversion weakness.

Subclinical Adaptation Complex—Shortened stride, landing on heel, no push-off on affected foot.

Treatment Considerations—Treatment should be designed to provide stability of the ankle mortis. In about 80% of cases, this can be done by appropriate muscle strengthening, proprioceptive exercises, agility workouts, and an ankle brace. If the athlete is functionally disabled in the face of this program, with episodes of instability or internal derangement, surgical stabilization is necessary.

Acute Phase Rehabilitation—In nonoperative cases, any residual swelling and deficits in range of motion should be normalized by rest, modalities, and protected motion. In operative cases, the stiffness from the surgery and immobilization should be worked on with short-arc passive and active assisted exercises.

Recovery Phase Rehabilitation—This will be basically the same as for the acute ankle sprain protocol but will have a larger emphasis on proprioceptive training and closed-chain strengthening of the entire lower leg. Minitrampoline exercises are an excellent way to achieve both goals (Figure 19–16). Jumping, one-legged jumping, crossover steps, and rotational jumps stimulate proprioception and require muscle contractions for joint stabilization.

Functional Phase Rehabilitation—Same as for acute ankle sprain protocol.

Criteria for Return to Play—Same as for acute ankle sprain.

Plantar Fasciitis (Heel Spur)

Plantar fasciitis involves a microtrauma overload injury to the plantar fascia as it inserts into the base of the calcaneus. Calcific deposits may form in this damaged area, giving rise to a heel spur on plain X-ray. This is a classic example of overload with associated biomechanical abnormalities.

Method of Presentation—Chronic overload, with gradual onset. This usually occurs in runners or other athletes who do long-distance, long-duration, and relatively low-intensity sports that involve repetitively landing on the foot. There may be a history of change in technique, alteration in distance or time, changes in shoes, or injury in other areas of the body.

Clinical Symptom Complex—The characteristic symptoms relate to tightness and lack of pliability of the tissues. There is soreness upon arising in the morning, pain upon getting up after sitting down, and soreness that increases with distance run or time spent on the feet. The symptoms are localized to the insertion of the plantar fascia.

Tissue Injury Complex—Plantar fascial insertion into the heel.

Tissue Overload Complex—Plantar flexor muscles, foot intrinsic muscles, plantar fascia.

Functional Biomechanical Deficit Complex—Plantar flexor muscle inflexibility and strength weakness, creating functional pronation, or excessive velocity of movement from supination to pronation upon heel strike. This functional pronation creates a tensile overload in the plantar fascia, leading to clinical symptoms. It may be exacerbated by hip abductor weakness, creating a functional Trendelenburg position of the pelvis, with consequent hip flexion, knee flexion, and ankle dorsiflexion (Figure 19–17).

Subclinical Adaptation Complex—Running with first contact on metatarsal heads, shortened strike length, foot inversion upon landing.

Treatment Considerations—A large majority of patients with plantar fasciitis may be successfully treated without surgery. Treatment should be directed toward reducing the tensile overload and increasing the compliance of the tissue to stretching. Any severe pes planus or pes cavus should be evaluated and supported by a proper orthotic. Assessment of ankle dorsiflexion, flexibility, with the knee both extended and flexed, will allow determination of the tightness of the posterior musculature. Tarsal tunnel syndrome should also be ruled out. About 10% of athletes will not respond to conservative treatment or rehabilitation. Surgical debridement

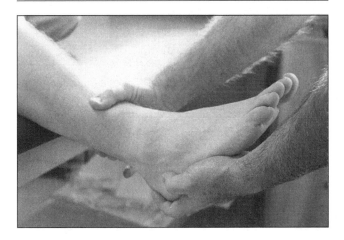

Figure 19–15 Anterior lateral rotary drawer test. Pressure is applied to the heel with the ankle in slight plantar flexion. More translation is noted on the lateral side.

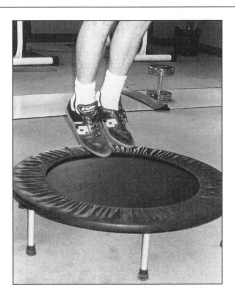

Figure 19–16 Minitrampoline jumping.

of the damaged tissue and bone spur may be necessary to allow the proper healing response.

Rehabilitation

Acute Phase Rehabilitation—Early rehabilitation efforts should allow decreased stress and should work on all of the clinical and biomechanical problems. Several specific techniques are helpful in this early phase (Exhibit 19–2 and Figures 19–18 through 19–20).

Recovery Phase Rehabilitation—Emphasis should be placed on strengthening of the calf musculature as it has been shown to be weak. Failure in eccentric loading seems to be the major factor as that allows extra load to be seen at the plantar fascial insertion, and it allows increased velocity of pronation. Closed-chain activities, including mini-trampoline jumping, hopping, and squats, are effective for rehabilitation. Neuromuscular and proprioceptive control activities, as demonstrated in the general outline, are also important.

Functional Phase Rehabilitation—Control of the entire leg should be emphasized. The ability to achieve stable one-legged stance is key to distributing loads over the entire leg. Trendelenburg position of the hip creates knee flexion and internal rotation. This position causes ankle dorsiflexion and heel valgus, creating functional pronation. Hip abduction exercises are very important to maintain proper leg posture.

Criteria for Return to Play—Full ankle dorsiflexion, good plantar flexor strength, and neuromuscular control of the entire lower extremity.

Posterior Tibial Tendinitis

The posterior tibial muscle and tendon are very important stabilizers of the midfoot, especially in foot strike and stance. In these functions, they are continually being placed under tensile load and are commonly injured.

Method of Presentation—Chronic microtrauma injury due to repetitive overload. Inciting factors include both anatomic and functional pronation of the foot and weak posterior calf musculature.

Clinical Symptom Complex—Tenderness behind and just proximal to the medial malleolus or inferior and distal to the malleolus as the tendon attaches at the apex of the arch of the foot (Figure 19–21). There may be crepitus, swelling, or nodularity along the tendon. There is usually soreness with activity and increasing symptoms with longer activities.

Tissue Injury Complex—Posterior tibial tendon, either along its tendon or at its distal insertion.

Tissue Overload Complex—Posterior calf muscles, posterior tibial muscle, longitudinal arch.

Functional Biomechanical Deficit Complex—Functional pronation due to posterior calf muscle weakness.

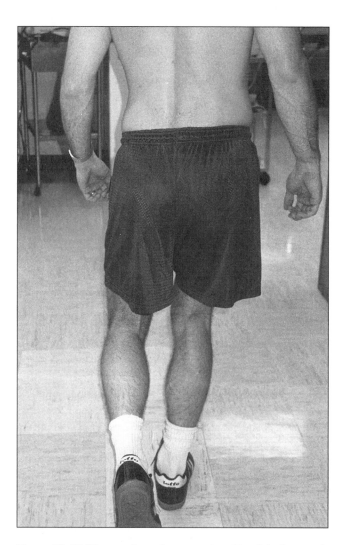

Figure 19–17 Hip muscle weakness creates a Trendelenburg position. This can create extra knee flexion and ankle dorsiflexion, with consequent foot pronation.

Subclinical Adaptation Complex—Shortened stride, foot supination, heel varus upon foot strike. These adaptations to produce supination in the face of calf muscle weakness create a larger range of pronation and velocity of pronation, making the functional pronation worse.

Treatment Considerations—Most of these injuries can be treated by correcting the biomechanical deficits and the subclinical adaptations through nonoperative rehabilitation. Surgical treatment should be reserved for recalcitrant tendinosis or tendon ruptures.

Rehabilitation

Rehabilitation should focus on reducing the tendinitis-related pain, allowing normal biomechanics, and strengthening the calf muscles. Most of the rehabilitation should follow the general ankle protocol.

Exhibit 19–2 Acute Phase Treatment

1. Rest from activities that irritate the plantar fascia.
2. Modalities:
   a. Ice massage—using a paper or styrofoam cup that has been three-quarters filled with water and frozen, peel down the top of the cup and rub the ice directly onto the sore heel for 5–10 minutes (or until numb)
   b. EGS
   c. Phonophoresis
3. Counterforce arch aid/supportive taping of the arch (Figure 19–18).
4. Deep friction massage—using the third finger over top of the second, apply pressure to tolerance over the inside aspect of the heel. Gently rub back and forth for 5 minutes, 3–5 times per day.
5. Toe curls—sit with feet resting on a towel on the floor. Curl toes and gather towel under the arch of the foot. Rest frequently to avoid cramping. Repeat three towel lengths (Figure 19–19).
6. Soda bottle rolling—patients with plantar fasciitis typically complain of pain in the morning when they awake and take their first steps. Therefore, we advise placing a soda bottle under the arch of the foot and having the patients gently roll it back and forth for 5 minutes in the morning before their feet hit the floor.
7. Stretching exercises:
   a. Calf stretch—with one foot up and another back, facing the wall and with the back leg straight, heel on the ground, lean hip toward wall until stretch is felt in calf (curl toes to maintain arch). Repeat with both the forward and back legs bent. Hold 20–30 seconds 3 times per leg 2–3 times per day (in the morning and before and after exercise) (Figure 19–20).
   b. Toe stretch—use hand to bend toes forward and hold 20–30 seconds and then backward. Repeat 5 times 2–3 times per day (in morning and before and after exercise).
8. Nighttime stretching—placing the foot and ankle in a nighttime splint allows correct positioning to maintain posterior muscle flexibility.
9. Strengthening exercises:
   a. Tubing exercises—draw the foot up toward the shin. Raise the foot up to the outside. Raise the foot up to the inside. Repeat 3 sets of 15 each motion. (Concentrate on slow return and do not let tubing rebound.)
   b. Toe raises—feet placed 12 inches apart, slowly raise to the balls of the feet, hold 3 seconds, and return to starting position. To make more difficult, drop heel off of step. Repeat 3 sets of 25.

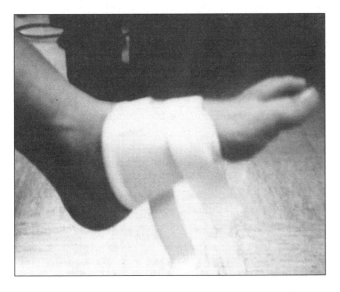

Figure 19–18 Counterforce arch brace (Medical Sports, Arlington, VA).

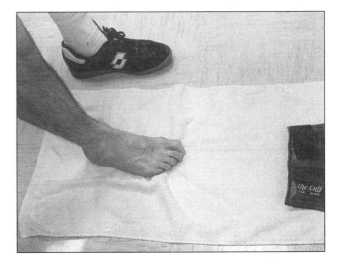

Figure 19–19 Toe curl exercises.

Acute Phase Rehabilitation—The tendon is rather superficial and can be treated with ultrasound or EGS orthotics to correct. Anatomic pronation may be necessary if Brody's Navicular Drop Test is greater than 1.5 cm (Figure 19–22).

Recovery Phase Rehabilitation—Loading should be done in eccentric fashion, with the heel in neutral. This will allow the tendon to work in its normal functional position. Closed-chain activities and progressions work best.

Functional Phase Rehabilitation—Power and agility must be restored by short-duration, high-intensity exercises such

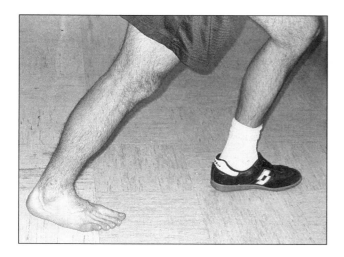

Figure 19–20 Calf stretches.

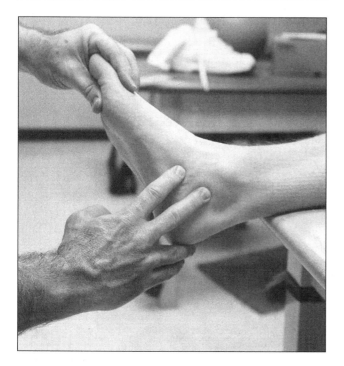

Figure 19–21 Posterior tibial tendon tenderness areas.

as jumping rope, trampoline, or jumping jacks. These exercises will also involve control of the entire leg.

Criteria for Return to Play—Full range of ankle motion, controlled heel position, and normal calf muscle strength.

Achilles Tendinitis

The Achilles tendon, the largest tendon in the body, experiences high loads in all sporting activities. It seems to toler-

ate these well in most instances. However, when injured, it is often difficult to treat.

Method of Presentation—Chronic tendinosis, with gradual onset of pain and dysfunction. Change in training or equipment is frequently an inciting cause. Occasionally, it may present acutely, due to a partial or complete tear.

Clinical Symptom Complex—Point-tender pain and/or swelling over the Achilles tendon, usually in its middle section proximal to its calcaneal insertion. It is characteristically quite sore upon rising and is stiff when first starting to run. Crepitus may be present. It is difficult to stand on tiptoe or to go up and down stairs.

Tissue Injury Complex—Achilles tendon, with either peritendinitis or insubstance tendinosis degeneration.

Tissue Overload Complex—Gastrocnemius and soleus muscles.

Functional Biomechanical Deficit Complex—Dorsiflexion inflexibility and calf muscle weakness, leading to tensile overload.

Subclinical Adaptation Complex—Shortened stride, landing on heel, jumping off opposite leg.

Treatment Considerations—Rest plays a major role in trying to allow healing of the tendon lesion. Local promotion of healing may also involve ultrasound and deep-friction massage. Short-term use of a heel lift may reduce tensile loading while allowing therapy. The heel lift should be eliminated after calf flexibility is improved by stretching because it will perpetuate the calf inflexibility. Because it takes a lot of repetitive tensile overload to cause this injury and because it is frequently associated with degenerative tendinosis, surgical treatment is more common.

Rehabilitation

Rehabilitation concerns for the operative and nonoperative cases are the same—improvement in flexibility and normalization of calf muscle strength. The rehabilitation protocol is the same as for the ankle rehabilitation.

Acute Phase Rehabilitation—Early range of motion of the ankle and foot is emphasized. An air cast or other pneumatic brace will protect the ankle and will keep the heel in neutral position. Wobble board exercises are good to stimulate proprioception.

Recovery Phase Rehabilitation—Concentric and eccentric loading in single and then multiple planes will encourage normal gastrocnemius and soleus function.

Functional Phase Rehabilitation—Sport-specific progressions, especially in single-leg stance, will allow normal motor patterns and normal control of the entire lower extremity.

SUMMARY

The ankle and foot work together as a functional unit. Even though specific anatomic areas may be major sites of

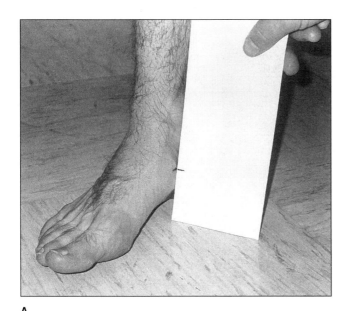

A

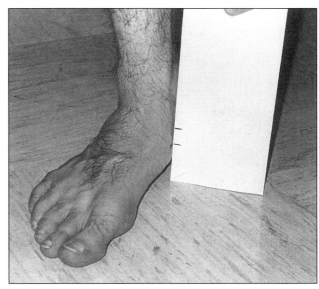

B

Figure 19–22 Navicular Drop Test. The distance between a mark on the tarsal navicular and the floor is measured in two positions—foot on the floor non–weight-bearing (*A*), and foot on the floor with weight-bearing (*B*). Measured difference greater than 1.2 cm is significant.

clinical symptoms, evaluation and rehabilitation must involve all of the functional units, including the hip and knee. Other clinical entities not specifically described are treated by the same protocol: (1) establish the complete and accurate diagnosis; (2) achieve anatomic normality and reduction of clinical symptoms; and (3) place patient in the general ankle and foot rehabilitation protocol.

SUGGESTED READING

Greenfield G, Stanish WD. Tendinitis and tendon ruptures. *OP Technique Sports Med.* 1994;2:9–17.

Kannus P, Renstrom P. Current concepts review: treatment for acute tears of the lateral ligaments of the ankle. *J Bone Joint Surg Am.* 1991;73:305–312.

Kibler WB, Goldberg C, Chandler TJ. Functional biomechanical deficits in running athletes with plantar fasciitis. *Am J Sports Med.* 1991;19:66–71.

Mann RA, Thompson FM. Rupture of the posterior tibial tendon causing flat foot. *J Bone Joint Surg Am.* 1985;67:556–561.

Stanish WD, Rubinovitch RM, Curwin S. Eccentric exercises in chronic tendinitis. *Clin Orthop.* 1986;208:65–68.

CHAPTER 20

Foot Injuries

Steve R. Geiringer

INTRODUCTION

For the majority of sports, repeated weight-bearing and impact on the foot are the final common denominators of the physical activities involved. The most apparent example is the long-distance runner, whose feet strike the often concrete ground thousands of times in one race. Although the overuse category of injuries would seem to dominate in such a setting, in fact, the natural "weeding-out" process results in a group of elite marathoners who have few such problems. Overuse foot injuries are common among joggers, recreational runners, and other athletes. Consider the variety of demands placed on the foot during activities as diverse as swimming, basketball, classical ballet, and rock climbing. Each presents a unique set of expectations and, although the human foot is generally well designed for those demands, it is not surprising that disorders of the foot rank high on the list of frequent sports-related injuries. Running, hiking, and all forms of dance are associated with high rates of foot injury, whereas football, weight lifting, and swimming have few associated foot problems.[1]

Two points are to be kept in mind when discussing the foot and its disorders. First, it is the only structure in the human body that routinely contacts the ground, sometimes with great force of impact. Second, the foot is basically a collection of bones, ligaments, and tendons. This distinguishes it from other areas of the body that receive significant functional contributions from muscles. Even the hand, most akin to the foot, has prominent thenar and hypothenar muscle masses responsible for some of the primary hand functions. These two points—one mechanical, one anatomic—are naturally related. It is difficult to conceptualize a fleshy, muscular structure that can withstand the repetitive impact of running. The lack of prominent muscle mass has implications for treatment of foot injuries as well. Unlike at the shoulder, hip, or knee, for example, muscle strengthening has a secondary role in the rehabilitation process of isolated foot injuries.

As in other areas of sports medicine, effective treatment and prevention of foot disorders rest on the foundation of an accurate, specific diagnosis; a detailed knowledge of general foot mechanics; and the pathomechanics of specific conditions.

ANATOMY

Bones

The skeletal foot [2(pp447,458)] is generally subdivided into three sections: the forefoot, the midfoot, and the hindfoot. The bones of the forefoot are the phalanges and the metatarsals (Figure 20–1). As in the hand, there are only two phalanges (and one interphalangeal joint) of the first digit, the large toe. The first metatarsal bone is the shortest and thickest, with the more lateral metatarsals becoming increasingly long and narrow. The midfoot includes a row of four bones, beginning with the laterally situated cuboid and the three cuneiforms. Together, these form the transverse arch of the foot. The medially placed navicular bone completes the midfoot (see Figure 20–1). The medial and lateral cuneiforms extend more distally than do the intermediate cuneiforms, leading to relative immobility of metatarsal II at its proximal end, with clinical implications to be discussed later.

The talus and calcaneus bones compose the hindfoot (see Figure 20–1). The talus has a complicated architecture. The distal aspect (the head) is convex for articulation with the navicular. Its most superior portion is the trochlea, narrower posteriorly than anteriorly for connection with the tibia. At the margins of the talus, smooth articular surfaces are present

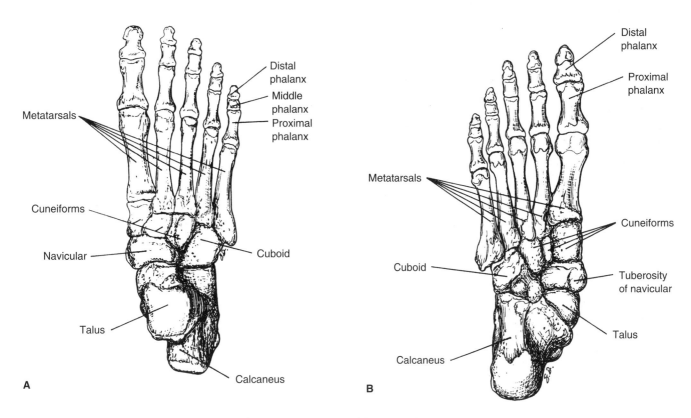

Figure 20–1 Bony anatomy of the foot. (*A*) Left—dorsal aspect. (*B*) Right—ventral aspect.

for the medial and lateral malleoli, and the plantar surface joins with the calcaneus. The calcaneus is the largest bone of the foot, with a thick, roughened posteroinferior portion for weight-bearing and three smooth surfaces on its anterior superior aspect for connection with the talus.

Soft Tissues

There are innumerable ligaments connecting the bones of the foot,[2(pp535–541)] most of which are not discussed in detail here. The intrinsic foot ligaments of greatest clinical importance lie on the plantar surface. The long plantar ligament connects the undersurfaces of the calcaneus, cuboid, and middle metatarsal bones. The short plantar ligament extends from the calcaneus to the cuboid, closely applied to the bony surfaces and very powerful. Together, these two ligaments play a major role in preserving the longitudinal arch of the foot.

The plantar fascia[2(pp652–654)] is a fibroaponeurotic complex that provides structure and support to the plantar aspect of the foot and an origin for muscles. It arises with substantial thickness from the medial tubercle of the calcaneus and continues distalward. At the level of the midfoot, the fascia broadens and subdivides into five components, each intermeshing with transverse and oblique fibers.

The only dorsal foot intrinsic muscle is the extensor digitorum brevis. The remainder are arranged in four layers on the ventral aspect.[2(pp654–656)] In the human, integrity of the basic structure of the foot, specifically, the transverse and longitudinal arches, is probably sufficiently maintained by plantar ligaments and the plantar fascia alone.

Of all the muscles arising in the leg, only the popliteus does not cross the ankle[2(pp645–651)]; the remainder insert onto the bones of the foot and, therefore, act on the intervening joints. The muscles of the anterior compartment of the leg cause inversion and ankle dorsiflexion. Lateral compartment muscles cause eversion and plantar flexion (except peroneus tertius, which functions as an extension of extensor digitorum longus). The superficial posterior calf group, the Achilles muscles, are nearly pure plantar flexors, although they do provide a valgus moment to the calcaneus, whereas the deep posterior muscles cause both inversion and plantar flexion. As clarified by the concept of closed-chain kinetics with regard to gait, some muscles are found to carry functions not listed in typical anatomy texts. Gastrocnemius, for example, is known to be a powerful plantar flexor, as just mentioned. During stance phase, however, and by virtue of its origin from the femur, the gastrocnemius contributes to knee stabilization.[3(p113)]

Biomechanics

The joint of the hindfoot is the subtalar joint, between the talus and calcaneus. Rotation occurs on an axis that is tilted, on average, 42 degrees up from horizontal, and 23 degrees from the midline.[3(pp15–21),4] This leads to the "mitered hinge" description of motion arising from the subtalar joint, with the following paired actions: flexion-extension, adduction-abduction, and supination-pronation. Two combinations of "linked" movements are thus possible: pronation, abduction, extension, and supination, adduction, and flexion.[5(p4)] Eversion is the functional correlate to the first combination, inversion to the second. These linked functional interrelationships of the foot carry significant implications in the practice of sports medicine. Midfoot overpronation is typically accompanied by tibial internal rotation, a valgus moment at the knee, internal rotation forces on the femur and hip joint, and a torquing stress on the lumbar region. A highly supinated foot often leads to tibial external rotation, varus at the knee, and external rotation at the thigh and hip (Figure 20–2). This type of biomechanical analysis illustrates the principles of kinetic chain theory. A dynamic musculoskeletal event anywhere in the body causes a ripple effect of linked secondary forces proximally and distally. This is particularly true when the foot is planted, with the resulting far-reaching secondary effects just detailed. Therefore, an athlete with foot overpronation or oversupination might present with symptoms in the leg, knee, thigh, hip, or back because of these kinetic chain implications.[6,7]

In the midfoot, the midtarsal joint comprises the calcaneocuboid (saddle joint—one convex, one concave surface) and talonavicular (condyloid joint—two convex surfaces) joints. With the foot in eversion, as with pronation, the axes of these two joints are aligned, allowing free, "unlocked" motion along their surfaces. When the foot is inverted, or "locked," the joint axes are not aligned, meaning less movement and more stability in the resulting supinated structure.

At the forefoot, during end stance phase in the gait cycle (push-off, if running), the metatarsophalangeal (MTP) joints are fully extended. Because of differential relative movements around the MTPs, this creates tautness of the plantar fascia and aponeurosis, with resultant elevation and rigidity of the longitudinal arch. Together, these effects are called the *windlass mechanism*[8] (Figure 20–3) and serve to stabilize the foot for push-off.

THE RUNNING CYCLE

The knowledge gained from careful study of foot anatomy and biomechanics can now be applied to running. By definition, running occurs when a "float" phase is introduced to gait, i.e., speed is enough that both feet are off the ground simultaneously for some portion of the cycle.[5(p2)] When a

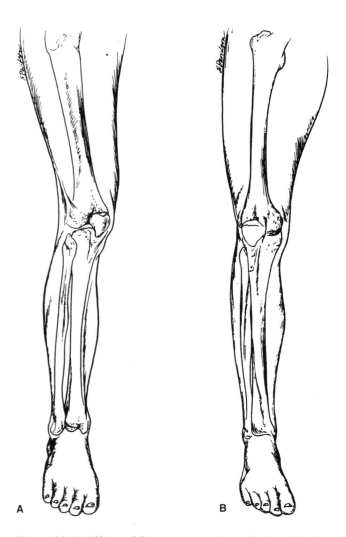

Figure 20–2 Effects of foot posture on lower limb mechanics. (*A*) Left—foot pronation leading to internal tibial and femoral rotations, valgus posture at the knee, and internal rotation at the hip. (*B*) Right—foot supination leading to external tibial and femoral rotations, varus posture at the knee, and external rotation at the hip.

foot strikes the ground, it enters stance phase, which is relatively shorter than during walking (33% with fast running versus 60% with walking).[5(p2)] At initial foot contact with the ground, it would be advantageous to land on a semirigid to rigid structure to avoid buckling of the limb. In fact, the kinetic chain allows for this, as the leg is slightly externally rotated, the foot inverted, at end swing. This results in the rigid, supinated foot making first ground contact.[3(pp15–22)] For the majority of stance phase, it would be ideal for the body's weight and the force of impact to be dispersed over a broader surface than would be allowed by the supinated posture. Immediately after contact, therefore, as the tibia progresses forward, it internally rotates over the planted foot, which itself makes the transition to the "unlocked," pronated-everted po-

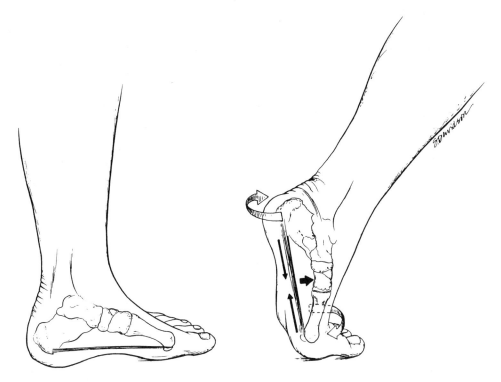

Figure 20–3 The windlass mechanism. At the end of stance phase, there is internal rotation around the head of the first metatarsal bone, with external rotation at the hindfoot. The resulting tension on the plantar fascia leads to heightening of the arch and relative stability of the foot for push-off.

sition, well suited for weight-bearing.[3(pp15–22)] At end stance (toe-off for joggers, push-off for sprinters), a somewhat rigid foot would again be preferred mechanically. Although frank inversion-supination does not take place, the windlass mechanism affords relative foot stability when the MTPs are fully extended.[8]

PLANTAR FASCIITIS

The plantar fascia, as described earlier, is a tough, fibrous, aponeurotic structure arising from the medial calcaneal tubercle and continuing distalward to the metatarsal area. It provides shape and support to the longitudinal arch and acts as a shock absorber on foot impact. The plantar fascia also plays an important role in the windlass mechanism, lending rigidity to the arch at end stance phase. Therefore, it repeatedly cycles through stretching and relaxation during walking or athletic activity, and, in doing so, is susceptible to tensile overload, particularly at its origin at the calcaneus. The overpronated foot seems more likely to develop symptomatic plantar fasciitis, perhaps from overstretching of the structure at midstance. Typical plantar fasciitis is also seen, however, in athletes with a rigid, supinated foot posture. Other factors, such as gastrocsoleus inflexibility and training errors, have also been implicated.[9–11(pp207–209)] Flexibility and strength deficits of the plantar flexors have been documented in athletes with plantar fasciitis.[12] Functional adaptations, such as running on the metatarsal heads or decreased stride length, can result from these biomechanical deficits. The major tissue overload along the medial arch of the foot occurs due to eccentric overload of the plantar flexor muscles.

Symptoms typically arise after a rapid increase in the distance, speed, intensity, or frequency of running or other sport, ie, with "overuse."[13–17] Pain is noticed directly at the medial heel and is often severe upon arising from sleep. A mild case will then hurt less during the day, except when running. More severe cases may cause intense pain throughout the day and curtailment of sports and other activities.

Physical examination abnormalities include tenderness, sometimes exquisite, to firm palpation over the medial calcaneal tubercle. In more advanced cases, the proximal medial longitudinal arch along the plantar aponeurosis is also tender. Rarely do the distal portions hurt. Secondary physical examination findings may include a pronated, everted foot posture (occasionally supination), as well as tightness of the gastrocsoleus complex, the hamstrings, and the gluteal groups. The patient's athletic shoes should be examined for characteristic signs of excessive wear.

The differential diagnosis of plantar fasciitis includes calcaneal bursitis, plantar ligament sprain, tarsal tunnel syndrome involving the calcaneal branch of the tibial nerve,[18] and sacral radiculopathy. Recalcitrant heel pain in the young athlete may signal Reiter's syndrome or another seronegative spondyloarthropathy.[19] Diagnostic testing in the routine case is rarely helpful. Radiographs often reveal a horizontally oriented bone spur projecting forward from the calcaneus; these are to be thought of as secondary to the pathomechanics of plantar fasciitis and not as a cause.[20] Nerve conduction studies may be performed if tarsal tunnel syndrome is a serious clinical consideration.[18]

Rehabilitation

Acute Phase

Ice, relative rest, and antiinflammatory medications comprise the acute treatment for plantar fasciitis. Ice is applied for 15–20 minutes, 3–4 times daily for 3–5 days, longer if significant irritation at the medial calcaneal tubercle persists.[21–23] Superficial application of heat will not warm the injured tissue and is, therefore, not useful at any point in the course of treatment.

Corticosteroid injections have long been recommended during the acute treatment phase of plantar fasciitis.[20] Whereas local corticosteroid installation can provide rapid symptomatic relief, its use is nonetheless best avoided. If subcutaneous fat atrophy were to occur in the specialized adipose compartments of the heel, the resulting lack of cushioning during the first half of stance phase could be detrimental.[24] More importantly, steroid injection too often replaces a careful search for the underlying intrinsic or extrinsic biomechanical factors leading to the heel pain of plantar fasciitis, and the opportunity for successful long-term treatment is missed.

For most athletes, complete rest from sports is not medically necessary and will not be adhered to, in any event. Relative rest[25] is advised; the patient is counseled to exercise pain free, or virtually so. If the plantar fasciitis arose from a rapid increase in activity, successful relative rest is usually achieved at about 80% of the previously pain-free level. Only in severe cases should total rest be suggested, and then only for a few days, while other measures are undertaken. If the degree of rest needed for adequate tissue healing would result in loss of aerobic conditioning, alternative exercise protocols are prescribed during the interim. Land-based nonimpact programs (e.g., exercise bicycle, rower, stair climber, cross-country ski machine) or water-based workouts are substituted as tolerated.[26]

If not otherwise contraindicated, full-dose nonsteroidal antiinflammatory medication can be given for 7–10 days.

Following that, as-needed dosing for analgesia is recommended.

Surgical approaches to plantar fasciitis are rarely needed. The horizontally oriented bone spur sometimes found on X-ray is a consequence, not a cause, of the problem. Section of the plantar fascia is the usual surgical approach but should not be considered in the routine case of plantar fasciitis.

Recovery Phase

There is no distinct time barrier between the various stages of rehabilitation of sports injuries. The measures recommended for plantar fasciitis and other conditions often overlap partially or totally. The recovery phase treatment for plantar fasciitis is tailored to the particular causative factors in an individual. Intervention might be as simple as education regarding a proper training schedule, running shoes, or surfaces. All contributing intrinsic biomechanical factors are addressed—for example, with a stretching program for the plantar fascia itself, as well as for the Achilles muscles, hamstrings, and gluteal groups.[27,28] If compensation for an overpronating foot is required, a commercially available orthosis is often satisfactory. Adequate arch support is the goal, along with limitation of hindfoot motion during the running cycle. Custom-made orthoses are seldom necessary for the recreational athlete. For the competitive or team athlete, low-dye taping for support of the arch may be helpful; the "weekend warrior" will rarely bother with taping.[29]

Concurrent with the above rehabilitative measures, the injured athlete is advised to slowly escalate the level of physical activity that led to the plantar fascia injury in the first place. Typically, a common-sense approach without rigid guidelines suffices. For the runner, mileage and speed will gradually increase over the course of several weeks, provided symptoms do not worsen. It is not medically necessary to wait for a completely pain-free situation before increasing exercise intensity, assuming that the athlete fully understands the inherent trade-off between more rapid healing and more rapid return to sport.

In the occasional recalcitrant case of plantar fasciitis, the symptoms may rapidly recur after modest activity gains. The physician can then oversee a conservative schedule of a weekly 10% increase in the daily duration of exercise, with at least two nonconsecutive days off from impact exercise each week. The prior level of duration of moderate activity should be accomplished before other parameters are advanced (speed, intensity, number of workouts weekly). The recovery phase of rehabilitation from a musculoskeletal injury ends when the athlete has returned to the full prior level of activity, pain free and without compromise in performance. By this time, the physician, therapist, or trainer has completed the education process regarding contributing extrinsic factors such as footwear, running surfaces, training errors, and such intrinsic factors as flexibility, strength, and muscle balance.

Maintenance and Prevention

Plantar fasciitis typically occurs as an overuse injury and is likely to recur intermittently. Many athletes need to live through two or more bouts of the same injury before accepting the necessity of a maintenance exercise program, with the goals of optimizing performance and preventing reinjury. As in the acute rehabilitation phase, a long-term exercise program for prevention is individualized for those factors causing the plantar fasciitis. Regular, effective stretching is mandatory for the plantar foot structures, as well as for the calf, hamstrings, and gluteal muscles. Stretching is done briefly before exercise or after light warm-up, with prolonged static stretching following exercise.[25] Stretching is recommended at least daily. Strengthening, if a component of the prescribed exercise program, should be logistically simple to perform and carried out three to four times weekly. Shoes and orthoses, if used, must be replaced as often as needed to maintain their structural integrity. The limit for a pair of running shoes is usually 300–400 miles. Rapid increases in the intensity or duration of exercise are avoided, and impact exercise, for the typical sports participant, should be performed no more than five times weekly, with the off days nonconsecutive. Finally, if symptoms of plantar fasciitis begin to recur despite adherence to these maintenance measures (or because they are occasionally ignored), the athlete is encouraged to seek expert professional help. In this way, the treatment course will be abbreviated, with little disruption of the exercise and sports routine. Plantar fasciitis may take 6–12 weeks to resolve. Running is typically resumed when tenderness over the plantar fascia, morning stiffness, and pain with weight-bearing have abated.[30] The circle of rehabilitation is completed with an individualized, effective maintenance exercise program for prevention of further injury and enhancement of future athletic performance.

STRESS FRACTURE

Pathomechanics

Fatigue stress fractures, the type most often occurring in athletes, arise from abnormal muscular stress to a previously normal bone.[31] Direct impact forces to the affected bone are not currently thought to play an important role in the pathophysiology of a typical stress fracture. As an athlete increases the intensity of exercise, adaptation of muscle occurs more quickly than that of bone.[32] This imbalance is accommodated when the exercise routine is advanced slowly. When advanced too quickly, vigorous muscular contractions can overwhelm the remodeling bony architecture, and a stress fracture may develop.

In the foot, the most common sites of stress fracture formation are the metatarsal bones II and III, although any of the metatarsals or other bones of the foot may be involved.[33–37] The proximal head of the second metatarsal bone is tucked between the medial and lateral cuneiform bones (see Figure 20–1). This leads to relative immobility of metatarsal II, with a consequent higher incidence of stress fractures there than in the other metatarsals. Involvement of the tarsal navicular is quite common in long-distance runners.[38(pp89–101)] The nearly universal cause in athletes is training error,[39] with a too-rapid increase in the duration, intensity, or difficulty of exercise.[40] Stress fracture, therefore, is characteristic of an overuse injury. Other extrinsic causes may play a role, such as poorly fitted or worn-out shoes, or a concrete running surface.[40] A cavus, oversupinated foot is an intrinsic biomechanical factor that has been related to an increased incidence of foot stress fractures.[41]

Method of Presentation

Localized pain with the offending activity, initially relieved by rest, is the primary symptom of a new stress fracture. Symptoms usually arise a few months after exercise intensity is increased,[42] but may develop within days. Rest pain will occur if training is not modified, as will mild local swelling and edema.[43]

The most prominent finding on physical examination is severe point tenderness over a short segment of the affected bone, usually at midshaft of metatarsals II or III. Swelling and erythema may also be present.[40] An inflexible foot with a supinated posture may be present. In a runner, the shoes should always be examined for signs of excessive or abnormal wear.

Plain radiographs may initially be normal; therefore, if necessary for confirmation of the diagnosis, radionuclide bone scanning may be performed. The initial phase of a three-phase scan is particularly sensitive early in the course, and the abnormality may persist for up to two years.[43]

Differential Diagnosis

Foot pain arising after a period of increased training may be related to ligament sprain, tendinitis, plantar fasciitis, or Morton's neuroma, among other causes. Frank bony fracture must be excluded. Elements of the history and physical examination, not detailed here, will allow for specific, accurate diagnosis. Particular attention should be paid to the fifth metatarsal, where a stress fracture must be differentiated from an acute fracture at the base, the so-called Jones fracture.[44] The acute fracture in that location may progress to become nonunion if not treated properly.[45,46]

Rehabilitation

Acute Phase

Standard physiatric measures of ice, oral antiinflammatory medications, and relative rest will successfully treat most stress fractures of the foot. Early in treatment, ice is applied for 15–20 minutes up to four times daily, with the beneficial effects of analgesia and control of swelling.[25] As symptoms improve, ice is used less often, although heat is not recommended.

A nonsteroidal antiinflammatory medication can be prescribed at full dose for up to several weeks, then tapered down or discontinued, depending on the need for ongoing analgesia.[40]

The prescription of relative rest[25] is indicated for metatarsal stress fractures. In this way, the athlete is asked to reduce activity to 80% or so of the previously pain-free level to allow for bone remodeling and healing.[40] In most cases, it is unnecessary to prescribe total rest for stress fractures of the foot.

Recovery Phase

The recovery phase of rehabilitation following a stress fracture of the foot starts whenever the athlete is able to exercise pain free, which may be within days of diagnosis if relative rest is successfully accomplished. From that point forward, a slow to moderate increase in duration of training is prescribed, as long as pain is absent or virtually so. Depending on the injured athlete's response, the allowable increment in exercise duration will range from 50% in mild cases to only 10% weekly in severe cases.[40] Using this formula in a case of a recalcitrant metatarsal stress fracture, a runner may jog pain free for 20 minutes at a time, three times in the first week, increasing to 22 minutes three times the second week, and so on.[25] Only when the desired duration of activity is achieved should the intensity of training slowly increase. This type of prescribed exercise schedule, modified as needed based on symptoms and physical examination findings, will allow for bone remodeling to accommodate the stepwise increases in activity. The practitioner should counsel the athlete on alternative, nonimpact forms of exercise, e.g., swimming or stair climber, to maintain aerobic conditioning during recovery.

Maintenance and Prevention

Two major areas comprise the ongoing treatment of a stress fracture of the foot. First is careful attention to any contributing underlying biomechanical factors such as an oversupinated foot. Orthoses, sometimes custom-fitted, may be needed in some cases, as athletic footwear does not adequately compensate for a high arch. Second, and typically more important, is a process of education of the athlete to avoid sudden increases in the duration or intensity of exercise. Cross-training, incorporating varied types of exercise into the weekly routine, may be helpful. Because force on the foot is common to many sports, swimming and other nonimpact activities are recommended after recurrent stress fractures of the foot.

METATARSALGIA

Pathomechanics

Metatarsalgia is pain at the plantar surface of the metatarsal heads, i.e., at the "ball of the foot." Although there are numerous orthopedic and podiatric surgical procedures to correct abnormalities in the metatarsophalangeal area, in most athletes, metatarsalgia is treated successfully with basic physiatric principles. Unless there is an underlying structural abnormality present, the nonoperative approach is indicated.[14–16]

In the mechanically normal foot, weight-bearing at mid- to end-stance phase is carried by the medial metatarsal head region.[5(pp9–10),47] A thickened callus typically forms in response to weight-bearing exercise. In the overpronated foot, pain can arise in this region as the first and second metatarsal heads accept exaggerated force of impact. This is the most common underlying biomechanical cause of metatarsalgia.

Method of Presentation

Once again, pain is the primary symptom, located directly under the first and/or second metatarsal heads. Metatarsalgia often occurs as the result of overuse, the training error whereby the athlete increases the duration or intensity of exercise too rapidly. Early in the course, pain will be noticed only during athletic activity; if left untreated, metatarsal pain will linger after exercise and will eventually be present even at rest.

There are two characteristic abnormalities in the physical examination of the patient with metatarsalgia: pain with palpation under the medial metatarsal heads and a pronated, everted posture to the foot. Inspection of the athletic footgear will usually confirm that the pronation seen statically translates to excessive medial forefoot weight-bearing. Because the athlete with a symptomatic overpronated foot is likely to experience problems elsewhere in the lower extremity, the examination also includes careful biomechanical consideration of the entire kinetic chain, including the ankle, knee, and hip girdle. Conversely, when athletes present with pain in those more proximal regions, the practitioner should include a careful foot examination. Radiographs and other diagnostic studies are not helpful in establishing the diagnosis of metatarsalgia.

Differential Diagnosis

As with heel pain, systemic arthritides should be considered, especially if pain is present in other joints or if signs of active synovitis are apparent. Morton's neuroma, which occasionally requires surgical treatment,[48] may present in similar fashion, although pain with neuroma is elicited with medial-lateral compression of the metatarsal heads, rather than on the plantar surface. Stress fractures may appear similar to metatarsalgia, although they are usually easily distinguished on physical examination by the more proximal and deep location of the tender areas.

Rehabilitation

Acute Phase

Ice three times daily can be used for acute metatarsalgia, although because of the local callus formation, this is less helpful than with other injuries. Relative rest, described in detail in earlier sections, is applicable here as well. Because the majority of athletes with metatarsalgia are overpronators, immediate attention must be paid to footwear and to orthoses, if needed. "Motion-control" shoes, with firmer midsole/arch support, are advised. It is often necessary to recommend commercially available longitudinal arch supports to replace those supplied with athletic shoes. Antiinflammatory medications are of adjunctive use, helpful mostly for analgesia on an as-needed basis.

Recovery Phase

The gradual increase in the duration and intensity of training following metatarsalgia is encouraged only after the contributing abnormal biomechanics are addressed. The physical examination will likely have highlighted not only forefoot pronation, but some of the following as well: hindfoot valgus; tight Achilles, hamstring, gluteal, or quadriceps muscles; inflexibility of the iliotibial band; improper muscle balance around the knee or hip girdle. For example, if hindfoot control is not accomplished with an off-the-shelf orthosis, along with calf/thigh stretching, a custom-casted orthosis may be helpful. As with other conditions, the duration and, eventually, the intensity of workouts are increased following metatarsalgia, once the acute flare is controlled and the causes addressed.

Maintenance and Prevention

By the time the athlete with metatarsalgia has returned to full sports activity, the physician or therapist will have completed instruction in an individualized stretching, strengthening, and fitness program, accounting for the entire kinetic chain from the foot proximalward. Naturally, it is then the responsibility of the athlete to incorporate this knowledge; human nature often dictates two or more injury recurrences before preventive exercises are taken seriously.

If orthotic devices were needed for the successful initial treatment of metatarsalgia, it is likely that they will be required for the long term. Whenever possible, it is best to avoid resorting to custom-made inserts except in high-level athletes, because of the time and expense incurred and the fact that they are not always precisely reproduced on refabrication.

OTHER INJURIES

Ligament Sprains

It has been mentioned that there are innumerable ligaments contributing to the structural integrity of the foot. These can be injured individually or collectively. In classical dancers, midtarsal ligament sprains or tears arise from strong valgus forces to the medial foot.[49(p151)] The long and short plantar ligaments are also susceptible to injury when high-impact forces are imparted to the foot. Professionally applied athletic taping may be helpful during the recovery phase of these injuries. Amateur athletes occasionally present with generalized aching of the foot, which can be quite severe, often after starting a new type of exercise. Physical examination will show no focal abnormality, but many areas may be painful with palpation or translation of adjacent bones. This may well represent generalized ligament sprain from overuse and is successfully treated with ice, analgesic medications, and a more gradual increase in training level.

Cuboid Syndrome

Cuboid syndrome[11(pp209–210),49(p165),50,51] is thought to result from subluxation of that bone plantarward, leading to pain with activity or weight-bearing. It is a somewhat ill-defined condition but thought to be more prevalent in the pronated foot.[51] Physical examination reveals pain and perhaps a slight indentation over the dorsal, lateral midfoot. Some therapists claim to be skilled in reduction of the subluxation, involving rapid plantar flexion of the midtarsal joint while the cuboid is displaced dorsally. Athletic taping may provide relief of pain, as well as structural integrity for recurrent cases.

Tendon Injuries

Tendon injuries involving the foot (Achilles tendinitis is not covered in this chapter) are generally of the acute, traumatic type or of the overuse type, with the former more common in high-level athletes and the latter more prevalent in recreational athletes. The laterally placed peroneal tendons, coursing in the fairly shallow sulcus in the posterior, distal fibula, are susceptible to subluxation, causing pain and instability. Recurrent subluxation may require operative repair,[52(pp107–110)] whereas peroneal tendinitis responds to relative rest, ice, and medication. The posterior tibial and the long digit flexor and extensor tendons are all subject to overuse.[45(pp110–116)]

SUMMARY

The foot is a complex bony and ligamentous structure, uniquely suited to the demands of weight-bearing and impact under varying circumstances. From the biomechanical viewpoint, it adapts remarkably well to become relatively rigid on landing, flattened and more shock-absorbing at midstance, then fairly rigid again in preparation for leaving the ground.

It pays the price for its repetitive striking the ground with an array of unfortunately common injuries in athletes.

As in other areas of musculoskeletal physical medicine, the mandatory precursor to successful rehabilitation of a foot injury is an accurate, specific diagnosis. The history and physical examination tools are generally sufficient for this, with radiographic and other studies called upon as needed. Careful attention is paid not only to the painful area itself, but full consideration is given to possibly contributing biomechanical factors elsewhere in the kinetic chain and to environmental and equipment issues.

Prescription of modalities, medications, relative rest, and an exercise and fitness program must be tailored to the individual athlete, accounting for those unique factors leading to the injury. Successful treatment includes recovery from the acute injury as well as prevention of future injury and enhancement of athletic performance through an education process that completes the circle of rehabilitation.

REFERENCES

1. Garrick JG, Requa RK. The epidemiology of foot and ankle injuries in sports. *Clin Sports Med*. 1988;7:29.

2. Williams PL, Warwick R, Dyson M, Bannister LH, eds. *Gray's Anatomy*. 37th ed. Edinburgh: Churchill Livingstone; 1989.

3. Rose J, Gamble JG, eds. *Human Walking*. 2nd ed. Baltimore: Williams & Wilkins; 1994.

4. Isman RE, Inman VT. *Anthropometric Studies of the Human Foot and Ankle*. Biomechanics Laboratory, University of California, Berkeley; May 1968. Technical Report.

5. Nuber GW. Biomechanics of the foot and ankle during gait. *Clin Sports Med*. 1988;7:1–13.

6. Pierrynowski MR, Smith SB. Rear foot inversion/eversion during gait relative to the subtalar joint neutral position. *Foot Ankle Int*. 1996;17:406–412.

7. Rodgers MM. Dynamic foot biomechanics. *J Orthop Sports Phys Ther*. 1995;21:306–316.

8. Hicks JH. The mechanics of the foot: II. The plantar aponeurosis and the arch. *J Anat*. 1954;88:25.

9. Tanner SM, Harvey JS. How we manage plantar fasciitis. *Phys Sports Med*. 1988;16:39.

10. Warren BC. Anatomical factors associated with predicting plantar fasciitis in long distance runners. *Med Sci Sports Exerc*. 1984;16:60.

11. Windsor RE, Dreyer SJ, Lester JP. Overuse injuries of the leg, ankle, and foot. *Phys Med Rehabil Clin North Am*. 1994;5:207–213.

12. Kibler WB, Goldberg C, Chandler TJ. Functional biomechanical deficits in running athletes with plantar fasciitis. *Am J Sports Med*. 1991;19:66–71.

13. Bauman PA, Gallagher SP, Hamilton WG. Common foot, ankle, and knee problems in professional dancers: orthopaedic and physical therapy evaluation and care. *Orthop Phys Ther Clin North Am*. 1996;5:497–513.

14. Khan K, Brown J, Way S, Vass N, Crichton K, Alexander R, et al. Overuse injuries in classical ballet. *Sports Med*. 1995;19:341–357.

15. Quirk R. Common foot and ankle injuries in dance. *Orthop Clin North Am*. 1994;25:123–133.

16. Standish WD. Lower leg, foot, and ankle injuries in young athletes. *Clin Sports Med*. 1995;14:651–668.

17. Zecher SB, Leach RE. Lower leg and foot injuries in tennis and other racquet sports. *Clin Sports Med*. 1995;14:223–239.

18. DeLisa JA, Saeed MA. The tarsal tunnel syndrome. *Muscle Nerve*. 1983;6:664–670.

19. Gerster JC. Plantar fasciitis and Achilles tendinitis among 150 cases of seronegative spondarthritis. *Rheum Rehabil*. 1980;19:218.

20. Reid DC. Ankle injuries in sports. *J Sports Med*. 1973;1:18.

21. Torg JS, Pavlov H, Torg E. Overuse injuries in sport: the foot. *Clin Sports Med*. 1987;6:291.

22. Newell SG, Miller SJ. Conservative treatment of plantar fascia strain. *Phys Sports Med*. 1977;11:68–73.

23. Roy S. How I manage plantar fasciitis. *Phys Sports Med*. 1983; 11(10):127–131.

24. Geiringer SR. Tendon sheath and insertion injections. In: Lennard TA, ed. *Physiatric Procedures in Clinical Practice*. Philadelphia: Hanley and Belfus; 1995:44–48.

25. Geiringer SR, Bowyer B, Press JM. Sports medicine: the physiatric approach. *Arch Phys Med Rehabil*. 1993;74:S428–S432.

26. Mascaro TB, Swanson LE. Rehabilitation of the foot and ankle. *Orthop Clin North Am*. 1994;25:147–160.

27. Andrews JR. Overuse syndromes of the lower extremity. *Clin Sports Med*. 1983;2:137.

28. Clancy WG. Runner's injuries. II. Evaluation and treatment of specific injuries. *Am J Sports Med*. 1980;8:287.

29. Tomaro JE, Butterfield SL. Biomechanical treatment of traumatic foot and ankle injuries with the use of foot orthotics. *J Orthop Sports Phys Ther*. 1995;21:373–380.

30. Singer KM, Fones DC. Soft tissue conditions of the ankle and foot. In: Nicholas JA, Hershman EB, eds. *The Upper Extremity in Sports Medicine*. St. Louis: CV Mosby; 1990:498.

31. Berquist TH, Cooper KL, Pritchard DJ. Stress fractures. In: Berquist TH, ed. *Imaging of Orthopedic Trauma*. 2nd ed. New York: Raven Press; 1992:881–894.

32. Daffner RH, Pavlov H. Stress fractures: current concepts. *AJR*. 1992; 159:245–252.

33. Childers RL, Meyers DH, Turner PR. Lesser metatarsal stress fractures: a study of 37 cases. *Clin Podiatr Med Surg*. 1990;7:633–644.

34. Greaney RB, Gerber FH, Laughlan RL. Distribution and natural history of stress fractures in US Marine recruits. *Radiology*. 1983; 146:339–346.

35. Orava S, Puranen J, Ala-Ketola L. Stress fractures caused by physical exercise. *Acta Orthop Scand*. 1978;49:19–27.

36. Pester S, Smith PC. Stress fractures in the lower extremities of soldiers in basic training. *Orthop Rev*. 1992;21:297–303.

37. Wilson ES, Katz FN. Stress fractures: an analysis of 250 consecutive cases. *Radiology*. 1969;92:481–486.

38. Ting A, King W, Yocum L, et al. Stress fractures of the tarsal navicular in long-distance runners. *Clin Sports Med*. 1988;7:89–101.

39. Gooch JL, Geiringer SR, Akau CK. Sports medicine: lower extremity injuries. *Arch Phys Med Rehabil*. 1993;74:S438–S442.

40. Geiringer SR. Stress fractures. In: Mehta A, ed. *Rehabilitation of Fractures*. Philadelphia: Hanley and Belfus; 1995:93–104.

41. Gilad M, Ahronson Z, Stein M, et al. The low arch, a protective factor in stress fractures. *Orthop Rev*. 1985;11(11):81–84.

42. Ha KI, Hahn SH, Chung MY, et al. A clinical study of stress fractures in sports activities. *Orthopedics*. 1991;14:1089–1095.

43. Keats TE. *Radiology of Musculoskeletal Stress Injury*. Chicago: Year Book Medical Publishers; 1990:4–9.

44. Jones R. Fracture of the base of the fifth metatarsal bone by indirect violence. *Ann Surg*. 1902;35:696–700.

45. Byrd T. Jones fracture: relearning an old injury. *South Med J*. 1992;85:748–750.

46. Seitz WH, Grantham SA. The Jones fracture in the nonathlete. *Foot Ankle*. 1985;6:97–100.

47. Hutton WC, Stott JRR, Stokes IAF. The mechanics of the foot. In: Klenerman L, ed. *The Foot and Its Disorders*. Oxford: Blackwell Scientific Publications; 1976:30.

48. Dellon AL. Treatment of Morton's neuroma as a nerve compression. The role for neurolysis. *J Am Podiatr Med Assoc*. 1992;82: 399–402.

49. Hamilton WG. Foot and ankle injuries in dancers. *Clin Sports Med*. 1988;7:143–173.

50. Beaman DN, Roeser WM, Holmes JR, Saltzman CL. Cuboid stress fractures: a report of two cases. *Foot Ankle*. 1993;14:525–528.

51. Newell SG, Woodle A. Cuboid syndrome. *Phys Sports Med*. 1981; 9:71.

52. Frey CC, Shereff MJ. Tendon injuries about the ankle in athletes. *Clin Sports Med*. 1988;7:103–118.

Index